Gerontology: New Frontiers

Gerontology: New Frontiers

Editor: Oliver Fincher

AMERICAN
MEDICAL PUBLISHERS
www.americanmedicalpublishers.com

AMERICAN
MEDICAL PUBLISHERS
www.americanmedicalpublishers.com

Cataloging-in-Publication Data

Gerontology : new frontiers / edited by Oliver Fincher.
p. cm.
Includes bibliographical references and index.
ISBN 978-1-63927-007-1
1. Gerontology. 2. Geriatrics. 3. Older people--Diseases. 4. Older people--Health and hygiene.
5. Older people--Medical care. 6. Aging. I. Fincher, Oliver.
RC952 .G47 2021
618.97--dc23

American Medical Publishers,
41 Flatbush Avenue,
1st Floor, New York,
NY 11217, USA

ISBN 978-1-63927-007-1 (Hardback)

Contents

Preface

The purpose of the book is to provide a glimpse into the dynamics and to present opinions and studies of some of the scientists engaged in the development of new ideas in the field from very different standpoints. This book will prove useful to students and researchers owing to its high content quality.

The study of social, cultural, psychological, cognitive and biological aspects of aging is known as gerontology. It aims to trace the progressive changes that take place with the passage of time in a cell, a tissue, an organ system, a total organism and a group of organisms. Gerontology deals with the changes that occur between the completion of maturity and the death of the individual. It has sub-fields like biogerontology, social gerontology, environmental gerontology, and jurisprudential gerontology. Biogerontology deals with the biological aging process, its potential means and evolutionary origins to interfere in the process. Social gerontology is a subset that has specialized in studying and working with older adults. Environmental gerontology is a specialty of gerontology that seeks to improve the relationship between aging persons and their physical and social environments. Jurisprudential gerontology deals with the ways, laws and legal structures that interact with the aging experience. This book unravels the recent studies in the field of gerontology. It aims to shed light on some of the unexplored aspects of gerontology and the recent researches in this field. This book is a resource guide for experts as well as students.

At the end, I would like to appreciate all the efforts made by the authors in completing their chapters professionally. I express my deepest gratitude to all of them for contributing to this book by sharing their valuable works. A special thanks to my family and friends for their constant support in this journey.

Editor

1

Revisiting the Role of Neighbourhood Change in Social Exclusion and Inclusion of Older People

Victoria F. Burns,[1,2] Jean-Pierre Lavoie,[1,2,3] and Damaris Rose[4]

[1] *Centre de Recherche et d'Expertise en Gérontologie Sociale (CREGÉS), C.S.S.S. Cavendish, 5800 Cavendish Boulevard, Montréal, QC, Canada H4W 2T5*
[2] *School of Social Work, McGill University, Montréal, QC, Canada H3A 2A7*
[3] *École de Travail social, Université du Québec à Montréal, Montréal, QC, Canada H2L 4Y2*
[4] *Centre Urbanisation Culture Société, Université INRS, 385 Rue Sherbrooke Est, Montréal, QC, Canada H2X 1E3*

Correspondence should be addressed to Victoria F. Burns, victoria.burns@mail.mcgill.ca

Academic Editor: Frank Oswald

Objective. To explore how older people who are "aging in place" are affected when the urban neighbourhoods in which they are aging are themselves undergoing socioeconomic and demographic change. *Methods.* A qualitative case study was conducted in two contrasting neighbourhoods in Montréal (Québec, Canada), the analysis drawing on concepts of social exclusion and attachment. *Results.* Participants express variable levels of attachment to neighbourhood. Gentrification triggered processes of social exclusion among older adults: loss of social spaces dedicated to older people led to social disconnectedness, invisibility, and loss of political influence on neighbourhood planning. Conversely, certain changes in a disadvantaged neighbourhood fostered their social inclusion. *Conclusion.* This study thus highlights the importance of examining the impacts of neighbourhood change when exploring the dynamics of aging in place and when considering interventions to maintain quality of life of those concerned.

1. Introduction

A number of researchers have suggested that with advancing age, a person's geographical area tends to become increasingly limited in space [1–6]. Research that has explored the question of the meaning of place in different groups indicates that proximity of neighbours has a greater importance in the lives of older residents [7]. The neighbourhood is more significant for older people and the disadvantaged than for the younger and more affluent, who tend to develop social networks more diffuse in space [8, 9]. (Following current conventions, we use the terms "older person" and "older adult" in reference to people aged 65 years and over.) Moreover, the neighbourhood and the "home" become key elements in social life—social relations gradually become limited to people who live nearby—and also in defining one's sense of self, because the neighbourhood provides a number of identity markers [10]. Older people tend to be more reliant on their immediate environment as they are less likely to be involved in employment and have greater chance of becoming physically dependent [11]. Despite the growing body of aging-in-place research, social gerontology, hampered by static "environmental fit" models [12] has paid relatively little attention to the changes taking place in the neighbourhoods within which older people are aging and to how they experience these changes (submit to? actively participate in?...). It has been largely up to researchers in the geographies of aging to demonstrate the importance of neighbourhood change. Moreover, the social gerontology literature on aging in place and on the role of place in aging in old urban neighbourhoods—including a notable recent UK-Canadian comparison [13]—still focuses predominantly on neighbourhoods experiencing observable physical decline or mounting criminality. The latter could have negative impacts on older people's comfort level in their homes or on their ability to appropriate and navigate local public spaces [14, 15]. This focus is not surprising given that living in neighbourhoods of "multiple deprivation" can potentially reinforce the social exclusion of older people. However, it is also important to uncover possible dynamics of social exclusion of older people who find themselves living amidst growing affluence where they experience forms of place reshaping largely beyond their control, as in the case of neighbourhoods undergoing gentrification [16].

Gentrification is simultaneously a physical, economic, social, and cultural phenomenon classically defined in the literature as involving the "invasion" of previously working-class neighbourhoods by middle or upper-income groups and the subsequent displacement of many of the original residents [17]. (The use of the term "invasion" intentionally evokes the notion of invasion and succession developed by the Chicago School of urban sociology.) Debates and empirical research surrounding this topic now amount to a vast body of scholarship in urban geography and cognate fields; indeed, gentrification is often seen as the most important type of urban change across the global North over the past three decades [18]. This process involves a change in population characteristics with the arrival of younger, better educated people with higher incomes, a significant increase in the cost of housing (including house values, rents, property taxes), particular styles of commercial revitalization, increased traffic on neighbourhood commercial streets, and finally, displacement of former residents to more affordable neighbourhoods.

Over the past 15 years or so, the forms taken by gentrification have diversified [19]. While private-sector actors (e.g., home renovators, landlords) still cause displacement, core city municipalities of large metropolitan areas are increasingly courting, even orchestrating gentrification. For example, they may facilitate new housing construction and the rebranding of neighbourhood commercial arteries [20, 21] so as to relaunch local economies, resolve fiscal crunches, and attract young and urbane singles and/or families, such that in some cases the long-standing trend for demographic aging of the innercity has been dramatically reversed. Consequently, scholarly debates are increasingly seeking to conceptualize and shed light on the various forms of "indirect" displacement that may be created when an existing population is not literally forced out of an area—because they live in social housing or are otherwise protected from displacement in the literal sense—but their local cultures and narratives of place, their access to familiar services, or their channels of local political representation are disrupted by the influx of younger, more educated and wealthier newcomers [22–25]. A complementary insight from the social determinants of health literature [26] is that discrepancies between personal income (low) and neighbourhood status (high) can be associated with poor health, especially for older people. These trends create a need to deepen our understandings of how gentrification can affect older people.

Empirical work on its indirect negative effects on older people is as yet very sparse, but with a few insightful exceptions, such as that of Lehman-Frisch [27] alluding to commercial gentrification's culturally and economically exclusionary impact on long-term older adult residents of San Francisco and findings from Toulouse, France showing how neighbourhood revitalization may generate among older adults a sense of being out of place to the point that they are reluctant to venture out of their house [3]. In contrast, little attention has been paid to the potentially positive experiences of some older people in contexts of gentrification [28]. For instance, with gentrification comes an increase in real estate assets and it may give a greater sense of security due to increased numbers of people on local shopping streets, improved public facilities and services, and more opportunities to meet people. For these reasons, we decided to launch a study to explore older adults' perceptions of gentrification and to determine its effects on both their social exclusion and inclusion. Drawing on concepts of social exclusion, direct and indirect displacement, and attachment, this paper addresses how older people experience change in two contrasting neighbourhoods in Montréal, Canada: (1) La Petite-Patrie, a rapidly gentrifying neighbourhood and (2) Lower Notre-Dame-de-Grâce (NDG), a disadvantaged neighbourhood. This study forms part of a larger qualitative research project aiming to better understand the ways in which gentrification can contribute to the dynamics of social exclusion and inclusion of older people. As well as the Montréal study areas, the research has an international comparative dimension embracing two neighbourhoods in Toulouse, France (Minimes and Marengo). (A comparison including the two French neighbourhoods is beyond the scope of this paper.) The aims of this study were to answer the following questions.

(1) What place does the neighbourhood have in the everyday lives of older residents? (What places do they frequent? Where are their social networks situated? What neighbourhood resources and services do they use?)

(2) What neighbourhood changes do older residents notice?

(3) How do neighbourhood changes affect older residents' experiences of social exclusion/inclusion?

2. Theoretical Framework

2.1. Social Exclusion. This research project is framed primarily by a conceptualization of the dynamics of social exclusion [29]. Social exclusion originated as a sociological concept, emerging from European policy circles, especially in the 1990s [30, 31] extending into gerontological research and public policy debates, especially within the context of the United Kingdom [14, 15, 32–34]. More recently, Billette and Lavoie [29] define social exclusion as a process of nonacknowledgement and deprivation of rights and resources of certain segments of the population (in this case, older adults) that takes the shape of power dynamics between groups with divergent visions and interests. Such processes result in inequities and lead eventually to isolation from society in seven dimensions: (1) symbolic exclusion (negative images, overrepresentations, and invisibility); (2) identity exclusion (multiple identities are dismissed and a person's identity is reduced to belonging to one singular group, for example, "old", "frail", "burdensome"); (3) sociopolitical exclusion (barriers to civic/political participation); (4) institutional exclusion (reduced access to services); (5) economic exclusion (lack of financial resources); (6) exclusion of significant social ties (absence/loss of social network); (7) territorial exclusion (reduced geographic living area, unsafe neighbourhood). Billette and Lavoie's definition puts forth two essential characteristics of social exclusion. First, it is a dynamic, fluid process rather than a static state. Second, since it is a multidimensional concept, it allows for a rich understanding of how social exclusion can be experienced across many facets of a person or population's life. For instance, in relation to gentrification, increases in rents and the changing commercial landscape may put financial strain on older people, especially those with modest incomes (economic exclusion). Older adults could also lose their political influence in relation to social planning (sociopolitical exclusion). The arrival of younger, more educated populations can reinforce certain stereotypes of older people, such as "slow"; "nosy"; "busy-bodies" of the neighbourhood (symbolic exclusion). Leaving a familiar neighbourhood or having friends and neighbours move away can also lead to social network exclusion. The dimension of territorial exclusion is of particular interest because neighbourhood change involving gentrification could lead to feelings of insecurity as familiar institutions disappear and the public spaces of everyday life take on a new look and "feel." Territorial exclusion also shares dimensions with the useful geographic concepts of direct displacement (physically forced out of one's neighbourhood) and indirect displacement, as described above.

2.2. Attachment to Place. The concept of attachment is central to understanding how urban change can affect older adults. An individual's level of attachment to their environment will have a direct impact on how changes are experienced and perceived. This is especially the case for older people because, as mentioned above, the immediate environment becomes more important with age [8, 9]. Older people develop a sense of self-attachment, personal identity, and social differentiation through the relationship they construct and maintain with daily, "ordinary" spaces [35]. Therefore, understanding older people's attachment to place becomes a crucial element to understanding how they experience neighbourhood change.

It is important to make the distinction between place and space. Space refers to the physical location, whereas place can be thought of as a process and includes an integration of physical, social, emotional and symbolic aspects, interacting in different degrees [6, 36]. Several authors have since written on attachment to place [37–41] dating back to the path-breaking work of Rowles [42, 43] who developed a theory of *insideness* to conceptualize attachment to place, using three components: (1) autobiographical; (2) physical; (3) social. For Rowles, physical insideness is associated with living somewhere for long periods of time—the resident establishes a sense of environmental control or mastery by creating an idiosyncratic rhythm and routine. Social insideness evolves not only from everyday social exchanges and relationships but also from a sense of being well known and knowing others. Third, autobiographical insideness has been suggested to be the most relevant to describe older people's attachment to place because it is embedded in memories. As we age, these memories are recalled selectively in the creation of one's identity. Older people with strong ties to place are also reported to feel more in control, more secure and to have a positive sense of self. Attachment to place has also been studied by Rubinstein and Parmelee [40] and more recently by Sugihara and Evans [44] who make the link between older people's attachment to their dwelling, maintaining a positive self-image and maintaining their independence. Overall, in the past 30 years the study of attachment to place has captured the attention of scholars from geographical, gerontological, and environmental psychology perspectives [6, 37, 39, 45, 46], yet to date little has been written on what occurs when older people, who are aging in place, experience a neighbourhood that is itself undergoing change [14].

3. Methods

3.1. Study Design and Sample. We situated our research in an explorative, qualitative case study design [47], cases being the changing neighbourhood, the unit of analysis being the older person's personal experience of neighbourhood change. Case study methodology is suitable for studying complex and multifaceted social phenomena embedded in specific contexts [48]. Our overarching research question is concerned with how older adults experience different types of neighbourhood change, especially those involving gentrification. Exploring this complex issue necessitates recourse to multiple sources of evidence (e.g., document analysis, interviews with older people, and key informants), which is typical of case study methodology in the social sciences. For the Montréal component of the research, we selected two inner-city neighbourhoods (see descriptions below) where local community stakeholders were concerned about current or impending gentrification and how it could affect older people. Following a complete ethics review process by two university ethics boards (covering informed consent, confidentiality, respect, risks, and benefits, etc.), we conducted 30 semistructured face-to-face interviews with autonomous and mobile older adults aged from 68 to 95 years. All of our participants had lived in one of the two Montréal neighbourhoods for at least 10 years or did live previously there but had moved away in the past five years. We included private renters, homeowners, and people living in residences for autonomous older adults. We also conducted 10 in-depth interviews with key informants (i.e., six in La Petite-Patrie and four in Lower NDG, who came from varied backgrounds (e.g., municipal councillor, priest, community workers, etc.). Table 1 summarizes some key characteristics of the older adults who participated in this study.

3.2. Data Collection. Participants were referred from a variety of community organizations (e.g., a tenant advocacy organization, the local community health care centre in both

Table 1: Profile of study participants ($n = 30$).

	La Petite-Patrie	Lower NDG	Total
Total participants	18	12	30
Men	6	5	11
Women	12	7	19
65–69	1	0	1
70–74	1	3	4
75–79	8	3	11
80–84	4	1	5
85–90	3	3	6
90+	1	2	3
Mother tongue			
French	12	0	12
English	0	5	5
Italian	6	7	13
*Highest level of education**			
Primary school (incomplete or complete)	8	7	15
Some high school	5	1	6
High school (completed)	2	1	3
Postsecondary	2	2	4
Socioeconomic status			
Low income#	9	3	12
Current residents			
Owners	5	9	14
Renters	13	3	16
Renters living in HLM (public housing)∞	4	1	5
Former residents	5	1	6
Years in neighbourhood $			
Less than 30 years	5	4	9
30 to 39 years	7	2	9
50 years and over	6	6	12
Total	18	12	30

*No information for two participants, one in each neighbourhood.

#For the study purposes, low-income participants are those receiving the guaranteed income supplement (GIS), which provides additional money to top off the Old Age Security Pension. The maximum annual income for a single person GIS recipient is $15,960 (Service Canada, Old Age Security Payment Rates, April-June 2011: http://www.servicecanada.gc.ca/eng/isp/oas/oasrates.shtml). This definition is more stringent than Statistics Canada's low-income cut-off of $22,229 before tax in 2009 for a single person living in a city of more than 100,000 inhabitants (Statistics Canada, Low Income Lines 2008-2009: http://www.statcan.gc.ca/pub/75f0002m/2010005/tbl/tbl02-eng.htm).

∞HLM (Habitations à loyer modique) are apartment complexes for low-to-modest income households, owned and managed by the public sector. Rent is set at 25% of household income and includes basic utilities. Tenants are selected from a waiting list according to needs-based criteria established by the provincial government. Those in our study are specifically for autonomous older adults.

$Lowest value of years in neighbourhood is 9 years followed by 12 years; all others resided in neighbourhood over 15 years.

neighbourhoods, and the NDG Senior Citizens Council). Our research assistants put up posters in businesses and distributed pamphlets and presented the project at various social events for older people. We encountered important challenges recruiting individuals displaced as a result of gentrification (this is a widespread problem in gentrification research [11]). Although we had partnered with a tenant advocacy organization in La Petite-Patrie that was willing to refer recently displaced clients, this strategy only generated one interview. In Lower NDG, the Senior Citizens Council had also hoped to refer recently displaced members but was unable to locate former residents who had maintained ties with the Council. Other prospective participants were ineligible or not interested for various reasons (e.g., did not meet age requirements, insufficient length of residency, poor health). Attempts to recruit displaced individuals using the snowball method were also unfruitful. We also contacted several autonomous residences for older people in adjacent areas of Montréal, but their administrators were not willing to participate in the study. In sum, in La Petite-Patrie we interviewed five displaced residents. In Lower NDG, we interviewed one long-term resident who had recently left.

However, only one of the displaced participants was forced to leave because of a housing takeover, all of the others moved due to declining health.

Interviews were conducted in English, French, and/or Italian, lasted between 60 minutes to two hours, were voice recorded and transcribed in their entirety, the Italian material being subsequently translated into French. The original French language interview guide was developed in collaboration with our French colleagues and upon completion was translated into English and Italian. Our interviews aimed to explore what changes older residents perceive as having occurred in the neighbourhood (e.g., new constructions, population, neighbourhood image, etc.) and what the effects have been on them. Some of the potential impacts were covered systematically: social networks, change in urban landscape (e.g., loss/gain of new businesses, new constructions). We also wanted to explore to what extent older people's social networks and activities were located inside and outside of their neighbourhood, to be able to evaluate the significance of the local neighbourhood. Finally, we were interested in what place older residents see for themselves in the neighbourhood, how they feel about aging in place, what keeps them in their home. The interview ended with a brief sociodemographic questionnaire to better contextualize their perspectives.

The key informants were interviewed using a semistructured interview guide and informed consent was obtained before each interview. The interviews lasted between 45 minutes to one hour and were voice recorded in their entirety. Participants were asked to describe the neighbourhood (types and cost of real estate and rentals, population, transportation, cultural activities, businesses, etc.). They were then asked about any changes they had noticed (new constructions, population, etc.). Finally, they were asked specifically about the role that older adults have in the neighbourhood and whether they believe the neighbourhood is a good place to age. The term "gentrification" was purposefully excluded from all recruitment material and the interview guides so as not to bias participants' responses.

3.3. Analysis. All interview transcripts were read, and an analytic summary was created for each participant to understand the situation and the dynamics of social inclusion/exclusion of each of the participants. The analysis employed both deductive and inductive approaches in identifying themes to generate an understanding of how neighbourhood change was experienced in the everyday lives of older adults. The seven dimensions of the social exclusion framework [29] (symbolic, identity, territorial, sociopolitical, social network, economic, and institutional) were employed for the first round of the deductive coding. To obtain a better understanding of the participants' perspective, we also used Rowles' three components of attachment (physical, social, and autobiographical). To avoid forcing material into predefined categories and to reflect themes emerging from the data, we generated codes inductively using the grounded theory approach of Glaser and Strauss [49]. These inductively generated codes were reviewed and discussed until the research team members arrived at a consensus. The entire analysis process was facilitated by using the qualitative software package QDA Miner.

4. The Two Study Neighbourhoods

Before moving on to the presentation of findings, we now briefly introduce the two neighbourhoods, referring to a summary table showing how their sociodemographic characteristics evolved over the decade preceding the start of our fieldwork (Table 2).

4.1. La Petite-Patrie. La Petite-Patrie is a working-class inner city district a few kilometres north of downtown Montréal and dating from the 1910s–1920s when it was considered part of a larger suburban district called Villeray. It is mainly French-Canadian in ethnocultural composition but is also home to one of the founding parishes of the city's Italian-origin community. In the 1970s and 1980s its ethnocultural profile diversified with the settlement of Latin American and Southeast Asian immigrants. It is known citywide today mainly for two major culinary attractions in its western sector: the Jean-Talon produce market and the Little Italy commercial strip on nearby St. Lawrence Boulevard, both of which have been the object of large municipally led revitalization initiatives in the past 10–15 years. Little Italy has undergone a "rebranding" through ethnic entrepreneurship and many of the traditional storefronts on the main shopping street have been renovated and given way to more luxurious boutiques. Although the resident population of Italian ethnic origin has shrunk by half from 1996 (5%) to 2006 (2.5%), the local Italian business community is still powerful and Little Italy remains a draw for Italian-origin residents of Montréal and upper-middle-class consumers alike. The market has been somewhat reoriented toward regionally produced and artisanal specialty foodstuffs although a vast array of fresh produce is still available.

Bucking the societal-scale trend of an aging population, this area is now home to fewer senior citizens than a decade or so ago, and their relative weight has also diminished (Table 2). It remains ethnically diverse, although the visible minority population has fallen, especially in the sectors most touched by the commercial gentrification that has been the key change in this area over the past 15 years or so. La Petite-Patrie has seen a rapid increase in residential gentrification activity since the early 2000s, in part due to an overspill from the city's two most gentrified districts, to which it is adjacent. Housing market changes symptomatic of this gentrification are increased rates of homeownership (Table 2), spiralling real estate values (especially since the mid-2000s, according to our key informants), mushrooming infill condominium construction, and conversions of rental units and nonresidential buildings (including an iconic church) to condominiums, including some up-market housing units. Our community-based key informants claim that transformations of existing rental units have generated displacement in spite of the safeguards of tenants that are in principle built into law. As well, the neighbourhood has

TABLE 2: Basic Sociodemographic data, Montréal Census Metropolitan Area (CMA), Lower NDG, and La Petite-Patrie, 1996 and 2006.

	Montréal CMA		Lower NDG		Petite-Patrie	
	1996	2006	1996	2006	1996	2006
Total population	3,326,510	3,635,571	9,553	10,284	15,792	15,423
Variation %		+9.3		+7.7		−2.3
Population 65 and over	400,135	495,690	1,110	1,120	2,025	1,740
% of total population	12.2	13.6	11.6	10.9	12.8	11.3
Population 20 to 44	1,338,110	1,313,615	4680	4995	7735	8225
% of total population	40,2	36,1	49,0	48,6	49,0	53,4
% with university degree	15.4	21.0	21.1	29.8	15.4	31.3
% low income households	27.3	21.1	45.6	41.8	58.6	40.4
Average total personal income ratio (CMA = 1.0)	1.0	1.0	0.75	0.74	0.60	0.72
% of private dwellings owned	48.5	53.4	19.0	20.3	15.5	18.5
Visible minority population	401,420	590,375	2,695	3,605	4,150	3,730
% of total population	12.2	16.5	28.7	35.8	26.5	24.4

Source: Statistics Canada, Censuses of 1996 and 2006, 20% sample data. The data for the case study neighbourhoods were calculated by aggregation of data published at the census tract level of geography.

seen an influx of a younger, highly educated population, the average incomes of its residents, while still modest overall, have increased relative to the metropolitan area average while the proportion of low-income households has fallen (Table 2). Two community organizations that have supported our project see these changes as creating pressures on low-income renters and are especially uneasy as to whether residents in their 70s and older will still have their place in the neighbourhood if current trends persist.

4.2. Lower NDG. Lower NDG, an interwar suburb in the city's west end, is mainly inhabited by an English-speaking and lower- to middle-income population, but like La Petite-Patrie, it was also a major area of settlement of Italian immigrants, the wave in this case beginning in the 1940s. In this case too, the Italian-origin population has halved in the decade 1996-2006 (6% to 3.2%). Unlike La Petite-Patrie, the main socioeconomic trend over the past decade or so has been one of stability, even stagnation relative to the metropolitan area, rather than increasing income levels (Table 2). However, a mega-hospital project, the new McGill University Health Centre (MUHC) campus, was planned over a decade ago and has been under construction since 2009 on a vast site immediately adjacent to a section of this neighbourhood, named after the Catholic parish of Saint-Raymond, which forms the core of our study area. This has already led to speculative construction of condominiums, although so far these have been low end of market. Significant revitalization of this working class neighbourhood is expected once the hospital is completed. Local community organizations have been highly proactive in warning about and trying to mitigate the potentially negative effects of gentrification on the area's low-income residents. Census data for 2006 (Table 2) show a neighbourhood whose older population is holding its own in absolute terms, but not in relative terms. A major change is that the absolute and relative numbers of people belonging to a visible minority have risen considerably, unlike in La Petite-Patrie (Table 2), most of the increase being concentrated in the St-Raymond sector. As to two of the classic precursors of gentrification, the proportion of university degree holders increased faster than in the CMA as a whole but there was no relative increase in the weight of the 20–44 age group; thus, signs of incipient gentrification were less marked than in La Petite-Patrie.

5. Results

5.1. La Petite-Patrie. Before addressing the perception of changes and their assessment, it is important to describe the two main populations of older people residing in La Petite-Patrie: (1) the Italian population, homeowners who live in Little Italy, a sector within La Petite-Patrie (western sector of the neighbourhood); (2) the French-Canadians, who are mainly renters, residing near the centre and east of the neighbourhood. The Italians have a strong sense of attachment to Little Italy because this is the sector to which they immigrated, bought their first home, and raised their families (strong sense of autobiographical insideness). Several interviewees expressed their attachment to the area of Little Italy, comparing it to a village, or rather "the village". Their lives are organized around this relatively small geographic space, and they are able to run all their daily errands on foot. Almost all of the Italians had dense social networks within the neighbourhood. They also demonstrated strong attachment to shops and cafés they frequented on a regular basis as well as the local parish and associations. The public Jean-Talon market and parks also emerged as significant places that were part of their routine. Contrary to the Italians, the French-Canadians' attachment was more instrumental: as an 85-year-old female renter pointed out, "*we appreciate the neighbourhood because everything is at your fingertips*" [translation]. Yet, some French Canadian participants expressed complex and deep-rooted attachment that went beyond the instrumental attachment to the neighbourhood. For example, the woman who was forced out of the neighbourhood because of a housing takeover continued to return frequently to shop in familiar stores. Other French Canadians felt attachment to La Petite-Patrie that went beyond having shops nearby; the attachment to their immediate environment became more evident as they expressed feeling threatened and uncomfortable with the arrival of new ethnic minorities.

For both populations, the perception of changes varied considerably among interviewees. Some participants perceived only very few changes, if any, while others perceived several. People living in social housing complexes or in older residents' apartment complexes generally perceived little change in the neighbourhood; many people living in these residences often only described the change in their individual residence. Moreover, the changes reported by participants focused on the immediate environs (one's neighbours, one's street, or at most a few surrounding streets). The most common change noticed was a perception of increasing ethnoracial diversity (which, as we saw in Table 2, is not supported by census data). Reactions to this varied from frank expressions of unease—a sense of strangeness in once-familiar public spaces which led some people not to frequent them any more—to discourses avowing tolerance and even a cosmopolitan mentality. For instance, one 79-year-old French-speaking woman stated, "*You have to go to McDonald's to see this. We don't feel at home, it's full of immigrants. I know. I don't understand how they let that many into the country! I just don't know*" [translation]. An 85-year-old French-Canadian woman said she felt "invaded," "*It's too crowded now (St-Hubert Street), and you hear all different languages. We ask ourselves where we are. I don't like it. They are invading us! I am scared that in 10 years, what other languages are we going to hear? They are going to take everything from us ... all the businesses; it's them who are running them*" [translation]. French Canadian interviewees also reported that local churches were increasingly being "taken over" by the Haitian population. Some told us they attend church much less often because they feel out of place, "*I'm the only white face in the room*" [translation], an 82-year-old woman reported. In contrast, a man of Italian descent viewed this newfound diversity positively, "*it helps to know new people, other cultures, to reduce prejudice, because we are all alike!*" [translation].

Several interviewees reported that real estate values and rents had increased substantially in recent years. Several also pointed out the spread of condominiums, some referring to the transformation of a local church into quite luxurious condominiums. Despite the documented increase in the number of residents with university degrees, very few study participants noted the arrival of a younger, better educated and wealthier population to the neighbourhood, with the exception of one 76-year-old French-speaking woman who welcomes the arrival of more "*refined people*" [translation]. While some owners appreciated the increased value of their homes, others saw the recent developments as negative because they did not meet the needs of families and low-income residents of the neighbourhood. An Italian-speaking owner noted that the neighbourhood has become prohibitively expensive, preventing members of his family to settle there.

As for the business changes, the positions were also very diverse. Some participants harshly critiqued the changes to two major commercial streets in the neighbourhood, notably St-Hubert Street where the variety of its stores had been lost and the new shops did not meet the needs of the older neighbourhood residents: "*All the stores we liked, they are all gone. They were all replaced by fabric stores, prom dresses, wedding boutiques .... "It is not at my age that I'll buy that!*" [translation] (71-year-old French-Canadian woman, renter). As for commercial shift of St-Lawrence Boulevard and the renovation of the Jean-Talon market, many appreciated the changes and the arrival of new businesses: "*there's a lot of progress in Little Italy, in shops, restaurants ... Many people are coming*" [translation] (71-year-old Italian man, homeowner). However, few say they regularly attend the new restaurants and cafés, preferring familiar places. Others lament the increased traffic in Little Italy and higher market prices that have forced them to do their shopping elsewhere. One 91-year-old Italian man (home owner) described his ambivalence about the changes: "*The Jean-Talon market used to be more traditional, now it has become very commercial, there are too many people, in the summer we can't go Fridays, Thursday evenings, and Saturday afternoon, there are just too many people! The market is working well, so for us; it is a good thing because the houses have doubled in value! To buy a home here, if I wanted to sell my house, they are going to pay!*" [translation].

A neighbourhood change that negatively affected a number of the French-Canadian residents was the disappearance of the Golden Age Clubs and bingos: "*Ah! It shocked me because it was the only fun we had. You know old people are not interested in going to bars to drink, I do not drink. That was the only place we had to go. So since it closed: "Stay home!" So we stay at home ... It's as if for older residents, we're just too old, they are just waiting for us to die!*" [translation] (71-year-old French-Canadian woman, renter). In recent years, three clubs catering to French-Canadians have closed their doors, while the Italian-speaking club continues to operate. According to two key informants, these closures are related to lack of leadership in the clubs, deficient financial support from the municipal borough, and to their declining popularity, especially as the aging population of the neighbourhood decreases. In this sense, the closure may be linked to the gentrification with the arrival of a younger and more educated population.

5.2. Lower NDG. The two main populations residing in Lower NDG are the Italian-Canadians, of whom those in our sample are all homeowners, and the English-speaking Canadians, of whom those we interviewed are both home owners and renters (Table 1). The scarcity of businesses in Lower NDG, especially in the St-Raymond sector, forces its residents to leave the neighbourhood regularly and frequently to meet most of their consumer, social, and in some cases, spiritual needs. As such, their instrumental attachment is low, especially compared to the residents of La Petite-Patrie. Some residents expressed indifference toward their neighbourhood, as one 90-year-old English-speaking woman made clear when asked why she decided to move to the neighbourhood and stay for so many years: "*I don't know, it's a place to live, you have to live some place!*" However, some homeowners demonstrated a strong sense of attachment linked to their deep-rooted history with the neighbourhood. For example, one 74-year-old woman who bought the house she grew up in from her mother explained: "*It's just home... My family they all stuck around, you know I got 4 children. And I have the 2 boys living here. I am very... My own son with his 2 kids down the street, it's great, it's great!*" However, compared to the Italian-origin residents, the social attachments among the English speaking Canadians were more family oriented around individual homes whereas the Italians met regularly to socialize at St-Raymond's Parish and the bocce courts located behind St-Raymond's Community Centre. ("Bocce" is a ball sport belonging to the boules sport family that is commonly played outdoors during the summer months among the Italian communities in Montréal.)

As in La Petite-Patrie, the most common change noticed in Lower NDG was the increase in ethnic minority populations (which in this case is more congruent with the census data—Table 2). Perceptions were also mixed, but several participants responded negatively toward the arrival of a medical transit house for Inuit people, as they felt the centre changed the image of the neighbourhood: "*I don't know what they are going to do. I mean they (Inuit) are laying on churches... Churches lawns and... Well just yesterday, at the bus one was sitting in the door steps... I mean that's not very nice when people pass on the bus and see it, it is not very nice for people living here either...*" (74-year-old English-speaking woman, homeowner). However, some residents, such as a 90-year-old English-speaking woman renter embraced the diversity: "*Now there is everything. There's Hindus and Jewish, but everyone gets along well.*"

Some of the residents also reported feeling less secure in the neighbourhood: "*Put it this way, you ask me, if I feel at home on my street, yes. Ask me if I could go down to Saint-James, after 9 o'clock, no!*" (74-year-old English-speaking woman, homeowner). An 85-year-old English-speaking homeowner also mentioned that the neighbourhood is becoming less safe, that there have been a couple of recent shootings and a "person was beat up" at the top of her street.

Similar to La Petite-Patrie, there were also reports of lost institutions; for example, a 74-year-old English-speaking woman regrets the loss of the church in which she was an active member for over 40 years: "*I like my new church but I mean I loved my old church. That was a surprise, but I can worship anywhere. You know, it is not like I was married there, my father or mother... No they weren't married there but... But all my kids were christened there..., you know, so I have a lot more attachment to that, I mean to that one.*" Despite this loss, there were no collective political movements to save this important institution. Some of the English-speaking interviewees expressed frustration and felt they did not have a political voice, especially compared to the Italian population: "*It's more difficult. First of all, the older residents' voices are all Italian, who is going to give... I don't think anyone really cares. I mean politicians pretend they do for five minutes to bet whatever bills they want passed; they make it look like they really care... Yes, but this is silly, but I think there is a place for giving people more of a say in life rather than just being consumers*" (73-year-old English-speaking woman, homeowner). Despite the generally reported deterioration of the neighbourhood, the arrival of the new community centre was unanimously viewed as a positive addition, as one 73-year-old woman owner pointed out: "*Oh! It is a beautiful place.*" Participants viewed the community centre as a new place to meet with their peers, "*At least now we have a place to go in the winter, where we can go for 2-3 hours during the evening.*" [translation] (70-year-old Italian woman, homeowner). Finally, interviewees expected important future changes with the construction of the new mega-hospital centre yet the opinions were mixed. Some consider the potential negative ramifications of the construction: "*I don't know they've been talking about it for the past 10 years and nothing has happened yet. They're talking about making it (main artery running through St-Raymond) a one way street.... I can't imagine that!*" (90-year-old English speaking woman, renter). While others viewed the new construction in a more positive light: "*I think because of the super hospital I think it has given people a boost, even though there's been lots of complaints about what's being done but the fact that at least there is some activity is making the place more... less of a forgotten area... Yes it is a place that will be convenient, and ah it will be fine. Rather before it was a place that you hardly knew it existed, so now it is coming into its own.*" (73 year-old English-speaking woman, homeowner).

6. Discussion

Through this study we obtained an improved understanding of how older residents who are aging in place experience neighbourhoods that are themselves undergoing change. The results show that even when older residents remain in place, they may experience feelings of strangeness, insecurity, and social exclusion.

The experiences of attachment to neighbourhood differed depending on the nature of the neighbourhood and the population at hand. Instrumental (or functional) attachment was not captured by Rowles' threefold typology, yet it was the most widely reported among both the Italians and French Canadians in La Petite-Patrie. It is not surprising that there was no reported instrumental attachment in Lower NDG since the neighbourhood is lacking in local services, which forces the residents to leave the area to meet the majority of their daily needs. Commercial and institutional deficiency in Lower NDG not only prevented the residents from "living" the neighbourhood, it also prohibited them from establishing a routine with it (Rowles' [38, 39] physical insideness). However, with the arrival of the new mega-hospital, residents may become more instrumentally attached, as some of the residents forecast that the construction will bring new businesses and services to their "forgotten" neighbourhood.

Two groups seem to stand out in both neighbourhoods, although we are cautious given the small number of participants: (1) the Italian homeowners, and (2) the English and French-speaking renters. First, neighbourhood attachment is recognized as being more prevalent for homeowners than it is for renters, the formers' symbolic as well as material investment being greater due to their likelihood of moving less frequently than renters [45]. Second, compared to the Italians, the French- and English-speaking Canadian interviewees had a widely dispersed social network in the city, and/or had moved several times during their adult lives, thereby not establishing the same sense of social connectedness (social insideness) as the Italians. The Italians' description of the neighbourhood as a "village" effectively portrays their warm feelings of connectedness with neighbours and their surroundings and seems to be related to their stronger sense of autobiographical insideness, as they had built their lives in the neighbourhood. In Lower NDG, some of the English-speaking Canadians were homeowners, yet there was much less a sense of social connectedness and autobiographical insideness beyond their individual homes and their immediate families.

We have alluded to the fact that the older residents' perceived changes do not necessarily reflect the reality of the neighbourhood changes, especially in regards to the proportion of the visible minority population (principally in La Petite-Patrie). Yet the first, and sometimes the only, type of change noted in both neighbourhoods was in terms of visible signs of an increasing ethnoracial diversity and physical signs such as new condos, commercial revitalisation, and so forth. On the other hand, new younger and better-educated populations went virtually unnoticed. This relative invisibility of the arrival of this new population suggests that social class change is less dramatic than ethnic distinctions. This finding draws a parallel to Alba's [50] Mexican study, where changes related to gentrification were not perceived by interviewees besides home renovations. Negative comments relating to the perceived increase in ethnic minorities were more common than were positive ones. The French Canadians in La Petite-Patrie and the English-speaking participants in Lower NDG felt especially "invaded," that they no longer belonged or felt "at home" among the new faces on their once familiar landscape. The negative feelings of "strangeness" in a well-known environment provide evidence of indirect displacement and symbolic exclusion [29] resonating with Nord's [51] "politics of resentment" in which the London shopkeepers who were interviewed blamed multiculturalism and cultural diversity in the neighbourhood for inequalities and feeling powerless. On the other hand, the Italians did not report the same negative experience, which is likely to be related to their strong sense of social insideness to the neighbourhood.

Among the reported changes, the greatest effect on older residents was related to the closure of the Golden Age Clubs and churches as well as the revamping of a commercial street (niche market of bridal and evening wear) and a public market (higher market prices). However, an important distinction between the English- and French-speaking populations was that the English-speaking residents of Lower NDG seemed less affected by changes, such as the closure of their Anglican church, because they were used to leaving the neighbourhood to meet their needs. In addition, an unexpected result was the implementation of a new community centre with activities catering to older people in Lower NDG, a deteriorating neighbourhood, whereas in La Petite-Patrie, a neighbourhood undergoing gentrification, we see the closure of important institutions for older adults. This surprising finding is at odds with the viewpoint of Bowling and Stratford (2007) [52] who suggest that increasing the affluence of an area may improve the social and physical functioning of older people who are aging in place. This was not the case in La Petite-Patrie, where the closure of French-Canadian Golden Age Clubs led to a form of "house arrest" for some of the participants. Yet, in Lower NDG, the English-speaking Canadians reported fear of crime, which prevented them from going out at night. As noted by Anne-Marie Séguin et al. [53], when one is confined to the home it becomes a place of isolation and invisibility. Feelings of insecurity and the disappearance of familiar institutions provided evidence of Billette and Lavoie's [29] dimension of territorial exclusion. Conversely, in both neighbourhoods, the Italians had managed to maintain their social and cultural institutions. For instance, at present, the Italian Parish in La Petite-Patrie has many members who attend very regularly, and a number of activities continue to be organized around the church. Similarly, the Italian Golden Age clubs of this community continue to operate, contrary to the French-Canadian clubs. A key informant even spoke of the older Italians wanting to open a residence catering specifically to Italian seniors in Little Italy. Similarly, in Lower NDG, the older Italians continued to meet regularly at St-Raymond's Church and the bocce courts located behind St-Raymond's Community Centre.

For a number of reasons, the residents of Italian descent in both neighbourhoods viewed the neighbourhood changes with more serenity and comfort than the French- and English-speaking Canadian residents. Similar to Pashup-Graham [28] whose Chicago-based study unveiled some of the positive consequences of gentrification, the Italians viewed the revitalization with enthusiasm; they recognized that the neighbourhood was becoming more attractive and that the value of their homes was increasing. While the Italians were mostly homeowners, giving them some protection against the gentrification of the neighbourhood, the French Canadians were all renters. It is thus not surprising that the renters we met, be they French or English-speaking, were at the same time less attached to their neighbourhood and possibly more vulnerable to perceived and objective local changes generating experiences of social exclusion. For instance, the French- and English- speaking Canadians were experiencing forms of symbolic exclusion, as was pointed out by two key informants who believed that these populations were no longer seen or heard, rendering them invisible. Similar to Martin [23] who looks at political displacement, the absence of the voices of this population in politics and decision making also suggests a form of sociopolitical exclusion. The visibility and political influence of the Italians were obvious to some of the other interviewees, which may have reinforced feelings of exclusion among the French- and English-speaking populations. This finding is supported by Phillipson [14] who writes, "variations in community attachments now illustrate significant inequalities within the older population: most notably between those able to make conscious decisions about where and with whom to live, and those who feel marginalised and alienated by changes in the communities in which they have "aged in place" (page 336). Finally, unlike the French- and English-speaking communities, the Italians had managed to maintain their cultural and social institutions. The reasons for this preservation are complex, and we are cautious given the small sample size; it appears that their strong sense of physical, social, and autobiographical insideness led to greater visibility, political power, and control over changes, which in turn protected them from some dynamics of social exclusion.

The first expected impact of gentrification is often financial [54]. An unexpected finding was that almost no respondents experienced economic exclusion. This appears to be related to the fact that La Petite-Patrie is undergoing incomplete gentrification [55]; that the neighbourhood is maintaining a certain social mix that is manifested by the heterogeneity of businesses, the cost of housing, and social status of the population. A second potentially protective element is that Québec has a system of rent regulation. The situation could be very different in other cities that do not have these protective measures in place; thus there is scope for further research.

7. Conclusion

The majority of environmental gerontology research has focused on how to provide security and strengthen an older person's sense of self while they age in place. There is a call for further research that considers how neighbourhood change affects older residents who age in place. This study goes beyond economic impacts of neighbourhood change and considers the importance of social, cultural, and political consequences that may affect people's quality of life. Our observations also support the relevance of examining the possible role of gentrification in the dynamics of social exclusion of older people who are living in a changing working class neighbourhood and, at the same time, have little control over local institutions and organizations that are essential to meet their needs. In addition, this study reinforces the importance of considering the heterogeneity of the older adult population; inequalities and social differences still exist, even within golden age cohorts. To this end, Manzo [56], citing Hummon [56], recalled that the rootedness of some members of the community involves the removal and exclusion of other members. Finally, our findings demonstrate the crucial role that social spaces play in order to maintain or develop social links, increase visibility and consequently feelings of inclusion. There is a need to maintain these social spaces for older residents, especially in changing environments, to ensure that older people have a space to be seen and heard.

Acknowledgments

This research is funded (2008–2011) by the Social Sciences and Humanities Research Council of Canada, Grant no. 410-2008–0224. We wish to thank all our interviewees and the various community organizations that provided guidance and assistance with recruitment. The usual disclaimers apply.

References

[1] S. Clément, J. Mantovani, and M. Membrado, "Localisation Urbaine et expression du vieillissement," *Sociologie Santé*, vol. 11, pp. 105–118, 1994.

[2] S. Clément, J. Mantovani, and M. Membrado, "Vivre la ville à la vieillesse: se ménager et se risquer," *Les Annales de la Recherche Urbaine*, vol. 73, 1996.

[3] S. Clément, J. Mantovani, and M. Membrado, "Expériences du vieillissement et formes urbaines," in *L'urbain dans Tous ses états. Faire, Vivre, Dire la Ville*, N. Haumont, Ed., pp. 231–242, L'Harmattan, Paris, France, 1998.

[4] C. Lalive d'Epinay, J. Christe, H. M. Coenen-Huther et al., *Vieillesses- Situations, Itinéraires et Modes de vie des Personnes Agées Aujourd'hui*, Georgi, Saint-Saphorin, Switzerland, 1983.

[5] F. Oswald, A. Hieber, H. W. Wahl, and H. Mollenkopf, "Ageing and person-environment fit in different urban neighbourhoods," *European Journal of Ageing*, vol. 2, no. 2, pp. 88–97, 2005.

[6] J. Wiles, "Conceptualizing place in the care of older people: the contributions of geographical gerontology," *Journal of Clinical Nursing*, vol. 14, no. 8 B, pp. 100–108, 2005.

[7] M. P. Cutchin, "Agenda for future spaces for inquiry into the role of place for older people's care," *Journal of Clinical Nursing*, vol. 14, no. 8 B, pp. 121–129, 2005.

[8] G. Bridge, R. Forrest, and E. Holland, *Neighbouring: A Review of the Evidence*, University of Bristol, ESRC Centre for Neighbourhood Research, Bristol, UK, 2004.

[9] A. M. Guest and S. K. Wierzbicki, "Social ties at the neighborhood level: two decades of GSS evidence," *Urban Affairs Review*, vol. 35, no. 1, pp. 92–111, 1999.

[10] S. Clément, J. Mantovani, and M. Membrado, "Bon voisinage aux solidarités de proximité," in *Solitude et Isolement des Personnes âgées. L'environnement Solidaire*, pp. 105–138, Erès, Toulouse, France, 2004.

[11] R. Atkinson and M. Wulff, *Gentrification and Displacement: A Review of Approaches and Findings in the Literature AHURI Positioning Paper no. 115*, Southern and Monash Research Centre: Australian Housing and Urban Research Institute, 2009.

[12] H.-W. Wahl and G. D. Weisman, "Environmental gerontology at the beginning of the new millennium: reflections on its historical, empirical, and theoretical development," *The Gerontologist*, vol. 43, no. 5, pp. 616–627, 2003.

[13] A. E. Smith, *Ageing in Urban Neighbourhoods: Place Attachment and Social Exclusion*, Policy Press, Bristol, UK, 2010.

[14] C. Phillipson, "The "elected" and the "excluded": sociological perspectives on the experience of place and community in old age," *Ageing & Society*, vol. 27, no. 3, pp. 321–342, 2007.

[15] T. Scharf, C. Phillipson, and A. E. Smith, *Multiple Exclusion and Quality of Life amongst Excluded Older People in Disadvantaged Neighbourhoods*, Office of the Deputy Prime Minister, Social Exclusion Unit, London, UK, 2005.

[16] C. Phillipson, "Ageing and urban society: growing old in the century of the city," in *The Sage Handbook of Social Gerontology*, D. Daffener and C. Phillipson, Eds., Sage, Thousand Oaks, Calif, USA, 2010.

[17] C. Hamnett, "Gentrification, postindustrialism, industrial and occupational restructuring in global cities," in *A Companion to the City*, G. Bridge and S. Watson, Eds., Blackwell, Oxford, UK, 2008.

[18] L. Lees, T. Slater, and E. Wyly, *Gentrification*, Routledge, London, UK, 2007.

[19] K. Shaw, "Gentrification: what it is, why it is, and what can be done about it," *Geography Compass*, vol. 2, pp. 1697–1728, 2008.

[20] J. Hackworth and J. Rekers, "Ethnic packaging and gentrification: the case of four neighborhoods in Toronto," *Urban Affairs Review*, vol. 41, no. 2, pp. 211–236, 2005.

[21] D. Rose, "Local state policy and "new-build gentrifi cation" in Montréal: the role of the "population factor" in a fragmented governance context," *Population, Space and Place*, vol. 16, no. 5, pp. 413–428, 2010.

[22] P. Marcuse, "Abandonment, gentrification and displacement: the linkages in New York City," in *Gentrification of the City*, N. Smith and P. Williams, Eds., pp. 153–177, Unwin Hyman, London, UK, 1986.

[23] L. Martin, "Fighting for control: political displacement in Atlanta's gentrifying neighborhoods," *Urban Affairs Review*, vol. 42, no. 5, pp. 603–628, 2007.

[24] M. Davidson and L. Lees, "New-build gentrification and London's riverside renaissance," *Environment and Planning A*, vol. 37, no. 7, pp. 1165–1190, 2005.

[25] N. Blomley, *Unsettling the City: Urban Land and the Politics of Property*, Routledge, London, UK, 2004.

[26] D. J. H. Deeg and G. C. F. Thomése, "Discrepancies between personal income and neighbourhood status: effects on physical and mental health," *European Journal of Ageing*, vol. 2, no. 2, pp. 98–108, 2005.

[27] S. Lehman-Frisch, "Like a village: les habitants et leur rue commerçante dans Noe Valley, un quartier gentrifié de San Francisco," *Espaces et Sociétés*, vol. 108-109, pp. 49–68, 2002.

[28] J. Pashup-Graham, *Coping with Changes in the Neighbourhood: Residential Capital, Aging and Neighbourhood Preferences*, Doctor of Philosophy Dissertation, Sociology, University of Chicago, Chicago, Ill, USA, 2003.

[29] V. Billette and J.-P. Lavoie, "Introduction. Vieillissements, exclusions sociales et solidarités," in *Vieillir au Pluriel. Perspectives Sociales*, M. N. Dans Charpentier, V. Billette, J.P. Lavoie, A. Grenier, and I. Olazabal, Eds., pp. 1–22, Presses de l'Université du Québec, Québec, Canada, 2010.

[30] S. Paugam, *L'Exclusion. L'État des Savoirs*, La Découverte, Paris, France, 1996.

[31] F. X. Merrien, "État-providence et lutte contre l'exclusion," in *L'Exclusion, L'État des Savoirs*, pp. 417–421, La Découverte, Paris, France, 1996.

[32] D. Byrne, *Social Exclusion*, Open University Press, Buckingham, UK, 1999.

[33] T. Scharf, C. Phillipson, P. Kingston, and A. E. Smith, "Social exclusion and older people: exploring the connections," *Education and Ageing*, vol. 16, pp. 303–320, 2001.

[34] C. Lessof and R. Jowell, *Measuring Social Exclusion*, University of Oxford, National Centre for Social Research and Department of Sociology, Centre for Research into Elections and Social Trends, Oxford, UK, 2000.

[35] C. Twigger-Ross and D. Uzzell, "Place and identity processes," *Journal of Environmental Psychology*, vol. 16, no. 3, pp. 205–220, 1996.

[36] D. Massey, *A Global Sense of Place*, Policy Press, Cambridge, Mass, USA, 1994.

[37] S. Peace and C. Holland, *Inclusive Housing in an Ageing Society, Innovative Approaches*, Policy Press, Bristol, UK, 2001.

[38] S. Peace, H.-W. Wahl, H. Mollenkopf, and F. Oswald, "Environment and ageing," in *Ageing in Society*, J. Bond, S. Peace, F. Dittman-Kohli, and G. Westerhof, Eds., 3rd edition, 2007.

[39] S. Peace, C. Holland, and L. Kellaher, *Environment and Identity in Later Life*, Open University Press, Maidenhead, UK, 2005.

[40] R. L. Rubinstein and P. A. Parmelee, "Attachment to place and representation of life course by the elderly," in *Place Attachment: Human Behavior and Environment*, I. Altman and S. M. Low, Eds., vol. 12, pp. 139–163, Plenum Press, New York, NY, USA, 1992.

[41] L. M. Vandemark, "Promoting the sense of self, place, and belonging in displaced persons: the example of homelessness," *Archives of Psychiatric Nursing*, vol. 21, no. 5, pp. 241–248, 2007.

[42] G. Rowles, *Prisoners of Space? Exploring the Geographical Experience of Older People*, Westview Press, Boulder, Colo, USA, 1978.

[43] G. Rowles, "Geographical dimensions of social support in rural Appalachian community," in *Aging and Milieu: Environmental Perspectives on Growing Old*, G. Rowles and R. Ohta, Eds., pp. 231–239, Academic Press, New York, NY, USA, 1983.

[44] S. Sugihara and G. W. Evans, "Place attachment and social support at continuing care retirement communities," *Environment and Behavior*, vol. 32, no. 3, pp. 400–409, 2000.

[45] B. Brown, D. D. Perkins, and G. Brown, "Place attachment in a revitalizing neighborhood: individual and block levels of analysis," *Journal of Environmental Psychology*, vol. 23, no. 3, pp. 259–271, 2003.

[46] S. M. Golant, *A Place to Grow Old: The Meaning of Environment in Old Age*, Colombia University Press, New York, NY, USA, 1984.

[47] R. Stake, *The Art of Case Study Research CA*, Sage, Thousand Oaks, Calif, USA, 1995.

[48] R. Yin, *Applications of Case Study Research*, Sage, Beverly Hills, Calif, USA, 1993.

[49] B. G. Glaser and A. L. Straus, *The Discovery of Grounded Theory*, Aldine, Chicago, Ill, USA, 1967.

[50] M. Alba, "Mémoire urbaine et représentations socio-spatiales: l'expérience du vieillir dans la métropole, le cas de la ville de Mexico," in *Proceedings of the Vivre le vieillir: des lieux, des mots, des actes*, Université de Toulouse II-Le Mirail, Toulouse, France, 2009.

[51] P. G. Nord, "The small shopkeepers movement and politics in France, 1888–1914," in *Shopkeepers and Master Artisans in Nineteenth Century Europe*, H.-G. H. Geoffrey Crossick, Ed., Methuen, London, UK, 1984.

[52] A. Bowling and M. Stafford, "How do objective and subjective assessments of neighbourhood influence social and physical functioning in older age? Findings from a British survey of ageing," *Social Science & Medicine*, vol. 64, no. 12, pp. 2533–2549, 2007.

[53] A.-M. Séguin, P. Apparicio, and P. Negron, *Évolution de la Distribution Spatiale de la Population âgée dans Huit Métropoles: Une Ségrégation qui s'amenuise ?* INRS Centre Urbanisation Culture Société, Montréal, Canada, 2008.

[54] S. M. Keigher, *Housing Risks and Homelessness among the Urban Elderly*, Haworth Press, New York, NY, USA, 1991.

[55] R. A. Walks and R. Maaranen, *The Timing, Patterning, & Forms of Gentrification & Neighbourhood Upgrading in Montreal, Toronto & Vancouver, 1961 to 2001*, Centre for Urban and Community Studies, Cities Centre, University of Toronto, Totonto, Canada, 2008.

[56] D. M. Hummon, "Community attachment," in *Place Attachment*, I. Altman and S. M. Low, Eds., pp. 253–278, Plenum Press, New York, NY, USA, 1992.

2

Montreal Cognitive Assessment and Modified Mini Mental State Examination in African Americans

Kaycee M. Sink,[1] Suzanne Craft,[1] S. Carrie Smith,[2] Joseph A. Maldjian,[3] Donald W. Bowden,[2] Jianzhao Xu,[2] Barry I. Freedman,[4] and Jasmin Divers[5]

[1]*Department of Internal Medicine (Geriatrics), Wake Forest School of Medicine, Winston-Salem, NC 27157, USA*
[2]*Department of Biochemistry, Wake Forest School of Medicine, Winston-Salem, NC 27157, USA*
[3]*Department of Radiology, University of Texas Southwestern Medical Center, Dallas, TX 75390, USA*
[4]*Department of Internal Medicine (Nephrology), Wake Forest School of Medicine, Winston-Salem, NC 27157, USA*
[5]*Department of Biostatistics, Wake Forest School of Medicine, Winston-Salem, NC 27157, USA*

Correspondence should be addressed to Kaycee M. Sink; kmsink@wakehealth.edu

Academic Editor: Elke Bromberg

Background. Sparse data limit the interpretation of Montreal Cognitive Assessment (MoCA) scores, particularly in minority populations. Additionally, there are no published data on how MoCA scores compare to the widely used Modified Mini Mental State Examination (3MSE). We provide performance data on the MoCA in a large cohort of African Americans and compare 3MSE and MoCA scores, providing a "crosswalk" for interpreting scores. *Methods.* Five hundred and thirty African Americans with type 2 diabetes were enrolled in African American-Diabetes Heart Study-MIND, a cross-sectional study of cognition and structural and functional brain imaging. After excluding participants with possible cognitive impairment (n = 115), mean (SD) MoCA and 3MSE scores are presented stratified by age and education. *Results.* Participant mean age was 58.2 years (range: 35-83); 61% were female; and 64.9% had >12 years of education. Mean (SD) 3MSE and MoCA scores were 86.9 (8.2) and 19.8 (3.8), respectively. 93.5% of the cohort had a "positive" screen on the MoCA, scoring <26 (education-adjusted), compared with 47.5% on the 3MSE (cut-point < 88). A 3MSE score of 88 corresponded to a MoCA score of 20 in this population. *Conclusion.* The present data suggest the need for caution when applying proposed MoCA cutoffs to African Americans.

1. Introduction

With the aging population there is a concomitant diversification of the United States such that, by 2050, it is predicted that the proportion of ethnic minority older adults (≥65) will nearly double (from 19.7% in 2012 to 39.1% in 2050) [1]. Thus, it is critical that cognitive screening tools be useful, applicable, and interpretable in a wide variety of settings and populations.

The Montreal Cognitive Assessment (MoCA) is a freely available screening test of global cognitive function that has been translated into 53 languages (http://www.mocatest.org/) [2]. Though increasingly used, interpretation of MoCA scores in research settings and in diverse populations remains limited by sparse data and lack of comparative data with other tests. The largest source of normative data on the MoCA for US populations comes from the Dallas Heart Study, where 2653 participants were tested [3]. The Dallas Heart Study cohort is ethnically diverse; however, the published data does not provide race-/ethnicity-specific norms based on age or education. This limits the usefulness of the MoCA in minority patients and research participants.

There is also little information regarding how MoCA scores relate to other commonly used cognitive screening tests. Only a few studies have compared the MoCA to the Mini Mental State Examination (MMSE) [4–6], and none, that we are aware of, compared it to the widely used Modified Mini Mental State Examination (3MSE) [7].

The objective of this report is to provide performance data on the MoCA in a large cohort of African Americans and to compare 3MSE and MoCA scores to provide a "crosswalk" for interpreting scores in middle-aged and older

African American-Diabetes Heart Study MIND (AA-DHS MIND) study enrollees. These data should help clinicians and researchers interpret MoCA scores in African Americans. They will also be useful for comparing MoCA scores to expected 3MSE scores for clinical assessment and/or inclusion/exclusion criteria in research studies.

2. Methods

2.1. Participants. The AA-DHS MIND enrolled 530 African Americans with type 2 diabetes (T2D) at the Wake Forest School of Medicine (WFSM). T2D was diagnosed in those with clinical disease onset after 30 years of age in the absence of diabetic ketoacidosis and in the setting of (a) active medical treatment (insulin and/or oral hypoglycemic agents), (b) fasting blood sugar > 126 mg/dL (7 mmol/L) or nonfasting blood sugar > 200 mg/dL (11.1 mmol/L), or (c) hemoglobin A1c (HbA1c) > 6.5%.

2.2. Measures/Assessments. Demographic data, medical history, current medications, and vital signs were recorded. Participants self-identified as African American. Participants had a fasting blood draw on which a variety of assays were performed including measures of serum creatinine, blood urea nitrogen, lipids, thyroid stimulating hormone, and vitamin B12 (LabCorp, Burlington, NC). After a morning snack, cognitive testing was performed. This study was approved by the WFSM Institutional Review Board and all participants provided written informed consent.

Cognition was assessed with a 45-minute battery of standard neuropsychological tests chosen to represent a broad variety of cognitive domains, with emphasis on executive function due to the known association between vascular cognitive impairment and executive dysfunction [8]. Global cognition was assessed with the 3MSE [9] and the MoCA [2]. The Rey Auditory Verbal Learning Test (RAVLT) [10] was used to assess learning and memory. Executive function was assessed with the WAIS-III Digit Symbol Coding (DSC) [11] (measuring speed of processing and working memory), the Stroop test [12] (measuring response inhibition), and verbal fluency for animals. Depression was assessed with the Center for Epidemiologic Studies Short Depression scale (CES-D 10) [13, 14]. Interviewers were trained, certified, and subsequently assessed for quality control in all cognitive tests by a single investigator (KMS).

2.3. Exclusions for Possible Cognitive Impairment. In an attempt to provide mean (SD) performance data as close to normative data as possible, we excluded participants from the analyses if they had conditions that could cause cognitive impairment or evidence of cognitive impairment on other tests in the neuropsychiatric battery. Participants were excluded from these analyses if they had evidence of hypothyroidism (TSH > 5.0 μIU/L; $n = 24$ excluded), vitamin B12 deficiency (B12 < 147.6 pmol/L; < 200 pg/mL; $n = 12$ excluded), or significant depression (defined as answering with "yes" to "I felt depressed" on 5–7 days of the last week; $n = 32$ excluded). Total CES-D 10 score was not used as a cutoff due to concerns that some of the items have been shown to be invalid in AA [15, 16]. Using published normative data, we also excluded participants who performed worse than 1.5 SD below the mean for their age/education on verbal fluency for animals ($n = 14$ excluded) or the RAVLT long delay ($n = 45$ people). Other tests in our cognitive battery were not able to be used for exclusion purposes because reliable normative data in AA could not be found. In total, 115 participants (of 530) were excluded, leaving a sample size of 415 for these analyses.

2.4. Analyses. To determine whether the ordering of tests impacted scores, the first 200 study participants were randomized to receive the 3MSE or the MoCA as either the first or last test in the cognitive battery. Wilcoxon two-sample tests were used to compare the distribution of the observed 3MSE and MoCA scores by randomization order. Poisson-gamma models were also fitted to test for association between these scores and randomization order after adjusting for age, gender, and education level. There was no impact of test order on performance for either the 3MSE or MoCA (p value of 0.58 for 3MSE and 0.82 for MoCA; data not shown); therefore, 3MSE was administered first after the 200th participant and all subsequent analyses and presentation of results were done without regard to test order.

Demographic characteristics are presented using descriptive statistics, mean (SD) and %, for continuous and categorical variables, respectively. Means, medians, and SDs are presented for the MoCA and 3MSE by age and education. MoCA and 3MSE scores were compared using the Wilcoxon rank order test. Equipercentile matching was used to create a functional relationship between MoCA and 3MSE. Briefly, a 4th-degree polynomial log-linear equation was used to smooth the observed MoCA and 3MSE scores to reduce irregularities in the score distributions [17]. Equipercentile equating was then performed by determining the percentile rank of a given MoCA score and identifying the corresponding 3MS score that leads to the same ranking. Equipercentile analyses were performed with R-package Equate [18].

3. Results

Demographic and health characteristics of the participants are presented in Table 1. Participants had a mean age of 58.2 years (range: 35–83) and 61% were women. Nearly 65% had some college education; 19.8% had at least a four-year degree. The mean (SD) HbA1c was 8.0% (2.0) and the average duration of T2D was 13.0 (7.7) years. Although 83% of the sample had a diagnosis of hypertension, they were under relatively good control with mean (SD) systolic blood pressure of 131.4 (17.7) mm Hg.

MoCA. The mean (SD) MoCA score was 19.8 (3.8). Utilizing the <26 cutoff for impairment [2], 93.5% of our participants would be considered impaired after correction for education. Table 2 provides MoCA score means (SD) and medians by age and education. These scores are not corrected for education, given the fact that we stratified by education. Mean

TABLE 1: Characteristics of 415 African Americans with type 2 diabetes mellitus.

Variable	Mean (SD) or %	Range
Demographics		
Age (years)	58.2 (9.3)	35–83
Female	61.3	
Education (years)		
<12	10.8	
12	24.3	
13–15	45.1	
≥16	19.8	
Health related characteristics		
Diabetes duration (years)	13.0 (7.7)	1.2–56.6
Body mass index (kg/m^2)	35.9 (8.8)	17.9–75.7
Systolic blood pressure (mm Hg)	131.4 (17.7)	78.5–194.0
Diastolic blood pressure (mm Hg)	76.9 (11.2)	48.0–110.0
Smoking		
Never	46.7	
Past	31.0	
Current	22.3	
Hypertension (%)	83.3	
Fasting glucose (mmol/L)	8.3 (3.6)	2.8–25.1
Hemoglobin A1c (%)	8.0 (2.0)	4.7–15.9
Serum creatinine (μmol/L)	88.4 (26.5)	40.7–388.1
Thyroid stimulating hormone (μIU/L)	1.7 (1.0)	0.01–4.98
Vitamin B12 (pmol/L)	487.1 (272.9)	152.8–1476
Cognitive function		
MoCA (0–30)	19.8 (3.8)	6–29
3MSE (0–100)	86.9 (8.2)	46–100
RAVLT delayed recall (0–15)	6.1 (2.9)	1–15
DSC (0–133)	51.1 (16.2)	2–96
Verbal fluency for animals (0–undefined)	16.1 (4.5)	8–31
Stroop interference (seconds)	37.1 (16.4)	−20–134

MoCA, Montreal Cognitive Assessment; 3MSE, Modified Mini Mental State Examination; RAVLT, Rey Auditory Verbal Learning Test; DSC, Digit Symbol Coding.

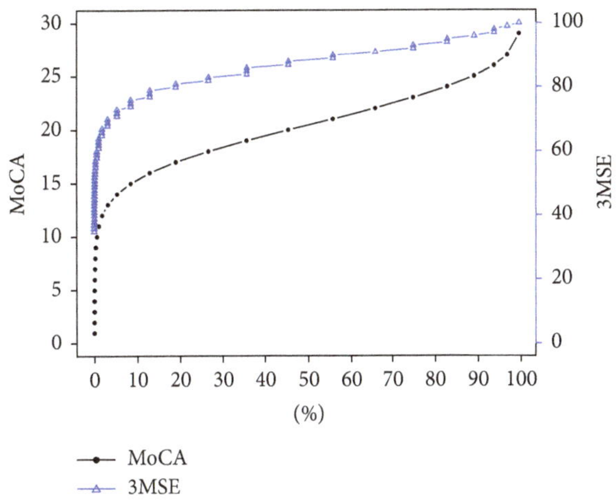

FIGURE 1: Equivalent MoCA score for a given 3MSE Score. To obtain a MoCA score for a given 3MSE score, find the relevant score on y-axis labeled 3MSE and draw a line until it intersects the 3MSE curve and then look down x-axis and note the percentile that the score corresponds to. Using that same percentile, draw a line upwards until it intersects the MoCA curve and then note the value on y-axis labeled MoCA that this point intersects with. That is the MoCA score that is equivalent to the selected 3MSE score. Reverse the process to find a 3MSE score corresponding to a given MoCA score. For example, 3MSE 80 is approximately the 18th percentile. The 18th percentile MoCA score is approximately 17.

scores decline with age (Spearman's rank correlation = −0.19, $p < 0.001$). For example, amongst those with a high school education (12 years), participants who are less than 55 years old had a mean MoCA score of 20.5 compared to 19.8 for those who are 55 to 65 years old and 18.7 for those who are 65 years old and older. Similarly, scores were higher for those with greater education (Spearman's rank correlation = 0.39, $p < 0.001$), with a 4–7-point spread between those with less than 12 years of education and those with a college degree or more (16+ years), depending on age (Table 2).

3MSE. The mean (SD) 3MSE score for the cohort was 86.9 (8.2). Using a cutoff of <88 to define suspected impairment [19, 20], 47.5% of participants would be considered impaired. Table 3 provides 3MSE means (SD) and medians by age and education. Similar to the MoCA, 3MSE scores were affected by age (Spearman's rank correlation = −0.20, $p < 0.001$) and education (Spearman's rank correlation = 0.41, $p < 0.001$).

Figure 1 and Table 4 display how the MoCA and 3MSE scores relate using models based on equipercentile performance. For example, a score of 88 on the 3MSE is equivalent to a score of 20 on the MoCA.

4. Discussion

This report provides age- and education-stratified data for the MoCA and the 3MSE in a large sample of middle-aged and older-aged African Americans with T2D. As expected, age and education were significantly associated with performance on the MoCA, emphasizing the importance of basing conclusions on stratified data. With these data, clinicians can now compare the MoCA performance of African Americans in their office to mean scores of African Americans of a similar age and education level. This is important, because African Americans are known to perform worse on a variety of cognitive tests than European Americans, potentially due

Table 2: Montreal Cognitive Assessment (MoCA) scores by age and education in 414 African Americans.

Age (years)	Education								All	
	<12 years		12 years		13–15 years		16+ years			
	N	Mean (SD) median	*N*	Mean (SD) median	*N*	Mean (SD) median	*N*	Mean (SD) median	*N*	Mean (SD) median
<55	15	18.8 (3.1) 19.0	50	19.3 (3.9) 19.5	66	20.7 (3.4) 20.0	28	23.4 (3.1) 24.0	159	20.5 (3.8) 20.0
55–65	15	18.0 (3.0) 18.0	38	18.4 (3.7) 18.5	74	19.8 (3.3) 20.0	36	22.3 (3.6) 23.0	163	19.8 (3.7) 20.0
>65	15	14.4 (3.3) 15.0	13	17.7 (4.2) 19.0	46	19.2 (2.9) 19.5	18	21.6 (3.1) 21.0	92	18.7 (3.9) 19.0
All	45	17.1 (3.6) 17.0	101	18.7 (3.8) 19.0	186	19.9 (3.3) 20.0	82	22.5 (3.4) 23.0	414	19.8 (3.8) 20.0

Note: MoCA scores are raw scores, with no extra point given for education ≤12 years. $N = 414$, not 415, because age was missing for one person. Range for age <55 is 35–54; range for >65 is 66–83 years. For participants with <12 years of education, 11 had 5–8 years and 34 had 9–11 years.

Table 3: Modified Mini Mental State Examination (3MSE) scores by age and education in 414 African Americans.

Age (years)	Education								All	
	<12 years		12 years		13–15 years		16+ years			
	N	Mean (SD) median	*N*	Mean (SD) median	*N*	Mean (SD) median	*N*	Mean (SD) median	*N*	Mean (SD) median
<55	15	82.7 (6.7) 85.0	50	86.6 (7.2) 88.0	66	89.0 (6.0) 89.5	28	94.2 (4.6) 95.0	159	88.5 (7.0) 89.0
55–65	15	79.7 (10.8) 84.0	38	84.1 (6.8) 84.0	74	87.9 (7.5) 89.0	36	90.1 (6.9) 92.0	163	86.7 (8.1) 87.0
>65	15	73.9 (11.0) 74.0	13	81.1 (8.2) 82.0	46	86.4 (6.6) 86.0	18	90.2 (8.0) 92.0	92	84.4 (9.4) 88.0
All	45	78.8 (10.2) 79.0	101	84.9 (7.4) 86.0	186	87.9 (6.8) 88.0	82	91.5 (6.7) 94.0	414	86.9 (8.2) 88.0

Note: $N = 414$, not 415, because age was missing for one person. Range for age <55 is 35–54; range for >65 is 66–83 years. For participants with <12 years of education, 11 had 5–8 years and 34 had 9–11 years.

to educational and socioeconomic factors, and thus race-specific normative data are critical for making accurate clinical assessments [21].

With that said, these results should not be considered strictly "normative" data as we did not clinically assess participants for cognitive impairment. When comparing the performance of AA-DHS MIND participants on the MoCA to African Americans in the Dallas Heart Study [3], AA-DHS MIND participants performed several points worse. The mean age of African Americans in the Dallas Heart Study was younger (49.9 years compared to 58.2 years in AA-DHS MIND), with similar mean levels of education, yet the mean (SD) MoCA score was 22 (4). Data specific to African Americans in the Dallas Heart Study were not presented by age/education. The youngest AA-DHS MIND group (age < 55 years) with 13–15 years of education had mean (SD) MoCA scores of 20.7 (3.4). Sixty-two percent of Dallas Heart Study participants fell below the education-corrected cut-point of 26, compared to 93.5% of AA-DHS MIND participants. Performance on the 3MSE was also lower in the AA-DHS MIND sample compared to 3MSE normative data published for a sample of 238 elderly African Americans residing in Tampa, FL [22]. The age strata presented were not the same, limiting direct comparisons between reports. However, mean 3MSE scores in AA-DHS MIND participants who are 55–65 years old were several points lower than those in the participants who are 60–71 years old in the Tampa-based Brown et al.'s study across all education groups but particularly for participants with high school or less education.

There are several reasons why AA-DHS MIND MoCA and 3MSE scores may have been lower than those in published norms. First, all participants have T2D and diabetes has been shown to adversely impact cognition [23]. Second, there may be regional variation in cognitive performance among African Americans, such that those residing in North Carolina may perform worse than those in other regions of the country due to differences in cognitive risk factors (North Carolina is in the stroke belt) [24] or quality of education, especially in the southern US where older participants may have been educated in segregated, rural schools [21, 25]. There are other methodological considerations to factor in when interpreting the current results, including the fact that this was a single center study and results may not generalize to all African Americans based on presence of T2D. However, African Americans have a lifetime risk for T2D that exceeds 50% [26]. These data should not be interpreted as strictly "normative" since no clinical evaluation to determine cognitive status (normal or impaired) was performed. Therefore, we did not provide ROC curves with suggested "cutoffs" for the MoCA as a screening test in African Americans. However, we did exclude participants with hypothyroidism, vitamin B12 deficiency, and depressed mood as all of these conditions could have impacted test scores negatively. In addition, we excluded participants with evidence of memory impairment and poor category fluency for animals in a further attempt to provide data on participants that could be considered free of significant cognitive impairment. In addition, these participants volunteered to be in a research study and study volunteers are typically healthier than the general population (healthy volunteer effect).

In spite of these methodological limitations, there are several noteworthy strengths. We have presented the first report of MoCA scores stratified by age and education in a large sample of African Americans. In addition, we present the first "crosswalk" that can be used to compare

Table 4: Conversion table between observed MoCA and 3MSE scores in African Americans.

MOCA	3MSE
1	0–37
2	38–40
3	41-42
4	43-44
5	45-46
6	47–49
7	50–52
8	53-54
9	55–57
10	58–60
11	61–64
12	65–67
13	68–70
14	71–73
15	74–76
16	77–79
17	80-81
18	82-83
19	84–86
20	87-88
21	89-90
22	91
23	92-93
24	94-95
25	96
26	97-98
27	99
29	100

scores between the MoCA and 3MSE. This is important because many large epidemiologic studies (examples include the Cardiovascular Health Study, Health ABC Study, Cache County Study, Women's Health Initiative, and Canadian Study of Health and Aging) and clinical trials (Women's Health Initiative Memory Study and Lifestyle Interventions and Independence for Elders (LIFE) Study) have used the 3MSE. In order to compare results in those studies with the more contemporary MoCA test, development of a crosswalk is necessary. This allows researchers to identify a MoCA score that would be comparable to a given 3MSE score for inclusion into or exclusion from a study based on previous studies and allows clinicians to translate risk associated with a specific 3MSE score to a MoCA score that they obtained in clinic in African Americans.

In conclusion, the present data suggests the need for caution when applying proposed MoCA cutoffs to African Americans. Based on the suggested cutoff of <26, 93.5% of AA-DHS MIND participants would have been classified as impaired, which is clearly unlikely. Additional studies using large, diverse populations, where MoCA scores can be stratified by race, age, and education, are needed. We also recommend that MoCA/3MSE comparisons be replicated in other cohorts to determine if our "crosswalk" of scores is applicable to other race/ethnicity groups.

Conflict of Interests

All authors declare that there is no conflict of interests related to this paper.

Authors' Contribution

Kaycee M. Sink participated in study design, interpretation of data, and drafting of the paper. Suzanne Craft participated in interpretation of data and critical revision of the paper. Carrie Smith took part in data acquisition, critical revision of the paper, and administrative support. Donald W. Bowden took part in study design, interpretation of data, and critical revision of the paper. Jianzhao Xu participated in data acquisition, critical revision of the paper, and administrative support. Joseph A. Maldjian had a role in study design, interpretation of data, critical revision of the paper, and obtaining funding. Barry I. Freedman took part in study design, interpretation of data, critical revision of the paper, and obtaining funding. Jasmin Divers had a role in study design, statistical analysis, interpretation of data, critical revision of the paper, and obtaining funding.

Acknowledgments

This study was funded by NIH R01 NS075107 (Jasmin Divers, Joseph A. Maldjian, and Barry I. Freedman), R01 NS-058700 (Donald W. Bowden), and R01 DK-071891 (Barry I. Freedman).

References

[1] J. M. Ortman, V. A. Velkoff, and H. Hogan, *An Aging Nation: The Older Population in the United States*, US Census Bureau, Washington, DC, USA, 2014.

[2] Z. S. Nasreddine, N. A. Phillips, V. Bédirian et al., "The Montreal Cognitive Assessment, MoCA: a brief screening tool for mild cognitive impairment," *Journal of the American Geriatrics Society*, vol. 53, no. 4, pp. 695–699, 2005.

[3] H. C. Rossetti, L. H. Lacritz, C. Munro Cullum, and M. F. Weiner, "Normative data for the Montreal Cognitive Assessment (MoCA) in a population-based sample," *Neurology*, vol. 77, no. 13, pp. 1272–1275, 2011.

[4] Y. Dong, W. Y. Lee, N. A. Basri et al., "The Montreal cognitive assessment is superior to the mini-mental state examination in detecting patients at higher risk of dementia," *International Psychogeriatrics*, vol. 24, no. 11, pp. 1749–1755, 2012.

[5] D. R. Roalf, P. J. Moberg, S. X. Xie, D. A. Wolk, S. T. Moelter, and S. E. Arnold, "Comparative accuracies of two common screening instruments for classification of Alzheimer's disease, mild cognitive impairment, and healthy aging," *Alzheimer's and Dementia*, vol. 9, no. 5, pp. 529–537, 2013.

[6] S. Freitas, M. R. Simões, L. Alves, and I. Santana, "Montreal cognitive assessment: validation study for mild cognitive impairment and alzheimer disease," *Alzheimer Disease and Associated Disorders*, vol. 27, no. 1, pp. 37–43, 2013.

[7] M. F. Folstein, S. E. Folstein, and P. R. McHugh, "'Mini-mental state'. a practical method for grading the cognitive state of patients for the clinician," *Journal of Psychiatric Research*, vol. 12, no. 3, pp. 189–198, 1975.

[8] S. T. Pendlebury, A. Markwick, C. A. de Jager, G. Zamboni, G. K. Wilcock, and P. M. Rothwell, "Differences in cognitive profile between TIA, stroke and elderly memory research subjects: a comparison of the MMSE and MoCA," *Cerebrovascular Diseases*, vol. 34, no. 1, pp. 48–54, 2012.

[9] E. L. Teng and H. C. Chui, "The Modified Mini-Mental State (3MS) examination," *Journal of Clinical Psychiatry*, vol. 48, no. 8, pp. 314–318, 1987.

[10] M. Lezak, *Neuropsychological Assessment*, Oxford University Press, New York, NY, USA, 1983.

[11] D. Wechsler, *WAIS-III Manual*, Psychological Corporation, New York, NY, USA, 1997.

[12] P. J. Houx, J. Jolles, and F. W. Vreeling, "Stroop interference: aging effects assessed with the Stroop Color-Word Test," *Experimental Aging Research*, vol. 19, no. 3, pp. 209–224, 1993.

[13] M. Irwin, K. H. Artin, and M. N. Oxman, "Screening for depression in the older adult: criterion validity of the 10-item Center for Epidemiological Studies Depression Scale (CES-D)," *Archives of Internal Medicine*, vol. 159, no. 15, pp. 1701–1704, 1999.

[14] E. M. Andresen, J. A. Malmgren, W. B. Carter, and D. L. Patrick, "Screening for depression in well older adults: evaluation of a short form of the CES-D (Center for Epidemiologic Studies Depression Scale)," *American Journal of Preventive Medicine*, vol. 10, no. 2, pp. 77–84, 1994.

[15] E. Torres, "Psychometric properties of the center for epidemiologic studies depression scale in African American and black caribbean us adults," *Issues in Mental Health Nursing*, vol. 33, no. 10, pp. 687–696, 2012.

[16] C. M. Callahan and F. D. Wolinsky, "The effect of gender and race on the measurement properties of the CES-D in older adults," *Medical Care*, vol. 32, no. 4, pp. 341–356, 1994.

[17] P. W. Holland and D. T. Thayer, "Univariate and bivariate loglinear models for discrete test score distributions," *Journal of Educational and Behavioral Statistics*, vol. 25, no. 2, pp. 133–183, 2000.

[18] A. Albano, *Equate: Observed-Score Linking and Equating. R Package Version 2.0-3*, 2014.

[19] S. R. Rapp, M. A. Espeland, P. Hogan, B. N. Jones, and E. Dugan, "Baseline experience with modified mini mental state exam: the Women's Health Initiative Memory Study (WHIMS)," *Aging & Mental Health*, vol. 7, no. 3, pp. 217–223, 2003.

[20] K. M. Sink, M. A. Espeland, J. Rushing et al., "The LIFE Cognition Study: design and baseline characteristics," *Clinical Interventions in Aging*, vol. 9, pp. 1425–1436, 2014.

[21] J. J. Manly, D. M. Jacobs, M. Sano et al., "Cognitive test performance among nondemented elderly African Americans and whites," *Neurology*, vol. 50, no. 5, pp. 1238–1245, 1998.

[22] L. M. Brown, J. A. Schinka, J. A. Mortimer, and A. B. Graves, "3MS normative data for elderly African Americans," *Journal of Clinical and Experimental Neuropsychology*, vol. 25, no. 2, pp. 234–241, 2003.

[23] S. Sadanand, R. Balachandar, and S. Bharath, "Memory and executive functions in persons with type 2 diabetes: a meta-analysis," *Diabetes/Metabolism Research and Reviews*, 2015.

[24] V. G. Wadley, F. W. Unverzagt, L. C. McGuire et al., "Incident cognitive impairment is elevated in the stroke belt: the REGARDS Study," *Annals of Neurology*, vol. 70, no. 2, pp. 229–236, 2011.

[25] J. J. Manly, D. A. Byrd, P. Touradji, and Y. Stern, "Acculturation, reading level, and neuropsychological test performance among African American elders," *Applied Neuropsychology*, vol. 11, no. 1, pp. 37–46, 2004.

[26] E. W. Gregg, X. Zhuo, Y. J. Cheng, A. L. Albright, K. M. V. Narayan, and T. J. Thompson, "Trends in lifetime risk and years of life lost due to diabetes in the USA, 1985–2011: a modelling study," *The Lancet Diabetes and Endocrinology*, vol. 2, no. 11, pp. 867–874, 2014.

3

Is Collective Efficacy Age Graded? The Development and Evaluation of a New Measure of Collective Efficacy for Older Adults

Adena M. Galinsky,[1] Kathleen A. Cagney,[2] and Christopher R. Browning[3]

[1] *Center on the Demography and Economics of Aging, NORC and the University of Chicago, 1155 E. 60th Street, Chicago, IL 60637, USA*
[2] *Departments of Sociology and Health Studies, University of Chicago, 1155 E. 60th Street, Rm 238, Chicago, IL 60637, USA*
[3] *Department of Sociology, Ohio State University, 214 Townshend Hall, 1885 Neil Avenue Mall, Columbus, OH 43210, USA*

Correspondence should be addressed to Kathleen A. Cagney, k-cagney@uchicago.edu

Academic Editor: Lindy Clemson

Objectives. Community processes are key determinants of older adults' ability to age in place, but existing scales measuring these constructs may not provide accurate, unbiased measurements among older adults because they were designed with the concerns of child-rearing respondents in mind. This study examines the properties of a new theory-based measure of collective efficacy (CE) that accounts for the perspectives of older residents. *Methods.* Data come from the population-based Chicago Neighborhood Organization, Aging and Health study ($N = 1,151$), which surveyed adults aged 65 to 95. Using descriptive statistics, correlations, and factor analysis, we explored the acceptability, reliability, and validity of the new measure. *Results.* Principal component analysis indicated that the new scale measures a single latent factor. It had good internal consistency reliability, was highly correlated with the original scale, and was similarly associated with neighborhood exchange and disorder, self-rated health, mobility, and loneliness. The new scale also showed less age-differentiated nonresponse compared to the original scale. *Discussion.* The older adult CE scale has reliability and validity equivalent to that of the existing measure but benefits from a more developed theoretical grounding and reduced likelihood of age-related differential nonresponse.

1. Introduction

Evidence suggests that community processes are important to older adults' ability to age in place [1, 2]. Of the eight factors identified in the World Health Organization's report on age-friendly cities [3], three seem fundamentally dependent on community processes. These three, *Age-Friendly Outdoor Spaces* (WHO factor 1), *Social Participation* (WHO factor 4), and *Respect and Social Inclusion* (WHO factor 5) may all be supported by structural innovations and resource infusion, but, in all likelihood, cannot be sustained without ongoing community involvement. Community-level behavior is important not only for the immediate results produced by discrete actions and social exchange, but also for its role in shaping the perceptions and norms of behavior held by the community's residents.

The perceptions and norms of behavior likely relevant to the three WHO factors fall under the rubric of a well-developed sociological construct, *collective efficacy*. Collective efficacy (CE) refers to perceptions and norms of two categories of social processes that represent two kinds of community social resources: trust and connection, commonly referred to as social cohesion, and expectations for action, commonly referred to as informal social control. Studies have shown the importance of CE for multiple aspects of well-being among older adults [4–7]. In particular, CE has been shown to play a role in enhancing older adults' physical health and neighborhood satisfaction, which may predict their intentions to move and actual migration [2, 5, 8–14]. Unfortunately, existing scales measuring this construct may not be ideal for use with older adults because they were designed with the concerns of child-rearing respondents in mind [15]. For example, scale items that ask about expectations of neighbor cooperation in monitoring children may be less relevant to adults whose children are grown. At the same time, the priorities of older adults are not necessarily reflected in these existing scales.

At the individual level, a number of scales measuring such constructs as anxiety and life satisfaction have been developed based on theory and evidence regarding the distinctiveness of older adults' experiences (e.g., [16–19]). These and similar scales are able to measure the constructs of interest among older adults more accurately and with less response bias because they take into account the unique concerns, challenges, and goals of adults in the later decades of their lives [20]. For example, scales that feature items that are more salient to older adults show increased instrument acceptability in the form of higher response rates and lower differential nonresponse [21]. Such scales, by providing more easily recognized and comprehended items, also reduce response burden [22]. By following the same principles, scales measuring neighborhood social processes can be designed such that they produce more accurate measurement among older adults.

In this study we describe and test a new measure of CE. This measure was developed specifically for use in older populations, taking into account the unique ways that people of their age and cohort interpret and respond to common environmental cues, and the particular cues that we hypothesized would be uniquely important to older adults. In the first part of this paper, we explain the theoretical framework guiding our identification of environmental cues for CE likely to be salient to older adults. In the second part of the paper, we test the new measure's instrument acceptability, dimensionality, reliability, and criterion validity in an older adult population. In the third part of the paper, we appraise the new measure's construct validity by examining its association with individual health-related outcomes. Our aim was to construct a scale that can be used in research on neighborhood social processes, the health of older adults, and other factors that relate to aging in place.

Our theoretical framework combines CE theory with a consideration of the particular challenges and opportunities of the older adult life stage. As alluded to above, CE theory attempts to explain the association between neighborhood structural factors, social processes, and individual-level outcomes by positing that the neighborhood processes of social cohesion and informal social control mediate the relationship between the structural factors and individual outcomes [23, 24]. For example, compositional socioeconomic status may impact social cohesion, which in turn affects self-rated health, asthma rates, and inflammatory marker levels by reducing stress and fear [4–7, 25]. CE is therefore likely to be a part of the societal system that supports healthy living, safeguards individuals against adverse health events, and thereby enables aging in place [26]. CE is related to, but distinct from, social network interaction and exchange and social and physical disorder. The first is concerned with norms and expectations, while the second and third refer to actual behavior and conditions.

A range of theories from the aging and life course literature provide us with a framework for generating a set of cues for social cohesion and informal social control that would be particularly salient to older adults [27–33]. A key focus of later life is to develop mechanisms to adapt to new challenges, including frailty and morbidity and decreased scope and density of social networks [30, 32, 34–37]. As applied to the CE framework, these perspectives suggest that perceptions of neighbors' willingness to assist older adults with tasks, and perceptions of neighborhood norms related to regulating behavior with the goal of enhancing neighborhood safety and traversability, will be particularly important. At the same time, older adults are not only concerned with compensating for losses and coping with challenges. Generativity is also a key component of later life, defined as helping the next generation by, for instance, passing on wisdom and thereby leaving a legacy [27–29]. Within the CE framework, this perspective incorporates the notion that intergenerational exchange may contribute to a prosocial orientation and a mutual respect for community contributions across the life course.

In the remainder of this section, we discuss the research literature underlying our selection of the four specific types of cues for CE that we believe would be particularly salient to older adults. The two types of social cohesion cues that we hypothesize to be particularly salient to older adults, based on theory in urban sociology and literature on aging, are those that relate to *active caretaking of vulnerable residents* and *age integration/lack of ageism*. The two types of informal social control cues that we hypothesize to be particularly salient to older adults, based on the theory and literature on aging, are those that relate to *minimizing social incivility* and *maximizing accessibility*.

Older adults may be particularly attuned to displays of solidarity in the form of social cohesion cues related to active caring and caretaking. Frailty and decreased mobility make some tasks that are easy in middle age significantly more difficult in later life [38, 39]. Simultaneously, many older adults experience a decrease in the scope and density of their social networks [40, 41]. As a result of this combination of changes, older adults are often more reliant on assistance from community members [42, 43]. Perceptions of the availability of neighbor assistance may be particularly important to the well-being of older women compared to older men and older single men compared to older married men, who are unlikely and unable, respectively, to rely on their spouses for help [44]. Older adults who believe that their neighbors will provide active caretaking may be more confident about their ability to stay in their homes. Our new measure of CE includes two items designed to capture the tendency toward active caretaking facet of the social cohesion construct.

Older adults may also be particularly attuned to, and able to benefit substantially from, social cohesions cues related to age integration and lack of ageism. Aging societies have experienced an increase in social separation of age groups, even as age heterogeneity within most neighborhoods has increased [45–48]. One reason for the persistence of social segregation by age despite decreased logistical barriers to socializing across age boundaries may be ageism, which may interfere with communication across agelines [49]. Another factor impeding such communication is the decrease in information processing speed and loss of hearing that commonly occurs at older ages [50–52]. These factors combine to create a situation in which sustained effort is required for cross-generational socializing.

Perceptions of opportunities for cross-generational interactions are relevant to older adults priorities, and ability to age in place, for a number of reasons. Communities in which older and younger people associate may be communities in which there are fewer age-based misunderstandings, biases, fears, and resentments, and greater empathy on the part of younger people for the challenges that come with later life [45, 48, 49, 53]. Older adults who perceive their communities as age integrated may therefore feel safer venturing outside to participate in community life, because they would have less reason to fear and more reason to feel connected to a wider range of their neighbors. Expectations of communication across age lines also encompass expectations for the ability to potentially pass on wisdom, neighborhood history, or practical advice and thereby feel and be useful [54]. Such opportunities for generativity are likely to be crucial to neighborhood satisfaction; being able to fill this social role has been associated with lower mortality [55]. Our new measure of CE includes three items designed to capture the age integration facet of the social cohesion construct.

Regarding the domain of informal social control, we expect that older adults pay increased attention to the community's expectations for behaviors that minimize social incivility, as a result of reverse ageism (prejudice of older people against younger people), the increase in frailty that often accompanies advancing age [48, 56]. Older people with impaired balance, reduced muscle strength, and limited gait speed may be more likely than spry younger adults to find the loud, unpredictable peregrinations of rowdy teenagers threatening [48]. Furthermore, as a result of reverse ageism, elderly residents may perceive even subdued teenagers as a threat [56]. Their perceptions of the neighborhood's expectations for protecting vulnerable residents from malicious young people may be particularly important for older residents' willingness to venture outside on a regular basis and for their neighborhood satisfaction. Our new measure of CE includes one item designed to capture the expectation for actions that minimize social incivility, a component of the informal social control construct.

Lastly, increased frailty and disability may also increase the salience of cues for informal social control in the form of expectations for behaviors that maximize accessibility. For many older adults, navigating their neighborhoods becomes more difficult as their mobility decreases and their vulnerability for adverse health outcomes resulting from interactions with environmental hazards increases [57–60]. Older frail adults may be more attuned to obstacles and hazards in the physical environment, particularly as those environments become dilapidated [61]. Increased expectations for actions aimed at improving the safety and integrity of the environment may be related to increased likelihood of maintaining and using physical abilities and competencies for two reasons: (1) it may be related to increased confidence about venturing outside, and (2) it may relate to actual improved conditions [8, 61, 62]. Maintenance of the environment can in turn prevent the adverse health events that constitute barriers to aging in place [13, 14, 26]. Our new measure of CE includes two items designed to capture the expectations for actions that maximize accessibility, a component of the informal social control construct.

2. Methods

2.1. Data and Sample. We used data from the Chicago Neighborhood, Organization, Aging and Health study (NOAH). This study surveyed 1,500 adults aged 65 and over living in 80 selected Chicago neighborhood clusters. Each cluster was defined by two to three census tracts consisting of approximately 4,000 housing units. The sample frame consisted of all households in the city of Chicago containing at least one member 65 years of age or older. The weighted response rate for households with a phone number was 55.3% while the rate for those households for which a phone number could not be identified was 12.4%. The overall weighted response rate for the survey was 44.3%, a good rate for a telephone interview by contemporary standards [63, 64]. Interviews were conducted over the phone in English and Spanish between August 2006 and September 2007. The NOAH study was approved by the institutional review boards of both NORC and the Division of Biological Sciences at the University of Chicago. All participants provided verbal consent.

The sample consisted of the 76.7% of the 1,507 respondents with complete demographic, health, and community process data ($N = 1,151$). Descriptive statistics are shown in Table 1. The mean age was 73 (range 65–95), and 68% were female. Over two fifths (44%) were non-Hispanic White, over a third were Non-Hispanic Black (35.8%), and the rest were Hispanic (14.9%) or Other (5%). About a third (32.6%) were married, and about a tenth (9.8%) lived with someone under the age of 18. About a quarter had less than 12 years of education, about another quarter had graduated from high school, and a little under half had some college or more. A little more than a tenth of the sample had lived in their neighborhood for less than 10 years, while a little less than three quarters had lived in their neighborhood for more than 20 years. Those missing data, who were therefore excluded from the sample as described above, were more likely to be White Non-Hispanic than to be any other race/ethnicity combination.

2.2. Measures of CE. The CE questions were presented to the respondent in two blocks. The first block was introduced with the sentences, "Now I'm going to read some statements about things that people in your neighborhood may or may not do. For each of these statements, please tell me whether you strongly agree, somewhat agree, somewhat disagree, or strongly disagree." The second block was introduced with the sentence, "For each of the following, please tell me if it is very likely, somewhat likely, somewhat unlikely, or very unlikely that people in your neighborhood would act in the following manner."

Table 1: Descriptive statistics.

	%
Age (years)	
65–74	59.7
75–84	31.4
85–95	8.6
Sex	
Female	67.7
Male	32.3
Race/ethnicity	
White Non-Hispanic	44.0
Black Non-Hispanic	35.8
Hispanic	14.9
Other	5.0
Married	32.6
Live with child under age 18	9.8
Education, in years	
<12	24.5
12	26.7
>12	48.7
Years in neighborhood	
<10	11.3
10–19	16.8
20–29	12.6
30–39	19.2
40+	40.1

2.2.1. Collective Efficacy—Original Scale Items. The original CE scale, composed of eight items, first appeared in the Project on Human Development in Chicago Neighborhoods [65]. In the NOAH survey, the items were administered alongside the new CE items. The following three items were in the first block: this is a close knit neighborhood; people around here are willing to help their neighbors; people in this neighborhood can be trusted. The next five items were in the second block: your neighbors would break up a fight in front of your house in which someone was being threatened or beaten; your neighbors would do something about it if a group of neighborhood children were skipping school and hanging out on a street corner; your neighbors would do something about it if some children were spray-painting graffiti on a local building; neighborhood residents would organize to try to do something to keep the fire station open if because of budget cuts the fire station closest to your home was going to be closed down by the city; people in your neighborhood would scold a child who was showing disrespect to an adult.

2.2.2. Collective Efficacy—New Scale Items. The new CE scale, composed of eight items, was created by two of the authors. The age integration facet of social cohesion was measured with three items in the first block: people in your neighborhood treat older people in this neighborhood with respect; younger adults and children generally know who the older people in the neighborhood are; older people in this neighborhood socialize with younger adults as well as people their own age. The answer options for each of these were strongly agree, somewhat agree, somewhat disagree, and strongly disagree. The active caretaking facet of social cohesion was measured with two items, one in each block: your neighbors would shop for groceries for you, if you were sick; people in your neighborhood would check on older or more vulnerable residents if there was a heat wave. The answer options for the first item were the same as those for the age integration items. The answer options for the second item were very likely, somewhat likely, somewhat unlikely, and very unlikely. The maximizing accessibility facet of informal social control was measured with two items in the second block: people in your neighborhood would help to keep the sidewalks and other public spaces clear if there was a snowstorm; people in the neighborhood would help to get the problem corrected, if there was a problem in the neighborhood that affected older adults, like crumbling sidewalks or unsafe parks. The answer options for both items ranged from very likely to very unlikely. The minimizing social incivility facet of informal social control was measured with a single item in the second block: neighborhood residents would intervene if an older person in your neighborhood was being threatened by a group of teenagers. The answer options for this item again ranged from very likely to very unlikely.

2.3. Demographic and Health Measures. Sociodemographic measures included age, race/ethnicity, and marital status. An indicator for the presence of a child under the age of 18 in the household of the respondent was constructed using the list generated by a household roster. Health was measured using a self-report measure that asked: overall, how would you rate your health in the past 4 weeks: excellent, very good, good, fair, poor, or very poor? We treated self-rated health as an ordinal categorical variable, collapsing the categories poor and very poor into one, because less than 2% of the sample answered "very poor". A measure of mobility was constructed using two measures taken from the Health and Retirement Survey (2002) and two measures adapted from the California Health and Interview Survey (CHIS). The resulting ordinal variable had the following categories: has difficulty walking across a room, has difficulty walking one block, walks less than 10 minutes or more each week, walks 10 minutes or more once or a few times each week, walks 10 minutes or more daily, walks 10 minutes or more multiple times a day. Loneliness was measured using Hughes et al. [66] three-item scale. It has a range of 0 to 3 and a mean of 1.4.

2.4. Neighborhood Process Measures. Besides CE, NOAH measured two other neighborhood processes. Neighborhood disorder was measured with a four-item scale from the PHDCN and was introduced with the sentence, "I'm going to read a list of things that are problems in some neighborhoods. For each, please tell me how much of a problem it is in your neighborhood—a big problem, somewhat of a problem, or not a problem." The four items asked about litter, graffiti, drug use and sale, and public drinking. The scale was reliable in this sample (Cronbach's alpha = 0.74) and had a range of 1 to 3, with a mean of 1.54. Neighborhood exchange was measured with a four-item scale from the PHDCN and was introduced with the sentence, "Now I am going to ask about some things you might do with people in your neighborhood. For each, please tell me if it happens often, sometimes, rarely or never." The four items asked about doing favors, watching over homes of absent neighbors, asking for advice, and visiting. The scale was reliable in this sample (Cronbach's alpha = 0.75) and had a range of 1 to 4, with a mean of 2.8.

2.5. Analysis. In the first section of the analysis, the properties of the new CE scale were examined. Instrument acceptability and item salience were examined by comparing response rates and differential nonresponse for each item in the original and new CE scales. Next, the new scale was examined for dimensionality using principal component analysis. Because only one factor was identified, the next step was to estimate internal consistency reliability by calculating Cronbach's alpha for the new scale. Criterion validity of the new scale was tested by calculating correlations with the original CE scale. Convergent validity of the new scale was tested by calculating the correlations of the new CE scale with other NOAH measures of neighborhood processes.

In the second section of the analysis, the construct validity of the new CE scale was tested in a two-step process. First, we examined the correlations between the new scale and the health, mobility and loneliness measures, comparing the results to those from identical analyses using the original CE scale. Second, we examined whether the new scale can predict well-being more accurately in certain demographic subgroups by comparing the fit statistics of regressions estimated in those subgroups.

3. Results

3.1. New Collective Efficacy Scale: Instrument Acceptability. We first examined percentage missing for each of the items in the original and new CE scales. The items most likely to be missing in the original CE scale were "do something about kids skipping school" (4.4%) and "scold child for showing adult disrespect" (3.7%). The items most likely to be missing in the new CE scale were "younger people know older people" (5%) and "older people socialize with younger adults" (4.6%). The percentage missing one or more item from the original CE scale was 10.9%, while the percentage missing one or more item from the new CE scale was 13.0%. No clear pattern emerged of one scale showing more missing than the other.

3.2. New Collective Efficacy Scale: Differential Nonresponse. The results of the differential nonresponse analysis are shown in Table 2. Consistent with previous research, respondents in the middle and oldest age categories were more likely than those in the youngest age category to be missing at least one item from both the original and older adult CE scales [22]. The extent of this differential nonresponse by age was not equal between scales, however. Those in the oldest age category were more likely to be missing *five* of the eight items in the old CE scale: the trustworthy neighbors item (7.9% versus 1.4%, $P < 0.01$), the scold a disrespectful child item (9.4% versus 2.4%, $P < 0.01$), the graffiti item (7.1% versus 1.7%, $P < 0.05$), the skipping school item (9.4% versus 3.1%, $P < 0.05$), and the break up a fight item (4.7% versus 0.7%, $P < 0.05$). In comparison, those in the oldest age category were only more likely to be missing *three* of the eight items in the new CE scale: the young people know older people item (11.0% versus 3.7%, $P < 0.05$), the older people socialize with young adults item (9.4% versus 3.7%, $P < 0.05$), and the neighbors intervene to protect threatened elder item (6.3% versus 1.7%, $P < 0.05$). Those in the middle age category did not differ from those in the youngest age category in their likelihood of missing any of the items in the new scale but did differ in their likelihood of missing one item in the original scale: the scold a disrespectful child item (4.9% versus 2.4%, $P < 0.05$). Because such a small percentage of the respondents were in the oldest age category (9%), we recalculated these percentages comparing the youngest old to the two older groups combined. In this case, those in the middle and oldest age categories were more likely to be missing four of the items from the original scale, but were only more likely to be missing two of the items from the new scale. In the old scale, these items were the trustworthy neighbors item (4.2% versus 1.4%, $P < 0.01$), the fire station item (3.7% versus 1.8%), the scold a disrespectful child item (5.8% versus 2.3%, $P < 0.01$), and the do something about a child skipping school item (6.3% versus 3.1%, $P < 0.01$). In the new scale, these items were the young people know older people item (7.0% versus 3.7%, $P < 0.01$) and the older people socialize with young adults item (6.0% versus 3.7%, $P < 0.05$).

3.3. New Collective Efficacy Scale: Dimensionality, Reliability, Criterion and Convergent Validity. The results from the principal component analysis suggested that the eight items in the new CE scale represented a single latent factor, since only one component had an eigenvalue greater than one. The internal consistency reliability of the scale, as measured by Cronbach's alpha, was 0.81. It was slightly higher for those over 77 and men (0.82 for both groups) and slightly lower for those 65–69 and women (0.79 and 0.80, resp.). The internal consistency reliability of the theoretically defined subscales was 0.65 (informal social control) and 0.72 (social cohesion).

To examine the criterion validity of the new scale, we calculated its correlation with the old CE scale. The correlation of the scales with each other was 0.81, the correlation of the theoretically defined old and new social cohesion subscales was 0.68, and the correlation of the theoretically defined old and new informal social control subscales was 0.72.

We next tested for convergent and divergent validity by examining the association of the new CE scale with the two other NOAH measures of neighborhood quality, neighborhood disorder and neighborhood exchange (Table 3). Neighborhood exchange was more highly correlated with the new CE scale than it was with the original scale,

Table 2: Percent missing each collective efficacy xcale item, by age group.

	Young old 65–74[a] $N = 60\%$ of the sample	Middle old 75–84[b] $N = 31\%$ of the sample	Oldest old 85–95[b] $N = 9\%$ of the sample
Original collective efficacy scale items			
Close knit neighborhood	0.9	0.1	0.3
Trustworthy neighbors	1.4**	3.2+	7.9**
Neighbors help	1.3	1.3	2.4
Fire station	1.8*	3.4+	4.7
Scold a disrespectful child	2.4**	4.9*	9.4**
Do something about children spraying graffiti	1.7	1.9	7.1*
Do something about children skipping school	3.1**	5.5+	9.4*
Break up a fight	0.7+	1.3	4.7*
Missing one or more item from the original CE scale	8.3***	13.6**	19.5**
New collective efficacy scale items			
Respect for old people	1.0	1.2	2.4
Groceries when sick	2.0	2.1	2.4
Young people know older people	3.7**	5.9+	11.0*
Older people socialize with young adults	3.7*	5.1	9.4*
Neighbors intervene to protect threatened elder	1.7	1.1	6.3*
Neighbors help fix issue affecting older adults	1.5	1.7	5.5+
Neighbors check on elders during heat wave	2.2	2.1	3.1
Neighbors shovel snow	1.7	2.5	0.8
Missing one or more item from the new CE scale	10.9***	14.4+	21.9**

[a]% missing differs from % missing among middle/oldest old, $^{**}P < 0.01^{*}P < 0.05 + P < 0.1$.
[b]% missing differs from % missing among young old, $^{**}P < 0.01^{*}P < 0.05 + P < 0.1$.

while neighborhood disorder was more highly (negatively) correlated with the original CE scale than the new CE scale. Also, disorder was more highly (negatively) correlated with the new theoretically defined CE subscale of informal control than with the new theoretically defined CE subscale of social cohesion, while the reverse was true for exchange.

3.4. New Collective Efficacy Scale: Construct Validity. In the second part of the analysis, we examined the construct validity of the new scale by comparing its correlation with various health measures with similar correlations between the original scale and those measures. The correlations between the original and the new CE scales and the self-rated health, mobility, and loneliness measures are shown in Table 4. The correlation between self-rated health and CE, whether measured with the original or the new scale, was -0.17 ($P < 0.0001$). The correlation between mobility and CE, whether measured with the original or the new scale, was 0.07 ($P < 0.05$). The correlations between loneliness and the original and new CE scales differed. The correlation with the original scale was -0.16 ($P < 0.0001$) while the correlation with the new scale was -0.20 ($P < 0.0001$).

Lastly, we regressed each of these three measures on the two CE measures one at a time and compared the fit statistics. The fit of the models, as measured by the r-squared statistic, was not better for one scale than for the other (not shown). We also compared the fit statistics of these models estimated for the male and female subsamples, the married and unmarried subsamples, each of the age subgroups, and the sub-samples with and without children in their households (not shown). There were no differences in fit.

4. Discussion

The aim of this paper was to describe the development and examine the properties of a new theory-based measure of CE that incorporates the perspectives of older residents. One motivation for creating a new scale customized for a particular subpopulation is that the increased instrument acceptability and salience of the customized items may increase the response rate for the scale items. The results from our examination of the percentage missing the individual items, as well as percentage missing one or more items from the old versus the new CE scales, did not show such effects. Neither at the individual item level, nor at the scale level, did it appear that one scale is less or more likely to have missing values.

However, another motivation for creating a new scale customized for a particular subpopulation is that the increased salience of the customized items may decrease or eliminate differential nonresponse by the variables that define the subpopulation. The results from our analysis suggest such an effect in our new CE scale. The likelihood

TABLE 3: Correlations of collective efficacy scales and subscales with other neighborhood scales.

	Original CE scale	New CE scale	New CE scale—social cohesion subscale	New CE scale—informal social control subscale
Disorder	−0.39	−0.33	−0.28	−0.33
Exchange	0.43	0.53	0.52	0.41

All correlations are significant at $P < 0.0001$, except that between disorder and exchange, which is significant at $P < 0.01$.

TABLE 4: Correlations of collective efficacy scales with health and well-being.

	Original CE scale	New CE scale
Self-reported health	−0.17***	−0.17***
Mobility	0.07*	0.07*
Loneliness	−0.16***	−0.20***

$^{***}P < 0.001^{**}P < 0.01^{*}P < 0.05 + P < 0.1$.

of missing was greater among the oldest old than the rest of the sample for five of the eight items in the original scale, but only three of the eight items in the new scale. The new scale is therefore better suited for use in older populations, because nonresponse will be less likely to be a function of age. This pattern was also in line with our hypothesis that items related to children would be less relevant and therefore harder to answer for older adults. Of the items with differential nonresponse, three of the five from the original scale and one of the three from the new older adult scale concerned young people.

The results of our dimensionality and reliability analysis suggest that the scale measures one factor, with good reliability. It has reasonable criterion validity, in that it was closely correlated with the original CE scale and the other two neighborhood scales, neighborhood exchange and disorder. It was perhaps to be expected that neighborhood exchange would be more highly correlated with the new CE scale than with the original scale, while neighborhood disorder would be more highly (negatively) correlated with the original CE scale than with the new CE scale, since the original CE scale has an equal number of social cohesion and informal social control items, while the new CE scale has 5 social cohesion items but only 3 informal social control items. This difference in the number of items measuring each part of CE may also explain why disorder was more highly (negatively) correlated with the new theoretically defined CE subscale of informal control than with the new theoretically defined CE subscale of social cohesion, while the reverse was true for exchange.

The results of the construct validity analysis suggest that the new CE scale predicts health and mobility just as well as does the original CE scale and may predict loneliness slightly better—an important finding given recent literature on the prevalence and salience of loneliness among older adults.

4.1. Limitations. The primary limitation of this study is its geographic specificity. Because it is limited to a single city, replication studies will need to examine the measure's psychometric properties in rural and suburban contexts, as well as in other urban areas. The other limitations of this study relate to its survey modality. Phone surveys are subject to sampling and response bias, the first exacerbated by increased use of call screening technology and the rapid growth of telephone marketing [64, 67]. However, the risk of social desirability bias inherent in the telephone survey administration modality should be relatively minor given the non-personal and therefore non-sensitive nature of most of the questions asked [68, 69]. Also, sampling or response bias due to hearing impairment is likely to be less significant than such bias due to vision and fine motor impairment in studies using self-administered questionnaires [22, 70].

5. Conclusions

The importance of neighborhood context, and in particular its potential ability to modify adverse health event risk, prevalence, and severity is being increasingly recognized. For example, the original measure of CE has just recently been added to the PhenX toolkit, a set of consensus measures intended to standardize genetic and epidemiological research (http://www.phenxtoolkit.org/-February 4 2011, Version 4.2). While the benefits to using standard measures include comparability across studies and the potential to easily combine results in meta-analyses, there are also benefits to using measures customized to particular populations. The new measure of CE presented in this study has reliability and validity equivalent to that of the existing measure but benefits from a stronger gerontology-related theoretical grounding and reduced likelihood of age-related differential nonresponse.

The two measures exhibited both high correlation and comparable effects on the health outcomes considered. These findings raise the larger question of the extent to which measures of distinct forms of CE are capturing an underlying latent neighborhood capacity.

CE theory underscores the goal-directed nature of mobilization capacity, suggesting that a given neighborhood may have differing levels of CE depending upon the specific challenge under consideration. In this view, communities with high levels of CE with respect to the social control of public space may or may not share a comparable willingness to maintain and promote the health and well-being of local older adults.

Yet, in practice, evidence suggests that high levels of CE across multiple objectives are likely to cluster together in the same communities. This may be due to the shared origins of distinct forms of CE in the structural (e.g., economic advantage, residential stability) and social (e.g., informal network density, voluntary organization participation) conditions of urban neighborhoods. Cohesive neighborhoods with high levels of mutual trust and solidarity may provide the conditions under which generalized prosocial norms emerge, benefiting a broad base of residential constituencies.

Although the current analysis offers evidence consistent with the notion of a generalized collective capacity, we do not view these results as grounds upon which we reject the hypothesis that CE exhibits distinct dimensions. First, CE with respect to the social control of public space may have indirect benefits for older adults. Fear and the associated withdrawal from neighborhood environments may have important health implications for older adults and may be strongly related to local norms regarding the social control of children (a significant component of the original CE scale). Thus it may be the case that the original CE operates, in part, indirectly to produce comparable associations with the health outcomes considered. Second, research on the dynamics of neighborhood collective capacities is incipient. Analyses of the association and impact of CE measures focused on other shared goals (e.g., expectations regarding influence of local institutions) may reveal different patterns, warranting more extensive research.

In the case of older adult's perceptions of their communities' association with the factors that predict whether and how older adults age in place, the strength and mechanisms are still not fully understood. For example, it may be that even before health deteriorates, specific expectations that neighbors will provide help when needed and will take steps to maintain the safety of the common areas are the particular perceptions that predict intentions to stay. Similarly, it may be that when health and functionality deteriorate, the specific perception that neighbors are assuming the caretaking role usually shouldered by family may be the particular perception that forestalls a move. This new measure of CE can be used to test these hypothesized pathways, as well as the others discussed in the introduction (Section 1), that may link CE to neighborhood satisfaction, health, and the other factors that predict intention to move and actual migration.

Author's Contribution

C. R. Browning and K. A. Cagney planned the study and designed the instrument. A. M. Galinsky performed the statistical analysis and wrote the paper. K. A. Cagney supervised the data analysis. K. A. Cagney and C. R. Browning contributed to the final draft.

Acknowledgments

The authors are grateful to Alma Kuby, who managed the project, Erin Wargo, who assisted in data collection tasks, Colm O'Muircheartaigh and Ned English, who conducted the project's sample design and management, and Martha Van Haitsma and Kelly Daley, who supervised and managed the telephone interviewing. They thank Robert Sampson for consultation on the development of the measures. This work was supported by a grant from the National Institute on Aging at the National Institutes of Health (Grant no. R01 AG022488-01 to K.A.Cagney).

References

[1] C. Cannuscio, J. Block, and I. Kawachi, "Social capital and successful aging: the role of senior housing," *Annals of Internal Medicine*, vol. 139, no. 5, pp. 395–399, 2003.

[2] J. H. Oh, "Social bonds and the migration intentions of elderly urban residents: the mediating effects of residential satisfaction," *Population Research and Policy Review*, vol. 22, no. 2, pp. 127–146, 2003.

[3] World Health Organization, *Global Age-Friendy Cities: A Guide*, WHO Press, Geneva, Switzerland, 2007.

[4] C. R. Browning and K. A. Cagney, "Neighborhood structural disadvantage, collective efficacy, and self-rated physical health in an urban setting," *Journal of Health and Social Behavior*, vol. 43, no. 4, pp. 383–399, 2002.

[5] K. A. Cagney and C. R. Browning, "Exploring neighborhood-level variation in asthma and other respiratory diseases: the contribution of neighborhood social context," *Journal of General Internal Medicine*, vol. 19, no. 3, pp. 229–236, 2004.

[6] I. Kawachi and L. F. Berkman, "Social cohesion, social capital, and health," in *Social Epidemiology*, L. F. Berkman and I. Kawachi, Eds., Oxford University Press, Oxford, UK, 2000.

[7] A. Nazmi, A. Diez Roux, N. Ranjit, T. E. Seeman, and N. S. Jenny, "Cross-sectional and longitudinal associations of neighborhood characteristics with inflammatory markers: findings from the multi-ethnic study of atherosclerosis," *Health and Place*, vol. 16, no. 6, pp. 1104–1112, 2010.

[8] J. L. Balfour and G. J. Kaplan, "Neighborhood environment and loss of physical function in older adults: evidence from the Alameda County Study," *American Journal of Epidemiology*, vol. 155, no. 6, pp. 507–515, 2002.

[9] C. E. Ross, "Walking, exercising, and smoking: does neighborhood matter?" *Social Science and Medicine*, vol. 51, no. 2, pp. 265–274, 2000.

[10] M. Wen and N. A. Christakis, "Neighborhood effects on post-hospitalization mortality: a population-based cohort study of the elderly in Chicago," *Health Services Research*, vol. 40, no. 4, pp. 1108–1127, 2005.

[11] E. Litwak and C. F. Longino, "Migration patterns among the elderly: a developmental perspective," *Gerontologist*, vol. 27, no. 3, pp. 266–272, 1987.

[12] D. E. Bradley, "Litwak and Longino's developmental model of later-life migration: evidence from the American community survey, 2005–2007," *Journal of Applied Gerontology*, vol. 30, no. 2, pp. 141–158, 2011.

[13] J. F. Sergeant, D. J. Ekerdt, and R. K. Chapin, "Older adults' expectations to move: do they predict actual community-based or nursing facility moves within 2 years?" *Journal of Aging and Health*, vol. 22, no. 7, pp. 1029–1053, 2010.

[14] K. J. Stoeckel and F. Porell, "Do older adults anticipate relocating? The relationship between housing relocation expectations and falls," *Journal of Applied Gerontology*, vol. 29, no. 2, pp. 231–250, 2010.

[15] F. Earls and S. L. Buka, "Project on human development in chicago neighborhoods," Technical Report, National Institute of Justice, Rockville, Md, USA, 1997.

[16] M. P. Lawton, "The Philadelphia geriatric center morale scale: a revision," *Journals of Gerontology*, vol. 30, no. 1, pp. 85–89, 1975.

[17] B. L. Neugarten, R. J. Havighurst, and S. S. Tobin, "The measurement of life satisfaction," *Journals of Gerontology*, vol. 16, pp. 134–143, 1961.

[18] D. L. Segal, A. June, M. Payne, F. L. Coolidge, and B. Yochim, "Development and initial validation of a self-report assessment tool for anxiety among older adults: the Geriatric Anxiety Scale," *Journal of Anxiety Disorders*, vol. 24, no. 7, pp. 709–714, 2010.

[19] J. A. Yesavage, T. L. Brink, T. L. Rose et al., "Development and validation of a geriatric depression screening scale: a preliminary report," *Journal of Psychiatric Research*, vol. 17, no. 1, pp. 37–49, 1983.

[20] L. Halvorsrud and M. Kalfoss, "The conceptualization and measurement of quality of life in older adults: a review of empirical studies published during 1994–2006," *European Journal of Ageing*, vol. 4, no. 4, pp. 229–246, 2007.

[21] R. Fitzpatrick, C. Davey, M. J. Buxton, and D. R. Jones, "Evaluating patient-based outcome measures for use in clinical trials: a review," *Health Technology Assessment*, vol. 2, no. 14, 1998.

[22] C. A. McHorney, "Measuring and monitoring general health status in elderly persons: practical and methodological issues in using the SF-36 health survey," *Gerontologist*, vol. 36, no. 5, pp. 571–583, 1996.

[23] R. J. Sampson, S. W. Raudenbush, and F. Earls, "Neighborhoods and violent crime: a multilevel study of collective efficacy," *Science*, vol. 277, no. 5328, pp. 918–924, 1997.

[24] S. W. Raudenbush and R. J. Sampson, "Ecometrics: toward a science of assessing ecological settings, with application to the systematic social observation of neighborhoods," *Sociological Methodology*, vol. 29, no. 1, pp. 1–41, 1999.

[25] K. A. Cagney, T. A. Glass, K. A. Skarupski, L. L. Barnes, B. S. Schwartz, and C. F. Mendes de Leon, "Neighborhood-level cohesion and disorder: measurement and validation in two older adult urban populations," *Journals of Gerontology B*, vol. 64, no. 3, pp. 415–424, 2009.

[26] D. T. Lau, K. G. Scandrett, M. Jarzebowski, K. Holman, and L. Emanuel, "Health-related safety: a framework to address barriers to aging in place," *Gerontologist*, vol. 47, no. 6, pp. 830–837, 2007.

[27] E. H. Erikson and J. M. Erikson, *The Life Cycle Completed*, Norton, New York, NY, USA, 1997.

[28] C. D. Ryff, "Psychological well-being in adult life," *Current Directions in Psychological Science*, vol. 4, pp. 99–104, 1995.

[29] C.D. Ryff, "Happiness is everything, or is it? Explorations on the meaning of psychological well-being," *Journal of Personality and Social Psychology*, vol. 57, no. 6, pp. 1069–1081, 1989.

[30] L. P. Fried, C. M. Tangen, J. Walston et al., "Frailty in older adults: evidence for a phenotype," *Journals of Gerontology*, vol. 56, no. 3, pp. M146–M156, 2001.

[31] K. Erikson, "Reflections on generativity and society: a sociologist's perspective," in *The Generative Society: Caring for Future Generations*, E. de St. Aubin, D. P. McAdams, and T. Kim, Eds., pp. 51–61, American Psychological Association, Washington, DC, USA, 2004.

[32] E. Pfeiffer, "Psychopathology and social pathology," in *Handbook of the Psychology of Aging*, J. E. Birren and K. W. Schaie, Eds., pp. 650–671, Academic Press, New York, NY, USA, 1977.

[33] C. D. Ryff, "Beyond Ponce de Leon and life satisfaction: new directions in quest of successful ageing," *International Journal of Behavioral Development*, vol. 12, p. 55, 1989.

[34] B. Cornwell, L. P. Schumm, E. O. Laumann, and J. Graber, "Social networks in the nshap study: rationale, measurement, and preliminary findings," *Journals of Gerontology B*, vol. 64, no. 1, pp. I47–I55, 2009.

[35] D. Dannefer, "Cumulative advantage/disadvantage and the life course: cross-fertilizing age and social science theory," *Journals of Gerontology B*, vol. 58, supplement 6, pp. S327–S337, 2003.

[36] G. H. Elder, M. K. Johnson, and R. Crosnoe, "The emergence and development of life course theory," in *Handbook of the Life Course*, J. T. Mortimer and M. J. Shanahan, Eds., pp. 3–22, Springer, New York, NY, USA, 2004.

[37] S. A. Robert, K. A. Cagney, and M. Weden, "A life course approach to the study of neighborhoods and health," in *Handbook of Medical Sociology*, C. Bird, P. Conrad, and A. M. Fremont, Eds., Vanderbilt University Press, Nashville, Tenn, USA, 2010.

[38] T. L. Gruenewald, T. E. Seeman, A. S. Karlamangla, and C. A. Sarkisian, "Allostatic load and frailty in older adults," *Journal of the American Geriatrics Society*, vol. 57, no. 9, pp. 1525–1531, 2009.

[39] C. O. Weiss, "Frailty and chronic diseases in older adults," *Clinics in Geriatric Medicine*, vol. 27, no. 1, pp. 39–52, 2011.

[40] R. O. Hansson and B. N. Carpenter, *Relationships in Old Age: Coping with the Challenge of Transition*, Guilford Press, New York, NY, USA, 1994.

[41] J. E. Lansford, A. M. Sherman, and T. C. Antonucci, "Satisfaction with social networks: an examination of socioemotional selectivity theory across cohorts," *Psychology and Aging*, vol. 13, no. 4, pp. 544–552, 1998.

[42] K. E. Campbell and B. A. Lee, "Sources of personal neighbor networks: social integration, need, or time?" *Social Forces*, vol. 70, pp. 77–100, 1992.

[43] M. H. Cantor, "Life space and the social support system of the inner city elderly of New York," *Gerontologist*, vol. 15, no. 1, pp. 23–27, 1975.

[44] R. A. R. Gurung, S. E. Taylor, and T. E. Seeman, "Accounting for changes in social support among married older adults: insights from the MacArthur studies of successful aging," *Psychology and Aging*, vol. 18, no. 3, pp. 487–496, 2003.

[45] M. W. Riley and J. W. Riley, "Age integration: conceptual and historical background," *Gerontologist*, vol. 40, no. 3, pp. 266–270, 2000.

[46] G. O. Hagestad, "Towards a society for all ages: new thinking, new language, new conversations," *United Nations Bulletin on Aging*, no. 2-3, 1998.

[47] G. O. Hagestad and D. Dannefer, "Concepts and theories of aging: beyond microfication in social science approaches," in *Handbook of Aging and the Social Sciences*, R. H. Binstock and L. K. George, Eds., pp. 3–21, Academic Press, New York, NY, USA, 5th edition, 2001.

[48] P. Uhlenberg, "Integration of old and young," *Gerontologist*, vol. 40, no. 3, pp. 276–279, 2000.

[49] G. O. Hagestad and P. Uhlenberg, "The social separation of old and young: a root of ageism," *Journal of Social Issues*, vol. 61, no. 2, pp. 343–360, 2005.

[50] E. Janse, "Processing of fast speech by elderly listeners," *Journal of the Acoustical Society of America*, vol. 125, no. 4, pp. 2361–2373, 2009.

[51] X. Z. Liu and D. Yan, "Ageing and hearing loss," *Journal of Pathology*, vol. 211, no. 2, pp. 188–197, 2007.

[52] N. Wild-Wall and M. Falkenstein, "Age-dependent impairment of auditory processing under spatially focused and divided attention: an electrophysiological study," *Biological Psychology*, vol. 83, no. 1, pp. 27–36, 2010.

[53] M. W. Riley and J. W. Riley, "Age integration and the lives of older people," *Gerontologist*, vol. 34, no. 1, pp. 110–115, 1994.

[54] M. W. Riley, "Successful aging," *The Gerontologist*, vol. 38, no. 2, p. 151, 1998.

[55] T. L. Gruenewald, A. S. Karlamangla, G. A. Greendale, B. H. Singer, and T. E. Seeman, "Increased mortality risk in older adults with persistently low or declining feelings of usefulness to others," *Journal of Aging and Health*, vol. 21, no. 2, pp. 398–425, 2009.

[56] B. Levy and M. R. Banaji, "Implicit ageism," in *Ageism: Stereotyping and Prejudice Against Older Persons*, T. Nelson, Ed., pp. 49–75, MIT Press, Cambridge, Mass, USA, 2002.

[57] P. F. Adams, G. E. Hendershot, and M. A. Marano, "Current estimates from the national health interview survey, United States, 1996," Tech. Rep. 200, National Center for Health Statistics, Hyattsville, Md, USA, 1999.

[58] L. P. Fried, L. Ferrucci, J. Darer, J. D. Williamson, and G. Anderson, "Untangling the concepts of disability, frailty, and comorbidity: implications for improved targeting and care," *Journals of Gerontology*, vol. 59, no. 3, pp. 255–263, 2004.

[59] L. P. Fried, C. M. Tangen, J. Walston et al., "Frailty in older adults: evidence for a phenotype," *Journals of Gerontology*, vol. 56, no. 3, pp. M146–M156, 2001.

[60] L. Ferrucci, J. M. Guralnik, S. Studenski, L. P. Fried, G. B. Cutler, and J. D. Walston, "Designing randomized, controlled trials aimed at preventing or delaying functional decline and disability in frail, older persons: a consensus report," *Journal of the American Geriatrics Society*, vol. 52, no. 4, pp. 625–634, 2004.

[61] C. R. Clark, I. Kawachi, L. Ryan, K. Ertel, M. E. Fay, and L. F. Berkman, "Perceived neighborhood safety and incident mobility disability among elders: the hazards of poverty," *BMC Public Health*, vol. 9, article 162, 2009.

[62] J. W. Reich, A. J. Zautra, and J. Hill, "Activity, event transactions, and quality of life in older adults," *Psychology and Aging*, vol. 2, no. 2, pp. 116–124, 1987.

[63] E. Wargo, N. English, and A. Kuby, *NOAH—Neighborhood, Organization, Aging and Health*, NORC/University of Chicago, Chicago, Ill, USA, 2008.

[64] R. Curtin, S. Presser, and E. Singer, "Changes in telephone survey nonresponse over the past quarter century," *Public Opinion Quarterly*, vol. 69, no. 1, pp. 87–98, 2005.

[65] M. Tonry, L. E. Ohlin, and D. P. Farrington, "Human development and criminal behavior: new ways of advancing knowledge," in *Research in Criminology*, A. Blumstein and D. P. Farrington, Eds., Springer, New York, NY, USA, 1991.

[66] M. E. Hughes, L. J. Waite, L. C. Hawkley, and J. T. Cacioppo, "A short scale for measuring loneliness in large surveys: results from two population-based studies," *Research on Aging*, vol. 26, no. 6, pp. 655–672, 2004.

[67] A. M. Kempf and P. L. Remington, "New challenges for telephone survey research in the twenty-first century," *Annual Review of Public Health*, vol. 28, pp. 113–126, 2007.

[68] A. L. Holbrook, M. C. Green, and J. A. Krosnick, "Telephone versus face-to-face interviewing of national probability samples with long questionnaires: comparisons of respondent satisficing and social desirability response bias," *Public Opinion Quarterly*, vol. 67, no. 1, pp. 79–125, 2003.

[69] A. R. Herzog and W. L. Rodgers, "Interviewing older adults: mode comparison using data from a face-to-face survey and a telephone resurvey," *Public Opinion Quarterly*, vol. 52, no. 1, pp. 84–99, 1988.

[70] D. O. Kaldenberg, H. F. Koenig, and B. W. Becker, "Mail survey response rate patterns in a population of the elderly: does response deteriorate with age?" *Public Opinion Quarterly*, vol. 58, no. 1, pp. 68–76, 1994.

4

White Blood Cell Count in Elderly is Clinically Useful in Predicting Long-Term Survival

Göran Nilsson,[1] Pär Hedberg,[2] and John Öhrvik[3]

[1] *Centre for Clinical Research, Västmanland County Hospital, Uppsala University, 721 89 Västerås, Sweden*
[2] *Department of Clinical Physiology, Västmanland County Hospital, 721 89 Västerås, Sweden*
[3] *Department of Medicine, Karolinska Institutet, 171 76 Stockholm, Sweden*

Correspondence should be addressed to John Öhrvik; john.ohrvik@ki.se

Academic Editor: Astrid E. Fletcher

Introduction. White blood cell (WBC) count is often included in routine clinical checkups. We determined the prognostic impact of WBC count on all-cause, cardiovascular, and noncardiovascular mortality during an 11-year followup in a general population of 75-year-olds. *Study Population.* The study included 207 men and 220 women comprising 69% of the invited 75-year-olds in a defined geographical area. *Main Results.* The median WBC count (in 10^9/L) was 6.3 (interquartile range 5.4–7.2) for men and 5.7 (4.9–6.8) for women, $P < 0.001$ for sex difference. The hazard ratio (HR) for all-cause mortality per 10^9/L increase in WBCs was 1.16 (95% confidence interval, 1.03–1.32; $P = 0.016$) in men and 1.28 (1.10–1.50; $P = 0.002$) in women. These HRs were essentially unchanged by adjustment for established risk factors (current smoking, known hypertension, prior myocardial infarction, known diabetes, total cholesterol, high-density lipoprotein cholesterol, and body mass index). Furthermore, increased WBC count was significantly associated with cardiovascular mortality in both sexes and with noncardiovascular mortality in women. *Conclusions.* The WBC count deserves attention as a potentially clinical useful predictor of survival in the 75-year-olds, especially among women.

1. Introduction

The white blood cell (WBC) count is marker of systemic inflammation. It is determined routinely by means of well-standardized automated methods at low cost and with high precision. Consequently, the WBC count is often included in routine clinical checkups. Data from multiple observational studies have demonstrated that WBC count has an independent ability to predict all-cause mortality [1–4], cancer mortality [5, 6] and cardiovascular diseases and mortality [7]. Reports [2, 8, 9] suggest that the predictive ability of the WBC counts also applies to the elderly but there is a need for further studies on this topic, particularly among elderly women.

The aim of the present study was to determine the prognostic impact of WBC count on all-cause, cardiovascular, and noncardiovascular mortality during an 11-year followup in a general population of 75-year-olds.

2. Methods

2.1. Study Population. The city of Västerås (130,000 inhabitants) situated in central Sweden has a population that is socioeconomically representative for the country. In 1997 a random sample of 618 of the 1,100 inhabitants born in 1922 (i.e., 75 year old) were invited to participate in a cardiovascular health survey. Four hundred thirty-two individuals (210 men and 222 women) finally accepted the invitation, corresponding to a participation rate of 70%. Reasons for nonparticipation were: Unknown ($n = 46$), never reached ($n = 29$), unwilling due to diseases under treatment ($n = 54$), locomotive impairment ($n = 28$), language difficulties or logistical problems ($n = 26$), or died before examination ($n = 2$). Due to missing values in WBC counts (4 subjects), the examined cohort finally comprised 208 men and 220 women (69% of invited individuals).

The study was approved by the research ethics committee of Uppsala University, Sweden, and was conducted in accordance with the Declaration of Helsinki. All subjects gave their informed consent.

2.2. Blood Analyses. The blood samples were collected in a fasting state in the morning. WBCs were counted with an automated blood cell counter, Cell-Dyn 3500 (Abbott). Serum triglycerides, total cholesterol, and high-density lipoprotein cholesterol (HDL-C) were determined enzymatically on an automated analyser system (Hitachi 717, Boehringer Mannheim). Low-density lipoprotein cholesterol (LDL-C) was calculated using the Friedewald formula [10]. The blood glucose samples were treated with a haemolytic reagent (Merck Diagnostica) and glucose was determined enzymatically with glucose dehydrogenase on a Cobas Mira analyser. Plasma glucose was computed from venous whole blood glucose using the formula: plasma glucose = 0.558 + 1.119* whole blood glucose [11].

Blood pressure (BP) was measured to the nearest five mm Hg with a mercury sphygmomanometer with the subjects in a supine position having rested for five minutes.

2.3. Prospective Followup. All-cause mortality served as the primary end point. By means of the Swedish population register, the study cohort was followed for all-cause mortality from the index examination in 1997 until November 1, 2008. Only one individual (a man) was lost to followup (reason: migration). Causes of death until November 1, 2008, were obtained from the Swedish Cause of Death Register. The 10th revision of the International Statistical Classification of Diseases (ICD) was used to identify causes of death. For the present analyses, causes of death were grouped into two categories: cardiovascular, ICD 10, I00-I99, or noncardiovascular comprising all other causes of death. The study was not powered for analyzing more detailed categories of death causes.

2.4. Statistical Analyses. Continuous variables were summarized by medians and interquartile ranges and categorical variables by numbers and proportions. The Wilcoxon-Mann-Whitney rank sum test was used to compare continuous variables and Fisher's exact test to compare categorical variables.

Crude and adjusted prospective associations of the WBC count with mortality were assessed by hazard ratios (HR) and corresponding 95% confidence intervals (CI) using uni- and multivariable Cox proportional hazard regression. For continuous variables, the assumption of proportional hazards (PH) was assessed by examining the variables' interaction with time or a function of time (e.g., log(time)) in a Cox model. The PH assumption for categorical variables was assessed by visual inspection of the log (−log(cumulative survival)). Cumulative survival was estimated by means of the Kaplan-Meier survival curves. Associations between continuous variables were assessed by Spearman's rank correlation. The sex disparity in the strength of the association between WBC count and other markers was assessed by including the interaction term between sex and WBC count in a regression model with the marker as dependent variable.

A two-sided P value <0.05 was regarded as statistically significant in all analyses. IBM SPSS version 20 was used for the analyses.

3. Results

The distribution of the WBC counts among the participants at baseline was positively skewed. The ranges of the WBC counts (in 10^9/L) were 3.0–12.0 for men and 2.9–10.6 for women. The median (interquartile range) was 6.3 (5.4–7.2) for men and 5.7 (4.9–6.8) for women. The mean (SD) was 6.36 (1.44) for men and 5.90 (1.46) for women. The sex disparity was statistically significant ($P < 0.001$).

Table 1 shows the baseline characteristics for men and women stratified by survival status. Of note only WBC count differed significantly between survivors and nonsurvivors in both sexes (higher in nonsurvivors); in addition known hypertension, prior myocardial infarction, and lower HDL-C levels were significantly more common in nonsurviving men and higher plasma glucose levels in nonsurviving women.

There were strong correlations between WBC count and plasma glucose and HDL-C, respectively, in women (Spearman correlation 0.29; $P < 0.001$ and Spearman correlation −0.25; $P < 0.001$) but not in men (Spearman correlation 0.09; $P = 0.22$ and Spearman correlation 0.01; $P = 0.88$). The sex disparity in the strength of these associations was significant ($P = 0.030$ and $P < 0.001$).

During a median followup of 11.4 years (range 0.2–11.8 years) 108 (52%) men and 67 (30%) women died. The total number of person-years with followup was 4088 implying 4.3 deaths per 100 person-years at risk (men 5.9; women 3.0). In men there were 48 deaths from cardiovascular causes and 60 from noncardiovascular causes (including 31 attributed to malignancy). The corresponding figures for women were 32 deaths from cardiovascular causes and 35 from noncardiovascular causes (including 13 attributed to malignancy). The cause of death was unknown in one man and three women.

The mortality among the 30% of invited individuals who did not participate in the investigation was considerably higher (67%) than among the participants.

Table 2 shows the Cox regression analyses of WBC count and all-cause, cardiovascular, and noncardiovascular mortality stratified by sex. Three different models were assessed: model 1 unadjusted HR for WBC count, model 2 HR for WBC count adjusted for current smoking and known hypertension, and model 3 HR for WBC count adjusted for current smoking, known hypertension, prior myocardial infarction, known diabetes, total cholesterol, HDL-C, and BMI. Model 2, which adjusts for the two most significant risk factors, was used for the cardiovascular and noncardiovascular mortality since the relatively few events in these categories did not allow further adjustments. The prognostic ability of the WBC count for all-cause mortality was considerably better in women than in men, but the sex disparity did not reach statistical significance ($P = 0.34$).

In an additional analysis we excluded deaths within 5 years, thereby reasonably excluding prevalent severe disease at the time of inclusion in the study. For all-cause mortality,

Table 1: Sex-specific baseline characteristics of the study cohort according to survival status. Categorical variables are shown as number (%) and continuous variables as median (interquartile range).

	Survivors		Nonsurvivors	
	Men ($n = 99$)	Women ($n = 153$)	Men ($n = 108$)	Women ($n = 67$)
Current smoker	9 (9)	8 (5)	18 (17)	8 (12)
Known hypertension	14 (14)†	39 (25)	41 (38)†	26 (39)
Known diabetes	6 (6)	9 (6)	9 (8)	8 (12)
Prior myocardial infarction	9 (9)†	4 (3)	22 (20)†	6 (9)
Statin medication	1 (1)	4 (3)	6 (6)	3 (4)
WBC count (10^9/L)	6.1 (5.4–6.8)†	5.6 (4.7–6.7)‡	6.4 (5.5–7.4)†	5.8 (5.1–7.1)‡
BMI (kg/m^2)	25.4 (23.1–26.8)	26.2 (23.7–29.3)	25.1 (23.7–27.3)	25.8 (23.4–28.3)
Plasma glucose (mmol/L)	5.8 (5.4–6.4)	5.9 (5.4–6.4)‡	5.9 (5.4–6.6)	6.0 (5.5–7.2)‡
Systolic BP (mmHg)	160 (144–180)	165 (150–190)	160 (150–180)	165 (150–180)
Diastolic BP (mmHg)	83 (75–90)	85 (80–90)	85 (80–91)	85 (75–90)
Total cholesterol (mmol/L)	6.0 (5.4–6.8)	6.6 (5.8–7.3)	5.9 (5.3–6.5)	6.5 (5.9–7.0)
LDL-cholesterol (mmol/L)	3.8 (3.2–4.7)	4.1 (3.4–4.8)	3.8 (2.9–4.3)	4.2 (3.6–4.8)
HDL-cholesterol (mmol/L)	1.4 (1.2–1.7)†	1.6 (1.4–2.0)	1.4 (1.2–1.5)†	1.5 (1.2–1.9)
Triglycerides (mmol/L)	1.4 (1.0–1.8)	1.4 (1.1–2.1)	1.6 (1.1–2.0)	1.5 (1.1–2.0)

†Significant difference between survivors and nonsurvivors in men.
‡Significant difference between survivors and nonsurvivors in women.

the HR (95%CI) was 1.11 (0.96–1.29; $P = 0.175$) in men and 1.27 (1.08–1.51; $P = 0.004$) in women.

Figure 1 shows the Kaplan-Meier curves for all-cause mortality according to sex-specific WBC count tertiles. Of note women with a WBC count in the two lowest tertiles ($\leq 6.4 \times 10^9$/L) had a considerably lower cumulative mortality during followup (27%) compared with the mortality among men (62%) in the highest tertile (WBC count $\geq 6.8 \times 10^9$/L).

4. Discussion

4.1. Principal Finding. The principal finding in the present community-based study of 75-year-olds is a considerable long-term prognostic significance of the basic WBC count, especially among women. Determination of the WBC count is a well standardized and cost-effective procedure with excellent precision and it is often included in routine checkups. Thus, the present finding is of potential clinical importance. We previously reported the poor prognostic value of serum cholesterol in the present population [12]. Evidently, the WBC count has a much stronger prognostic ability with regard to total mortality and cardiovascular mortality than total cholesterol and LDL-C among the elderly.

4.2. Strengths and Limitations. The restriction of the present investigation to one age class made it possible to leave age out of account as covariate, thereby enabling us to draw conclusions about WBC counts and mortality despite a relatively low number of participants in the study. This advantage, of course, was obtained at the cost of generalizing our conclusions to people not 75 years of age and to people living in other geographical areas. However, our conclusions seem reasonably applicable to north Europeans and white North Americans in their seventies. The strength of the present study is increased by a relatively long time of followup.

The examined communitybased cohort was well defined and the participation rate was rather high. Reasons for nonparticipation were accounted for and included a substantial fraction of individuals already under medical attention. This is a likely explanation for the higher mortality among nonparticipants than among participants. Similar studies from other centers need to confirm the results from the present study.

4.3. Comparison with Other Studies. It is well known that the WBC count is higher among men than among women [3, 13]. The reason for this sex disparity is unknown. Modification of inflammatory reaction owing to the necessity of female acceptance of the genetically different fetal tissue during pregnancy may be one speculative reason for the sex disparity.

Multiple observational studies have demonstrated that WBC counts have substantial ability to predict all-cause mortality [1–4, 14], cardiovascular mortality [14, 15], cerebrovascular mortality [7], and cancer mortality [5, 6, 14] as well as incident coronary heart diseases [15, 16]. Only a few of these studies have included women [3, 6, 15]. In these observational studies broad age categories of mainly middle-aged people have been evaluated as homogenous groups with no opportunity to distinguish prognoses for distinct age classes, such as the 75-year-olds of the present study.

The sex difference in WBC count found in the present study corresponds to that found in people over 75 years of age in the United States National Health and Nutrition Examination Survey (NHANES) [17]. Furthermore the NHANES

TABLE 2: Cox regression analyses of all-cause, cardiovascular, and noncardiovascular mortality according to WBC count stratified by sex ($n = 207$ men and $n = 220$ women).

	HR	95% CI	*P* value
Men			
All-cause mortality			
Model 1	1.16	1.03–1.32	0.016
Model 3	1.12	0.98–1.28	0.092
Cardiovascular mortality			
Model 1	1.21	1.01–1.45	0.038
Model 2	1.13	0.95–1.35	0.181
Noncardiovascular mortality			
Model 1	1.12	0.95–1.33	0.171
Model 2	1.09	0.92–1.30	0.331
Women			
All-cause mortality			
Model 1	1.28	1.10–1.50	0.002
Model 3	1.23	1.03–1.47	0.020
Cardiovascular mortality			
Model 1	1.30	1.04–1.62	0.021
Model 2	1.21	0.96–1.53	0.110
Noncardiovascular mortality			
Model 1	1.27	1.03–1.58	0.028
Model 2	1.20	0.95–1.52	0.119

All hazard ratios (HR) are per 10^9/L increase in WBC count. Model 1: crude HR, model 2: HR adjusted for current smoking and known hypertension, and model 3: HR adjusted for current smoking, known hypertension, prior myocardial infarction, known diabetes, total cholesterol, HDL-cholesterol, and BMI.

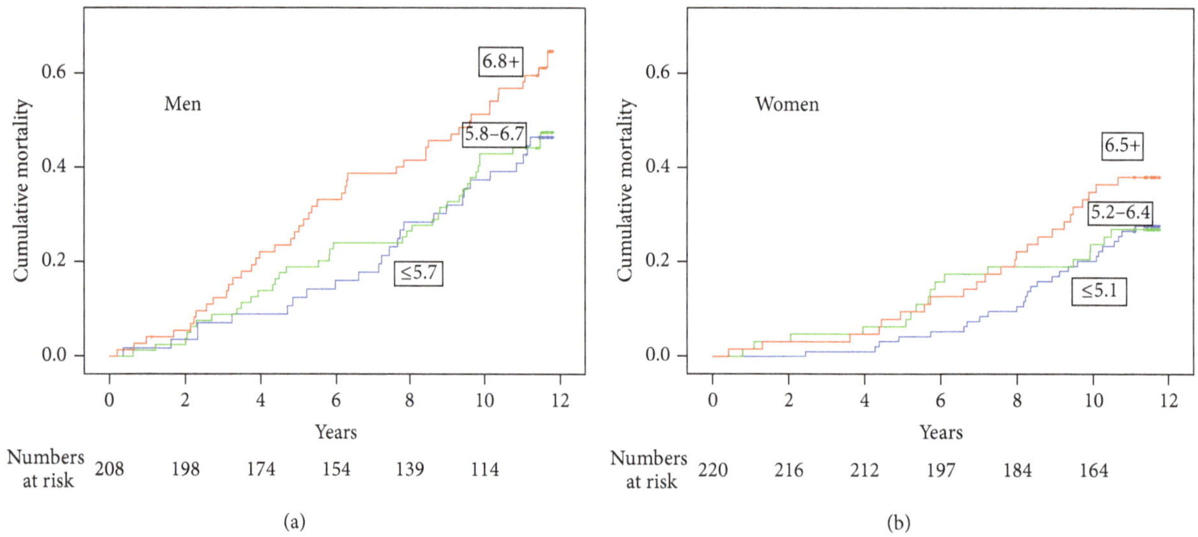

FIGURE 1: Kaplan-Meier curves showing cumulative all-cause mortality according to sex-specific WBC count tertiles.

study demonstrated a mean WBC count slightly on the rise in those above 65 years of age [17].

Each age class represents survivors from younger age classes. Consequently, clinically established risk factors among middle-aged people may not be applicable to elderly people, whereas other factors, exemplified by the WBC count, may assume greater importance. Our finding of this test's relatively strong prognostic ability among the elderly is clinically important.

Concerning the prognostic aspect of the WBC count, two past studies have included elderly women. In a 10-year followup of 705 men and women, more than 85 years old, in Leiden in The Netherlands, Willems et al. [8] found results similar to ours. However, their analyses were not stratified by sex.

Margolis et al. [15] reported a followup of 72,000 women from the Women's Health Initiative Observational Study. Higher WBC counts predicted cardiovascular events and total mortality during a mean followup of 6.1 years also after multifactor adjustment including age. The oldest group (70–79 years) comprised 22% of the cohort, but no separate analyses were performed for this age group. Women in the top quartile ($\geq 6.7 \times 10^9$, cells/L) had 50% higher risk for total mortality than women in the lowest quartile ($\leq 4.7 \times 10^9$, cells/L).

Concerning elderly men, Weijenberg et al. [2] reported 5-year survival among 884 randomly selected men, aged 65–84 years, from the general population. The excess mortality risk with increasing WBC count was similar to our results. Notably, the followup time for Weijenberg et al. [2] was considerably shorter than that of the present study (5 versus 11 years). In the present study we observed a significantly higher risk of mortality among women even if deaths within 5 years were excluded.

4.4. Possible Mechanisms. The WBC count tends to cluster with other established risk factors such as tobacco smoking [14, 18] as well as HDL-cholesterol and triglycerides [9, 13]. However, the risk excess found in the present analyses was practically unchanged after adjustment for these factors.

The pathophysiological mechanisms that link elevated WBC count to increased mortality are not well understood. Thus, it is not known whether elevated WBC count is involved directly in the pathogenesis of vascular diseases or is merely a risk indicator of other factors causing vascular damage [19]. The same uncertainty applies also to the well-known relation between elevated WBC count and diabetes [20]. There is clear evidence that neutrophil is the subgroup of WBC that is most strongly associated with coronary risk [16]. This finding might provide clues as to the association between WBC counts and cardiovascular death.

4.5. Clinical Implications. By means of our data, the mortality risk among elderly people at different levels of basal WBC counts (Figure 1) can be estimated in a cost-effective manner during clinical checkups.

Of note, this prognostic ability contrasts with the serum cholesterol's lack of ability to predict all-cause mortality among the elderly [12]. The within-subject variability compared with the between-subject variability is similar to WBC count and serum cholesterol [21]. Thus, determination of the WBC count seems more useful than the determination of the serum cholesterol in a clinical geriatric context.

Conflict of Interests

The authors declare that there is no conflict of interests regarding the publication of this paper.

Acknowledgments

The authors are grateful to Marja-Leena Ojutkangas for her excellent care of the study participants and data management. The authors are also grateful to Mattias Rehn for excellent technical support. This work was supported by Västmanland County Council Research foundation.

References

[1] R. F. Gillum, D. D. Ingram, and D. M. Makuc, "White blood cell count, coronary heart disease, and death: the NHANES I epidemiologic follow-up study," *American Heart Journal*, vol. 125, no. 3, pp. 855–863, 1993.

[2] M. P. Weijenberg, E. J. M. Feskens, and D. Kromhout, "White blood cell count and the risk of coronary heart disease and all-cause mortality in elderly men," *Arteriosclerosis, Thrombosis, and Vascular Biology*, vol. 16, no. 4, pp. 499–503, 1996.

[3] C. Ruggiero, E. J. Metter, A. Cherubini et al., "White blood cell count and mortality in the Baltimore Longitudinal Study of Aging," *Journal of the American College of Cardiology*, vol. 49, no. 18, pp. 1841–1850, 2007.

[4] S. T. Weiss, M. R. Segal, D. Sparrow, and C. Wager, "Relation of FEV1 and peripheral blood leukocyte count to total mortality. The Normative Aging Study," *American Journal of Epidemiology*, vol. 142, no. 5, pp. 493–503, 1995.

[5] T. P. Erlinger, P. Muntner, and K. J. Helzlsouer, "WBC count and the risk of cancer mortality in a national sample of U.S. adults: results from the Second National Health and Nutrition Examination Survey mortality study," *Cancer Epidemiology Biomarkers and Prevention*, vol. 13, no. 6, pp. 1052–1056, 2004.

[6] K. L. Margolis, R. J. Rodabough, C. A. Thomson, A. M. Lopez, and A. McTiernan, "Prospective study of leukocyte count as a predictor of incident breast, colorectal, endometrial, and lung cancer and mortality in postmenopausal women," *Archives of Internal Medicine*, vol. 167, no. 17, pp. 1837–1844, 2007.

[7] D. W. Brown, E. S. Ford, W. H. Giles, J. B. Croft, L. S. Balluz, and A. H. Mokdad, "Associations between white blood cell count and risk for cerebrovascular disease mortality: NHANES II Mortality Study, 1976—1992," *Annals of Epidemiology*, vol. 14, no. 6, pp. 425–430, 2004.

[8] J. M. Willems, S. Trompet, G. J. Blauw, R. G. J. Westendorp, and A. J. M. de Craen, "White blood cell count and c-reactive protein are independent predictors of mortality in the oldest old," *Journals of Gerontology A*, vol. 65, no. 7, pp. 764–768, 2010.

[9] G. Nilsson, P. Hedberg, and J. Ohrvik, "Inflammation and the metabolic syndrome: clustering and impact on survival in a Swedish community-based cohort of 75 year olds," *Metabolic Syndrome and Related Disorders*, vol. 11, no. 2, pp. 92–101, 2013.

[10] W. T. Friedewald, R. I. Levy, and D. S. Fredrickson, "Estimation of the concentration of low-density lipoprotein cholesterol in plasma, without use of the preparative ultracentrifuge," *Clinical Chemistry*, vol. 18, no. 6, pp. 499–502, 1972.

[11] "Age- and sex-specific prevalences of diabetes and impaired glucose regulation in 13 European cohorts," *Diabetes Care*, vol. 26, no. 1, pp. 61–69, 2003.

[12] G. Nilsson, J. Ohrvik, I. Lonnberg, and P. Hedberg, "Ten-year survival in 75-year-old men and women: predictive ability of total cholesterol, HDL-C, and LDL-C," *Current Gerontology and Geriatrics Research*, vol. 2009, Article ID 158425, 7 pages, 2009.

[13] G. Nilsson, P. Hedberg, T. Jonason, I. Lönnberg, Å. Tenerz, and J. Öhrvik, "White blood cell counts associate more strongly to the metabolic syndrome in 75-year-old women than in men: a population based study," *Metabolic Syndrome and Related Disorders*, vol. 5, no. 4, pp. 359–364, 2007.

[14] R. H. Grimm Jr., J. D. Neaton, and W. Ludwig, "Prognostic importance of the white blood cell count for coronary, cancer,

and all-cause mortality," *Journal of the American Medical Association*, vol. 254, no. 14, pp. 1932–1937, 1985.

[15] K. L. Margolis, J. E. Manson, P. Greenland et al., "Leukocyte count as a predictor of cardiovascular events and mortality in postmenopausal women: the Women's Health Initiative Observational Study," *Archives of Internal Medicine*, vol. 165, no. 5, pp. 500–508, 2005.

[16] J. G. Wheeler, M. E. Mussolino, R. F. Gillum, and J. Danesh, "Associations between differential leucocyte count and incident coronary heart disease: 1764 Incident cases from seven prospective studies of 30,374 individuals," *European Heart Journal*, vol. 25, no. 15, pp. 1287–1292, 2004.

[17] C. K.-W. Cheng, J. Chan, G. S. Cembrowski, and O. W. van Assendelft, "Complete blood count reference interval diagrams derived from NHANES III: stratification by age, sex, and race," *Laboratory Hematology*, vol. 10, no. 1, pp. 42–53, 2004.

[18] F. Corre, J. Lellouch, and D. Schwartz, "Smoking and leucocyte-counts. Results of an epidemiological survey," *The Lancet*, vol. 2, no. 7725, pp. 632–634, 1971.

[19] R. W. Alexander, "Inflammation and coronary artery disease," *The New England Journal of Medicine*, vol. 331, no. 7, pp. 468–469, 1994.

[20] E. Gkrania-Klotsas, Z. Ye, A. J. Cooper et al., "Differential white blood cell count and type 2 diabetes: systematic review and meta-analysis of cross-sectional and prospective studies," *PLoS ONE*, vol. 5, no. 10, Article ID e13405, 2010.

[21] D. W. Ross, L. H. Ayscue, J. Watson, and S. A. Bentley, "Stability of hematologic parameters in healthy subjects. Intraindividual versus interindividual variation," *American Journal of Clinical Pathology*, vol. 90, no. 3, pp. 262–267, 1988.

5

Using Structured Observation and Content Analysis to Explore the Presence of Older People in Public Fora in Developing Countries

Geraldine Nosowska,[1] Kevin McKee,[2] and Lena Dahlberg[2,3]

[1]*Effective Practice Ltd., 8 Bridgetown, Totnes, Devon TQ95AB, UK*
[2]*School of Education, Health and Social Studies, Dalarna University, 791 88 Falun, Sweden*
[3]*Aging Research Centre, Karolinska Institutet and Stockholm University, Gävlegatan 16, 113 30 Stockholm, Sweden*

Correspondence should be addressed to Lena Dahlberg; ldh@du.se

Academic Editor: F. R. Ferraro

There is a lack of research on the everyday lives of older people in developing countries. This exploratory study used structured observation and content analysis to examine the presence of older people in public fora and considered the methods' potential for understanding older people's social integration and inclusion. Structured observation occurred of public social spaces in six cities each located in a different developing country and in one city in the United Kingdom, together with content analysis of the presence of people in newspaper pictures and on television in the selected countries. Results indicated that across all fieldwork sites and data sources, there was a low presence of older people, with women considerably less present than men in developing countries. There was variation across fieldwork sites in older people's presence by place and time of day and in their accompanied status. The presence of older people in images drawn from newspapers was associated with the news/non-news nature of the source. The utility of the study's methodological approach is considered, as is the degree to which the presence of older people in public fora might relate to social integration and inclusion in different cultural contexts.

1. Introduction

By 2050, there will be approximately 2 billion people aged 60 years or more and the number of older people will outnumber the young. The most rapid changes will take place in developing countries, and projections indicate that by then four of five older people will live in developing countries [1]. This demographic change has implications not only for the delivery of health and social care and for age-related policy issues, such as pensions, but also for the everyday life of citizens both young and old. Our capacity to understand how demographic changes in developing countries will impact on older people's lives is limited by the relative lack of research on the everyday lives of older people in such countries [2]. In this paper, we describe an exploratory study that examines the public presence of older people, with consideration of differences between women and men. This is done via the structured observation of social spaces in selected cities in six developing countries and one city in a developed county and content analysis of examples of the countries' respective print and broadcast media, specifically images in newspapers and on television channels. The potential of such data for understanding the social integration and inclusion of older people is discussed.

When proposing a need for more social research on older people in developing countries, the methodological approach to be adopted requires particularly careful consideration. Applying conventional research methods might be problematic. Using survey methods and instruments created for use in developed countries raises issues of validity, if concepts and language are simply imported without thought for differing cultural contexts. Difficulties in accessing older people and the use of standardised but culturally biased procedures and formats for delivering questions and eliciting responses threaten reliability and representativeness (cf. [3]). Qualitative methods are suitable for developing understanding and theory and are arguably more sensitive than quantitative studies to cultural issues. However, studies using such methods have limitations as their (usually) small and unrepresentative samples prevent generalization of their findings to target populations, and the studies' findings are additionally often difficult to reproduce [4].

Observational methods and content analysis might circumvent some of the problems that arise in using conventional research methods in the context of developing countries. It can be argued that the actual presence or absence of older people in public fora, such as social and cultural spaces, is a good marker of their level of social integration (cf. [5]). The use of social spaces can influence societal attitudes to different groups and the degree to which they belong in society [6]. Also, it can direct us towards the way space works to include or exclude people [7]. Presence or absence can also be considered through visibility in different media such as newspapers, films, or television. Mass media are a force for shaping attitudes and images of older people in media shape perceptions and self-perceptions of ageing [8–11]. Underrepresentation in media could lead to a perception that groups of the population are of little significance to society (cf. [12]). Thus, how far older people are visible in such cultural spaces and the nature of their presentation are both reflections and drivers of social norms, becoming both measures of social integration and factors that affect social integration.

Studies that document the presence or absence of older people in public fora might therefore provide valuable data that will contribute to our understanding of the place of older people in their respective societies. However, there are a very limited number of such studies, particularly in developing countries. There is some information, primarily from developed countries, about places that are important to older people. For example, Londoners identified a religious building as an important place in their lives [13] and different ethnic groups identified varying benefits in using parks in the United States of America (US) [14], while older people in Hong Kong found that poor health, lack of time, and issues with other users reduced their use of parks, despite their health and social and psychological benefits ([15]; cf. [16]).

With regard to the presence and form of presentation of older people in broadcast and print media there is a considerable body of work available, but there is a knowledge gap around images of older people in non-Western cultures with cross-cultural research extremely limited [17]. In the available research from developed countries, there is a consensus that older people have been and continue to be less present than expected with regard to their prevalence in the population. For example, an extensive observational study of German television networks found that people over 60 were very underrepresented, particularly women and those of advanced old age [18]. Research on prime time US television echoes this [19–21]. Similarly, US [22] and German studies [23] have found an underrepresentation of older people in television and printed advertisements, respectively. Content analysis of print media in one area in the USA found that stories that could be illustrated by pictures of people of any age tended to feature younger people [24]. Older people were also underrepresented in the United Kingdom (UK) magazine advertisements, Canadian television advertisement, and Irish newspapers [25–27]. Although there are positive images on older people in aspirational advertising (for a discussion, see [27]), when present in media older people are frequently constructed as victims and being frail, vulnerable, and so forth [28], not the least when mentioned in the context of population ageing [9].

Considering developing or non-Western countries, a study on the presentation of older people on Taiwanese television [29] produced findings similar to those obtained in the USA, while studies looking at the presentation of older people in the media in India and Japan found that there was an underrepresentation of older people, particularly of older women, in magazine and television announcements, respectively [30, 31].

When studying older people's presence in public fora, it is important to consider the differing life situations of older women and men in developing and developed countries. First, there are health differences between women and men, with greater healthy life expectancy among women in both developing and developed countries [32]. Second, there are social differences. Studies in both developed and developing countries have established that social contacts and social support are positively associated with health and wellbeing (e.g., [33–38]) and that older women have higher levels of social contacts and social support than older men (e.g., [1, 33, 39, 40]). However, as women live longer and tend to marry older men, they are more likely to enter widowhood than men and at a younger age [41]. These gender differences in health and social support would be anticipated to influence the extent to which older women and men are present in public spaces.

Furthermore, there are gender differences with regard to media representation. As indicated above, research has shown that older women are particularly underrepresented across a range of media. Feminist critique of media representations suggests that underrepresentation may play a significant role in how women interpret and experience ageing [42]. In addition, in both developing and developed countries, women are generally shown in traditionally feminine and stereotyped roles, and they are often portrayed in a negative and circumscribed manner [43]. For example, one study of Arabic television found that women are more often shown in domestic roles and indoor settings, whereas men are shown in professional roles and outdoors settings (see [44]).

Our primary research question is: how present are older people in public fora in developing countries? A secondary research question is: is the presence of older people in public fora related to their gender? Our site selection, of six cities in six developing countries and one city in a developed country, and the use of two data collection methods were motivated by several considerations. First, as this was an exploratory study it was important to examine the validity, reliability, and feasibility of the methods adopted across a wide range of settings. The selection of a range of developing countries

TABLE 1: Observations of older people in public places and in media.

	Data source									
	Public spaces		Newspapers			Television				
	Observations		Read	Pictures examined		Channels watched	Observation periods	Total time	Scenes examined	
	Periods	Time								
	n	%	n	n	%	n	n	%	n	%
City/country										
Haleb/Syria	42	15.9	3	114	7.96	8	6	22.2	165	27.6
Amman/Jordan	42	15.9	3	136	9.49	5	5	18.5	77	12.9
Luxor/Egypt	42	15.9	3	236	16.5	4	5	18.5	50	8.35
Bangkok/Thailand	36	13.6	3	450	31.4	0	0	0	0	0
Nairobi/Kenya	30	11.4	2	170	11.9	0	0	0	0	0
Arusha/Tanzania	30	11.4	2	93	6.49	6	5	18.5	111	18.5
Sheffield/UK	42	15.9	2	234	16.3	4	6	22.2	196	32.7
Total	**264**	**100**	**18**	**1433**	**100**	**27**	**27**	**100**	**599**	**100**

fulfilled this consideration, as such countries would provide challenges and contexts as fieldwork sites that would contrast with those found in the developed country; there would also likely be differences between the selected developing countries themselves. Second, there is a tremendous gap between our understanding of the demographic changes affecting older people in the developing world and our understanding of the public lives of older people in such countries. Our study, with its primary focus on developing countries, would thus both increase the amount of data available on the presence of older women and men in social spaces and in the media in such countries and offer some insight into how their presence in public fora in developing countries contrasts with their presence in similar fora in a developed country, with opportunity for cautious comparison due to the use of standardised methods across fieldwork sites. Finally, the use of three different data sources—non-participant structured observation in social spaces and content analysis of images of older people both in newspapers and on television—would allow for triangulation of data as a way of evaluating the robustness of findings.

2. Method

2.1. Country Selection. This study involved gathering data in six developing countries—Syria, Jordan, Egypt, Thailand, Kenya, and Tanzania—and in one Western country—the UK—over the course of 2007. In each of these countries, structured observations were carried out in public social places where people were likely to be present and content analysis was performed of images in newspapers and television programmes in which they were likely to be depicted.

Country selection was guided by a need for variation in geographical location, political structures, and ethnic and social mixes, as well as demography. The chosen developing countries offer diversity of cultures, with varying degrees of contrast and comparison with the selected site in the UK. The selected countries represent, respectively, the overwhelmingly Arabic Muslim Syria and Jordan and Hamitic Muslim Egypt; the multiplicity of ethnic groups in Black East Africa, with a predominantly Christian culture and minority Muslim culture in Kenya, and strong Christian and Muslim cultures in Tanzania; and the distinctive, largely Buddhist Thai culture of the Indian subcontinent, with its Chinese and Malay subpopulations. The UK has predominantly a white population with strong Christian heritage but has increasingly diverse ethnic and religious minorities [45, 46]. At the time of data collection, Syria, Egypt, Kenya, and Tanzania had presidential and parliamentary government and Jordan and Thailand had constitutional monarchies with parliamentary government, as did the UK. The urban population is 90 per cent in the UK, 82 per cent in Jordan, 50 per cent in Syria, 43 per cent in Egypt, 33 per cent in Thailand, 23 per cent in Tanzania, and 19 per cent in Kenya [47]. Life expectancy in the selected countries varies considerably. In 2006, it was 79 years in the UK, 72 in Syria and Thailand, 71 in Jordan, and 68 in Egypt, but only 53 in Kenya and 50 in Tanzania. Twenty-two percent of the UK population is over 60, compared to 12 per cent in Thailand, 7 per cent in Egypt, and 5 per cent or less in other countries [48].

2.2. Data Collection. The procedures used for structured observation and content analysis are described in detail below. For all data sources, an older person was defined as a person whose appearance suggested an age of 60 or more. For all procedures, weekends in non-Muslim countries and Fridays in Muslim countries were not used for data collection in order to avoid "atypical" days producing biased data.

2.3. Structured Observations. A site selection frame was developed for the structured observations of older people. As detailed in Table 1, seven large cities were chosen for observation of social spaces: Sheffield (UK), Haleb (Syria),

Amman (Jordan), Luxor (Egypt), Bangkok (Thailand), Nairobi (Kenya), and Arusha (Tanzania). The smallest city observed was Arusha with a population of around 140,000; the largest city was Bangkok with 966,000 [49]. Within each city a central area featuring the main public buildings was selected to ensure that fieldwork sites for observation would be within walking distance of each other. In each city, observations were carried out in seven social spaces: a market, a religious building (e.g., a Christian church/cathedral, Muslim mosque, or Hindu temple, representing the largest denomination in each city), a park, a bus station, a post office, a hotel, and a café. Social spaces were selected to reflect divergence in function, physical layout, open versus enclosed aspect, and expected use by differing subgroups of the population.

A time sampling frame for recording of data from observations was developed based on previous work on the observation of older people in residential care environments [50, 51] and adapted through piloting. For religious buildings, post offices, cafes, and hotels, people going in or out were counted. For markets, parks, and transport stations, people were counted as they passed a particular point including, where appropriate, counting people going on and off buses. Observations were carried out during six phases of the day: 7 am–9 am, 9 am–12 noon, 12 noon–2 pm, 2 pm–5 pm, 5 pm–8 pm, and 8 pm–11 pm. A five-minute period was randomly selected within each phase, during which continuous observation occurred and data was recorded. In each five-minute period, the number and gender of any observed older people were recorded, as were the age and gender constitution of groups involving older people. The five- minute period of data recording balances two conflicting needs: the first is the requirement for a long enough period of behaviour observation to capture the continuous nature of life's ebb and flow and identify the context for activity so as to support the reliable coding of events; the second is the need to restrain the time for observation so as to allow for the accurate recording of often significant amounts of data with accompanying field notes. Breaking up the day into periods also ensured that reliability of the recorded information is not compromised by tiredness, while the overall pattern of life is retained through sampling across an entire day. Information on the validity and reliability of this specific observational data time sampling framework is published elsewhere [50, 51], although it is derived from standard procedures for structured observation methods [4].

Due to local circumstances, some adjustments were made to the site selection frame. Where the city center was non-residential, as in Amman and Bangkok, the old center and the area around the railway station were chosen, respectively, as they are focal points of city life. In Nairobi, the city center was not residential but it was not safe to observe outside this area. In Luxor and Arusha, a main bus stop was selected as the bus station was out of town; in Bangkok the train station was used, as the bus station was in a different area; in Bangkok, Nairobi, and Arusha there were no parks within the area observed so this part of the observation schedule could not be carried out. Some adjustments to the sampling frame were also required to reflect local circumstances. In Nairobi and Arusha, tourists are advised not to go out on foot after dark, so observations could not be done after 8 pm. If a building was not open during a given phase of the day, data could not be collected. Religious buildings, cafes, and post offices were affected by closure. Public spaces selected for observation were in total closed on 11 occasions between 7 and 9 am, on 10 occasions between 8 and 11 pm, on 8 occasions between 5 and 8 pm, and on 1 occasion between 9 and 12 am.

2.4. Content Analysis. Media content analysis was undertaken of newspaper pictures and television channels, as detailed in Table 1. Because our study focuses on the visibility of older people, we selected newspapers and television as mass media genres containing a significant component of visual information (as opposed to, say, literature or radio).

2.4.1. Newspapers. A sampling frame was developed in which for each country two local language papers and one English language paper were chosen, unless English was the local language (UK, Kenya, and Tanzania) where two English papers were chosen only. Within this frame, as the researchers had restricted prior knowledge of the countries' media, the newspapers were arbitrarily selected from amongst those papers prominently displayed on at least two news stalls on a given day in each city. Eighteen papers in total were selected. All were dailies and all were published within the relevant country. Circulation and ownership varied.

Within each newspaper, every picture was examined and data extracted on people represented in terms of gender, age group, and number. Where older people were depicted, a brief description of their activity was recorded. The page number and section were noted, together with the headline for English papers and a brief description for other language papers, except when the picture contained only a face with no indication of context. Pictures advertising a product were recorded as adverts and the products were identified where possible. The sections in which the picture appeared were used as base categories for the analysis and finally combined into two superordinate categories: news and non-news.

2.4.2. Television. Within the sampling frame developed for television, terrestrial television channels were prioritized, followed by channels from the region in which the country was situated, and if this was insufficient, a sample of the remaining channels was chosen. Television channels were recorded in all countries but Thailand and Kenya, as in these two countries the researcher was not able to access them within a context that allowed for reliable data recording. In Syria, eight channels were selected, all Arabic. In Jordan, five channels were selected, three of which were Arabic and the other two are Canadian and Turkish. In Egypt, four channels were selected, two Arabic and one American and there was one other channel of unknown origin. In Tanzania, six channels were selected: these were Tanzanian, French African, South African, Indian, British, and American. In the UK, four of the five British terrestrial channels were selected. In total, 27 channels were selected.

The time sampling frame for recording of data from television was developed via adaptation of the frame used for the observation of social spaces described above and via extensive piloting. Each selected channel in a country was studied for a five-minute period during each of the same six phases of the day used for social space observations. A five-minute period was judged, a useful time frame for coding television material as it provides sufficient time to avoid the whole period being taken up by advertisements or credits and to establish reliably the type of programme being broadcast.

During these five-minute periods, every scene was recorded and data extracted on people represented in terms of gender, age group, and number. By "scene," what is meant is a linear representation or presentation of events or narrative, commencing and ending on an edit or camera switch. Where older people were depicted, a brief description of their activity was recorded. The programme type and where possible the name of the programme were recorded. For programmes in English, the programme type was generally evident through the language. For other channels, the type was decided based on the action and appearance of the scenes. Analytic categories were decided by identifying common programme types in UK and finally combined into two superordinate categories: news or non-news.

As with observations of social spaces, some adjustments to the sampling frame had to be made. It was not possible to observe television from 12 to 2 pm in Jordan, 8 to 11 pm in Egypt, and 7 to 9 am in Tanzania, due to pragmatic constraints on the researcher's access to media during these phases.

2.5. Data Analysis. As the data collected was largely non-normal in distribution, nonparametric analytic techniques were used. Parametric analyses were used only where they provided valuable additional descriptive information. Where repeated testing of the same sample occurred, Bonferroni corrections to reduce Type I errors were applied, with an appropriate reduction in alpha for each analysis. Where category cell n was too low to enable reliable analysis, combination of categories occurred.

3. Results

3.1. Social Spaces. In total, 310 older people were observed in social spaces. This was a mean of 1.17 (SD = 4.16, range 0–39) older people per observation period and a median value of 0 (IQR = 0-1) older people per observation period. The number of observed older people per period was therefore greatly skewed toward low values, and older people were observed in only 26.1% of the 264 observation periods. With regard to gender, 184 (59.4%) men and 126 (40.6%) women were observed. In all cities in developing countries, more men than women were observed (developing countries combined: men $n = 96$, women $n = 7$), whereas in Sheffield more women than men were observed (women $n = 119$, men $n = 88$).

The number of older people observed per period varied considerably across cities (see Table 2). Although Sheffield had by far the highest mean number of older people observed per period, this value was inflated by a small number of observation periods with relatively large number of older people. Thus, excluding Arusha (no older people observed), the median number of older people observed per period was highest in Amman (.50, IQR = 0–2.00) and joint lowest in Luxor and Nairobi (0, IQR = 0-0). Due to the very small number of women observed in cities in developing countries and thus the confounding of city status (developed versus developing) with gender, all following statistical comparison between developing country cities and Sheffield was carried out using cases of observed males only.

There was significant variation across cities in the number of older men observed per period ($H(6) = 38.3$, $p < .001$). With regard to the social spaces in which older people were observed, a market was the location in which most older people were observed ($n = 121$), followed by a bus/train station ($n = 70$), a post office ($n = 67$) through to a hotel being the location in which fewest older people were observed ($n = 4$). There was significant variation across social spaces in the number of older men observed per period ($H(6) = 26.3$, $p < .001$); this variation is found in Haleb ($H(3) = 18.7$, $p < .001$) and in Bangkok, Nairobi, Luxor, and Arusha combined ($H(3) = 14.2$, $p = .003$), but not in Sheffield ($H(3) = 8.80$, $p = .032$) or Amman ($H(3) = 2.30$, $p = .514$).

With regard to older people observed per phase of day, the largest number of older people was observed between noon and 2 pm ($n = 115$), followed by 2–5 pm ($n = 96$) and 9 am noon ($n = 63$), with fewer older people observed in the early morning (7–9 am, $n = 12$) and early and late evening (5–8 pm, $n = 18$; 8–11 pm, $n = 6$). There was significant variation across phases of the day in the number of older men observed per period ($H(5) = 15.4$, $p = .009$), but this association was only true for Sheffield ($H(3) = 17.1$, $p = .001$).

There was also considerable variation across cities in the proportion of older people observed who were accompanied as opposed to observed ones alone. While nearly half of the older people observed in Luxor, Nairobi, and Sheffield were accompanied, only 15.8 per cent of older people observed in Bangkok were accompanied, 14.3 per cent in Haleb, and 8.89 per cent in Amman. There was a significant association between the accompanied versus alone status of older men and city ($\chi^2(3) = 18.0$, $p < .001$), with Sheffield having by far the highest proportion of accompanied older men (42.0%).

Of those observed older people who were accompanied, 84 (79.2%) were accompanied by older people only, while 20 (18.9%) were accompanied by people of other age groups only and two (1.89%) accompanied by mixed age groups of younger and older people. There was a significant association between city status (developed versus developing) and whether or not the accompanying person was old (Sheffield 94.6%, developing cities 40.0%, $\varphi = -.66$, $p < .001$) with accompanied older people in Sheffield predominantly accompanied by other older people.

3.2. Newspapers. A total of 1433 pictures were extracted from newspapers. With regard to the images of people whose ages could be reliably determined, 217 older people were observed in total, in comparison to 513 children or babies, 988 middle-aged people, and 2109 young people. There was thus significant variation in the absolute level of presence of

Table 2: Observations of older people by gender in seven cities.

	City															
	Haleb		Amman		Luxor		Bangkok		Nairobi		Arusha		Sheffield		Total	
	n	%	*n*	%	*n*	%	*n*	%	*n*	%	*n*	%	*n*	%	*n*	%
Men	24	85.7	44	97.8	9	100	17	89.5	2	100	0	0	88	42.5	184	59.4
Women	4	14.3	1	2.22	0	0	2	10.5	0	0	0	0	119	57.5	126	40.6
Total	**28**	**100**	**45**	**100**	**9**	**100**	**19**	**100**	**2**	**100**	**0**	**100**	**207**	**100**	**310**	**100**
Observation period																
Mean	0.64		1.07		0.21		0.53		0.07		0		4.93		1.17	
(SD, range)	(1.45, 0–7)		(1.56, 0–7)		(0.47, 0–2)		(1.06, 0–4)		(0.25, 0-1)		(0.00, 0-0)		(9.32, 0–39)		(4.16, 0–39)	
Median	0		0.50		0		0		0		0		0		0	
(IQR)	(0–0.25)		(0–2.00)		(0-0)		(0–0.75)		(0-0)		(0-0)		(0–5.25)		(0-1.00)	

TABLE 3: Images of people by age and gender in pictures in newspapers from seven cities.

	City							
	Haleb	Amman	Luxor	Bangkok	Nairobi	Arusha	Sheffield	Total
	n (%)	*n* (%)	*n* (%)	*n* (%)	*n* (%)	*n* (%)	*n* (%)	*n* (%)
Pictures examined	114 (7.96)	136 (9.49)	236 (16.5)	450 (31.4)	170 (11.9)	93 (6.49)	234 (16.3)	1433 (100)
Picture content								
Older men	9 (7.89)	3 (2.21)	23 (9.75)	30 (6.67)	15 (8.82)	4 (4.30)	4 (1.71)	88 (6.14)
Older women	0 (0.0)	0 (0.0)	2 (0.85)	9 (2.00)	11 (6.47)	1 (1.08)	4 (1.71)	27 (1.88)
Non-older men	69 (60.5)	98 (72.1)	177 (75.0)	293 (65.1)	114 (67.1)	61 (65.6)	126 (53.8)	938 (65.6)
Non-older women	14 (12.3)	27 (19.9)	45 (19.1)	172 (38.2)	49 (28.8)	20 (21.5)	58 (24.8)	385 (26.9)

Note: percentages do not total 100 within countries as some pictures contained images of people from more than one age/gender category while age/gender category could not be determined in other pictures.

the different age groups (Friedman $\chi^2 = 798.2(3)$, $p < .001$). This variation was significant both for males (Friedman $\chi^2 = 336.3(2)$, $p < .001$) and for females (Friedman $\chi^2 = 265.5(2)$, $p < .001$), excluding children and babies from the analysis (gender not recorded). In terms of the proportion of pictures examined that contained images of people by age group and gender, 88 (6.14%) pictures depicted older men, 27 (1.88%) depicted older women, 938 (65.5%) depicted non-older men, and 385 (26.9%) depicted non-older women. There was thus significant variation in the proportional presence of the different age groups (Cochrane's Q = 1616.1(3), $p < .001$). This variation was significant both for males (McNemar's $\chi^2 = 747.7(1)$, $p < .001$) and for females (McNemar's $\chi^2 = 317.0(1)$, $p < .001$).

The proportion of pictures containing older people varied significantly across countries (see Table 3), from 15.3 per cent in Kenya to 2.21 per cent in Jordan ($\chi^2(6) = 28.7$, $p < .001$). There was also significant variation by country in the proportion of pictures depicting non-old people ($\chi^2(6) = 39.6$, $p < .001$). For men, there was significant association between country status and depiction in pictures, both for older men (developing country 7.01%, UK 1.71%, $\varphi = -.08$, $p = .002$) and for non-older men (developing country 67.7%, UK 53.8%, $\varphi = -.11$, $p < .001$). For women, the association between country status and depiction in pictures was non-significant, both for older women (developing country 1.92%, UK 1.71%, $\varphi = -.06$, $p = .830$) and for non-older women (developing country 27.3%, UK 24.8%, $\varphi = -.02$, $p = .433$).

We examined the association between picture content (news or non-news material) and the gender and age of the person depicted. Significant associations were obtained for depiction of an older woman (news 1.51%, non-news 3.43%, $\varphi = -.06$, $p = .028$) and depiction of a non-old man (news 65.9%, non-news 52.6%, $\varphi = .13$, $p < .001$). These associations remained significant when controlling for country status.

3.3. Television. Content analysis was undertaken of a total of 599 television scenes. With regard to the images of people whose ages could be reliably determined, 106 older people were observed in total, in comparison to 170 children or babies, 370 middle-aged people, and 855 young people. There was thus significant variation in the absolute presence of the different age groups (Friedman $\chi^2 = 343.2(3)$, $p < .001$). This variation was significant both for males (Friedman $\chi^2 = 129.8(2)$, $p < .001$) and for females (Friedman $\chi^2 = 177.3(2)$, $p < .001$), excluding children and babies from the analysis (gender not recorded). Overall, few of the scenes analysed contained older people. Of the 599 analysed scenes, 47 (7.85%) contained older people, while in comparison, 533 scenes (89.0%) contained non-old people. Thirty-four scenes (5.68%) contained older men, while 17 scenes (2.84%) contained older women, and 340 (56.8%) scenes contained non-old men while 252 (42.1%) contained non-old women. There was thus significant variation in the proportional presence of the different age groups (Cochrane's Q = 579.3(3), $p < .001$). This variation was significant both for males (McNemar's $\chi^2 = 261.3(1)$, $p < .001$) and for females (McNemar's $\chi^2 = 211.4(1)$, $p < .001$).

The proportion of scenes containing older people varied significantly across countries (see Table 4), from 18.0 per cent in Egypt to 4.24 per cent in Syria ($\chi^2(4) = 12.0$, $p = .017$). There was also significant variation by country in the proportion of pictures depicting non-old people ($\chi^2(4) = 18.3$, $p = .001$). Due to the small number of scenes containing older women, developing countries were considered as a whole before examining the association between country status and depiction of people in scenes by age and gender. There were no significant associations between country status and the frequency with which old and non-old people, either males or females, were depicted in scenes.

There was no significant association between presence of older people in scenes and the period of day in which the scenes were broadcast, and there is no significant association between programme type and presence of older people.

4. Discussion

Our data, drawn from the structured observations of public social spaces and from the content analysis of images in newspapers and on television channels, is mutually reinforcing: data from all sources indicated a low presence of older people in public fora. Overall, this low presence was particularly true for the developed country sites relative to the developed country site in our study, with women additionally considerably less present than men in developing countries.

Table 4: Images of people by age and gender in scenes on television from five cities.

	City					
	Haleb	Amman	Luxor	Arusha	Sheffield	Total
	n (%)	*n* (%)	*n* (%)	*n* (%)	*n* (%)	*n* (%)
Scenes examined	165 (27.6)	77 (12.9)	50 (8.35)	111 (18.5)	196 (32.7)	599 (100)
Scene content						
Older men	5 (3.03)	7 (9.09)	7 (14.0)	3 (2.70)	12 (6.12)	34 (5.68)
Older women	2 (1.21)	3 (3.90)	3 (6.00)	4 (3.60)	5 (2.55)	17 (2.84)
Non-older men	76 (46.1)	48 (62.3)	26 (52.0)	68 (61.3)	122 (62.2)	340 (56.8)
Non-older women	61 (37.0)	22 (28.6)	22 (44.0)	63 (56.8)	84 (42.9)	252 (42.1)

Note: percentages do not total 100 within countries as some scenes contained images of people from more than one age/gender category while age/gender category could not be determined in other scenes.

These findings support the other work that suggests that older people are infrequently visible in social spaces (e.g., [13–15]) and our data echo the claims of a UK Government report that older people are excluded from neighborhoods and leisure activities [35]. There is comparability also with research on media in developed countries that shows older people being underrepresented in advertisements and television (e.g., [18–20, 22, 23, 27, 29]).

One would expect a lower presence of older people in cities in developing countries due to the lower proportions of older people in these countries compared to developed countries. However, when the median number of older people per observation period is considered as the benchmark, Sheffield had a lower median of older people observed in social spaces than Amman. Thus, older people were generally absent from social spaces in both Sheffield and the developing country cities, but only for Sheffield there were a small number of periods when older people were frequently observed. Social spaces were not evenly used by the older people observed, with most older people observed in markets, transport hubs, and post offices. The fact that so few older people were seen in locations more associated with leisure, such as cafes and hotels, is interesting. Research in Western countries indicates that economic and health factors impact older people's leisure activities [52], while being older, being female, and having a limited social network combined with poor finances and poor health reduce participation in activities [53]. While finances may not influence use of parks, poor weather conditions may impact more substantially on the use of open spaces by older, frailer users. It is also interesting that few older people were observed in religious buildings, as churches have been identified as places that are important to older people [13].

Older people in our sample of developing country cities, in comparison to those in Sheffield, are less likely to be accompanied when in public. Leaving aside the very low absolute level of presence of older people in the developing country cities sampled, the finding that older people in these cities are relatively unaccompanied when observed is intriguing. Being unaccompanied may indicate that an older person has a low availability of family relationships, which would place that person at higher risk of poor health, difficulty in accessing social care, and mistreatment and abuse [33–37, 54]. However, being unaccompanied in public may also be interpreted as a sign of social independence and a high level of functioning—no support is sought or needed, rather than being needed and unavailable. Where public social interaction did occur in our study, it was more intergenerational in our sampled developing cities than in Sheffield. This suggests a degree of social segregation by age group in Sheffield. An apparent reliance on age peers for public social activity could place older people at risk of a reduced social network with advancing age. For example, there is a link between spousal bereavement and social exclusion [55]. Older people in Sheffield were significantly more often observed around the middle of the day than in the morning, late afternoon, or evening, but this variation was not present in our sampled developing cities. The relative absence of older people at the beginning and end of the day might be due to older people's fear of the dark and of crime, as identified in previous research in developed countries (e.g., [56, 57]; see also [58], who discuss fear of crime as a domain of social exclusion). Taken overall, the data drawn from observation of social spaces are suggestive of segregation of older people from other age groups (see [59, 60]), a segregation related to place, time, and companionship.

4.1. Gender and Presence. When considering older women, 94.4 per cent of those observed were recorded in Sheffield. This confounding of gender with developing versus developed country city status prevented a more nuanced examination of how gender influences women's visibility in social spaces when comparing developed and developing contexts. However, this extremely low level of visibility of older women in our sampled developing country cities does reflect the predominant finding of gender inequalities in such countries (e.g., [61–63]). For example, Lloyd-Sherlock [64] argues that the relative deprivation of older women covers a wide range of aspects, such as entitlements to social policies, increased burdens of care and domestic responsibility, greater likelihood of living alone, and sometimes also discrimination against widows. Research also suggests that women tend to report greater fear of crime than men and that consequences of such fear in terms of the limitation of activities are particularly serious for women and older people [65].

The finding that older men were significantly more likely to be depicted in newspapers from developing countries in comparison to those from the UK, especially when taking population composition into account, suggests less media discrimination against older men in developing countries than in the UK. Previous research on the representation of older people in the media supports our finding that older women were less likely to be present than older men [18–20, 29]. Our finding that younger men were more likely to be depicted in news stories in newspapers and older women more likely to be depicted in non-news items could be seen as a double discrimination of age and gender and points again to older women having very low status within the media, if one accepts the argument that the news underrepresents people of lower status and that this is a gendered imbalance (see also [42, 66]). This finding could also be interpreted in the light of news value theory, in which it is argued that certain factors are associated with events that become news [67]. Most of the "news factors" identified tend to be characteristics of the new event itself rather than characteristics of those individuals involved in the events. However, within news value theory it is argued that an event is more likely to be rendered newsworthy if it involves people belonging to elite groups, who are likely to possess a substantial degree of fame and thereby attract audiences. The low presence of older people, particularly older women, in the media images in our study could thus be indicative of their exclusion from "elite groups" in society, as well as (or alternatively) their exclusion from newsworthy events. Either interpretation connects with an argument that older people and older women in particularly are an excluded social group [68].

4.2. Study Strengths and Weaknesses. The most valuable feature of this study is its uniqueness. There are no other directly comparable studies and extremely few of any kind concerned with social integration and exclusion of older people that present data from several countries with differing cultural, political, demographic, and socioeconomical profiles. As this is an exploratory study, it is essential that there is transparency about its methodological successes and limitations so that future research can improve upon this work. Many factors will have influenced the validity and reliability of the data collected and it is important to review these factors.

As mentioned in Section 2, aspects of the sampling frame had to be altered from those originally planned. Such adjustments, made due to local factors in different countries, will have affected the comparability of the data across sites. The choice of fieldwork countries, we have previously argued, reflected a diversity of geographic, ethnic, political, and demographic structures. Pragmatic considerations, such as the resources available to the study, also influenced the selection process, and there is clearly an argument that a different selection of countries (and indeed the selection of different cities within countries) could have produced a different set of findings. Similarly, the selection of social spaces within cities will have produced a unique set of findings—a different set of locations will have presented a different data profile. Nevertheless, the site selection was arrived at following careful deliberation about the meaning of places and their purpose in the lives of individuals and society and represents a sample of locations that are tightly defined both geographically and functionally. As much as any sampling of social spaces drawn from hugely different cultures, we would suggest that there is good reason to think we have attained a reasonable degree of comparability across sites and a robust reflection of the "life" of a city and its peoples. The resources available to the study also required that we emphasize those countries where less research has been carried out—the developing countries. Sheffield, as the single site for data collection in developed countries, should be thought of primarily as a comparator for the data collected from the developing country sites. There is, then, a need for reflection on the extent to which a relatively small number of observations of a few different social spaces, newspapers, and television channels can be interpreted in relation to social integration and exclusion processes on a global scale. Furthermore, while our selection of several different developing countries might have offered an opportunity for disaggregating the effects of ethnicity, religion, and political ideologies on the presence of older people, the small number of older people observed via the three data sources militated against any sophisticated unravelling of such effects, and in many cases in our analysis the data collected from the developing country locations had to be combined.

While acknowledging that carrying out observations in a different set of places within the same cities may well have produced a different data profile, a strength of the study is its capacity to triangulate the data from the three different sources of social spaces, newspaper pictures, and television. The first data source is indeed geographically very tightly defined and therefore highly suspect with regard to any claim for representation of the population from which it is selected. However, the second two data sources are national/regional, not local, and therefore can be argued to be reasonably robust with regard to how they reflect the cultures from which they are drawn. The information that emerges from all three data sources is mutually reinforcing such that the credibility of the data profile drawn from observation of social spaces is strengthened due to its similarity to those drawn from newspapers and television.

Our researcher will have approached the data collection process with conscious and unconscious assumptions and beliefs, which will have been embedded within that researcher's own cultural framework. This cultural anchoring will have affected the data collection process across the different cultures in which it occurred in fundamental and unquantifiable ways. For our study, all data was collected by the same individual. This approach was decided upon partly out of financial necessity and partly to ensure consistency of observations across all sites/countries. The researcher was well prepared through briefing, training, and piloting, and the use of a highly structured observation protocol will have maximized reliability during data collection. However, traditional indices of reliability available when more than one researcher is used during data collection (e.g., interrater reliability) cannot be determined for our study [69]; for further discussion on reliability and validity in observational studies, see [70]. A further limitation arising from our use of a single researcher was that during the observations of social spaces, while the absolute number, gender, and accompanied status of older people were recorded, it was not possible to record the presence of non-old people, or the specific behaviours of the older people observed, as there would have been too many data events to record. Thus, the structured observation method was not used to its full capacity, as has been the case in, for example, research regarding residential care facilities [51].

For all observations, there were difficulties in estimating age. Anyone appearing over the age of 60 was recorded as an older person, and where there was any uncertainty the person was excluded from the "older person" category. Estimates of age were further affected by the distance in observations used to limit the impact of the observer on the observed for social spaces data collection, the researcher's relative unfamiliarity with people from certain ethnic groups, and clothing that obscured faces. Thus, age estimation might be anticipated to be more reliable in the UK than in some of the developing country fieldwork sites. A further issue is whether the age of 60 was a suitable age at which to draw the boundary of old age, given the discrepancy in life expectancy across the sampled countries noted in Section 2. As noted previously, what may at a first glance seem like an absence of older people in developing countries can to some extent be explained by the low proportion of older people in the population, although this does not satisfactorily explain the relative absence of older women compared to older men in public fora. There is an argument that a different boundary for old age should have been set for each country, to reflect variation in life expectancy. Alternatively, a retrospective weighting could have been applied to adjust for life expectancy in the data analysis. We decided that it was preferable to avoid such data transformation and rather present the data as collected but placed within a detailed interpretative context to enable the reader to reach his/her own conclusions.

4.3. Conclusions and Implications for Policy. Overall, despite the challenges encountered in this study, it has produced interesting and original findings, which suggest that observational methods and content analysis have utility as ways of exploring social integration and inclusion of older people in both developed and developing countries. While again emphasizing the exploratory nature of our study, there are still broad implications of our findings for policy around older people. Firstly, a lack of presence of older people in public fora implies a lack of representation also in other areas of society such as policy and planning. There is awareness that more engagement is needed with older people in policy and planning, and there have been efforts to achieve this [71, 72]. It should be recognised that a lack of public presence of older people does not preclude a high status for older people in non-public fora or high levels of inclusion in non-public social networks, and this point might be especially pertinent in non-Western and traditional cultures. The role and status of the older person in family networks, for example, cannot be discerned through our data but will vary in nature and significance from culture to culture. Similarly, our study has little insight to offer on the place of older people in rural communities (cf. [73]).

Nevertheless, we would reinforce the notion that a lack of visibility of older people, a public absence of those in later life, has been identified as a form of exclusion [5] and has consequences for how a society configures and represents itself, which in turn will have ramifications for how the role of older people is constructed. Furthermore, this study shows that the exclusion of older people from public fora is not a uniform experience. The emphasis here is that women are more invisible than men, and women in our sample of developing country cities are especially invisible. This suggests exclusion not only by age but also by gender and finally by location, with its variations in demographic, socioeconomic, and cultural factors. If policy needs to address the absence of older people from public spheres, such policy must focus especially on the exclusion of older women.

There may be some concern that moving from a demonstration of the public presence or absence of a social group to the inference that such a group is socially excluded is too great leap. It may be unwise to apply a single model of social exclusion in vastly different cultural contexts without adaption to the local setting (see [74]). Nevertheless, if we accept the United Nation definition of social exclusion as the "involuntary exclusion of individuals and groups from society's political, economic, and societal processes, which prevents their full participation in the society in which they live" [75], then a relative absence from public fora must suggest at the very least a vulnerability to social exclusion, if not actual exclusion itself. We would offer this exploratory study as a starting point for reflection on how best social integration and inclusion can be measured and explored, particularly in locations such as developing countries that are underresearched and which differ in so many respects from the more usual Western sites of social research.

Conflict of Interests

The authors declare that there is no conflict of interests regarding the publication of this paper.

References

[1] UNFPA and HelpAge International, *Ageing in the Twenty-First Century: a Celebration and a Challenge*, United Nations Population Fund (UNFPA), New York, NY, USA, HelpAge International, London, UK, 2012.

[2] P. Lloyd-Sherlock, "Population ageing in developed and developing regions: Implications for health policy," *Social Science and Medicine*, vol. 51, no. 6, pp. 887–895, 2000.

[3] F. van de Vijver and K. Leung, *Methods and Data Analysis for Cross-Cultural Research*, SAGE, London, UK, 1997.

[4] A. Bryman, *Social Research Methods*, Oxford University Press, Oxford, UK, 4th edition, 2012.

[5] A. M. Grenier and N. Guberman, "Creating and sustaining disadvantage: the relevance of a social exclusion framework," *Health and Social Care in the Community*, vol. 17, no. 2, pp. 116–124, 2009.

[6] G. Laws, "Spatiality and age relations," in *Critical Approaches to Ageing and Later Life*, A. Jamieson, S. Harper, and C. Victor, Eds., pp. 90–101, Open University Press, Buckingham, UK, 1997.

[7] C. Phillipson and T. Scharf, "Rural and urban perspectives on growing old: developing a new research agenda," *European Journal of Ageing*, vol. 2, no. 2, pp. 67–75, 2005.

[8] M. Featherstone and M. Hepworth, "Images of ageing: cultural representations of later life," in *The Cambridge Handbook of Age and Ageing*, M. Johnson and V. Bengtson, Eds., pp. 258–362, Cambridge University Press, Cambridge, UK, 2005.

[9] A. S. Lundgren and K. Ljuslinder, "Problematic demography: representations of population ageing in the Swedish daily press," *Journal of Population Ageing*, vol. 4, no. 3, pp. 165–183, 2011.

[10] A. E. Barrett, A. Raphael, and J. Gunderson, "Reflections of old age, constructions of aging selves: drawing links between media images and views of aging," in *Aging, Media and Culture*, C. L. Harrington, D. D. Bielby, and A. R. Bardo, Eds., pp. 39–50, Lexington Books, London, UK, 2014.

[11] L. Vasil and H. Wass, "Portrayal of the elderly in the media: a literature review and implications for educational gerontologists," *Educational Gerontology*, vol. 19, no. 1, pp. 71–85, 1993.

[12] E. Noelle-Neumann, Ed., *The Spiral of Silence: Public Opinion—Our Social Skin*, The University of Chicago Press, Chicago, Ill, USA, 1986.

[13] T. Scharf, C. Phillipson, and A. E. Smith, "Social exclusion of older people in deprived urban communities of England," *European Journal of Ageing*, vol. 2, no. 2, pp. 76–87, 2005.

[14] H. E. A. Tinsley, D. J. Tinsley, and C. E. Croskeys, "Park usage, social milieu, and psychosocial benefits of park use reported by older urban park users from four ethnic groups," *Leisure Sciences*, vol. 24, no. 2, pp. 199–218, 2002.

[15] K. Hung and J. Crompton, "Benefits and constraints associated with the use of an urban park reported by a sample of elderly in Hong Kong," *Leisure Studies*, vol. 25, no. 3, pp. 291–311, 2006.

[16] C. Holland, A. Clark, J. Katz, and S. M. Peace, *Social Interactions in Urban Public Places*, Joseph Rowntree Foundation, London, UK, 2007.

[17] S. Wray, "Women growing older: agency, ethnicity and culture," *Sociology: The Journal of the British Sociological Association*, vol. 37, no. 3, pp. 511–527, 2003.

[18] E. M. Kessler, K. Rakoczy, and U. M. Staudinger, "The portrayal of older people in prime time television series: the match with gerontological evidence," *Ageing and Society*, vol. 24, no. 4, pp. 531–552, 2004.

[19] D. G. Bazzini, W. D. McIntosh, S. M. Smith, S. Cook, and C. Harris, "The aging woman in popular film: underrepresented, unattractive, unfriendly, and unintelligent," *Sex Roles*, vol. 36, no. 7-8, pp. 531–543, 1997.

[20] M. Sanders, "Older women and the media," *Women in Action*, vol. 3, p. 56, 2002.

[21] N. Signorielli, "Aging on television: messages relating to gender, race, and occupation in prime time," *Journal of Broadcasting & Electronic Media*, vol. 48, no. 2, pp. 279–301, 2004.

[22] M. M. Lee, B. Carpenter, and L. S. Meyers, "Representations of older adults in television advertisements," *Journal of Aging Studies*, vol. 21, no. 1, pp. 23–30, 2007.

[23] U. M. Röhr-Sendlmeier and S. Ueing, "Images of the elderly in printed advertisements in a time change perspective," *Zeitschrift fur Gerontologie und Geriatrie*, vol. 37, no. 1, pp. 56–62, 2004.

[24] E. Dozois, *Ageism: A Review of the Literature*, Calgary Health Region, Healthy Aging Committee, Calgary, Canada, 2005.

[25] National Centre for the Protection of Older People, *Constructing Ageing and Age Identity: A Case Study of Newspaper Discourses. Study 1*, NCPOP, Dublin, Ireland, 2009.

[26] V. Ylänne, A. Williams, and P. M. Wadleigh, "Ageing well? Older people's health and well-being as portrayed in UK magazine advertisements," *International Journal of Ageing and Later Life*, vol. 4, no. 2, pp. 33–62, 2009.

[27] S. Baumann and K. de Laat, "Aspiration and compromise: portrayals of older adults in television advertising," in *Aging, Media and Culture*, C. L. Harrington, D. D. Bielby, and A. R. Bardo, Eds., pp. 13–24, Lexington Books, London, UK, 2014.

[28] G. Fealy, M. McNamara, M. P. Treacy, and I. Lyons, "Constructing ageing and age identities: a case study of newspaper discourses," *Ageing and Society*, vol. 32, no. 1, pp. 85–102, 2012.

[29] L. Shu-Chin, *Older Adults on Prime-Time Television in Taiwan: Prevalence, Portrayal, and Communcation Interaction*, University of Kansas, Lawrence, Kan, USA, 2005.

[30] M. Prieler, F. Kohlbacher, S. Hagiwara, and A. Arima, "Gender representation of older people in Japanese television advertisements," *Sex Roles*, vol. 64, no. 5-6, pp. 405–415, 2011.

[31] P. Raman, J. Harwood, D. Weis, J. L. Anderson, and G. Miller, "Portrayals of older adults in U.S. and Indian magazine advertisements: a cross-cultural comparison," *Howard Journal of Communications*, vol. 19, no. 3, pp. 221–240, 2008.

[32] J. A. Salomon, H. Wang, M. K. Freeman et al., "Healthy life expectancy for 187 countries, 1990–2010: a systematic analysis for the Global Burden Disease Study 2010," *The Lancet*, vol. 380, no. 9859, pp. 2144–2162, 2012.

[33] T. C. Antonucci and H. Akiyama, "An examination of sex differences in social support among older men and women," *Sex Roles*, vol. 17, no. 11-12, pp. 737–749, 1987.

[34] S. C. Caetano, C. M. Silva, and M. V. Vettore, "Gender differences in the association of perceived social support and social network with self-rated health status among older adults: a population-based study in Brazil," *BMC Geriatrics*, vol. 13, no. 1, article 122, 2013.

[35] M. Barnes, A. Blom, K. Cox, and C. Lessof, *The Social Exclusion of Older People: Evidence from the First Wave of the English Longitudinal Study of Ageing (ELSA): Final Report*, Office of the Deputy Prime Minister, Social Exclusion Unit, London, UK, 2006.

[36] A. Motel-Klingebiel, C. Tesch-Roemer, and H. J. von Kondratowitz, "The role of family for quality of life in old age: a comparative perspective," in *Global Aging and Challenges to Families*, V. Bengtson and and A. Lowenstein, Eds., pp. 323–354, de Gruyter, New York, NY, USA, 2003.

[37] P. Van Eeuwijk, "Old-age vulnerability, ill-health and care support in urban areas of Indonesia," *Ageing and Society*, vol. 26, no. 1, pp. 61–80, 2006.

[38] J. A. Thiyagarajan, M. Prince, and W. Martin, "Social support network typologies and health outcomes of older people in low and middle income countries—a 10/66 Dementia Research Group population-based study," *International Review of Psychiatry*, vol. 26, no. 4, pp. 476–485, 2014.

[39] C. R. Victor, S. J. Scambler, L. Marston, J. Bond, and A. Bowling, "Older people's experiences of loneliness in the UK: does gender matter?" *Social Policy and Society*, vol. 5, no. 1, pp. 27–38, 2006.

[40] P. A. Dykstra and T. Fokkema, "Social and emotional loneliness among divorced and married men and women: comparing the deficit and cognitive perspectives," *Basic and Applied Social Psychology*, vol. 29, no. 1, pp. 1–12, 2007.

[41] J. B. Casterline, L. Williams, and P. McDonald, "The age difference between spouses: variations among developing countries," *Population Studies*, vol. 40, no. 3, pp. 353–374, 1986.

[42] D. Lemish and V. Muhlbauer, ""Can't have it all": representations of older women in popular culture," *Women and Therapy*, vol. 35, no. 3-4, pp. 165–180, 2012.

[43] R. L. Collins, "Content analysis of gender roles in media: Where are we now and where should we go?" *Sex Roles*, vol. 64, no. 3, pp. 290–298, 2011.

[44] T. Kharroub and A. J. Weaver, "Portrayals of women in transnational Arab television drama series," *Journal of Broadcasting & Electronic Media*, vol. 58, no. 2, pp. 179–195, 2014.

[45] US Department of State, *Background Notes*, 2008.

[46] Foreign and Commonwealth Office, *Country Profiles*, Foreign and Commonwealth Office, London, UK, 2008.

[47] Population Reference Bureau, *Data by Geography*, 2008.

[48] World Health Organization, *World Health Statistics 2008*, World Health Organization, Geneva, Switzerland, 2008.

[49] City Populations, November 2008, http://www.citypopulation.de/.

[50] K. J. McKee, G. Harrison, and K. Lee, "Activity, friendships and wellbeing in residential settings for older people," *Aging and Mental Health*, vol. 3, no. 2, pp. 143–152, 1999.

[51] K. J. McKee, D. M. Houston, and S. Barnes, "Methods for assessing quality of life and well-being in frail older people," *Psychology and Health*, vol. 17, no. 6, pp. 737–751, 2002.

[52] C. Gagliardi, L. Spazzafumo, F. Marcellini et al., "The outdoor mobility and leisure activities of older people in five European countries," *Ageing and Society*, vol. 27, no. 5, pp. 683–700, 2007.

[53] S. Paillard-Borg, H.-X. Wang, B. Winblad, and L. Fratiglioni, "Pattern of participation in leisure activities among older people in relation to their health conditions and contextual factors: a survey in a Swedish urban area," *Ageing & Society*, vol. 29, no. 5, pp. 803–821, 2009.

[54] R. Wolf, L. Daichman, and G. Bennett, "Abuse of the elderly," in *World Report on Violence and Health*, E. G. Krug, L. L. Dahlberg, J. A. Mercy, A. Zwi, and R. Lozano, Eds., pp. 123–145, World Health Organization, Geneva, Switzerland, 2002.

[55] R. Findlay and C. Cartwright, *Social Isolation and Older People: A Literature Review*, Australasian Centre on Ageing, The University of Queensland, Brisbane, Australia, 2002.

[56] K. McKee and C. Milner, "Health, fear of crime and psychosocial functioning in older people," *Journal of Health Psychology*, vol. 5, no. 4, pp. 473–486, 2000.

[57] C. Waterhouse and P. Angley, *Social Exclusion among Older People: a Preliminary Study from Inner-City Melbourne*, Brotherhood of St Laurence, Melbourne, Australia, 2005.

[58] R. Levitas, C. Pantazis, E. Fahmy, D. Gordon, E. Lloyd, and D. Patsios, *The Multi-Dimensional Analysis of Social Exclusion*, Task Force, London, UK, 2007.

[59] P. Uhlenberg and J. De Jong Gierveld, "Age-segregation in later life: an examination of personal networks," *Ageing and Society*, vol. 24, no. 1, pp. 5–28, 2004.

[60] A. Walker, "Public policy and the construction of old age in Europe," *Gerontologist*, vol. 40, no. 3, pp. 304–308, 2000.

[61] C. J. Mba, "Gender disparities in living arrangements of older people in Ghana: evidence from the 2003 Ghana demographic and health survey," *Journal of International Women's Studies*, vol. 9, no. 1, pp. 153–166, 2007.

[62] T. Sobieszczyk, J. Knodel, and N. Chayovan, "Gender and wellbeing among older people: evidence from Thailand," *Ageing and Society*, vol. 23, no. 6, pp. 701–735, 2003.

[63] K. M. Yount and E. M. Agree, "The power of older women and men in Egyptian and Tunisian families," *Journal of Marriage and Family*, vol. 66, no. 1, pp. 126–146, 2004.

[64] P. Lloyd-Sherlock, "Formal social protection for older people in developing countries: three different approaches," *Journal of Social Policy*, vol. 31, no. 4, pp. 695–713, 2002.

[65] T. Lorenc, M. Petticrew, M. Whitehead et al., "Fear of crime and the environment: systematic review of UK qualitative evidence," *BMC Public Health*, vol. 13, no. 1, article 496, 2013.

[66] S. Fountaine, "Are we there yet? The long ride to gender equity in the news," in *What's News? Reclaiming Journalism in New Zealand*, J. McGregor and M. Comrie, Eds., pp. 244–258, Dunmore Press, Palmerstone North, New Zealand, 2002.

[67] D. O'Neill and T. Harcup, "News values and selectivity," in *Handbook of Journalism Studies*, K. Wahl-Jorgensen and T. Hanitzsch, Eds., pp. 161–174, Routledge, New York, NY, USA, 2009.

[68] E. Becker and R. Boreham, *Understanding the Risks of Social Exclusion Across the Life Course: Older Age*, Cabinet Office and National Centre for Social Research, London, UK, 2009.

[69] M. Denscombe, *The Good Research Guide for Small-Scale Social Research Projects*, Open University Press, Maidenhead, UK, 4th edition, 2010.

[70] C. Robson, *Real World Reserach. A Resource for Social Scientists and Practitioner-Researchers*, Blackwell, Oxford, UK, 1997.

[71] Social Exclusion Unit, *A New Direction for the Social Exclusion Unit 2004-2005. Improving Service Delivery to the Most Disadvantaged*, Social Exclusion Unit, London, UK, 2004.

[72] A. Swan, "Improving engagement with older people," *British Journal of Community Nursing*, vol. 12, no. 8, pp. 372–373, 2007.

[73] J. Nilsson, M. Grafström, S. Zaman, and Z. N. Kabir, "Role and function: aspects of quality of life of older people in rural Bangladesh," *Journal of Aging Studies*, vol. 19, no. 3, pp. 363–374, 2005.

[74] P. Lloyd-Sherlock, A. Barrientos, and J. Mase, "Social inclusion of older people in developing countries: re lations and resources," in *From Exclusion to Inclusion in Old Age: A Global Challenge*, T. Scharf and and N. C. Keating, Eds., pp. 51–69, The Policy Press, Bristol, UK, 2012.

[75] United Nations, *Analysing and Measuring Social Inclusion in a Global Context*, United Nations, New York, NY, USA, 2010.

6

The Importance of Social Connectedness in Building Age-Friendly Communities

Charles A. Emlet[1] and Joane T. Moceri[2]

[1] *Social Work Program, University of Washington Tacoma, Tacoma, WA 98401, USA*
[2] *Nursing Program, University of Washington Tacoma, Tacoma, WA 98401, USA*

Correspondence should be addressed to Charles A. Emlet, caemlet@u.washington.edu

Academic Editor: Frank Oswald

The purpose of this paper is to further elucidate the importance of social relationships and social connectedness with aging in place and in developing elder-friendly communities. The process used in this study was inclusive of younger adults (age 40–65) as well as older adults (65+) in order to further understand how they envision a community that could support their own aging in place. A community forum, using the World Café format, was conducted in order to engage community members, 40 years and older, in conversation about the importance of social connectedness in elder-friendly communities. A second purpose of this forum was to obtain data on what would keep aging boomers in their community as they age. Three major themes emerged from qualitative analysis of the forum: *social reciprocity*, *meaningful interactions*, and *structural needs/barriers*. The results of this study reinforce the importance of social connectedness in creating and maintaining elder-friendly communities for older adults, as well as soon-to-be retired individuals, wishing to maintain life connectedness to their community. The study suggests the possibility of using more nontraditional research techniques (such as the World Café process) for gathering community level data.

1. Introduction

Increasingly, gerontological researchers, practitioners, policy makers, and planners are concerning themselves with the growing importance of aging in place. Aging in place does not have one single definition but broadly is considered to be the ability to continue to live in the environment of one's choice, even when declining competence reduces or threatens independence [1], while allowing for consumer choice in the types of services delivered [2]. Lawler [3] suggests that aging in place strategies can minimize inappropriate care and work best as a comprehensive and holistic approach to the needs of aging individuals and communities. Lau and colleagues [4] have conceptualized a framework for aging in place safely and acknowledge the importance of multiple factors, including the biological and psychological characteristics of the individual, the network of social support, formal services, the need for medical services, and the structure of the home and neighborhood. This and other frameworks clearly recognize that aging in place strategies must consider not only the personal (micro) environment, including housing, but also community and structural components as well [4, 5].

2. Theoretical Frameworks

Before embarking on a discussion of elder-friendly communities, it is important to discuss a number of theoretical frameworks and conceptualizations from gerontology that help inform our understanding of aging in place. There are numerous frameworks that are relevant to aging in place including ecological theory, person in environment, and social inclusion/exclusion. In addition, the area of environmental gerontology has specific relevance to this discussion.

Ecological theory [6] suggests that there is a mutual relationship and mutual reciprocity between individuals and their environment and that this interaction occurs at multiple levels, including the micro-, exo-, mezzo-, macro-, and chronosystems levels [6]. Ecological theory is important for the concept of aging in place as it suggests that individuals interact with multiple "levels" of environment in their day-to-day lives. Older people must not only interact with microenvironments such as their home and immediate family, but also with broader systems that can equally influence their ability to age in place. Another theoretical perspective that informs our discussion is that of person in environment [1]. This perspective, like ecological theory, acknowledges that the environment interacts with individuals at multiple levels and suggests that the environment is not a static backdrop but rather continually changes. From the person-in-environment perspective, the older person must continually take from the environment what he or she needs, control what can be modified, and adapt to conditions that cannot be changed [1].

Also of relevance to this discussion is the theory of social inclusion/exclusion. In social gerontology, the theory of social inclusion/exclusion examines the role of older people and highlights the social costs when individuals, families, or communities are excluded from or become disengaged from larger society due to characteristics such as poverty, gender, ethnicity, or neighborhood [7]. Scharf and colleagues [8] conceptualize the inclusion and exclusion of older people as associated with three key themes: participation and integration (beyond the labor market), spatial segregation, and institutional disengagement. Of particular interest in our exploration of aging in place is the thematic area of participation and integration. Scharf et al. [8] posit that participation and integration not only include older people's involvement in community life, but also are associated with their social capital, including civic participation, and the nature of social networks and mutuality/reciprocity. An elder-friendly community can support these concepts.

In addition to several theoretical frameworks, the field of environmental gerontology has specific relevance to the topic of aging in place. Wahl and Weisman [9] suggest that environmental gerontology's (EG) theories and findings can and should influence the development of age-friendly communities. For example, EG is concerned with the role of neighborhoods and the influence those neighborhoods have on opportunities and constraints of residents [10]. At a more macrolevel, EG recognizes the community as a locus of aging with a sociophysical and policy perspective [11].

With regard to elder-friendly communities, we can draw upon the work of Lawton [12] who posited that the environment has three major functions of maintenance, stimulation, and support [9]. Maintenance is concerned with the consistency and predictability of one's environment, while stimulation is concerned with the effect of stimuli on behavior. Finally, support is concerned with the environment's potential to compensate for diminished or lost competencies [13].

3. Elder-Friendly Communities

In recent years, the concept of elder-friendly communities has become central to the notion of aging in place. Described in various ways, an elder-friendly community is a place where "people can live their entire lives, if they so desire, rather than having to relocate and lose their social capital" [14, page 6]. An elder-friendly community examines the environment in more macro-level terms as places where older people are actively involved, valued, and supported by an infrastructure that accommodates their needs [15]. In what was perhaps the first on-line conference focusing on elder-friendly communities, the Sierra Health Foundation suggested that elder-friendly communities are those communities in which age is not considered a barrier to improving lifelong interests and activities, where support and accommodations exist to meet the basic health and social needs of those with age-related disabilities, and where opportunities exist for older adults to develop new sources of fulfillment and engagement [16].

While the literature on elder-friendly communities is to a degree embryonic, several models have been developed in recent years. Among these models created in the United States, Canada, and Europe, the interrelatedness of social and structural factors is found to be consistently important. For example, Feldman and Oberlink's [17] work on the *AdvantAge Initiative* demonstrated that elder-friendly communities must address basic needs, optimize well-being, maximize independence, and promote civic engagement. The City of Calgary Elder-Friendly Community Project noted that feeling safe, being valued and respected, staying active, and building community were important elements of an elder-friendly community [18]. The World Health Organization (WHO) has established international guidelines for age-friendly communities that include the encouragement of active aging by optimizing opportunities for health, participation, and security in order to enhance people's quality of life as they age [19]. According to the WHO, an age-friendly city adapts its structures and services to be accessible to, and inclusive of, older people with varying needs and capacities.

While various models have emerged identifying aspects key to the concept of elder-friendliness, a consistent theme found in the literature is associated with social interaction or social connectedness. Scharlach [14] suggests that an elder-friendly community fosters both *connection* and *contribution*. An elder-friendly community will assist older adults to maintain social connectedness while deepening existing relationships. Such a community will recognize the social capital of these relationships that in turn result in *contribution*. The concept of contribution recognizes the wisdom and experience of older citizens and sees them as more than clients, but rather as active contributors to community well-being [14]. Similarly, The Calgary Project identified as important the active participation of older people in their communities. This premise is consistent with the work of Rubinstein and colleagues [20] who found that the ability to actively manage one's environment was a source of well-being for older adults. Similarly, the model of age-friendly communities developed by the WHO clearly recognizes that social participation and social support are strongly associated with overall well-being, allowing elders to exercise their competence and enjoy the respect and esteem of their community [19]. Alley and colleagues [15] remind us that a community's respect for older adults, which includes available opportunities, contributes significantly to their quality of life.

While social participation and connectedness are important in an elder-friendly community, there is a need for reciprocity between older adults and their community. For example, the *AdvantAge Initiative* [17] promotes the importance of civic engagement, including meaningful connections, volunteer and paid opportunities, and the prioritization of aging issues. The WHO acknowledges that an age-friendly community provides the option for older adults to continue to contribute to their community through civic engagement with both paid and volunteer opportunities and to have the ability to be active in the political process. The benefits of such reciprocity are many, such as an increased sense of purpose and satisfaction for older adults as they engage with the community, while younger community members may benefit from the knowledge and experience older adults bring to the community. As an example, intergenerational programs recognize the knowledge and skills possessed by older adults that can be shared with youth, while providing opportunities for civic engagement for the older person [1]. The key here is mutual benefit while recognizing that each segment benefits differentially.

Much of the research on elder-friendly communities has highlighted the multidimensional nature of community life and has not focused primary attention on social connectedness despite the importance of interdependence and engagement as primary qualities of aging in community [21]. For example, the *AdvantAge Initiative* identifies social and civic engagement but used quantitative measures to evaluate communities in three preordained realms [17]. Additionally, age-friendly community projects often obtain views from current elders. If an age-friendly community is a positive place to "grow" old, then the views of younger citizens (baby boomers, for example) need to be taken into account. Alley and colleagues [15] suggest that in an age-prepared community, processes of planning and advocacy are utilized to foster aging in place, which may be a prospective view of what is needed in planning for future community needs. This process must take into account the views and needs of the citizens who are not yet defined as older adults, but who will bring their own needs and views to the community.

The purpose of this paper is to further elucidate the importance of social relationships and social connectedness in developing an elder-friendly community. The process used in the project described here was inclusive of younger adults (age 40–65) as well as older adults (65+) in order to help understand how they envision a community that could support their own aging. Alley et al. [15] describe the importance of an "age-prepared" community [15, page 8] as one which has assessed its current services and is planning for the needs of future populations. Second, the qualitative methodology used in this study allowed for a more naturalistic and personal narrative. Padgett [22] acknowledges the importance of "meaning making" in the narrative process that includes storytelling, conversation, and discourse of naturally occurring speech. This study, therefore, was informed by the perspective of narrative analysis and the use of the spoken and written word in narrating the meaning of social connectedness as we age.

4. Background

In April of 2002, surveys related to assessing the elder friendliness of communities were completed by 5.100 individuals, 65 and over, throughout 10 cities across the United States [23]. In one participating community in Western Washington, a total of 514 surveys were completed. Findings suggested that older adults in that community were satisfied with their neighborhoods and participated in religious or cultural activities, and the majority of respondents were engaged in health screening [24]. The vast majority of these respondents had participated in some type of social activity in the past week and slightly fewer than one in three people volunteered [23]. The survey results were promising and positive, yet are now dated and do not reflect the opinions of members of the aging baby boom generation. Second, the original survey did not focus specifically on the issue of social connectedness but limited the focus to volunteering and participation in cultural and religious activities.

Recognizing the need to better refine and focus attention on the importance of social connectedness as part of elder-friendly communities, a city committee responsible for the continuation of the elder-friendly community agenda sponsored a community forum in October of 2009. A community forum using the World Café format [25] was conducted in order to engage community members, 40 years and older, in conversation about the importance of social connectedness in elder-friendly communities. Previous research in this area has approached the topic of social connectedness through an a priori definition of social engagement, primarily utilizing quantitative methods for measurement and evaluation [23]. This forum, however, sought to understand social connectedness from those approaching retirement using a more naturalistic method. A second purpose of this forum was to obtain data on what would keep aging boomers in their community as they age. The results of the forum and its applicability to elder-friendly communities and aging in place research are being presented here.

4.1. World Café as a Research Strategy. The World Café is a concept that was born out of *Appreciative Inquiry* [26], which is a form of research that emphasizes the positive aspects of an experience, particularly how that experience can foster creativity among people [26]. The World Café format involves exchanging ideas and sharing different points of view in a safe, intimate setting with the purpose of coalescing wisdom and experience into learning. A foundational component of the World Café concept is conversations, purposeful conversations that have a reason for taking place, "conversations that matter" [25, page 4]. They may be initiated to solve a community problem or to envision a preferred future, in this case an elder-friendly community, with a focus on social connectedness. The World Café format places an emphasis on moving from simply talking to taking action. This movement takes place as participants are able to understand the connection between talking and acting, or conversation as action [25]. It was in this context of "sharing collective discoveries" [25, page 138] that the community forum took place. This study provided an opportunity to test the value of the World Café format as a method for future research.

5. Methods

This study was determined to be an exempt study by the University of Washington Human Subjects Division. The method employed for this study involved a melding of the World Café format as the structure of the study with a focus group format as the process that informed data collection in the study. Qualitative methodology was then used for data analysis. The data collection procedures differed from traditional focus groups in some significant ways. First, groups formed, discussed, and reformed with different participants for each of the three main questions that were posed at the forum. Second, instead of the more customary audio or video taping of the groups, each table was covered with paper on which participants wrote and/or drew as they discussed the topic at hand. These notes and doodles became the transcript along with notes taken by each table leader. This is consistent with narrative analysis in which both spoken and written words are used in meaning making [22]. Finally, groups were given great latitude as to how they addressed the discussion topic for their table. Some groups created action plans, and others were more reflective. The discussion leaders at each table helped to keep the group on topic and were careful not to inject their opinions into the group discussion.

The setting for the study was a community forum for those over 40 years of age living within the school district boundaries of a suburban community in Western Washington with a population of approximately 37.000, whose residents are predominately Caucasian (87%). Approximately 32% are ages 45 and over [27]. The forum included refreshments, and people were invited to sit at one of several round tables covered with paper for writing thoughts as they occurred to the participants. The conversation at each table began with the posing of one of three questions, with ample time allowed for each table group to discuss, strategize, and imagine a preferred future in an elder-friendly community. The three questions were as follows (1) What does it mean to you to be socially connected? (2) How can our city help with life transitions that would keep you in this community? (3) What do I have to offer my community? These three questions were developed through consensus by the city level committee charged with examining issues and processes that enhance an age-friendly community. The questions were designed to determine how people define and make meaning of being socially connected, to identify aspects of community life that would reinforce continuity with the community versus relocation to another community after retirement, and to ask participants to think about their own value to the community, thereby initiating thought around the idea of social reciprocity. Conversation was not limited to only the question at hand, and participants were invited to speak, draw, and write about the broader topic throughout the session. At set times, participants were asked to move to a different table, to be with a different group of people, and to consider a different question, until all three main questions were answered by most of the participants. One member from each table stayed behind during the rotation in order to serve as an ambassador for the previous members, thus assisting in continuity of conversation. A goal was to allow participants to engage creatively as they tackled the questions together. So, rather than gather individual feedback, table leaders encouraged participants to converse with each other and to spend time thinking together about potential solutions to dilemmas as they were raised by group members. Once the group session was completed, participants were invited to gather into a large group to debrief and discuss the most important topics from the perspectives of the participants. This conversation was also guided, and notes were recorded.

5.1. Sample. A purposive sample of people over age 40 was recruited through newspaper ads and invitations from the city Parks and Recreation Department and through the Aging in Place Committee (AIP) membership. Membership lists from the Senior Activity Center and local faith communities also served as sources for potential participants. The invitation requested community members to participate in a community forum to discuss how to create, promote, and maintain a more elder-friendly community. Ultimately, 23 individuals participated in the community forum and ranged in age from midforties to late eighties. Participants therefore represented both those who might be identified as baby boomers as well as those who are currently retired and may be defined more traditionally as older adults. We did not collect specific data on age, but some participants offered their age as part of the conversations. The majority of participants were female and Caucasian. Since this was originally conceived by the AIP committee as a community forum and not a research project, no additional sociodemographic data were collected on socioeconomic status, education, or other typical variables associated with creating a demographic profile.

5.2. Data Analysis. Following the World Café community forum, researchers were asked to analyze the data from the event in order for the AIP committee to present findings and make recommendations to city government officials. No identifying information about participants was included with the data provided for analysis. Using an approach consistent with grounded theory [28], the researchers analyzed the data for common categories and themes. First, they met together and carefully reviewed the data from each of the questions. They used an open coding process for notes of verbal exchanges, drawings and notes from participants, and memos from group leaders. The few illegible writings and unrecognizable doodles were dismissed from the analysis process. As categories began to emerge, coding became more selective until three main themes were identified. Throughout analysis, the researchers engaged in conversation about meanings and interpretations, until they were satisfied they had a clear understanding of the data. In order to confirm that trustworthiness of the data was maintained, once the themes were identified, the AIP committee reviewed the findings and then invited all of the original forum participants to attend a focus group to discuss the findings. The focus group was held in the same location as the community forum approximately two months after the forum was convened and was made up of five individuals (approximately 20% of forum members). Like the forum participants, most focus group participants were female and Caucasian, with one or two individuals representing communities of color. Focus group participants also ranged in age from early 50s to mid-70s. The focus group participants reviewed, clarified, and added data to the transcripts and confirmed that the themes identified by the researchers were reflective of the community meeting. The review by the focus groups provided credibility and trustworthiness (validity) to the qualitative findings, reinforcing a fit between the respondents' views and the researchers' interpretation as well as being confirmatory, for example, demonstrating that the study's findings were not imagined [22]. This process, known as member checking, not only serves to validate findings but is empowering to the participants and reinforces the close relationship between the researchers and the informants in qualitative research [22].

6. Results

The researchers identified three major themes that emanated directly from the data and were confirmed by the focus group. All three themes emerged from the open coding and were ultimately labeled as follows: *social reciprocity*, *meaningful interactions*, and *structural needs/barriers*. The three themes were identified and confirmed by both boomers and older participants.

6.1. Social Reciprocity. This theme was directly related to the overarching focus on social connectedness but illustrated the importance of added value in these relationships. Within the theme of social reciprocity, giving and receiving to/from one's community were both seen to be of equal importance. Some participants were currently volunteering or communicated an interest in doing so (giving). While exact ages were not available, it appeared that older adults (65+) were more likely to be active volunteers than their younger counterparts. Baby boomers expressed interest in volunteerism, while older adults may have already engaged in that process if they were interested. Many participants expressed an interest in receiving through such things as enhanced educational opportunities (e.g., more age-friendly options from the local community college and public university). The idea of educational opportunities at no or low cost was initially mentioned by younger participants. Participants also indicated that venues for creating social connectedness could come from both *formal* and *informal* entities. Formal entities are those which would require some infrastructure involving an organization or business, such as theater, outdoor concerts, or free movie nights. An example might be the initiation of social activities through city government, the local Chamber of Commerce, or even a local business. Informal entities would include activities that require limited resources, such as the creation of book clubs or neighborhood gatherings. Participants also suggested that such activities aimed at increasing social connectedness could be *sponsored* or *influenced* by community resources. For example, through the Senior Activity Center, the city might sponsor a new boomer or senior walking group. Communities also could advocate for the development of social venues through influence. The city government, for example, could attempt to influence the policy of a not- for-profit community organization regarding how cumbersome and degrading the process is for older adults with limited income to obtain reduced membership fees.

Reciprocity between formal and informal systems could also occur. For example, a nongovernmental organization such as a church could recruit older volunteers from their congregation to volunteer in local schools. The theme of social reciprocity can and should conceptually occur at multiple levels, such as between governmental and non-governmental organizations, as well as between individuals and their community. In all aspects of the data, reciprocity (the mutual exchange of commercial or other privileges) was exemplified as the willingness to give and receive in order to foster social connectedness. No one suggested getting something for nothing. Inherent in the discussion of social reciprocity was the notion that the relationship between the individual older persons may occur at multiple levels of community and environment. Relationships and mutual exchange might occur at the level of neighborhood, a community organization, or at the level of city government or policy advocacy. For example, some forum participants suggested helping others by providing space for a communal garden (neighborhood), while some suggested that developing a volunteer position to work as a senior ombudsman related to negotiating city services would be beneficial to the whole (city government level). This exchange improves the well-being of those being helped while fostering a sense of accomplishment and service.

6.2. Meaningful Interactions. While participants discussed the desire to give and receive in order to maintain social connectedness, they were clear, however, that these experiences should be meaningful both to themselves and others. While a high number of forum participants expressed a desire to volunteer in their community, they clearly stated that the activity should be meaningful to them and important to the community. This sentiment communicates the view that these individuals see themselves as having social capital (whether or not it is recognized by others). Volunteerism was seen as an important way to give back to the community. As one participant put it, "we should all volunteer, even if it is in the home—respite, visitor, chores." The participants shared a collective view that the purpose of volunteering was not to kill time. Rather, participants were interested in sharing their passions, time, sense of history, and even sharing personal space to accomplish this end. One participant suggested that people share their gardens with others or help others to do crafts in their homes. Participants also viewed volunteering as a way they could advocate for others and for their community. Finally, if participants were to be involved in meaningful interactions through volunteering, they wanted to feel appreciated for the work they did. They voiced the concern that organizations often diminished or ignored the value of their time as volunteers and took volunteers for granted. It is important to note here that forum participants did not suggest they wanted to volunteer for the sake of recognition, but rather they felt the need to be valued—not taken for granted. The message that was communicated by forum participants was that they desired both the organization/community in which they served as well as themselves to view their contributions as meaningful. While speculative due to a lack of specific data on age, the older participants appeared more settled in their roles as volunteers, as many of them had held these roles for some time. Younger adults (boomers) appeared to have more concerns about the meaning they derived from volunteer opportunities and how that may be accomplished.

6.3. Structural Needs/Barriers. While the majority of participants provided feedback on what or how they could contribute to their community to enhance social connectedness, a similar number of people voiced substantial frustration with the lack of either organized opportunities or communication with potential organizations with which to volunteer. These issues were impediments to social reciprocity as well as to meaningful interaction, and as such were labeled as structural needs or barriers. Structural (infrastructural) needs or barriers were those things participants viewed as currently lacking in the community but, if present, would facilitate social reciprocity both in terms of physical and social venues. For example, many forum participants expressed the need for improved methods by which potential volunteers could be connected to opportunities (community entities). These sentiments were expressed more strongly by younger participants. The examples that were given included organizations that needed volunteers should return phone calls more promptly to potential volunteers, as well as the need for more personal connections between those requesting volunteers and the people who might be willing to give of their time. Again, the importance of the value of time was communicated by the participants. They were not interested in having to make numerous inquiries to potential organizations in order to volunteer. The feeling expressed was that there was a lack of reciprocity from the very beginning on the part of agencies or organizations with which these individuals might wish to volunteer.

Transportation was described as an additional structural barrier and was mentioned frequently in all table conversations. Transportation was viewed as an essential element of social connectedness. In areas of both volunteerism as well as overall social connectedness, transportation issues associated with public transit and walkable communities were voiced. Issues concerning transportation included that a lack of reliable, frequent, and accessible transportation created barriers for participants within the community. As one individual said, "[a] lack of transportation isolates seniors." The view communicated by these participants was that improved transportation can foster and enhance social connectedness by decreasing barriers of distance and reducing the need for use of one's personal vehicle. One important distinction between younger and older participants was noted relevant to transportation. While younger participants voiced interest in improved transportation as a means toward improved social connectedness and as an environmentally friendly alternative to automobiles, older participants expressed a more urgent need for improved transportation, as well as having a more specific personal need. For example, one couple who was likely in their 70s expressed the need for improved transportation services for their parents (in their 90s) as they identified gaps in transportation services as personally problematic.

7. Discussion

The purpose of this research project was to analyze data gathered from aging individuals (including baby boomers) on the importance of social connectedness in the creation of elder-friendly communities through a naturalistic method of inquiry. By engaging in a more naturalistic conversation utilizing the World Café format, the participants in the study were able to utilize conversation in meaning making without the confines of any a priori assumptions about social connectedness.

The findings from this community forum and the subsequent focus group reinforce earlier data from the original *AdvantAge Initiative* as well as other literature on elder-friendly communities and point to the utility of several important theories. First, these findings echo the original framework from the *AdvantAge Initiative* [17], which emphasizes the importance of social and civic engagement. The individuals from this community forum, as well as the elder counterparts in the original study, underscored the importance of meaningful connections to family, friends, and neighbors as part of civic engagement. An elder-friendly community needs to find new ways to promote active and continual engagement in community life. The findings from this study parallel the view of Scharlach [14] who suggests that as "we get older and ever closer to the end of our lives, maintaining social connectedness and deepening existing relationships becomes a priority" [14, page 9]. These findings also reinforce the importance of participation and integration, which is a critical element of social exclusion theory [8]. Forum participants identified multiple activities associated with social inclusion/exclusion including production (economic or socially valued) activity, political activity to improve or protect the social environment, and social activity that involved engagement with family, friends, and community. Scharf and colleagues [8] define participation and integration as "older people's embeddedness in social networks and the extent to which older people contribute to or draw upon social capital that exists in their neighborhoods" [8, page 316]. Thus, our findings related to social reciprocity appear consistent with the major theme from social inclusion/exclusion theory. Our findings also reinforce the importance of Lawton's [12] environmental function of support. A community needs to be dynamic in order to support changes in the older citizenry. While the concept of support is typically relevant to adjustment to altered or lost competencies, the concept of support can be extended to include the need for continued and changing modes of social and civic engagement.

This study also reinforces both the importance of volunteer opportunities and that those opportunities be purposeful and meaningful. As suggested by Scharlach [14], in an elder-friendly community, older adults are not just seen as clients or passive recipients of services, but "active contributors to the well-being of the community" [14, page 9]. In the original *AdvantAge* survey, residents from this community volunteered at a rate substantially lower than the national average for the 10 *AdvantAge* communities [23]. What we learned from this study was that aging community members held interest and motivation to volunteer or otherwise be engaged in their community. We believe they see themselves as having social capital [29], but as Putnam [29] points out, others may not always share their view. The environmental function of stimulation [12] is relevant here as participants seemed to look to their community for stimuli for enhanced social well-being and to elicit new and relevant social and leisure behaviors [9]. Older participants appeared more likely to have volunteer and community activities in place, while younger adults (boomers) were perhaps seeking out methods for accomplishing that goal. Both younger and older participants also noted structural barriers to social connectedness and social integration, supporting Alley et al. [15] who suggest that while communities may be able to support aging in place, they may also contain barriers that make community living difficult for older residents. A recent study of 253 older adults reinforces the importance of organizational structure in volunteerism. Tang et al. [30] found organizational support (defined as choice of volunteer activity, training, and ongoing support) to be associated with socioemotional benefits, including perceived contribution and personal benefits. These researchers concluded that the "psychological well-being of older adults can be improved through engagement in meaningful volunteer activities and contribution to others" [30, page 603], again reinforcing what Rubinstein and colleagues [20] noted concerning the connection between well-being and active environmental management. In order for these benefits to occur, however, an elder-friendly community must work to eliminate structural and organizational barriers to volunteerism and social connectedness. As Scharf and colleagues [8] assert, participation and integration are enhanced by good public service such as access to reliable transportation. To not provide such services serves to reinforce the social exclusion of older people. The identification of structural barriers also reinforces the person-in-environment perspective that the needs of older people change over time and must be successfully navigated in order to maintain social integration. Lawton's [12] environmental function of maintenance is relevant here. If a community is to be elder-friendly, the infrastructure needs to be consistent and predictable at the very least, while at the same time dynamic in its ability to provide stimulation and support.

Community-based research is particularly useful when it is able to identify problems and move toward a resolution of that issue. Researchers can partner with communities to study areas of interest, interpret results [31], and assist in the empowerment of community members to make changes [32]. The findings from this study have already resulted in community level change efforts related to volunteerism. An annual volunteer fair was initiated in 2010 with the goal of creating a venue to match older volunteers with community level volunteer opportunities. This newly formed activity grew directly out of the identification of structural barriers in this research and was created through a partnership of senior advocates, the community's AIP committee, and local organizations, including the area hospital. In the first year of operation, 30 community organizations and programs participated along with 120 attendees. More than 80% of older adults were successfully matched with local organizations, thus improving social connectedness, integration, and reciprocity in a direct and clear way. This event has now been established as an annual event sponsored by seniors, city government, and other community entities. Its goal is to improve civic engagement among older residents, thus fostering the connectedness between older residents and organizations that serve the community.

In addition to the importance of civic engagement, the philosophy of aging in place supports the continued importance of maximizing independence for not only the frail and disabled, but for aging adults of all abilities. In particular, these findings point to the need for accessible and available transportation, an issue that city officials and community advocates should attempt to improve through partnerships. As Feldman and Oberlink [17] noted in their original findings, "transportation and safety are fundamental factors that enable older adults to stay connected to the community" [17, page 5]. Rosenbloom [33] suggests that transportation in elder-friendly communities will need to be planned to provide more customized services, linking residential concentrations with important destinations, including volunteer opportunity destinations. The project findings noted that while all participants voiced the need for improved transportation services, the kinds of services desired may change with age. The lack of this kind of transportation was clearly identified as a major structural barrier reinforcing social exclusion and needs to be considered as future planning takes place. With impending cuts to public transportation, the aging in place committee is examining potential alternatives to improve transportation through private and voluntary means.

7.1. Limitations. The results of this study provide important information on social connectedness in elder-friendly communities. Still, this study has several limitations that must be acknowledged. First, as a qualitative and naturalistic study, the findings are the specific views of those individuals involved and cannot be generalized to any larger population of aging adults. Second, a further limitation is that those who responded to the invitation to participate in the community forum may have had a greater interest in the topic, or a vested interest in having their voices heard as compared to those who did not or could not attend. However, the study results provide a new dimension to the subject area and support previous studies and theories on aging in place, thus adding to the picture of what needs to be done to support the creation of elder-friendly communities. Because of the homogeneous makeup of forum participants, the voices of other communities such as communities of color were not clearly heard. It must be acknowledged that the opinions and concerns of this group do not likely represent all older adults in this community. Finally, because sociodemographic data was not collected on individuals, distinctions between older (65+) and younger participants are based upon educated guesses about participant's age.

8. Conclusion and Implications

The results of this study reinforce the importance of social connectedness, participation, and integration in creating and maintaining elder-friendly communities and suggest that the findings are areas of concern not just for the old-old, but for recent and soon-to-be retired individuals wishing to maintain life satisfaction. The study suggests the possibility of using more nontraditional research techniques for gathering community level data such as the kinds of findings generated from the World Café process. While creating and fostering elder-friendly communities can be a long and ongoing process, small incremental change can occur from such studies as is illustrated by the case of the annual volunteer fair now established in this community.

If a national agenda of enabling our aging population to age in place is to be accomplished, creating elder-friendly communities has a logical and important role. Scharf et al. [7] suggest an important association between social connectedness and quality of life. They found that older people who rated their quality of life as "good" were less likely to experience social exclusion. For aging in place to happen successfully, with older adults being continually valued and integrated into community life, city officials, policy makers, and gerontological researchers will need to collaborate in order to move these ideas from research to reality.

References

[1] N. R. Hooyman and H. A. Kiyak, *Social Gerontology: A Multidisciplinary Perspective*, Allyn and Bacon, Boston, Mass, USA, 2011.

[2] G. E. Alkema, K. H. Wilber, and S. M. Enguidanos, "Community and facility based care," in *Handbook of Gerontology: Evidence Based Approaches to Theory, Practice, and Policy*, J. A. Blackburn and C. N. Dalmus, Eds., pp. 455–498, John Wiley and Sons, New York, NY, USA, 2007.

[3] K. Lawler, *Aging in Place: Coordinating Housing and Health Care Provision for America's Growing Elderly Population*, Harvard University, Cambridge, Mass, USA, 2001.

[4] D. T. Lau, K. G. Scandrett, M. Jarzebowski, K. Holman, and L. Emanuel, "Health-related safety: a framework to address barriers to aging in place," *Gerontologist*, vol. 47, no. 6, pp. 830–837, 2007.

[5] F. Oswald, D. Jopp, C. Rott, and H. Wahl, "Is aging in place a resource for or risk to life satisfaction?" *Gerontologist*, vol. 51, no. 2, pp. 238–250, 2011.

[6] K. J. Swick and R. D. Williams, "An analysis of Bronfenbrenner's bio-ecological perspective for early childhood educators: implications for working with families experiencing stress," *Early Childhood Education Journal*, vol. 33, no. 5, pp. 371–378, 2006.

[7] T. Scharf, C. Phillipson, and A. E. Smith, "Poverty and social exclusion—growing older in deprived social neighborhoods," in *Growing Older: Quality of Life in Old Age*, A. Walker and C. H. Hennessy, Eds., pp. 81–106, Open University Press, 2004.

[8] T. Scharf, C. Phillipson, P. Kingston, and A. E. Smith, "Social exclusion and older people: exploring the connections," *Education and Ageing*, vol. 16, no. 3, pp. 303–320, 2001.

[9] H.-W. Wahl and G. D. Weisman, "Environmental gerontology at the beginning of the new millennium: reflections on its historical, empirical, and theoretical development," *Gerontologist*, vol. 43, no. 5, pp. 616–627, 2003.

[10] R. J. Scheidt and P. G. Windley, "The ecology of aging," in *Handbook of the Psychology of Aging*, J. E. Birren and K. W. Schaie, Eds., pp. 245–258, Van Nostrand, 1985.

[11] M. P. Lawton, "The impact of the environment on aging and behavior," in *Handbook of the Psychology of Aging*, J. E. Birren and K. W. Schaie, Eds., pp. 276–301, Van Nostrand, 1977.

[12] M. P. Lawton, "Three functions of the residential environment," *Journal of Housing for the Elderly*, vol. 5, no. 1, pp. 35–50, 1989.

[13] H.-W. Wahl, "Environmental influences on aging and behavior," in *Handbook of the Psychology of Aging*, J. E. Birren and K. W. Schaie, Eds., pp. 215–232, Academic Press, New York, NY, USA, 2001.

[14] A. E. Scharlach, "Creating aging-friendly communities," *Generations*, vol. 33, no. 2, pp. 5–11, 2009.

[15] D. Alley, P. Liebig, J. Pynoos, T. Banerjee, and I. Choi, "Creating elder-friendly communities: preparations for an aging society," *Journal of Gerontological Social Work*, vol. 49, no. 1-2, pp. 1–18, 2007.

[16] Center for Advanced Studies of Aging Services, *Creating Aging-Friendly Communities: Final Report*, U. C. Berkeley, Berkeley, Calif, USA, 2009.

[17] P. H. Feldman and M. R. Oberlink, "The advantage initiative: developing community indicators to promote the health and well-being of older people," *Family & Community Health*, vol. 26, no. 4, pp. 268–274, 2003.

[18] C. D. Austin, E. des Camp, D. Flux, R. W. McClelland, and J. Sieppert, "Community development with older adults in their neighborhoods: the elder friendly communities program," *Families in Society*, vol. 86, no. 3, pp. 401–409, 2009.

[19] World Health Organization, *Global Age-friendly Cities: A Guide*, World Health Organization Publications, 2007.

[20] R. L. Rubinstein, J. C. Kilbride, and S. Nagy, *Elders Living Alone*, Walter de Gruyter, Berlin, Germany, 1992.

[21] W. H. Thomas and J. M. Blanchard, "Moving beyond place: aging in community," *Generations*, vol. 33, no. 2, pp. 12–17, 2009.

[22] D. Padgett, *Qualitative Methods in Social Work Research*, Sage, 2008.

[23] P. H. Feldman, M. R. Oberlink, E. Simantov, and M. D. Gursen, "A Tale of two americas: community opportunities and challenges," in *Center for Home Care Policy and Research*, Visiting Nurse Service of New York, New York, NY, USA, 2004.

[24] D. Hanson and C. A. Emlet, "Assessing a community's elder friendliness: a case example of the advantage initiative," *Family & Community Health*, vol. 29, no. 4, pp. 266–278, 2006.

[25] J. Brown and D. Isaacs, *The World Cafe: Shaping our Futures through Conversations that Matter*, Barrett-Koehler Publishers, San Francisco, Calif, USA, 2005.

[26] D. L. Cooperrider, D. K. Whitney, and J. M. Stavros, *Appreciative Inquiry Handbook: For Leaders of Change*, Crown Custom Publishing, Brunswick, Australia, 2008.

[27] U.S. Census Bureau, American Factfinder, http://factfinder.census.gov/home/saff/main.html?_lang=en, 2011.

[28] A. L. Strauss and J. M. Corbin, *Basics of Qualitative Research: Techniques and Procedures for Developing Grounded Theory*, Sage, 1998.

[29] R. D. Putnam, "Tuning in, tuning out: the strange disappearance of social capital in America," *Political Science and Politics*, vol. 28, no. 4, pp. 664–683, 1995.

[30] F. Tang, E. Choi, and N. Morrow-Howell, "Organizational support and volunteering benefits for older adults," *Gerontologist*, vol. 50, no. 5, pp. 603–612, 2010.

[31] J. Krysik and J. Finn, *Research for Effective Social Work Practice*, Routledge, London, UK, 2nd edition, 2010.

[32] C. Marlow and S. Boone, *Research Methods for Generalist Social Work*, Brooks/Cole, 4th edition, 2005.

[33] S. Rosenbloom, "Meeting transportation needs in an aging-friendly community," *Generations*, vol. 33, no. 2, pp. 33–43, 2009.

7

The Relationship between Intramuscular Adipose Tissue, Functional Mobility, and Strength in Postmenopausal Women with and without Type 2 Diabetes

Janet M. Pritchard,[1,2] Sarah Karampatos,[1,2] Karen A. Beattie,[2,3] Lora M. Giangregorio,[4] George Ioannidis,[1,2,3] Stephanie A. Atkinson,[5] Lehana Thabane,[6] Hertzel Gerstein,[2,6] Zubin Punthakee,[2] Jonathan D. Adachi,[2,3] and Alexandra Papaioannou[1,2]

[1]*Geriatric Education and Research in Aging Sciences (GERAS) Centre, St. Peter's Hospital, 88 Maplewood Avenue, Hamilton, ON, Canada L8M 1W9*
[2]*Department of Medicine, McMaster University, 1280 Main Street West, Hamilton, ON, Canada L8S 4K1*
[3]*Charlton Medical Centre, 25 Charlton Avenue East, Hamilton, ON, Canada L8N 1Y2*
[4]*Department of Kinesiology, University of Waterloo, 200 University Avenue West, Waterloo, ON, Canada N2L 3G1*
[5]*Department of Pediatrics, McMaster University, 1280 Main Street West, Hamilton, ON, Canada L8S 4K1*
[6]*Department of Clinical Epidemiology and Biostatistics, McMaster University, 1280 Main Street West, Hamilton, ON, Canada L8S 4K1*

Correspondence should be addressed to Janet M. Pritchard; pritchar@hhsc.ca

Academic Editor: Simone Reppermund

Objectives. To determine (1) whether intramuscular adipose tissue (IntraMAT) differs between women with and without type 2 diabetes and (2) the association between IntraMAT and mobility and strength. *Methods.* 59 women ≥ 65 years with and without type 2 diabetes were included. A 1-Tesla MRI was used to acquire images of the leg. Timed-up-and-go (TUG) and grip strength were measured. Regression was used to determine associations between the following: (1) type 2 diabetes and IntraMAT (covariates: age, ethnicity, BMI, waist : hip ratio, and energy expenditure), (2) IntraMAT and TUG (covariates: diabetes, age, BMI, and energy expenditure), and (3) IntraMAT and grip strength (covariates: diabetes, age, height, and lean mass). *Results.* Women with diabetes had more IntraMAT. After adjustment, IntraMAT was similar between groups (diabetes mean [SD] = 13.2 [1.4]%, controls 11.8 [1.3]%, $P = 0.515$). IntraMAT was related to TUG and grip strength, but the relationships became nonsignificant after adjustment for covariates (difference/percent IntraMAT [95% CI]: TUG = 0.041 seconds [−0.079–0.161], $P = 0.498$, grip strength = −0.144 kg [−0.335–0.066], $P = 0.175$). *Conclusions.* IntraMAT alone may not be a clinically important predictor of functional mobility and strength; however, whether losses in functional mobility and strength are promoted by IntraMAT accumulation should be explored.

1. Background

Most adults with type 2 diabetes experience accelerated musculoskeletal aging and a higher prevalence of frailty than people without diabetes of a comparable age [1, 2]. This leads to a greater risk of falls and fractures [3], greater healthcare expenditures, and increased morbidity and mortality [4]. Skeletal muscle atrophy and obesity, known as sarcopenic obesity, seem to be important contributing factors but do not entirely explain the variance in functional mobility and strength [5]. Skeletal muscle quality, which is influenced by the infiltration of adipose tissue into skeletal muscle, may also play a role.

Adipose tissue infiltration of the thigh, assessed with the computed tomography- (CT-) derived muscle density measurement [6], is related to lower muscle strength [7] and greater hip fracture risk [8]. However, assessing infiltration of adipose tissue into skeletal muscle with CT is limited.

It is an indirect measurement of muscle adiposity and does not differentiate between adipose tissue within the muscle and adipose tissue between the muscle bellies, which may be physiologically different depots of adipose tissue [9]. Compared to CT, studies using magnetic resonance imaging (MRI) are better able to assess adipose tissue within the muscle due to better image resolution and contrast [10]. Various terms have been used to describe these depots of adipose tissue beneath the subcutaneous adipose tissue and fascia of the muscle. For example, *intermuscular adipose tissue* (InterMAT) has been used to describe adipose tissue beneath the fascia and between and within muscle bellies [11–14]. However, others have used the same term to describe adipose tissue beneath the fascia and between the muscle bellies and not within the muscle bellies [15, 16]. Conversely, *intramuscular adipose tissue* (IntraMAT) has been defined by some groups as adipose tissue within the muscle bellies [17–20]. There are limited studies that examine InterMAT and IntraMAT separately using image analysis software, which is important considering that these depots of adipose tissue may have different effects on musculoskeletal health [9, 11].

Functional mobility and muscular strength are important determinants of healthy aging and preserving independence. The time taken to complete a timed-up-and-go (TUG) test is indicative of an older adult's level of function, with higher test scores linked to poor balance, slow gait speed, and difficulty with activities of daily living [21]. Likewise, older adults with poor grip strength are at higher risk of losing independence in activities of daily living [22] and mortality [23, 24]. Both TUG test and grip strength scores have been used to differentiate between frail and nonfrail older adults in the community [25] and are strong independent predictors of physical frailty [26].

The objectives of this study were to (1) determine whether lower leg percent IntraMAT differs between women with and without type 2 diabetes, (2) determine the association between percent IntraMAT and both functional mobility (TUG) and strength (grip strength), and (3) determine whether the relationships are affected by adjusting for type 2 diabetes and other potential covariates.

2. Methods

2.1. Study Participants. This cross-sectional study was conducted with postmenopausal women of age ≥65 years. Participants were recruited from outpatient diabetes clinics and by community advertisements. Participants with type 2 diabetes had a diagnosis of type 2 diabetes for ≥5 years. This study included participants recruited for the purpose of a study on bone health [27]; therefore exclusion criteria were (1) use of medications in the past 24 months known to affect bone (bisphosphonates, parathyroid hormone, calcitonin, selective estrogen receptor modulator, and hormone therapy); (2) chronic systemic glucocorticoid exposure (≥3 months at a prednisone equivalent dosage ≥ 7.5 mg/day); (3) Paget's disease; (4) hyperparathyroidism or hypoparathyroidism; (5) metastatic cancer in the past 5 years; and (6) severe renal impairment, defined as CrCl < 30 mL/min, which is the National Kidney Foundation cutoff for severe renal impairment or kidney failure [28]. Participants with ferromagnetic implants were excluded from the study. Study approval was granted by the Hamilton Integrated Research Ethics Board.

2.2. Magnetic Resonance Imaging (MRI). One researcher imaged each participant's nondominant lower leg with a peripheral 1-Tesla MRI system (OrthOne, GE Healthcare). The standard 66% tibia site (i.e., distance from the distal end of the medial malleolus to the medial knee joint cleft × 0.66) was marked on each participant's leg. Participants inserted their lower leg into a 160 mm diameter transmit/receive coil and padding was applied around the leg to reduce the potential of motion artifact. A 2-dimensional sagittal fast spin echo (FSE) localizer was used to position the participant's leg in the system and ten axial T_1-weighted images were obtained (Figures 1(a), 1(b)). Scan parameters were as follows: TR = 600 milliseconds (ms), TE = 22.9 ms, gap = 0 mm, flip angle = 90°, bandwidth = 25 kHz, acquisition matrix = 320 × 320, field of view = 16 cm, and scan time = 9:42 minutes.

2.3. MRI Analysis. Prior to image analysis, 2 authors (Janet M. Pritchard, Sarah Karampatos) independently reviewed all axial slices for image blurring, and participants with significant motion artifact (graded as 0 for no motion artifact or 1 for motion artifact) were excluded from analysis. Post-processing of all axial slices was performed using sliceOmatic version 4.3 rev. 7c (Tomovision, Montreal, Canada) (Figures 1(c), 1(d)). One person who was unaware of diabetes status (Sarah Karampatos) completed image analysis on the same workstation. Images were gamma corrected to calibrate the grey level of the images for slice-by-slice segmentation. We segmented the compartments of the lower leg according to the following definitions:

(i) subcutaneous adipose tissue: any tissue or component outside of the fascia, including vessels and skin;

(ii) total muscle: nonadipose tissue beneath the fascia, excluding bone;

(iii) tibia and fibula bone: cortical bone, excluding marrow;

(iv) intermuscular adipose tissue (InterMAT): adipose tissue beneath the fascia and between the following: (1) soleus and medial head of gastrocnemius, (2) lateral head of the gastrocnemius and medial head of gastrocnemius, and (3) lateral head of gastrocnemius and soleus; if vessels were contained in this compartment, they were included in the segmentation;

(v) intramuscular adipose tissue (IntraMAT): adipose tissue within the total muscle compartment (belly), including vessels.

The semiautomatic segmentation tools were used to segment the subcutaneous adipose tissue, total muscle, tibia, fibula, and intermuscular adipose tissue. Mathematical morphology was used to compute the watershed of the image and create a water parting mesh of the image. This step distinguishes between tissues with different grey level values, such as muscle and subcutaneous adipose tissue. The images were edited sparingly to refine the segmentation. Region

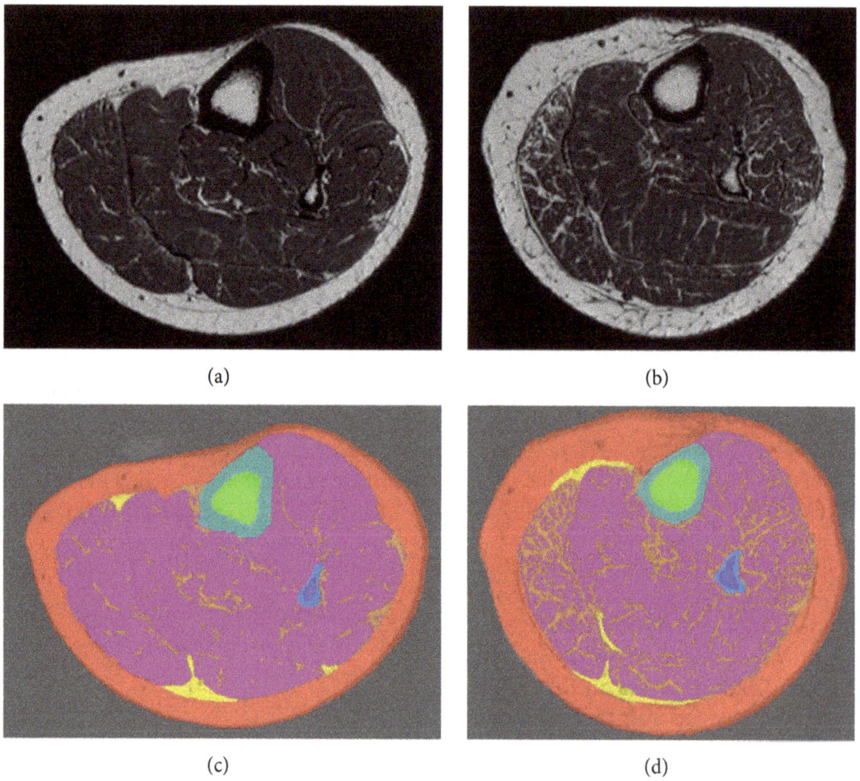

FIGURE 1: Axial MRI images of the lower leg from a Caucasian postmenopausal woman without type 2 diabetes (age 68 years, percent IntraMAT = 8%) (a) and with type 2 diabetes (age 67 years, percent IntraMAT = 14%) (b). Segmented images of the lower leg from the participant without type 2 diabetes (c) and with type 2 diabetes (d). Subcutaneous adipose tissue (red), muscle (fuchsia), intermuscular adipose tissue (InterMAT) (yellow), intramuscular adipose tissue (IntraMAT) (orange), tibia cortical bone (blue), tibia bone marrow (green), fibula cortical bone (royal blue), and fibula bone marrow (purple).

growing was used within the muscle to segment IntraMAT. A threshold was set to exclude pixels belonging to muscle and include pixels belonging to adipose tissue. A slicewise comparison between the original image and segmented image was completed to ensure that the segmentation was sensible. IntraMAT was normalized to the total muscle cross-sectional area (percent IntraMAT = [IntraMAT (mm^2) ÷ total muscle area (mm^2)] × 100%). To determine the short-term intrarater reliability of the segmentation protocol, one researcher (Sarah Karampatos) analyzed 21 anonymized randomly selected participants' scans in duplicate [29]. The time between the repeated analyses of a participant's scan was 2 weeks. Previous studies have validated the use of this software for the assessment of adipose tissue within the muscle [30, 31].

2.4. Additional Data Collection. Anthropometric, medical history, nutrition, and physical activity data were collected. A whole-body dual X-ray absorptiometry (DXA) (Hologic, Discovery QDR4500A) scan was used to ascertain total body mass, lean mass, and fat mass, from which percent lean and fat mass were derived. Height was measured using a wall-mounted stadiometer and BMI was calculated. Waist and hip circumference were measured to the nearest 0.1 cm. The age-adjusted Charlson Index, a commonly used measure of comorbidity, was calculated for each participant based on the presence of diseases. Weekly energy expenditure in habitual activities was estimated using the modified Paffenbarger Physical Activity Questionnaire, which quantifies kilocalorie (kcal) expenditure based on stair climbing, walking, and participation in activities [32, 33]. Dietary calcium and vitamin D intakes were quantified using a validated food frequency questionnaire [34] and supplemental calcium and vitamin D were captured to calculate total (diet + supplement) intake. Participant's ethnicity was recorded as Caucasian or non-Caucasian.

2.5. Functional Mobility and Strength Assessments. The TUG test was used to assess functional mobility [21]. This objective test has good interrater and intrarater reliability and is correlated with Berg Balance Scale scores, gait speed, and the Barthel Index of activities of daily living (ADLs) [21]. For the TUG test, participants were instructed to stand from a chair, walk 3 meters, turn, walk back to the chair, and sit down [21]. Gait aids were used when needed. To assess muscle strength, an isometric grip strength dynamometer was used (Takei T.T.K 5001 Isometric Grip A Dynamometer, Takei Scientific Instruments). Grip strength is a quick, objective measure of muscular strength and is correlated with quadriceps strength [35]. Grip strength was recorded with the dominant arm to the nearest kilogram for 3 trials, and the average grip strength was calculated for each participant. Arm specific force, a normalized measure of muscle quality, was calculated by taking the ratio of grip strength to arm muscle mass acquired with the DXA whole-body scan [2].

2.6. Statistical Analysis. To determine the relative intrarater reliability of the image analysis protocol, type 2,1 intraclass correlation coefficient (ICC) and 95% confidence intervals (CI) were calculated. All data were tested for normality using the Shapiro-Wilk test, and the mean (standard deviation (SD)) or median (interquartile range (25th and 75th percentiles)) was computed. Student's *t*-test was used to determine between-group differences in cross-sectional area of lower leg compartments. To determine whether percent IntraMAT (percent IntraMAT = [IntraMAT (mm^2) ÷ total muscle area (mm^2)] × 100%) differed for women with and without type 2 diabetes, unadjusted and adjusted parameter estimates were calculated for percent IntraMAT using an analysis of covariance (ANCOVA) model. Covariates for the adjusted model included age, ethnicity, BMI, waist-to-hip ratio, and energy expenditure in activities, as these variables are related to measures of muscle adiposity [13, 36–38]. Separate linear regression analyses were conducted to determine the relationships between the following: (1) TUG (dependent variable) and IntraMAT (independent variable) and (2) grip strength (dependent variable) and IntraMAT (independent variable). For each dependent variable, three models were produced and included (1) an unadjusted model, (2) a model adjusted for only diagnosis of type 2 diabetes, and (3) a model adjusted for covariates. For the TUG analysis, the covariates included age, diagnosis of type 2 diabetes, BMI, and weekly energy expenditure [39, 40]. For the grip strength analysis, the covariates included age, diagnosis of type 2 diabetes, height, and percent lean mass [2, 41]. The interaction term, IntraMAT*diabetes, was removed from the final models once it was shown not to be significant. The coefficient of determination (R^2) was used to determine the explained variance of the models. Covariates for the ANCOVA and linear regression models were selected on the basis of previous research showing an association with the dependent variable. In addition, all covariates were significantly ($P < 0.05$) related to both the dependent and independent variable in Pearson correlation analyses and had a Pearson correlation coefficient ≥ 0.30 [42]. Linear regression assumptions were checked and met for the models, including (1) linear relationship between dependent and predictor variable, (2) homoscedasticity, (3) normal distribution and independence of errors, and (4) multicollinearity (variance inflation factor ≤ 2). Analyses were performed with SPSS version 20 and an alpha level of ≤0.05 was considered statistically significant.

3. Results

29 participants with type 2 diabetes and 30 participants without type 2 diabetes (controls) completed the study visits. After reviewing the MRI scans for motion, 2 participants' scans were discarded (1 participant with type 2 diabetes, 1 control). Descriptive and anthropometric data are presented in Table 1. Most participants with type 2 diabetes were taking insulin (64% [18/28]) or metformin (39% [11/28]).

3.1. Type 2 Diabetes and IntraMAT. Unadjusted analyses revealed that the absolute amount of IntraMAT was greater in women with type 2 diabetes compared to controls, and there was no between-group difference in the amounts of InterMAT, subcutaneous adipose tissue, total muscle, or bone (Table 2). Unadjusted percent IntraMAT was greater in women with type 2 diabetes (mean [SD], 15.8 [1.5]%) compared to controls (8.9 [1.4]%, $P = 0.002$) (Figure 2(a)); however, after adjustment for age, ethnicity, BMI, waist: hip ratio, and energy expenditure, the between-group difference was reduced (13.2 [1.4]% versus 11.8 [1.3]%, $P = 0.515$) (Figure 2(b)).

3.2. Relationship between IntraMAT and Functional Mobility and Strength. Results of the linear regression models are presented in Table 3. There was a significant relationship between IntraMAT and TUG, where IntraMAT alone explained 18.9% of the variance in TUG result (Table 3, $P = 0.001$). Independent of type 2 diabetes, IntraMAT was still related to TUG ($P = 0.019$). After adjusting for type 2 diabetes, age, BMI, and energy expenditure, there was no statistically significant independent relationship between IntraMAT and TUG ($P = 0.378$). The model including IntraMAT, type 2 diabetes, age, BMI, and estimated energy expenditure explained 50.5% of the variance in TUG result ($P < 0.001$). There was no interaction between IntraMAT and diabetes ($P = 0.754$).

There was an inverse relationship between IntraMAT and grip strength, where IntraMAT alone explained 11.2% of the variance in grip strength (Table 3, $P = 0.012$). After adjusting for diagnosis of type 2 diabetes, the relationship between IntraMAT and grip strength remained significant ($P = 0.049$). Adjustment for type 2 diabetes, age, height, and percent lean mass revealed no statistically independent relationship between IntraMAT and grip strength ($P = 0.120$). There was no interaction between IntraMAT and diabetes ($P = 0.993$). The model including IntraMAT, type 2 diabetes, age, height, and percent lean mass explained 28.8% of the variance in grip strength ($P < 0.001$).

3.3. Intrarater Reliability. The intrarater reliability for the image analysis protocol was acceptable for segmentation of each compartment. The ICC estimates were as follows: IntraMAT ICC = 0.999 (95% CI, 0.997–0.999, $P < 0.001$), InterMAT ICC = 0.981 (95% CI, 0.953–0.992, $P < 0.001$), subcutaneous adipose tissue ICC = 0.999 (95% CI, 0.997–1.00, $P < 0.001$), total muscle ICC = 0.994 (95% CI, 0.986–0.998, $P < 0.001$), tibia ICC = 0.994 (95% CI, 0.986–0.998, $P < 0.001$), and fibula ICC = 0.972 (95% CI, 0.932–0.989, $P < 0.001$).

4. Discussion

This study demonstrated that women with type 2 diabetes have more IntraMAT in the lower leg compared to women without type 2 diabetes, according to the unadjusted analysis. However, adjustment for potential covariates attenuated this difference, suggesting that there may be other factors,

TABLE 1: Characteristics of study participants.

	Type 2 diabetes $n = 28$	Control $n = 29$	P value
Age, years	70.0 (68.0–74.0)	70.0 (68.0–73.5)	0.885
Years since diabetes diagnosis, years	17 (11)	—	—
Caucasian, n (%)	23 (82.1)	29 (100.0)	0.023*
Uses walking aid, n (%)	6 (21.4)	2 (6.9)	0.115
BMI, kg/m^2	34.3 (7.5)	28.0 (5.6)	<0.001*
Waist : hip ratio	0.89 (0.07)	0.83 (0.06)	0.005*
Percent body fat, %	39.3 (36.5–45.0)	38.5 (34.3–41.7)	0.693
Percent lean mass, %	57.9 (53.1–61.2)	60.8 (55.8–63.6)	0.550
Energy expenditure[a], kcal/week	1003 (302–2120)	1597 (1129–3865)	0.684
Age-adjusted Charlson Index	4.4 (1.6)	0.4 (1.3)	<0.001*
Number of years since menopause	20 (20–25)	20 (19–26)	0.857
Number of prescribed medications	6 (3)	2 (2)	<0.001*
Total calcium intake, mg/day	1594 (709)	2048 (589)	<0.001*
Total vitamin D intake, IU/day	794 (631)	1204 (938)	0.062
Current smoker, n (%)	2 (7.1)	0	0.237
Hip or knee osteoarthritis, n (%)	15 (53.6)	5 (17.2)	0.006*
TUG, seconds	11.8 (6.2–17.4)	9.0 (6.0–12.0)	<0.001*
Grip strength, kg	18.8 (4.9)	21.5 (6.3)	0.059
Specific force, $kg_{force}/kg_{arm\ mass}$	7.5 (2.7)	10.1 (3.4)	0.002*

Data are mean (SD) or median (25th–75th percentiles) unless indicated otherwise.
*$P < 0.05$ considered significant.
BMI: body mass index; TUG: timed-up-and-go.
[a]Energy expenditure based on habitual stair climbing, walking, and participation in recreational activities.

TABLE 2: Unadjusted comparison of cross-sectional area of lower leg compartments in women with and without type 2 diabetes.

	Type 2 diabetes $n = 28$	Control $n = 29$	P value
IntraMAT, mm^2	608.2 (463.5–1131.7)	393.4 (282.4–506.1)	0.012*
InterMAT, mm^2	96.8 (66.9–175.8)	80.6 (55.4–148.9)	0.146
Subcutaneous adipose tissue, mm^2	3724.9 (1587.3)	3538.6 (1156.1)	0.614
Total muscle, mm^2	5120.5 (845.2)	5072.3 (780.8)	0.824
Tibia, mm^2	302.5 (52.0)	289.6 (37.7)	0.285
Fibula, mm^2	64.9 (14.7)	60.1 (13.1)	0.202

Data are mean (SD) or median (interquartile range). *$P < 0.05$ considered significant.
IntraMAT: intramuscular adipose tissue; InterMAT: intermuscular adipose tissue.

TABLE 3: Unadjusted and adjusted relationships among IntraMAT, functional mobility, and strength.

	Unadjusted			Adjusted for diabetes status			Adjusted for other covariates		
	Incremental difference per percent IntraMAT (95% CI)	P value	R^2	Incremental difference per percent IntraMAT (95% CI)	P value	R^2	Incremental difference per percent IntraMAT (95% CI)	P value	R^2
TUG (sec)	0.188 (0.082 to 0.295)*	**<0.001**	0.189*	0.137 (0.023 to 0.250)*	**0.019**	0.219*	0.048 (−0.061 to 0.158)[a]	0.378	0.505*
Grip strength (kg)	−0.225 (−0.400 to −0.051)*	**0.012**	0.112*	−0.193 (−0.385 to −0.001)*	**0.049**	0.123*	−0.145 (−0.328 to 0.039)[b]	0.120	0.288*

*$P < 0.05$ considered significant.
IntraMAT: intramuscular adipose tissue.
[a]Adjusted model including the following covariates: type 2 diabetes, age, BMI, and energy expenditure.
[b]Adjusted model including the following covariates: type 2 diabetes, age, height, and percent lean mass.

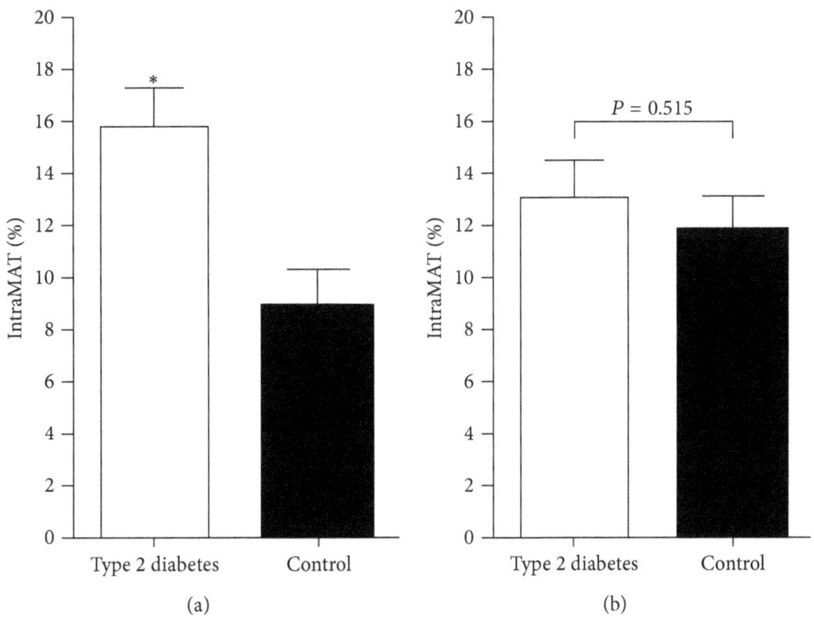

FIGURE 2: Unadjusted (a) and adjusted (b) comparison of percent IntraMAT in women with and without type 2 diabetes. IntraMAT: intramuscular adipose tissue. $^{*}P < 0.05$ considered significant. Percent IntraMAT = [IntraMAT (mm^2) ÷ total muscle area (mm^2)] × 100%. Covariates: age, ethnicity, BMI, waist : hip ratio, and weekly energy expenditure.

such as greater age, ethnicity, BMI, waist : hip ratio, and energy expenditure, which contributed to the difference in IntraMAT between groups. Regarding functional mobility and strength, unadjusted analyses showed that, for each 5% increase in IntraMAT, there was a 1-second increase in TUG result and approximately 1 kg decrease in grip strength. However, following adjustment for potential covariates, a 5% increase in IntraMAT only translated to a 0.20-second increase in TUG result and a 0.70 kg decrease in grip strength, and these associations were not statistically significant. This study also revealed that when considering IntraMAT in disease states, such as type 2 diabetes, covariates should also be considered and that IntraMAT alone is not strongly associated with functional mobility and strength.

This study sought to determine whether percent IntraMAT in the lower leg was different among women with and without type 2 diabetes, as IntraMAT may be one of the mediating factors responsible for the accelerated musculoskeletal aging observed in people with type 2 diabetes [1]. In agreement with other studies [2, 43, 44], we found that our cohort of women with type 2 diabetes had greater TUG test scores indicating poorer functional mobility, lower grip strength, and lower specific force, an indirect measure of muscle quality. Various mechanisms for poor functional mobility and strength in adults with type 2 diabetes have been proposed and include reduced muscle fibre size and number [45] and reduced α-motor neuron innervation [46]; however we hypothesized that IntraMAT might also be a likely mediator. On the microscopic level, intramyocellular lipid inhibits skeletal muscle oxidative phosphorylation ability [36, 47], and inflammatory cytokines secreted by adipose tissue in the skeletal muscle microenvironment [48] may lead to proteolysis and muscle catabolism [49]. Previous studies investigating muscle adiposity in adults with type 2 diabetes have used CT to indirectly assess muscle adiposity [37] or did not separate the depots of adipose tissue within the muscle from adipose tissue between the muscle bellies [12, 15, 17]. One study did elegantly separate the adipose tissue within the muscle bellies and adipose tissue between muscle bellies using MRI and also investigated diabetes-related differences in these compartments [17]. However, the authors reported no difference in the absolute amount of adipose tissue within muscle bellies in women with type 2 diabetes compared to controls [17], whereas we did find that women with type 2 diabetes had more IntraMAT in the lower leg. The discrepancy in results may be due to the fact that the mean age and BMI of participants with type 2 diabetes were lower compared to our study cohort, which may have blunted the difference in IntraMAT between groups, as IntraMAT is related to age and BMI [36]. Given that our image segmentation technique differentiates between the adipose tissue within the muscle bellies (IntraMAT) and that between the muscle bellies (InterMAT), two depots of adipose tissue which may be physiologically distinct, our findings may be used as rationale for further noninvasive studies on whether exercise interventions modify IntraMAT in adults with type 2 diabetes and whether modification results in improved metabolic control of diabetes, functional mobility, and strength. It may be important to consider other variables, such as age, ethnicity, energy expenditure in activities, and anthropometrics, as these variables blunted the association between IntraMAT and type 2 diabetes. However, it should be noted that lower energy expenditure, obesity, and abdominal adiposity are common characteristics of adults with type 2 diabetes.

Similar to other studies using MRI, our unadjusted analysis revealed that IntraMAT is related to functional mobility and strength [14, 18]. After adjusting for diabetes, the relationships were weakened but remained significant suggesting that this relationship is not unique to older adults with type 2 diabetes and rather may be a characteristic of aging. This may be explained in part by the idea that IntraMAT may diminish the activation of skeletal muscle, thus worsening functional mobility and strength [19]. Our study makes an important contribution to the literature because, unlike previous studies that have examined the relationships between muscle adiposity, function, and strength [14, 18], our analyses included potential covariates. In the study by Tuttle and colleagues, 78% of study participants had type 2 diabetes and 69% of the participants with type 2 diabetes had peripheral neuropathy [14], findings that were unaccounted for in the analysis making it difficult to conclude whether the reported relationships between muscle adiposity, function, and strength were driven by diabetes or neuropathy. In addition, the image segmentation techniques that were employed in both studies did not clearly distinguish between adipose tissue within muscle bellies and that between muscle bellies. Our study suggests that if IntraMAT is used as an outcome in future studies, investigators should consider possible confounding factors such as age, BMI, and energy expenditure in activities when assessing TUG as the dependent variable and age, height, and percent lean mass when assessing grip strength as the dependent variable. While IntraMAT alone was not strongly associated with functional mobility and strength in this study, larger studies should investigate whether assessing IntraMAT in conjunction with measures of sarcopenia, such as appendicular lean mass, would help clinicians discriminate those who are at risk of declines in functional mobility and muscular strength and may benefit from pharmacologic or lifestyle intervention. Promising results have been published suggesting that aerobic and eccentric resistance training may reduce the amount of IntraMAT and increase lean mass in the thigh and improve functional outcomes in older adults [50].

There are study limitations to acknowledge. First, participants in this study were recruited for the purposes of a study on skeletal health, and participants with diabetes were recruited from an outpatient clinic. Therefore, exclusion criteria were specific to that study and selection bias may have occurred, limiting the generalizability of our findings. Second, the study was powered to examine trabecular bone hole size in women with and without type 2 diabetes [27]. Future adequately powered studies should be conducted to confirm our results. Third, although the Paffenbarger Physical Activity Questionnaire has been validated [33, 51], we recognize that participants tend to overestimate physical activity levels by questionnaire, and assessment by accelerometer is superior. Fourth, peripheral neuropathy was not assessed for this study, and previous studies have suggested that adults with type 2 diabetes and peripheral neuropathy have more IntraMAT compared to controls [15]. Fifth, while others have validated the use of sliceOmatic software for the quantification of muscle adiposity, we have not yet validated our own method against a gold standard [30, 31]. Finally, due to the cross-sectional nature of our study, we were not able to determine whether IntraMAT causes poor functional mobility or strength. A longitudinal analysis of IntraMAT, functional mobility, and strength changes may help discern the directionality of the relationships.

5. Conclusion

In conclusion, our study makes a unique contribution to research examining IntraMAT, diabetes status, functional mobility, and strength because we employed an image segmentation methodology that differentiated between adipose tissue within the muscle bellies (IntraMAT) and that between the muscle bellies (InterMAT) and accounted for potential confounders in multiple linear regression analyses. While the unadjusted analysis demonstrated that women with type 2 diabetes have more IntraMAT within the muscle bellies, after considering other factors that could influence IntraMAT, women with type 2 diabetes did not have more IntraMAT compared to women without diabetes. In addition, IntraMAT alone is not associated with functional mobility and strength but in combination with other covariates may serve as a noninvasive biomarker of physical frailty in older adults.

Conflict of Interests

Janet M. Pritchard, Sarah Karampatos, Karen A. Beattie, George Ioannidis, Stephanie A. Atkinson, Lehana Thabane, and Zubin Punthakee have nothing to declare. Hertzel Gerstein has received consulting fees from Sanofi, Novo Nordisk, Lilly, Bristol-Myers-Squibb, Roche, AstraZeneca, GlaxoSmithKline, and Bayer, lecture fees from Sanofi-Aventis and Bayer, and support for research or continuing education through his institution from Sanofi-Aventis, Lilly, Merck, Novo Nordisk, Boehringer Ingelheim, Bristol-Myers-Squibb, and AstraZeneca. Lora M. Giangregorio has received a research grant from Merck Canada. Jonathan D. Adachi consults for and has received lecture fees from Amgen, Eli Lilly, Merck, Novartis, and Warner Chilcott. Alexandra Papaioannou has received grants and research support from Amgen, Eli Lilly, Merck Canada Inc., Novartis, and Warner Chilcott and consults for Amgen, Eli Lilly, Merck Canada Inc., Novartis, and Warner Chilcott.

Authors' Contribution

Janet M. Pritchard, Lora M. Giangregorio, Stephanie A. Atkinson, Karen A. Beattie, Hertzel Gerstein, Zubin Punthakee, Jonathan D. Adachi, and Alexandra Papaioannou were involved in the study conception, design, and interpretation of results. Janet M. Pritchard conducted study visits, collected data, and drafted the paper. Sarah Karampatos completed image analysis. Janet Pritchard, George Ioannidis, and Lehana Thabane conducted statistical analyses and interpreted results. All authors edited, read, and approved the final paper.

Acknowledgments

The authors would like to acknowledge study participants for volunteering their time and staff at the Hamilton Health Sciences Well-Health Centre and McMaster University Medical Centre Diabetes Outpatient Clinic for supporting the study and assisting with recruitment. The authors would also like to thank Dr. Dean Inglis for developing the MRI imaging protocol and Yves Martel (Tomovision), Amanda Lorbergs, Mike Davison, and Sami Shaker for providing valuable feedback on the segmentation protocol. Funding was generously provided by the Lloyd Carr Harris Foundation and the Hamilton Health Sciences Foundation.

References

[1] R. E. Hubbard, M. K. Andrew, N. Fallah, and K. Rockwood, "Comparison of the prognostic importance of diagnosed diabetes, co-morbidity and frailty in older people," *Diabetic Medicine*, vol. 27, no. 5, pp. 603–606, 2010.

[2] S. W. Park, B. H. Goodpaster, E. S. Strotmeyer et al., "Accelerated loss of skeletal muscle strength in older adults with type 2 diabetes: the health, aging, and body composition study," *Diabetes Care*, vol. 30, no. 6, pp. 1507–1512, 2007.

[3] P. Vestergaard, L. Rejnmark, and L. Mosekilde, "Diabetes and its complications and their relationship with risk of fractures in type 1 and 2 diabetes," *Calcified Tissue International*, vol. 84, no. 1, pp. 45–55, 2009.

[4] N. E. Gulcelik, M. Bayraktar, O. Caglar, M. Alpaslan, and J. Karakaya, "Mortality after hip fracture in diabetic patients," *Experimental and Clinical Endocrinology & Diabetes*, vol. 119, no. 7, pp. 414–418, 2011.

[5] M. Visser, A. B. Newman, M. C. Nevitt et al., "Reexamining the sarcopenia hypothesis. Muscle mass versus muscle strength," *Annals of the New York Academy of Sciences*, vol. 904, pp. 456–461, 2000.

[6] B. H. Goodpaster, D. E. Kelley, F. L. Thaete, J. He, and R. Ross, "Skeletal muscle attenuation determined by computed tomography is associated with skeletal muscle lipid content," *Journal of Applied Physiology*, vol. 89, no. 1, pp. 104–110, 2000.

[7] B. H. Goodpaster, C. L. Carlson, M. Visser et al., "Attenuation of skeletal muscle and strength in the elderly: the health ABC study," *Journal of Applied Physiology*, vol. 90, no. 6, pp. 2157–2165, 2001.

[8] T. Lang, J. A. Cauley, F. Tylavsky, D. Bauer, S. Cummings, and T. B. Harris, "Computed tomographic measurements of thigh muscle cross-sectional area and attenuation coefficient predict hip fracture: the Health, Aging, and Body Composition Study," *Journal of Bone and Mineral Research*, vol. 25, no. 3, pp. 513–519, 2010.

[9] R. Vettor, G. Milan, C. Franzin et al., "The origin of intermuscular adipose tissue and its pathophysiological implications," *American Journal of Physiology—Endocrinology and Metabolism*, vol. 297, no. 5, pp. E987–E998, 2009.

[10] J. C. Seidell, C. J. G. Bakker, and K. van der Kooy, "Imaging techniques for measuring adipose-tissue distribution—a comparison between computed tomography and 1.5-T magnetic resonance," *The American Journal of Clinical Nutrition*, vol. 51, no. 6, pp. 953–957, 1990.

[11] D. Gallagher, S. Heshka, D. E. Kelley et al., "Changes in adipose tissue depots and metabolic markers following 1-year diet and exercise intervention in overweight and obese patients with type 2 diabetes," *Diabetes Care*, vol. 37, no. 12, pp. 3325–3332, 2014.

[12] D. Gallagher, D. E. Kelley, J.-E. Yim et al., "Adipose tissue distribution is different in type 2 diabetes," *The American Journal of Clinical Nutrition*, vol. 89, no. 3, pp. 807–814, 2009.

[13] L. J. Tuttle, D. R. Sinacore, W. T. Cade, and M. J. Mueller, "Lower physical activity is associated with higher intermuscular adipose tissue in people with type 2 diabetes and peripheral neuropathy," *Physical Therapy*, vol. 91, no. 6, pp. 923–930, 2011.

[14] L. J. Tuttle, D. R. Sinacore, and M. J. Mueller, "Intermuscular adipose tissue is muscle specific and associated with poor functional performance," *Journal of Aging Research*, vol. 2012, Article ID 172957, 7 pages, 2012.

[15] T. N. Hilton, L. J. Tuttle, K. L. Bohnert, M. J. Mueller, and D. R. Sinacore, "Excessive adipose tissue infiltration in skeletal muscle in individuals with obesity, diabetes mellitus, and peripheral neuropathy: association with performance and function," *Physical Therapy*, vol. 88, no. 11, pp. 1336–1344, 2008.

[16] K. A. Beattie, N. J. MacIntyre, K. Ramadan, D. Inglis, and M. R. Maly, "Longitudinal changes in intermuscular fat volume and quadriceps muscle volume in the thighs of women with knee osteoarthritis," *Arthritis Care & Research*, vol. 64, no. 1, pp. 22–29, 2012.

[17] D. C. Karampinos, T. Baum, L. Nardo et al., "Characterization of the regional distribution of skeletal muscle adipose tissue in type 2 diabetes using chemical shift-based water/fat separation," *Journal of Magnetic Resonance Imaging*, vol. 35, no. 4, pp. 899–907, 2012.

[18] R. L. Marcus, O. Addison, L. E. Dibble, K. B. Foreman, G. Morrell, and P. Lastayo, "Intramuscular adipose tissue, sarcopenia, and mobility function in older individuals," *Journal of Aging Research*, vol. 2012, Article ID 629637, 6 pages, 2012.

[19] Y. Yoshida, R. L. Marcus, and P. C. Lastayo, "Intramuscular adipose tissue and central activation in older adults," *Muscle & Nerve*, vol. 46, no. 5, pp. 813–816, 2012.

[20] A. S. Gorgey and G. A. Dudley, "Skeletal muscle atrophy and increased intramuscular fat after incomplete spinal cord injury," *Spinal Cord*, vol. 45, no. 4, pp. 304–309, 2007.

[21] D. Podsiadlo and S. Richardson, "The timed 'Up & Go': a test of basic functional mobility for frail elderly persons," *Journal of the American Geriatrics Society*, vol. 39, no. 2, pp. 142–148, 1991.

[22] S. Giampaoli, L. Ferrucci, F. Cecchi et al., "Hand-grip strength predicts incident disability in non-disabled older men," *Age and Ageing*, vol. 28, no. 3, pp. 283–288, 1999.

[23] R. W. Bohannon, "Hand-grip dynamometry predicts future outcomes in aging adults," *Journal of Geriatric Physical Therapy*, vol. 31, no. 1, pp. 3–10, 2008.

[24] C. H. Y. Ling, D. Taekema, A. J. M. de Craen, J. Gussekloo, R. G. J. Westendorp, and A. B. Maier, "Handgrip strength and mortality in the oldest old population: the Leiden 85-plus study," *Canadian Medical Association Journal*, vol. 182, no. 5, pp. 429–435, 2010.

[25] G. M. Savva, O. A. Donoghue, F. Horgan, C. O'Regan, H. Cronin, and R. A. Kenny, "Using timed up-and-go to identify frail members of the older population," *The Journals of Gerontology Series A—Biological Sciences and Medical Sciences*, vol. 68, no. 4, pp. 441–446, 2013.

[26] B. R. Greene, E. P. Doheny, A. O'Halloran, and R. Anne Kenny, "Frailty status can be accurately assessed using inertial sensors and the TUG test," *Age and Ageing*, vol. 43, no. 3, pp. 406–411, 2014.

[27] J. M. Pritchard, L. M. Giangregorio, S. A. Atkinson et al., "Association of larger holes in the trabecular bone at the distal radius in postmenopausal women with type 2 diabetes mellitus compared to controls," *Arthritis Care & Research*, vol. 64, no. 1, pp. 83–91, 2012.

[28] A. S. Levey, J. Coresh, E. Balk et al., "National Kidney Foundation practice guidelines for chronic kidney disease: evaluation, classification, and stratification," *Annals of Internal Medicine*, vol. 139, no. 2, pp. 137–147, 2003.

[29] D. G. Bonett, "Sample size requirements for estimating intraclass correlations with desired precision," *Statistics in Medicine*, vol. 21, no. 9, pp. 1331–1335, 2002.

[30] N. Mitsiopoulos, R. N. Baumgartner, S. B. Heymsfield, W. Lyons, D. Gallagher, and R. Ross, "Cadaver validation of skeletal muscle measurement by magnetic resonance imaging and computerized tomography," *Journal of Applied Physiology*, vol. 85, no. 1, pp. 115–122, 1998.

[31] O. Demontiero, W. Li, E. Thembani, and G. Duque, "Validation of noninvasive quantification of bone marrow fat volume with microCT in aging rats," *Experimental Gerontology*, vol. 46, no. 6, pp. 435–440, 2011.

[32] R. S. Paffenbarger Jr., A. L. Wing, and R. T. Hyde, "Physical activity as an index of heart attack risk in college alumni," *The American Journal of Epidemiology*, vol. 108, no. 3, pp. 161–175, 1978.

[33] S. Mahabir, D. J. Baer, C. Giffen et al., "Comparison of energy expenditure estimates from 4 physical activity questionnaires with doubly labeled water estimates in postmenopausal women," *The American Journal of Clinical Nutrition*, vol. 84, no. 1, pp. 230–236, 2006.

[34] J. M. Pritchard, T. Seechurn, and S. A. Atkinson, "A food frequency questionnaire for the assessment of calcium, vitamin D and vitamin K: a pilot validation study," *Nutrients*, vol. 2, no. 8, pp. 805–819, 2010.

[35] H. J. Martin, V. Yule, H. E. Syddall, E. M. Dennison, C. Cooper, and A. A. Sayer, "Is hand-held dynamometry useful for the measurement of quadriceps strength in older people? A comparison with the gold standard biodex dynamometry," *Gerontology*, vol. 52, no. 3, pp. 154–159, 2006.

[36] M. Boettcher, J. Machann, N. Stefan et al., "Intermuscular adipose tissue (IMAT): association with other adipose tissue compartments and insulin sensitivity," *Journal of Magnetic Resonance Imaging*, vol. 29, no. 6, pp. 1340–1345, 2009.

[37] I. Miljkovic-Gacic, C. L. Gordon, B. H. Goodpaster et al., "Adipose tissue infiltration in skeletal muscle: age patterns and association with diabetes among men of African ancestry," *The American Journal of Clinical Nutrition*, vol. 87, no. 6, pp. 1590–1595, 2008.

[38] G. Mazzali, V. Di Francesco, E. Zoico et al., "Interrelations between fat distribution, muscle lipid content, adipocytokines, and insulin resistance: effect of moderate weight loss in older women," *The American Journal of Clinical Nutrition*, vol. 84, no. 5, pp. 1193–1199, 2006.

[39] H. A. Bischoff, H. B. Stähelin, A. U. Monsch et al., "Identifying a cut-off point for normal mobility: a comparison of the timed 'up and go' test in community-dwelling and institutionalised elderly women," *Age and Ageing*, vol. 32, no. 3, pp. 315–320, 2003.

[40] C. E. Garber, M. L. Greaney, D. Riebe, C. R. Nigg, P. A. Burbank, and P. G. Clark, "Physical and mental health-related correlates of physical function in community dwelling older adults: a cross sectional study," *BMC Geriatrics*, vol. 10, article 6, 2010.

[41] C. R. Gale, C. N. Martyn, C. Cooper, and A. A. Sayer, "Grip strength, body composition, and mortality," *International Journal of Epidemiology*, vol. 36, no. 1, pp. 228–235, 2007.

[42] G. R. Norman and D. L. Streiner, "Advanced topics in regression and ANOVA," in *Biostatistics: The Bare Essentials*, D. A. Farmer, Ed., pp. 167–176, BC Decker, Hamilton, Canada, 3rd edition, 2008.

[43] P. P. de Oliveira, S. M. Fachin, J. Tozatti, M. C. Ferreira, and L. P. F. Marinheiro, "Comparative analysis of risk for falls in patients with and without type 2 diabetes mellitus," *Revista da Associação Médica Brasileira*, vol. 58, no. 2, pp. 234–239, 2012.

[44] M. Leenders, L. B. Verdijk, L. van der Hoeven et al., "Patients with type 2 diabetes show a greater decline in muscle mass, muscle strength, and functional capacity with aging," *Journal of the American Medical Directors Association*, vol. 14, no. 8, pp. 585–592, 2013.

[45] M. Cesari, M. Pahor, F. Lauretani et al., "Skeletal muscle and mortality results from the InCHIANTI study," *The Journals of Gerontology Series A: Biological Sciences and Medical Sciences*, vol. 64, no. 3, pp. 377–384, 2009.

[46] A. B. Newman, V. Kupelian, M. Visser et al., "Sarcopenia: alternative definitions and associations with lower extremity function," *Journal of the American Geriatrics Society*, vol. 51, no. 11, pp. 1602–1609, 2003.

[47] M. E. Patti, A. J. Butte, S. Crunkhorn et al., "Coordinated reduction of genes of oxidative metabolism in humans with insulin resistance and diabetes: potential role of PGC1 and NRF1," *Proceedings of the National Academy of Sciences of the United States of America*, vol. 100, no. 14, pp. 8466–8471, 2003.

[48] E. Zoico, A. Rossi, V. Di Francesco et al., "Adipose tissue infiltration in skeletal muscle of healthy elderly men: relationships with body composition, insulin resistance, and inflammation at the systemic and tissue level," *The Journals of Gerontology Series A: Biological Sciences and Medical Sciences*, vol. 65, no. 3, pp. 295–299, 2010.

[49] C. Ebisui, T. Tsujinaka, T. Morimoto et al., "Interleukin-6 induces proteolysis by activating intracellular proteases (cathepsins B and L, proteasome) in C2C12 myotubes," *Clinical Science*, vol. 89, no. 4, pp. 431–439, 1995.

[50] R. L. Marcus, S. Smith, G. Morrell et al., "Comparison of combined aerobic and high-force eccentric resistance exercise with aerobic exercise only for people with type 2 diabetes mellitus," *Physical Therapy*, vol. 88, no. 11, pp. 1345–1354, 2008.

[51] B. E. Ainsworth, A. S. Leon, M. T. Richardson, D. R. Jacobs, and R. S. Paffenbarger Jr., "Accuracy of the college alumnus physical activity questionnaire," *Journal of Clinical Epidemiology*, vol. 46, no. 12, pp. 1403–1411, 1993.

8

Relationships between Social Resources and Healthful Behaviors across the Age Spectrum

Kristina H. Lewis,[1] Matthew W. Gillman,[1] Mary L. Greaney,[2] Elaine Puleo,[3] Gary G. Bennett,[4] and Karen M. Emmons[2]

[1] *Obesity Prevention Program, Department of Population Medicine, Harvard Medical School, Harvard Pilgrim Health Care Institute, Boston, MA 02215, USA*
[2] *Department of Medical Oncology/Population Sciences, Dana-Farber Cancer Institute, Boston, MA, USA*
[3] *Division of Biostatistics, Department of Public Health, University of Massachusetts, Amherst, MA 01003, USA*
[4] *Department of Psychology and Neuroscience, Duke Global Health Institute, Duke University, Durham, NC 27708, USA*

Correspondence should be addressed to Kristina H. Lewis, kristina.h.lewis@gmail.com

Academic Editor: Thomas M. Hess

Background. We examined cross-sectional relationships of social resources with health behaviors in adults ages 18–93 years. *Methods.* Baseline data from a 2009 risk behavior intervention trial were used to measure social resources, physical activity, and fruit and vegetable intake in 2,440 adults. To evaluate associations overall and within 4 age groups (18–34, 35–49, 50–64, and 65–93 y), we used multivariable regression. *Results.* Mean (SD) age was 49.4 (15) years, physical activity was 346 (304) minutes/week, and fruit and vegetable intake was 3.4 (2.4) servings/day. Mean social resource score was 1.2 (0–4 scale) in 18–34 year olds, 1.1 in all other age groups ($P = 0.04$). In multivariable models, for each one-point increment in social resource score, the odds ratio for getting 150–959 minutes of physical activity/wk (compared to <150 min/wk) was 3.7 (95% CI 3.0–4.6). Each one-point increment in score was also associated with 29% (95% CI: 23–35%) more servings of fruit and vegetables. We did not observe effect modification by age group. *Conclusions.* Although younger adults reported slightly higher resources than older adults, the magnitude of association between social resources and healthful behaviors did not differ between them.

1. Introduction

Chronic illness causes much of the morbidity, mortality, and rising cost of medical care in the United States [1, 2]. Healthful behaviors, such as having a diet rich in fruits and vegetables and getting regular physical activity, can prevent or delay the onset and progression of chronic disease [3]. Higher fruit and vegetable intake is associated with decreased mortality from cardiovascular disease [4], prevention or delay of neurodegenerative disease [5], and improved cognitive function [6]. Physical activity decreases the risk of cardiovascular disease, cancer, and obesity [7] and is associated with decreased rates of incident dementia [8] and hip fracture [9, 10], as well as improved quality of life [11].

A substantial literature emphasizes the importance of the social and environmental determinants of healthful behaviors and health outcomes [12–20]. For instance, weight gain in a person's social network is associated with his or her own risk of obesity, through changes in behavioral norms and unconscious behavior imitation [21]. The frequency with which the elderly participate in social events correlates with their rate of motor decline [22]. Components of the neighborhood environment, such as walkability, access to parkland, and safety also influence personal health behaviors [12]. Even the work environment has an influence on health behaviors and outcomes, and employers are struggling to make their workers less sedentary through onsite wellness programs and other initiatives [23–25].

As adults age, their social and physical environments undergo a transformation. An exit from the working world, gradual physical and cognitive decline, and the loss of friends and loved ones may all contribute to smaller social and geographic circles [26, 27]. Further, the loss of structure and routines that accompanies retirement and household downsizing may reduce opportunities for social influence and personal commitment to healthy habits. Along with reducing access to social resources, a gradual decrease in financial flexibility or physical and mental well being could also reduce the ability of older adults to capitalize on such resources through decreased mobility or decreased ability to perform one's activities of daily living. For example, even if an 80-year-old woman receives advice on healthy recipes or sees an advertisement for a new fitness club in her neighborhood (both forms of social resources available to her), she might be less able to benefit from these resources than her 35-year-old healthy neighbor, because she does not do her own grocery shopping and she no longer drives a car.

In the aging literature, there is a growing emphasis on the idea of "aging in place" or allowing people to remain in their home environments for as long as they wish and are safely able to do so [28]. For aging in place to produce the best possible health outcomes and contribute to longevity, a clear understanding of the relationship between social resources and health behaviors across the age spectrum is necessary. It is possible that the shrinking geographic environment, changing nature of relationships, and physiologic transitions associated with aging may both decrease the availability of social resources and lessen the impact of resources such as active neighbors, a seniors group at the local health club, or family members who visit to share recipes for healthy dishes.

The United States population is growing older [2], meaning that the burden of chronic illness will continue to rise. To address this problem, program developers and policy makers will benefit from understanding how social resources affect physical activity and dietary choices at different life stages.

In this study of adults from across the age spectrum, we examined the relationship between social resources (from neighbors, friends, family, and local organizations) and the health behaviors of fruit and vegetable intake and physical activity. We hypothesized that social resources in older adults would be fewer than in younger adults and would have less correlation with physical activity and fruit and vegetable intake.

2. Methods

2.1. Study Design and Participants. Study participants were enrollees in "Healthy Directions 2," a randomized trial of a multiple risk behavior intervention. We recruited participants at their annual well visit or chronic disease management appointment during 2009 in one of 2 urban primary care centers in the Boston area. Eligibility requirements included being 18 years or older and having the ability to read and write in English. Patients were excluded if they had received cancer therapy within the past year or carried a diagnosis of dementia or other neurodegenerative disorder or major psychiatric condition within the past 5 years.

Participants were approached first with a mailing, then enrolled in person at a medical appointment. At that visit, enrollees completed a self-administered baseline questionnaire detailing their health habits, perceived level of social support for healthful behavior and demographics. We obtained participant age, sex, and primary care provider (PCP) identity from electronic medical records. Of all approached to participate in the trial, 52% ($n = 2,440$) enrolled and completed the baseline survey. For our analyses, 123 participants were excluded due to incomplete data on the social resources measure, 185 for missing physical activity data, and 208 for missing fruit and vegetable intake data.

2.2. Main Measures. Our primary exposure measure was the level of social resources reported by participants in the baseline survey, as assessed by 3 subscales from the "Chronic Illness Resources Survey" (CIRS). The original CIRS was a 22-item instrument used to evaluate support for chronic illnesses and healthful behaviors. This instrument was designed to be adapted and modified for other populations or research questions [29]. The CIRS includes a number of support resources that reflect a range of processes by which social support may influence behavior, including engaging together in a specific behavior and providing support or actions that facilitate a behavior. The purpose of using the CIRS in this context was to determine the extent to which social resources are effective promoters for the target behaviors. Our survey for this study included the family and friends, neighborhood, and organizational subscales from the original CIRS, for a total of 9 items, each measured on a 5-point scale (ranging from 0, not at all to 4, very often). The specific items we used are provided verbatim in Table 1 of this paper.

We summed the points associated with each participant's responses and averaged by their number of completed items, to yield a total CIRS score of 0–4 points. We excluded participants who answered fewer than 7 of the 9 items ($n = 123$). Because socioeconomic position may be intricately linked to social resources, we did assess this as well (described below under other measures).

There were two outcome measures in this study—weekly minutes of moderate and vigorous physical activity and daily servings of fruit and vegetables. We assessed physical activity using four questions adapted from CDC's Behavioral Risk Factor Surveillance Survey (BRFSS) [30], which included descriptions of moderate (e.g., brisk walking, biking, or anything that causes small increases in breathing or heart rate) and vigorous (e.g., running, aerobics, or anything else that causes large increases in breathing or heart rate) activities. We summed reported moderate and vigorous physical activity into a total number of weekly minutes and assigned each participant to one of 3 categories, less than 150, 150–959, or 960 or more minutes per week. We set the lower cutoff at 150 minutes because that is the minimum weekly amount of moderate and vigorous physical activity recommended by the CDC [31]. We chose 960 minutes per week (corresponding to just over 2 hours per day) as the upper cutoff, as suggested in the literature [32], and because we felt this group of respondents were extreme in their level of reported physical activity.

We assessed fruit and vegetable intake using the National Cancer Institute's "5 A Day for Better Health" tool, a 7-item

Table 1: Items from the CIRS used in our baseline survey* [29].

CIRS subscale identity	Items used
Family and friends	"Family members or friends exercised with you"
	"You shared healthy low-fat recipes with friends or family members"
	"Family or friends bought foods or prepared foods for you that were especially healthy or recommended"
Neighborhood	"You walked or exercised outdoors in your neighborhood"
	"You ate at a restaurant that offered a variety of tasty, low-fat food choices"
	"You walked or did other exercise activities with neighbors"
Organizational	"You attended free or low-cost meetings (e.g., walking groups/clubs, Weight Watchers, church groups, to support healthy habits")
	"You volunteered your time for local organizations or causes"
	"You attended wellness programs or fitness facilities (e.g., the YMCA, Reggie Lewis Center, Gold's Gym, or Total Fitness)"

*Items were preceded with the following prompt: "For each question, please mark the response that best indicates your experience over the past 6 months." Participants could then choose to mark one of the following options: "Not at all," "A little," "A moderate amount," "Quite a bit," or "Very often."

instrument assessing frequency of intake for orange juice, other fruit juices, fruit, green salad, French fried potatoes, other kinds of potatoes, and other vegetables [33]. Using the responses to 6 of the 7 items (we excluded French fried potatoes), we calculated a total number of daily servings of fruits and vegetables for each participant.

2.3. Other Measures. Covariates from the medical record included sex and age, with age at enrollment categorized into the following groups: 18–34, 35–49, 50–64, or 65 years or older. We used survey data to obtain information on race/ethnicity (white, black, Hispanic, Asian, or other) and education (did not graduate from high school, high school graduate/GED, some college or 2-year degree, or 4-year college degree or more). We assessed financial situation by having participants rate the money situation in their household ("comfortable with extras," "enough but no extras," "have to cut back," or "cannot make ends meet"), which, as opposed to household income, minimized missing data and is relevant for use in retirement-age participants. Participants also reported current weight and height from which we calculated body mass index (BMI) using the formula weight (kg) divided by the square of height (m). Self-reported health status was determined using the one-item assessment from the Medical Outcomes Study Short-Form [34]. We also included a covariate corresponding to the PCP ID for each participant.

2.4. Statistical Analysis. We first examined the bivariate associations between age group and physical activity and fruit and vegetable intake. We also examined how CIRS score (and subscales) varied by age. We then used regression models to evaluate the relationship between CIRS score and the two outcomes. We modeled the relationship between CIRS and physical activity using multinomial logistic regression among the 2,155 participants with data on these 2 variables and the CIRS and fruit and vegetable intake relationship using negative binomial regression among the 2,134 participants with data on these 2 variables. Rather than reporting the negative binomial regression estimate as the log odds of changing fruit and vegetable intake, we calculated the antilog of the parameter estimate to show the predicted change in the ratio of fruit and vegetable intake per one point increment in CIRS score. We created multivariable models adjusted for sex, age group, race/ethnicity, education, financial status, BMI category, self-reported health status, and primary care provider. To assess whether age group had a modifying effect on the relationship between social support and healthful behaviors, we included interaction terms for "age group × CIRS score" in each of our final models. We conducted all analyses using SAS, V.9.2. (Cary, North Carolina).

3. Results

3.1. Population Characteristics. The majority of participants (65.7%) were women, with a mean (SD) age of all participants at baseline of 49.4 (15) years, ranging from 18 to 93 (Table 2). Just over half (54.7%) of participants were white. Sixty percent had a college degree, and about 46% rated their financial status as comfortable. Mean (SD) BMI was 28.1 (6.2) kg/m^2, and participants were about evenly split between the normal, overweight, and obese BMI ranges. Slightly over one-half (56%) rated their health as very good or excellent.

The mean CIRS score was 1.09 (SD 0.64, range 0–4). The youngest participants (age 18–35) reported slightly higher levels of social resources (mean 1.17) than those in the older age groups (mean 1.06) (one-way ANOVA $P = 0.04$) (Figure 1). Among the 3 CIRS subscales, only the level of family and friends support differed by age: the score was 1.32 in the youngest age group, 1.21 among 35–49 year olds, 1.26 among 50–64 year olds, and 1.10 among the 65–93 year olds (one-way ANOVA $P = .0005$).

Mean SD reported moderate and vigorous physical activity was 346 (304) minutes per week (Table 2). Reported PA levels did not differ substantially across age groups (Figure 2), with those 65 years and older actually reporting a mean of 353 minutes weekly and a one-way ANOVA test showing no significant variability across age groups (p 0.07). Participants reported a mean (SD) intake of 3.4 (2.5) servings of fruits and vegetables per day, with increasing mean number of servings by age group, such that the oldest adults reported 0.8 more servings per day (3.8) than the youngest (3.0) (one-way ANOVA $P < 0.0001$) (Figure 3).

3.2. Relationships between Social Resources and Healthful Behaviors. The crude multinomial logistic regression model

TABLE 2: Characteristics of participants (n = 2,440).

Characteristic (N respondents)	N (%)
Sex (2,440)	
Female	1603 (65.7%)
Age (years) (2,440)	
18–34	494 (20.2%)
35–49	679 (27.8%)
50–64	921 (37.8%)
≥65	345 (14.1%)
Race/Ethnicity (2,350)	
White	1307 (54.7%)
Black	667 (27.9%)
Hispanic	215 (9%)
Asian	107 (4.5%)
Other	54 (2.2%)
Education (2,403)	
Less than high school	89 (3.7%)
High school graduate/GED	296 (12.3%)
Some college or 2-year degree	577 (24%)
≥4-year college degree	1441 (60%)
Money situation in household (2,367)	
"Comfortable with extras"	1083 (45.8%)
"Enough but no extras"	683 (28.9%)
"Have to cut back"	476 (20.1%)
"Cannot make ends meet"	125 (5.3%)
BMI (kg/m^2) (2,327)	
Normal (18.5–24.9)	771 (33.1%)
Overweight (25–29.9)	785 (33.7%)
Obese (≥30)	771 (33.1%)
Health status (2,440)	
Very good/excellent	1282 (52.5%)
Good	860 (35.2%)
Fair/poor	298 (12.2%)
Moderate and vigorous physical activity category (2255)	
<150 min/wk	735 (32.6%)
150–959 min/wk	1289 (57.2%)
≥960 min/wk	231 (10.2%)
Fruit and vegetable intake (servings/day) (2232)	Mean (SD)
	3.4 (2.5)
CIRS scores (0–4 scale) (2317)	
Overall	1.09 (0.64)
Family and friends	1.19 (0.91)
Neighborhood	1.36 (0.83)
Organizational	0.74 (0.78)

of the relationship between CIRS score and physical activity showed that each one-point increment in CIRS score was associated with greater odds of reporting higher physical

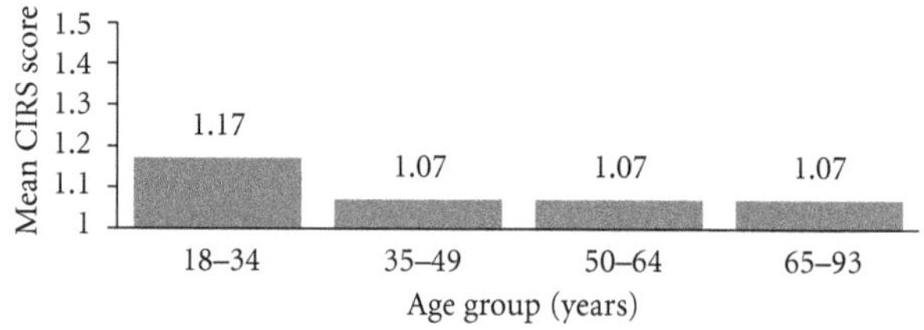

FIGURE 1: Mean score on 9 items of the CIRS (0–4 point scale) according to age group. one-way ANOVA P value across age groups = 0.04.

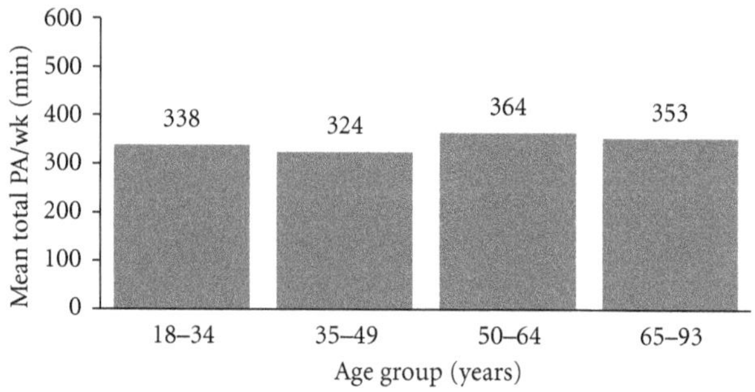

FIGURE 2: Self-reported mean moderate and vigorous physical activity, according to age group. One-way ANOVA P value across age groups = 0.07.

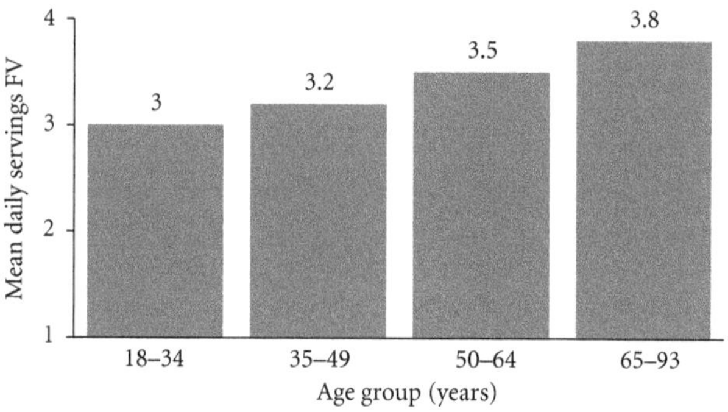

FIGURE 3: Self-reported mean fruit and vegetable intake, according to age group. one-way ANOVA P-value across age groups < 0.0001.

activity levels (relative to reporting <150 minutes/wk) (Table 3). Specifically, the OR (95% CI) for reporting 150–959 minutes of moderate and vigorous physical activity per week was 4.1 (3.4–4.9), and it was 4.4 (3.4–5.8) for reporting ≥960 min/wk. The results of multivariable models were similar to those in the crude models. The fully adjusted multinomial regression model for the CIRS physical activity relationship also showed increasing odds of higher physical activity for each one-point increment in CIRS score (3.7 (3.0–4.6) for 150–959 min/wk and 4.7 (3.5–6.3) for ≥960 min/wk, compared to <150 min/wk) (Table 3).

The crude negative binomial regression model of the CIRS fruit and vegetable relationship showed that each one-point increment in CIRS score was associated with 34% (95%CI 28–40%) more daily fruit and vegetable intake

TABLE 3: Associations of score on 9 items of the CIRS (0–4 scale) with self-reported moderate and vigorous physical activity and self-reported fruit and vegetable intake.

Moderate and vigorous physical activity category (min/wk)	*N*	Crude	Adjusted
		OR (95% CI) for one-point increment in CIRS score*	
<150	707	1.0 (Ref)	1.0 (Ref)
150–959	1233	4.1 (3.4, 4.9)	3.7 (3.0, 4.6)
≥960	215	4.4 (3.4, 5.8)	4.7 (3.5, 6.3)
Fruit and vegetable intake count data		Expected ratio of increase in FVI count (servings/day) (95% CI) per one-point increment in CIRS score**	
	2134	1.34 (1.28, 1.40)	1.29 (1.23, 1.35)

*Multinomial logistic model adjusted for sex, age, health, education, financial situation, race/ethnicity, primary care provider, and BMI.
**Negative binomial model adjusted for sex, age, health, education, financial situation, race/ethnicity, primary care provider, and BMI.

(Table 3). When this model was adjusted for our covariates, we found little change in the outcome, with the adjusted percent increase in fruit and vegetable servings at 29% (95% CI 23–35%) for each one-point increment in CIRS score (Table 3).

In order to test for effect modification by age, interaction terms for "age group × CIRS score" were introduced into the models. In the case of the physical activity outcome, the interaction terms were nonsignificant, with *P* 0.8 for 150–969 min/wk and *P* 0.9 for ≥960 min/week. For fruits and vegetables, the interaction terms were in ascending order of age group: 0.18, 0.95, 0.97 (>65 year olds as comparison group). This was also indicative of a lack of effect modification of the resource-behavior relationship by age group.

4. Discussion

In this large study with participants representing a wide age range and considerable racial/ethnic diversity, we found that greater social resources correlated with higher levels of physical activity and higher fruit and vegetable intake in adults of all age groups. Levels of social resources were slightly higher among younger participants, mainly due to greater support from friends and family, but, contrary to our hypothesis, older age did not appear to lessen the impact of social resources on behavior.

Although few data exist on how to interpret the CIRS score, our mean score of 1.09 was lower than the mean CIRS score of 2.7 previously reported in work by Glasgow et al. among a group of older women with diabetes [29]. Their score of 2.7, however, was based on the complete 22-item CIRS instrument, and in that study the average scores for the 3 subscales used here were also lower than for other CIRS subscales measured (family and friends 2.37, neighborhood 2.14, organizational 1.71) [29]. Even accounting for that difference, our subscale scores seemed low, a surprising finding given that a large percentage of our group was highly educated and financially comfortable [35].

The slightly higher CIRS scores in younger participants within this study were due to higher levels of resources from family and friends, which may reflect that older adults in our sample have fewer social contacts or that these family members and friends were simply less likely to encourage things like physical activity and fruit and vegetable consumption in older persons. Although statistically significant, the clinical impact of these different levels of social resources is unclear, given that adults 65 and older were just as likely as young adults to be physically active and more likely to meet recommended levels of fruit and vegetable intake.

The participants in our study reported high levels of physical activity, but, when viewed categorically (less than 150 min/wk versus more than 150 min/wk), these numbers may be on par with national samples relying on self-reported information. The 2007 nationwide BRFSS, for example, estimated that 60.4% of women and 68.9% of men met recommendations for "regular physical activity" [36]. In our sample, 67% of respondents reported at least 150 minutes per week, with many reporting substantially higher levels. Unlike the BRFSS nationwide sample, we did not find that weekly physical activity decreased with age [36]. When viewed as a continuous variable, our participants reported a mean of 346 minutes of total (moderate + vigorous) physical activity per week. The "Walk Kansas" study by Estabrooks et al. relied on the same items we used to assess physical activity, and within their most active group at baseline, the mean total (moderate + vigorous) physical activity reported was 308 minutes/week, not substantially different from our overall mean [30]. To guard against bias from potential overreporting, we analyzed physical activity as a categorical rather than continuous variable.

Study participants reported eating an average of 3.4 servings of fruits and vegetables daily, less than the recommended 5 servings, but consistent with previous research on adult patterns of fruit and vegetable intake in the US [37–39]. Older adults in our study reported higher levels of fruit and vegetable intake than younger adults. This finding could be due to unmeasured factors such as older adults eating more meals cooked at home [40] or to other diet-related lifestyle choices that may differ between age groups.

The direct relationship we observed between the social resource score and physical activity was consistent with our expectations. Previous work by Glasgow has shown a high degree of correlation between CIRS scores and physical activity levels [29]. The strength of this relationship could have a lot to do with how social resources are being measured in the instrument. For example, a 2009 systematic review concluded that subjective evaluations of social resources had greater correlation with physical activity than objective measures [27]. Other instruments using subjective measures of social resources have also shown strong links to physical activity behavior. For example, a 2003 cross-sectional study of Australian adults found that higher levels of subjective social resources from friends and family and membership in organizations that promote physical activity did correlate with higher levels of walking [41].

The direct relationship between social resources and fruit and vegetable intake has also been explored in the literature among different populations [18, 42–44]. Relating to our study, Glasgow and colleagues studied the link between CIRS scores and dietary behaviors and found that there was a high degree of correlation between the two and that changes in CIRS score predicted changes in behaviors in the setting of a longitudinal study [29]. The findings in our cross-sectional study support those noted by Glasgow et al. but our population is novel in that it includes people from across the age spectrum, showing that influences at the family and friends, neighborhood, and organizational levels directly correlate with increased fruit and vegetable intake behavior in adults of all ages.

We questioned whether the relationship between social resources and health behaviors would be different between older and younger adults and found that these relationships did not vary by age. Our hypothesis was based on the idea that older adults may be less able to capitalize on available resources than younger adults, due to physical, financial, and other limitations. Although other papers have examined the social support-behavior relationship exclusively in older adults [16] or compared its effects across racial/ethnic groups [17], this particular research question has not been previously explored in any paper of which we are aware. The lack of effect modification we observed suggests that, regardless of age, improved social resources from family and friends, neighborhood, and local organizations correlate equally with more healthful behavior. This could be because social resources act through different, but equally effective, mechanisms in the different age groups. For example, it could be that older adults are more likely to take advice and support from their offspring, whereas younger adults are more likely to achieve behavior change due to pressures from friends and colleagues. Furthermore, the relationship between social resources and behavior is complex and likely modified by factors that were unmeasured in our study, such as features of the built environment and self-efficacy [16]. However, our findings could also be due to a relatively small number of the "oldest old" within our sample. Although we did enroll participants as old as 93 years, those of advanced age were relatively few (only about 5% of those 65 and up were 85 years or older).

5. Limitations

Our study was cross-sectional, limiting causal inference. As is typical of large population level studies, most measures were based on self-report, which can lead to misclassification of exposure or outcome. As we would not expect the misclassification in this case to be differential, our estimates of effect are probably either closer to the null or associated with larger standard errors, both conservative biases. Residual confounding is possible in any observational study, but the relative lack of attenuation from crude to multivariable models argues against it as a major threat to validity. With regard to physical activity, we assessed only moderate and vigorous activity. Though we asked participants to include brisk walking in their estimates of physical activity, we did not analyze it separately, which could have added to the strength of our measure. Additionally, although we had an overall measure of health status, we did not specifically assess functional mobility of the participants or have an exact measure of ability to perform ADLs. Finally, our analyses did not examine for possible three-way interactions between things like race/ethnicity or gender, with age and social resources. This could potentially have masked underlying differences between races or between men and women with respect to the aging-social resources-health behaviors continuum.

Although our cohort is diverse in terms of race/ethnicity and age, the participants were also generally financially comfortable and well educated, which may limit the generalizability of our findings.

6. Conclusions

As the US population ages, the burden of chronic illness will undoubtedly increase. Although cross-sectional, our findings support the hypothesis that higher levels of social resources at the family, neighborhood, and organizational levels are associated with higher physical activity and fruit and vegetable intake in older as well as younger adults. Longitudinal studies and interventions are necessary to understand how programs and policies to bolster social resources can result in improved health-related behaviors and outcomes. Supporting such social resources may promote longevity and independence and decrease the need for costly medical services.

Conflict of Interests

The authors of this paper have no conflicts of interest to disclose.

Acknowledgments

The authors thank Harvard Vanguard Medical Associates for the opportunity to conduct their research in their clinical sites. This work was funded by NIH grants *R01 CA123228 and K05 CA124415*(Emmons, PI) and *K24 HL068041* (Gillman, PI), with support for Dr. Lewis's time from HRSA training grant *T32HP12706-02-01*. An abstract of the study was presented orally at the 2011 New England SGIM in Boston, MA. Poster presentations of the work took place at the 2011 Society of Behavioral Medicine Meeting in Washington DC and at the 2011 SGIM National Meeting in Phoenix AZ.

References

[1] D. E. Arterburn, P. K. Crane, and S. D. Sullivan, "The coming epidemic of obesity in elderly Americans," *Journal of the American Geriatrics Society*, vol. 52, no. 11, pp. 1907–1912, 2004.

[2] G. Anderson and J. Horvath, "The growing burden of chronic disease in America," *Public Health Reports*, vol. 119, no. 3, pp. 263–270, 2004.

[3] R. J. Ozminkowski, R. Z. Goetzel, F. Wang et al., "The savings gained from participation in health promotion programs for medicare beneficiaries," *Journal of Occupational and Environmental Medicine*, vol. 48, no. 11, pp. 1125–1132, 2006.

[4] F. J. He, C. A. Nowson, M. Lucas, and G. A. MacGregor, "Increased consumption of fruit and vegetables is related to a reduced risk of coronary heart disease: meta-analysis of cohort studies," *Journal of Human Hypertension*, vol. 21, no. 9, pp. 717–728, 2007.

[5] J. Joseph, G. Cole, E. Head, and D. Ingram, "Nutrition, brain aging, and neurodegeneration," *Journal of Neuroscience*, vol. 29, no. 41, pp. 12795–12801, 2009.

[6] M. C. Polidori, D. Praticó, F. Mangialasche et al., "Hiigh fruit and vegetable intake is positively correlated with antioxidant status and cognitive performance in healthy subjects," *Journal of Alzheimer's Disease*, vol. 17, no. 4, pp. 921–927, 2009.

[7] Centers for Disease Control and Prevention, "Physical Activity for Everyone: Physical Activity for Health," 2011, http://www.cdc.gov/physicalactivity/everyone/health/index.html.

[8] E. B. Larson, L. Wang, J. D. Bowen et al., "Exercise is associated with reduced risk for incident dementia among persons 65 years of age and older," *Annals of Internal Medicine*, vol. 144, no. 2, pp. 73–81, 2006.

[9] D. Feskanich, W. Willett, and G. Colditz, "Walking and leisure-time activity and risk of hip fracture in postmenopausal women," *Journal of the American Medical Association*, vol. 288, no. 18, pp. 2300–2306, 2002.

[10] E. W. Gregg, M. A. Pereira, and C. J. Caspersen, "Physical activity, falls, and fractures among older adults: a review of the epidemiologic evidence," *Journal of the American Geriatrics Society*, vol. 48, no. 8, pp. 883–893, 2000.

[11] A. Drewnowski and W. J. Evans, "Nutrition, physical activity, and quality of life in older adults: summary," *Journals of Gerontology Series A*, vol. 56, no. 2, pp. 89–94, 2001.

[12] W. Wendel-Vos, M. Droomers, S. Kremers, J. Brug, and F. Van Lenthe, "Potential environmental determinants of physical activity in adults: a systematic review," *Obesity Reviews*, vol. 8, no. 5, pp. 425–440, 2007.

[13] R. C. Brownson, E. A. Baker, R. A. Housemann, L. K. Brennan, and S. J. Bacak, "Environmental and policy determinants of physical activity in the United States," *American Journal of Public Health*, vol. 91, no. 12, pp. 1995–2003, 2001.

[14] B. M. Popkin, "What can public health nutritionists do to curb the epidemic of nutrition-related noncommunicable disease?" *Nutrition Reviews*, vol. 67, no. 1, supplement, pp. S79–S82, 2009.

[15] E. B. Kahn, L. T. Ramsey, R. C. Brownson et al., "The effectiveness of interventions to increase physical activity. A systematic review," *American Journal of Preventive Medicine*, vol. 22, no. 4, supplement, pp. 73–107, 2002.

[16] J.A. Carlson, J. F. Sallis, T. L. Conway et al., "Interactions between psychosocial and built environment factors in explaining older adults' physical activity," *Preventive Medicine*, vol. 54, no. 1, pp. 68–73, 2012.

[17] A. A. Eyler, R. C. Brownson, R. J. Donatelle, A. C. King, D. Brown, and J. F. Sallis, "Physical activity social support and middle- and older-aged minority women: results from a US survey," *Social Science and Medicine*, vol. 49, no. 6, pp. 781–789, 1999.

[18] A. R. Shaikh, A. L. Yaroch, L. Nebeling, M. C. Yeh, and K. Resnicow, "Psychosocial predictors of fruit and vegetable consumption in adults. A review of the literature," *American Journal of Preventive Medicine*, vol. 34, no. 6, pp. 535–543, 2008.

[19] S. Croezen, H. S. J. Picavet, A. Haveman-Nies, W. M. Verschuren, L. C. De Groot, and P. Van'T Veer, "Do positive or negative experiences of social support relate to current and future health? Results from the Doetinchem Cohort Study," *BMC Public Health*, vol. 12, no. 1, article 65, 2012.

[20] A. M. White, G. S. Philogene, L. Fine, and S. Sinha, "Social support and self-reported health status of older adults in the United States," *American Journal of Public Health*, vol. 99, no. 10, pp. 1872–1878, 2009.

[21] N. A. Christakis and J. H. Fowler, "The spread of obesity in a large social network over 32 years," *New England Journal of Medicine*, vol. 357, no. 4, pp. 370–379, 2007.

[22] A. S. Buchman, P. A. Boyle, R. S. Wilson, D. A. Fleischman, S. Leurgans, and D. A. Bennett, "Association between late-life social activity and motor decline in older adults," *Archives of Internal Medicine*, vol. 169, no. 12, pp. 1139–1146, 2009.

[23] H. K. Koh and K. G. Sebelius, "Promoting prevention through the affordable care act," *New England Journal of Medicine*, vol. 363, no. 14, pp. 1296–1299, 2010.

[24] L. M. Anderson, T. A. Quinn, K. Glanz et al., "The effectiveness of worksite nutrition and physical activity interventions for controlling employee overweight and obesity. A systematic review," *American Journal of Preventive Medicine*, vol. 37, no. 4, pp. 340–357, 2009.

[25] S. L. Tamers, S. A. A. Beresford, A. D. Cheadle, Y. Zheng, S. K. Bishop, and B. Thompson, "The association between worksite social support, diet, physical activity and body mass index," *Preventive Medicine*, vol. 53, no. 1-2, pp. 53–56, 2011.

[26] P. Clarke and E. R. Nieuwenhuijsen, "Environments for healthy ageing: a critical review," *Maturitas*, vol. 64, no. 1, pp. 14–19, 2009.

[27] I. H. Yen, Y. L. Michael, and L. Perdue, "Neighborhood environment in studies of health of older adults: a systematic review," *American Journal of Preventive Medicine*, vol. 37, no. 5, pp. 455–463, 2009.

[28] I. H. Yen, J. K. Shim, A. D. Martinez, and J. C. Barker, "Older people and social connectedness: how place and activities keep

people engaged," *Journal of Aging Research*, vol. 2012, Article ID 139523, 10 pages, 2012.

[29] R. E. Glasgow, D. J. Toobert, M. Barrera, and L. A. Strycker, "The chronic illness resources survey: cross-validation and sensitivity to intervention," *Health Education Research*, vol. 20, no. 4, pp. 402–409, 2005.

[30] P. A. Estabrooks, M. Bradshaw, D. A. Dzewaltowski, and R. L. Smith-Ray, "Determining the impact of walk Kansas: applying a team-building approach to community physical activity promotion," *Annals of Behavioral Medicine*, vol. 36, no. 1, pp. 1–12, 2008.

[31] Centers for Disease Control and Prevention, "Physical Activity for Everyone: How much physical activity do older adults need?" 2010, http://www.cdc.gov/physicalactivity/everyone/guidelines/olderadults.html.

[32] IPAQ Research Committee, "Guidelines for Data Processing and Analysis of the International Physical Activity Questionnaire (IPAQ)—Short and Long Forms," 2005, http://www.ipaq.ki.se/scoring.pdf.

[33] M. Serdula, R. Coates, T. Byers et al., "Evaluation of a brief telephone questionnaire to estimate fruit and vegetable consumption in diverse study populations," *Epidemiology*, vol. 4, no. 5, pp. 455–463, 1993.

[34] J. E. Ware Jr. and C. D. Sherbourne, "The MOS 36-item short-form health survey (SF-36)—I. Conceptual framework and item selection," *Medical Care*, vol. 30, no. 6, pp. 473–483, 1992.

[35] S. Weyers, N. Dragano, M. Richter, and H. Bosma, "How does socio economic position link to health behaviour? Sociological pathways and perspectives for health promotion," *Global Health Promotion*, vol. 17, no. 2, pp. 25–33, 2010.

[36] S. A. Carlson, J. E. Fulton, D. A. Galuska, J. Kruger, F. Lobelo, and F. V. Loustalot, "Prevalence of self-reported physically active adults—United States, 2007," *Morbidity and Mortality Weekly Report*, vol. 57, no. 48, pp. 1297–1300, 2008.

[37] J. Kruger, M. M. Yore, M. Solera, and R. Moeti, "Prevalence of fruit and vegetable consumption and physical activity by race/ethnicity - United States, 2005," *Morbidity and Mortality Weekly Report*, vol. 56, no. 13, pp. 301–304, 2007.

[38] J. Kimmons, C. Gillespie, J. Seymour, M. Serdula, and H. M. Blanck, "Fruit and vegetable intake among adolescents and adults in the United States: percentage meeting individualized recommendations," *MedGenMed Medscape General Medicine*, vol. 11, no. 1, article 26, 2009.

[39] S. L. Tamers, T. Agurs-Collins, K. W. Dodd, and L. Nebeling, "US and France adult fruit and vegetable consumption patterns: an international comparison," *European Journal of Clinical Nutrition*, vol. 63, no. 1, pp. 11–17, 2009.

[40] USDA Agricultural Research Service, "Away from home: Percentages of Selected Nutrients Contributed by Foods Eaten Away from Home by Gender and Age, What We Eat in America," NHANES 2007, 2008, and 2010, http://www.ars.usda.gov/ba/bhnrc/fsrg.

[41] B. Giles-Corti and R. J. Donovan, "Relative influences of individual, social environmental, and physical environmental correlates of walking," *American Journal of Public Health*, vol. 93, no. 9, pp. 1583–1589, 2003.

[42] J. E. Boyington, B. Schoster, K. Remmes Martin, J. Shreffler, and L. F. Callahan, "Perceptions of individual and community environmental influences on fruit and vegetable intake, North Carolina, 2004," *Preventing Chronic Disease*, vol. 6, no. 1, article A04, 2009.

[43] M. Baruth, S. Wilcox, and M. D. Condrasky, "Perceived environmental church support is associated with dietary practices among African-American adults," *Journal of the American Dietetic Association*, vol. 111, no. 6, pp. 889–893, 2011.

[44] G. J. Cutler, A. Flood, P. Hannan, and D. Neumark-Sztainer, "Multiple sociodemographic and socioenvironmental characteristics are correlated with major patterns of dietary intake in adolescents," *Journal of the American Dietetic Association*, vol. 111, no. 2, pp. 230–240, 2011.

9

Aging, Neuromuscular Decline, and the Change in Physiological and Behavioral Complexity of Upper-Limb Movement Dynamics

S. Morrison[1] and K. M. Newell[2]

[1] *School of Physical Therapy, Old Dominion University, Norfolk, VA 23529, USA*
[2] *Department of Kinesiology, Pennsylvania State University, State College, PA 16801, USA*

Correspondence should be addressed to S. Morrison, smorriso@odu.edu

Academic Editor: Wojtek Chodzko-Zajko

Aging is characterized by a general decline in physiological and behavioral function that has been widely interpreted within the context of the loss of complexity hypothesis. In this paper, we examine the relation between aging, neuromuscular function and physiological-behavioral complexity in the arm-hand effector system, specifically with reference to physiological tremor and isometric force production. Experimental findings reveal that the adaptive behavioral consequences of the aging-related functional decline in neurophysiological processes are less pronounced in simple motor tasks which provides support for the proposition that the motor output is influenced by both extrinsic (e.g., task related) and intrinsic (e.g., coordination, weakness) factors. Moreover, the aging-related change in complexity can be bidirectional (increase or decrease) according to the influence of task constraints on the adaptation required of the intrinsic properties of the effector system.

1. Introduction

A hallmark feature of aging and the onset of disease is a general decline in physiological function and behavioral capacity [1]. This decline can be manifested in different levels and functions of the biological system, including skeletal muscle [2–4], cardiovascular processes [5, 6], central nervous system activity [7–9], and respiratory function [10], leading to detriments in the behavioral capacity of activities of daily living, including increased tremor, loss of balance control, and a decline in walking ability [5, 6, 11–13]. Understanding the potential reason(s) for decline in function is a challenging undertaking, however, as there are numerous variables that can, either singularly or in combination, affect physiological function in the aging adult. For example, factors related to (but not limited to) biological, behavioral, socioeconomic, nutritional, and/or lifestyle/career choices can all impact on the general process of aging and have implications for physiological function [14–16].

The broad range of variables which can negatively affect function in the older adult makes a comprehensive understanding of the direct effect of aging very difficult. In the last decade, the functional deficits in aging have been investigated in the context of changes in the complexity and variability of the output of physiological system(s) [6, 12, 17, 18]. Specifically, the effects of aging are viewed to result in a deficit in physiological function that arises from a progressive "loss of complexity" of the physiological system. This deficit is postulated to arise from a decrease in the functioning number of components or elements of a given system and/or a decrease in the interaction/coupling between components [6, 12, 19].

There is not a single definition of a complex system but there is considerable agreement on the properties of complex systems that include (a) many degrees of freedom and interconnections between them and (b) the exhibition of spontaneous self-organization that is adaptive, nonlinear, and dynamic in that it evolves in time, and where order evolves and dissolves without a controller [6, 12, 17, 20]. This theoretical backdrop has led to the experimental emphasis on the time- and frequency-domain structure of variability as opposed to the traditional approach of only considering the dispersion properties of variables through the assumptions about central tendency properties of distributions. Central to this approach has been the use of nonlinear measures of physiological and behavioral time series [20–22]. These tools have revealed changes in complexity with healthy aging and/or age-related diseases like essential tremor, type 2 diabetes, and Parkinson's disease [23–29].

2. Measuring Physiological Complexity

Given the inherent complexity of many physiological outputs, there has been a concerted effort to develop appropriate nonlinear tools that can quantify the specific signal of interest [30, 31]. To this end, a variety of measures have been developed and utilized to assess the dynamic properties of specific physiological signals. While a complete review of the differing assessment tools is beyond the scope of this paper, there are certain tools that have been commonly used to assess time series related to physiological processes (a more comprehensive review of the various measures, their use and limitations, is provided by Stergiou and Decker [31, 32] and Bravi et al. [30]). A few of the analyses used include time-frequency analysis, wavelet analysis, recurrence plots, poincare plots, measures of signal entropy (e.g., approximate entropy (ApEn), sample entropy (SampEn), and multiscale entropy (MSE)), correlation dimension, detrended fluctuation analysis (DFA), and Lyapunov exponent [9, 32–43].

Each analytic technique has been designed to assess different aspects of the signal and, in many cases, produces a single outcome measure of the attractor dynamics [18, 30]. One advantage of using such measures to assess complexity is that they are typically dimensionless to the scale of systems and define conditions for dynamic similarities [44]. This allows for the comparison of signal complexity arising from different physiological systems and processes. However, the reliance on any one measure can potentially give a misleading representation of physiological complexity [19]. Therefore, it is recommended that the measurement of physiological complexity be based on multiple measures of system dynamics to increase the sensitivity of complexity assessment under both healthy and pathological conditions [18, 19, 30]. Despite the range of selected measures that can be used to capture the dynamics of a given signal and their limitations, as is highlighted in Figure 1, it is clear that changes in the dynamics of signals are more readily distinguished using nonlinear measures of pattern complexity than the standard dispersion measures (SD, CV) of a variable.

While there is growing evidence to support the view that aging can be characterized by a general loss of physiological and behavioral complexity, there are findings that challenge the universal nature of the direction of change in complexity with aging. The focus of this paper is to evaluate recent experimental findings as to the effect aging has on neuromuscular function and its relation to changes in physiological and behavioral complexity. While examples for the effects of aging on complexity will be provided for a number of different movement forms, the emphasis is on the neuromuscular function of the arm-hand effector complex given that, for any individual, an optimal degree of hand control is required to perform everyday fine motor skills involving precision, grasping, and/or manipulating small objects [45]. One factor that can negatively impact general hand function is the degree of tremulous oscillations observed during fine motor tasks involving a degree of precision or force control. While these tremors are usually of small amplitude in young adults so that they rarely impact on hand control, these oscillations tend to increase with aging and can severely influence the performance of fine motor skills in older persons [46–50]. Here, we provide an overview of the major aging-related changes in physiological tremor and isometric force production.

3. Functional and Structural Adaptations in Skeletal Muscle with Aging

It is widely held that aging is associated with a general decline in skeletal muscle function [3, 4, 51, 52]. One consequence of this decline is that older people lose the capacity to generate task-relevant and/or precise levels of muscle force in the context of action. This decline has been attributed to a loss of overall muscle function [4, 53] and has been associated with changes in a number of mechanisms involving those intrinsic to the muscle and through its neural interface. The specific muscle changes found in the elderly include increases in average muscle force [54, 55], increased motor unit (MU) firing rate variability [56], modulation of MU firing rate [57, 58], altered synchrony between MU recruitment and MU firing rate [51], and reduced sensitivity [59]. Structural changes in the muscle properties associated with aging include a loss (atrophy) of fast twitch motor units and/or switch to slow twitch units (referred to as MU remodeling), altered MU size, and/or a decline in the number of alpha motor neurons within the spinal cord [3, 51, 52, 56, 57, 60]. Consequences of these changes include an overall decrease in muscle cross-sectional area, a reduction in muscle mass, and a decline in strength [4, 16, 61, 62].

Generally, the term sarcopenia has been used to describe the loss of muscle mass and low muscle function (strength or performance) associated with aging [63–65]. However, given the diverse range of age-related changes that occur in muscle, which can span basic structural changes to functional changes impacting on the overall "muscle quality," it has been proposed that the term dynapenia be used to denote those alterations in contractile properties and/or neuromuscular function while sarcopenia be used to describe any age-related loss of muscle mass [15, 16, 66]. It has been proposed that such a distinction would provide a framework for independently assessing those age-related factors which affect muscle mass separately from those variables which impact on neuromuscular function [15].

The consequences of these age-related changes in function and mass are that the capacity of skeletal muscle to produce force is compromised in the older adult [4, 62, 67]. Indeed, the muscle responses of older adults are often characterized by prolonged contraction time, an increase

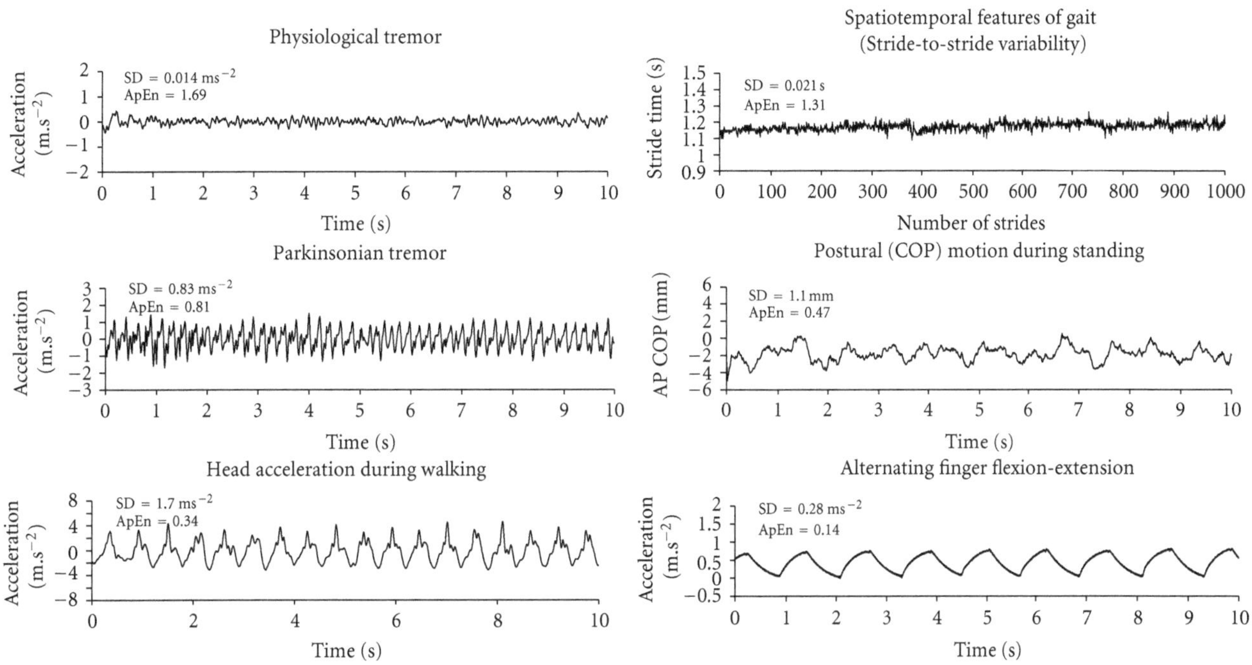

FIGURE 1: Examples of various physiological signals related to tremor, postural motion, and gait. For each example, an index of the variation in regards to amplitude (SD) and for changes in the variation over the time course of the signal (using approximate entropy (ApEn) analysis) is shown. As this figure illustrates, the more semirhythmical and repeatable signals (e.g., head acceleration, finger motion) were characterized by lower ApEn values, which implies increased regularity (decreased complexity) of the movement signal. Furthermore, the signals that appear more noiselike and irregular (e.g., physiological tremor, stride-to-stride variability) have higher ApEn values implying greater complexity. In contrast, a standard measure of variation (SD) provides little distinction between signals, illustrating that such assessments of variability, by themselves, may be less useful in determining the inherent variability across different movement signals.

in the level of muscle activity for a given level of force production, a decrease in the steadiness at which force can be produced, and a decline in overall muscle force producing capacity [4, 53, 57, 62, 68, 69]. It is clear that there are many types of change that can occur with the normal aging process and that ultimately affect muscle function.

While aging has been associated with a number of changes at the muscle level, the impact that these changes have on overall movement performance is less well understood. Here we will focus on the relation between aging, neuromuscular function, and physiological-behavioral complexity in the arm-hand effector unit. Aging is associated with a general decline in hand function [46, 47, 70] and there have been numerous investigations of the effect of aging on physiological tremor [49, 50, 71, 72] and isometric force production [47, 57, 69]. This paper will address these changes in physiological tremor and isometric force control within the context of the loss of complexity hypothesis [6, 12, 19], which holds that the process of healthy aging is reflected by a loss of complexity of the respective physiological system. This hypothesis is, in part, derived from the broader construct of dynamical disease [73, 74] and a dynamical systems approach to aging [75, 76], in which physiological systems change due to aberrations in the temporal organization of the evolving dynamics.

4. Physiological Tremor with Aging

Physiological tremor is an intrinsic feature of the neuromuscular system reflecting the combined output of multiple oscillatory sources, including the mechanical resonant properties of the specific limb segment, cardiac mechanics, peripheral neural mechanisms (that include contributions from stretch reflexes), and central neural processes [45, 77]. As highlighted in Figure 2, the neural component of a typical tremor signal has most power between 8–12 Hz and represents input from the basal ganglia, inferior olive, deep cerebellar nuclei, thalamus, and, at the spinal cord, alpha motor neurons [45, 78]. One motor symptom linked with aging is an increase in the amplitude of the 8–12 Hz component of physiological tremor, a behavioral consequence that can have negative implications for the ability of an individual to perform everyday fine motor skills. This increase in tremor amplitude is believed to primarily derive from altered central neural output and reflects the more general decline in the functional capacity of the aging neuromuscular system [24, 48–50, 71, 72, 79].

Given that physiological tremor is, in part, derived from neuromuscular mechanisms, it is important to isolate the basis of any age-related changes and how they fit within the more general context of our understanding of muscle adaptations with aging. In particular, it is important to

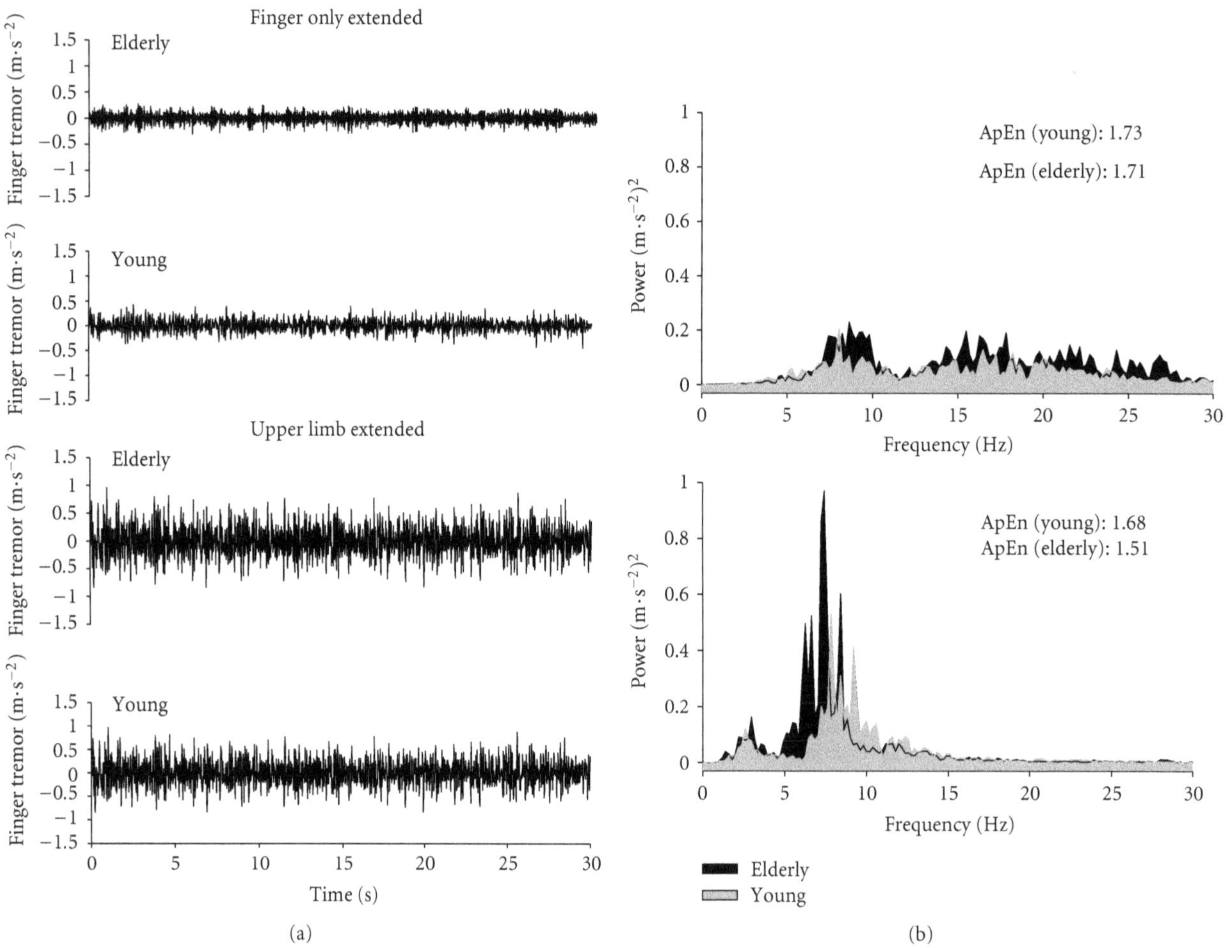

FIGURE 2: Representative postural acceleration (tremor) traces and power spectral profiles from the index finger of a healthy young and an elderly subject. Traces for each person are shown for conditions where (a) only the finger was extended (the rest of the upper limb was externally supported) and (b) when the entire upper arm was unsupported. Tremor traces were obtained from a single trial for the index finger of each individual. Measures of the degree of regularity (ApEn) of each tremor signal are also shown for each condition. For this analysis, higher values reflect greater complexity within the tremor time series. This example highlights that the age-related differences in finger tremor were only present under conditions where the entire arm was held against gravity.

determine whether the increases in tremor amplitude are due to a specific decline in aspects of neuromuscular function associated with aging or to a diminished ability of the older neuromuscular system to adapt to more challenging and/or physically demanding task demands. Furthermore, while a long standing view is that tremor tends to increase with aging [49, 71, 72], this position has not been universally supported by contemporary experimental research [48, 50]. For example, several studies have observed no age-related increase in tremor amplitude and only subtle changes in the frequency of the 8–12 Hz neural tremor peak [41, 50, 80]. The significance of these findings cannot be understated, because if the established changes in muscle physiology with aging do not translate to increases in physiological tremor, then the reasons for this dissociation remain to be fully elucidated. One suggestion as to why these studies have not reported aging-related increase in physiological tremor is that the changes may only be detectable in the oldest-old members of the population (e.g., for persons aged 80 years or older [41]). An alternative reason for the lack of aging-related change in tremor amplitude may be due to the conditions or tasks under which physiological tremor is assessed [81].

In the majority of studies of age-tremor effects, the common practice has been to limit the assessment of these oscillations to the tremor within a single (usually the finger) segment [41, 50, 79, 82]. In this situation, the more proximal segments are supported externally and do not contribute to the oscillations seen distally. This experimental approach has been employed in an effort to tease out and isolate the specific age-related adaptations in muscle physiology since the action is restricted to a single segment, joint, and/or muscle group. However, while this approach allows a more direct evaluation of the responses of an individual muscle, it has been argued that this protocol is somewhat artificial, since there are few (if any) instances during everyday tasks where persons are required to perform a functional, goal-directed action involving a single muscle and/or segment. Conversely, under more real world conditions where individuals need to maintain the postural position of the entire limb, tremor is rarely localized to a single segment. Consequently, while single joint movements provide insight as to the intrinsic function of a specific, isolated muscle, it remains an open question as to what these findings reveal about the challenges the aging neuromuscular system faces when performing everyday actions involving multiple limb segments.

An alternative experimental approach has been to examine postural tremor when the entire upper arm is unsupported. This protocol provides a more realistic evaluation of the tremor responses apparent in the performance of everyday actions and insight into differences due to aging or disease [24, 83–86]. Tasks of this nature are inherently more challenging as there is now a more substantive strength requirement (e.g., to sustain limb position against gravity) and the need to adaptively compensate for the tremor in multiple segments so they do not all sequentially magnify the oscillations at the more distal segments [72, 87]. Given that these tasks place increased demands for control on the neuromotor system, it has been suggested that examining tremor from different segments when the entire arm is unsupported may prove to be useful in discerning between neurologically healthy and clinical populations [83, 84, 86].

Indeed, when this approach has been adopted, very clear and notable differences in tremor are found as a function of normal aging [24, 72], Parkinson's disease [27, 85, 86, 88, 89], and multiple sclerosis [83]. The typical pattern of results for this type of approach, as shown in Figures 2 and 3, is that older persons tend to exhibit greater hand and finger tremor coupled with increased muscle activity in the forearm extensors when required to hold the entire arm against gravity, compared to the EMG/tremor responses when only the finger is extended (the other segments were supported externally). For the healthy elderly individuals, where tremor increases were reported, these were limited to the more distal segments only (e.g., the hand and finger), with no notable changes in the tremor from the forearm or upper arm [24, 72]. Further, the age-related increases appear to be exacerbated when the older person performs the task in a standing position compared to sitting [24], which supports the view that relatively simple postural adjustments can also influence tremor dynamics [87]. In both situations, however, the tremor increase is primarily restricted to the neural 8–12 Hz component and related muscle activity, indicating that changes in the output of those central neural processes underlying tremor genesis were responsible for the aging-related differences.

These contrasting findings on single versus multiple segment tremor invite the question as to the relative difficulty of movements performed about a single joint/segment. For comparison, the amplitude of physiological tremor observed from the finger under single segment conditions has been reported to be within the range of 1–3 mm [90], whereas, for tasks requiring individuals to hold their entire arm up against gravity, oscillations of the order of 10–20 mm have been reported for the index finger [24, 72]. If one considers the task goal during these actions was to minimize limb postural motion (tremor), there is a higher degree of difficulty in controlling the muscles about an entire limb to minimize oscillations (and hence the greatest potential for actually being able to reduce tremor) under conditions where the entire arm must be coordinated and controlled, and not just the oscillations in a single distal segment. However, optimal performance for task of this nature is not simply the result of increasing muscle activity. Previous research has demonstrated that when subjects actively cocontracted the muscles of the arm to stiffen the arm, the degree of tremor at the finger increased significantly [91]. Consequently, individuals need to find a balance between required levels of muscle activity to hold the limb against gravity while also be able to achieve a necessary degree of control to ensure limb oscillations are kept to a minimum. It is likely that a combination of a loss of muscle function and control (dynapenia) and muscle strength (sacropenia) in older adults contributes significantly to their increased tremor responses.

The age-related adaptive changes in the tremor tasks show that the aging neuromuscular system is less able to adapt to the constraints of performing more challenging and/or physically demanding everyday tasks. Under these situations, the capacity of the older person is stressed more and so the effects of the changes at the individual muscle level are aggregated in some way that is reflected by an increase in physiological tremor. In comparison to single-joint tremor actions, older participants find multiple segment tremor tasks more demanding and so the increased tremor reflects the greater demands of holding the entire limb unsupported. Furthermore, the selective changes in EMG activity and the 8–12 Hz neural component of tremor for this type of action support the position that increased neuromuscular drive generated in response to the more challenging task conditions is a contributing factor to revealing the aging-related increases in oscillatory outputs [51, 58].

5. Aging Changes in Physiological Complexity of Tremor

In addition to the challenges about the theoretical relevance of examining tremor in single joint versus multiple joint postural tasks, there is still, as noted previously, ambiguity as to whether tremor variability actually increases with the process of aging. In an effort to provide greater insight as to the effects of aging and/or disease on physiological and behavioral processes, there has been an evaluation of the spatial/temporal pattern of the given tremor signal using measures of complexity [6, 12, 17].

This experimental approach to aging is based on the proposition that there is a deficit in physiological function that results from a progressive loss of complexity (i.e., dynamic variability) of the physiological system. This deficit has been phrased "loss of complexity" and is postulated to arise from the general decrease in the number of elements of a given system and/or decrease in the interaction/coupling between control processes [6, 12, 19]. Given the complex nature of the oscillatory output that is physiological tremor, it is natural that the theoretical perspective of complexity has been drawn on to examine the questions of the dynamics of aging and disease with associated measures that are beyond

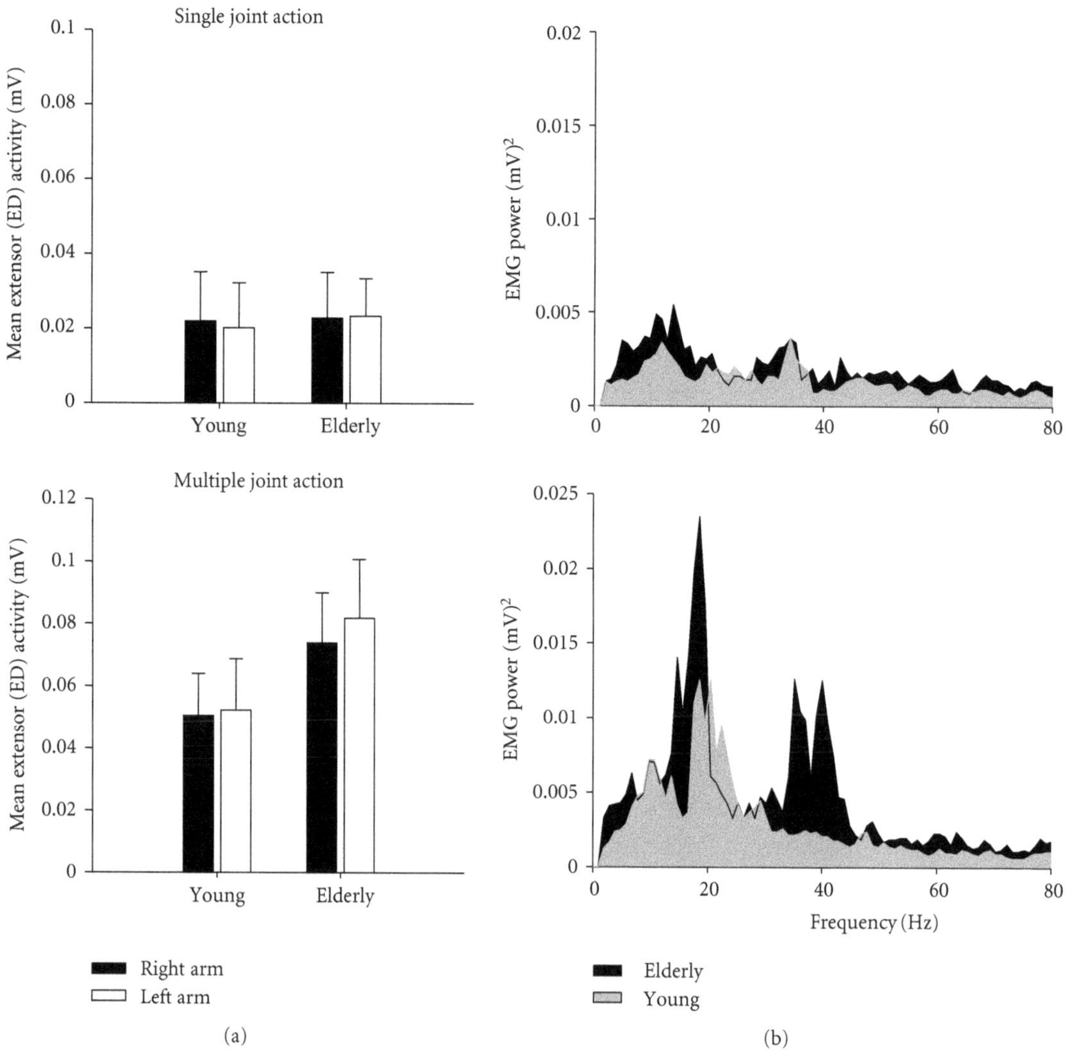

FIGURE 3: Overall changes in mean RMS EMG activity from the extensor muscles of the forearm and examples of the power spectral profiles for a healthy young and elderly individual. Traces for each person are shown for conditions where only the finger was extended (the rest of the upper limb was externally supported) and when the entire upper arm was unsupported. As with Figure 2, any age-related differences in muscle activity were only seen under physically demanding task conditions.

the standard dispersion indices of variability (e.g., standard deviation).

Central to this approach has been the use of dynamical nonlinear measures of a physiological and behavioral time series [20–22]. These tools have revealed changes in complexity with healthy aging and/or age-related diseases including essential tremor and Parkinson's disease [23–27, 85]. One of the more commonly used measures has been approximate entropy (ApEn), which has also been employed to assess complexity changes for a variety of physiological related signals including hormone secretion, isometric force outputs, muscle activity, heart rate, postural motion, and gait [37–40, 92, 93]. ApEn measures the probability that runs of patterns that are close for m observations remain close on the next $(m + 1)$ incremental comparisons. This analysis produces a single value (range of 0–2) with higher values reflecting greater irregularity while lower values represent a greater repeatability or higher regularity in the time series. For example, using approximate entropy (ApEn) measures, Sturman and associates [41] reported that there was an increase in the time-dependent structure of physiological tremor with advanced age, despite there being no differences in tremor amplitude between the respective age groups. Other studies have reported similar age-related differences in physiological tremor using the same analyses [24, 72, 81]. Interestingly, Hong et al. [81] conducted a study to examine whether there were any age-related differences for tremor in the frontal and transverse planes of motion. While no aging-related effects were observed for tremor in the vertical direction, changes in the tremor ApEn values for motion in the mediolateral axis between the young and older adults were reported.

Together, these results support the view that aging and disease can be reflected by a change in the time-dependent pattern or structure of the specific tremor signal output. This result, combined with the lack of any age differences in signal regularity during the finger only conditions (see Figure 2), is consistent with the proposition that the neuromuscular system of older individuals is typically not challenged enough under the single segment condition to necessarily reveal any appreciable change in the system dynamics. The added strength and coordination demands placed on the older individual of having to hold their upper arm against gravity and minimize tremor support the general premise of the loss of complexity hypothesis.

While it has been proposed that the general aging process is accompanied by a decrease in physiological complexity [6, 12], it is important to note that, with regard to physiological tremor, the results of previous studies do not universally support this perspective since there appears to be no consistent difference in the structure of tremor signal under single segment conditions. The fact that several studies have either reported no change or a decline in physiological complexity for tremor signal dynamics in older people lends support to the proposition that the hypothesis of a unidirectional nature of the loss of complexity hypotheses is too narrow [18]. A contrasting perspective is that there can be an increase or decrease in a given signal's pattern over time depending on the interaction between components of the biological system and the inherent task dynamics [18].

There is empirical evidence to support the position that the aging-related changes in signal complexity can be bi-directional. In a recent study [85], it was reported that the physiological tremor of older persons with Parkinson's disease (PD) exhibited a loss of complexity compared to the healthy individuals of a similar age. However, the whole body motion (COP) of these same PD individuals was characterized by an *increase* in signal complexity when compared to the healthy elderly. This reciprocal pattern of change in these oscillatory signals within the same subjects supports the bi-directional perspective on changes in complexity with aging. Similarly, Hong et al. [81] reported that the only significant aging-related change in finger tremor was for side-to-side motion, while tremor in the vertical plane exhibited no difference between young, old (60–65 yrs), and older-old (70–75 yrs) individuals. It would seem that a strong contributor to the observed age differences in signal complexity is the older individual's need to increase their neuromuscular output so as to realize the specific demands of the task being performed [17].

The bi-directional hypothesis for the change of complexity in the movement dynamics with aging is based on the framework that the confluence of organismic, environmental, and task constraints channels the coordination and control of the system degrees of freedom [17, 18, 94]. In this view, the aging and loss of complexity effect will hold when an increase in the dimension of behavior is required from the intrinsic dynamics to realize the task demands. And the bi-directional effect of an increment in complexity will be prevalent when the confluence of constraints channels a reduction in the functional degrees of freedom of the system. As we note later, a good example of this bi-directional hypothesis is in isometric force control [94] where aging leads to a loss of complexity in the control of a constant force level (where better performance is realized by increasing the functional degrees of freedom) and an increment in complexity in a sine wave force tacking (where better performance is realized by reducing the degrees of freedom of the intrinsic dynamics). In this framework, the aging effect is more generally a loss of adaptation of the functional degrees of freedom rather than universally loss of complexity.

6. Isometric Force Production with Aging

In grasping actions, individuals need to produce a certain degree of isometric force in order to hold and/or manipulate a given object [95, 96]. When producing this action, one consequence is the production of small fluctuations in the force output, that have been referred to as reflecting force steadiness or isometric force tremor [68, 97]. Healthy older individuals, in comparison to young adults, often exhibit reduced control in force production, as quantified by an increase in these fluctuations [59, 98, 99]. Interestingly, this age-related decline in force producing capacity has typically been interpreted to reflect changes in motor unit (MU) control and sensorimotor function rather than in terms of more macro the constraints such as muscle strength per se. The consequence of these changes is that elderly adults exhibit greater targeting error and isometric force variability. As illustrated in Figure 4, both of these features of variability tend to be more pronounced when producing lower maximum voluntary contraction (MVC) forces in comparison to higher maximal forces [57, 68, 100–102] and during force tracking tasks where a sinusoidal target is displayed in comparison to a constant force target [103].

Given the prevailing view that overall muscle strength declines with aging [3, 4, 13, 67], the finding that it is more difficult to produce accurate levels of force output at lower MVC levels seems somewhat counterintuitive. If a decline in force producing capacity was to be the principal mitigating factor in the loss of muscle function in the older adult, then it would be predicted that producing higher forces would be more difficult. What these studies demonstrate is that any age-related changes in movement ability are not merely the product of alteration within the older muscle itself. Indeed, similar to the findings shown previously for physiological tremor tasks, it would appear that the effects of aging are amplified under more challenging actions (e.g., sinusoidal versus constant force production).

However, one important distinction can be made regarding the age-related changes in both physiological and isometric tremor. For physiological tremor, the argument often made is that the increased tremor amplitude reported where the entire arm is held against gravity primarily reflects the diminished strength of the older person. However, the same argument cannot be made for isometric force tremor, since here the greatest difference is in performing tasks of lower force levels. Under isometric conditions, the suggested

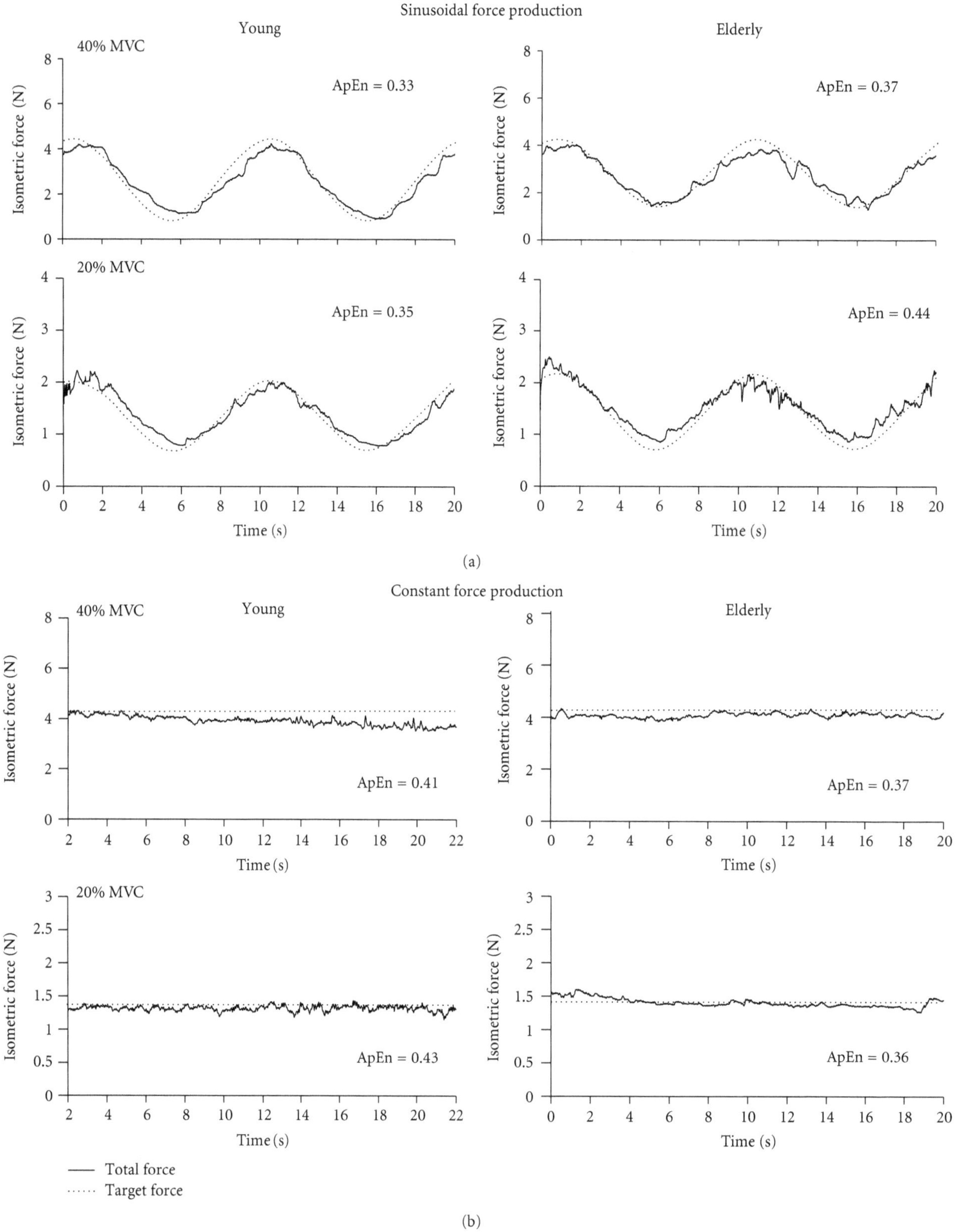

FIGURE 4: Representative examples of isometric force production trace (40% and 20% MVC) for a single young and older person. Examples are shown as individuals tracked a sinusoidal and constant target force. All traces were attained from a single subject during a single trial within each condition.

reason(s) for the age-related differences in performance at lower force levels typically draws on the manner in which the neuromuscular system modulates MU recruitment and firing rate(s) in order to accurately grade force output [51, 94, 104]. Within this context, it would appear that the age-related variation in isometric force production dynamics is driven more by task-specific control and coordination constraints rather than the ability to produce (and sustain) high absolute force levels [69].

Further support for the notion that chronological age *per se* does not always drive the changes seen in force production comes from a study by Sosnoff and Newell [105]. They reported that when differences in the maximal voluntary contraction (MVC) force of young and older individuals were controlled for, there was no performance difference in terms of the isometric force variability between age groups. From these findings it was argued that chronological age is not, by itself, a sufficient indicator of the decline in isometric force control, but rather that the relative degree of weakness, irrespective of age, is a more appropriate biological index. This result is of some importance since it would indicate that any age-related declines in isometric force control maybe more a function of inactivity, and so is modifiable by training, rather than simply the inevitable process of decline associated with chronological aging. Indeed, subsequent studies have demonstrated that improvements in isometric force control can be elicited with specific exercise interventions [55, 106].

7. Aging and Complexity in Isometric Force Control

As with the assessment of physiological tremor, additional insight as the any age-related changes in force production has been reported when measures of complexity have been applied to the time series. In addition to the straightforward assessments of changes in force variability or targeting error, many studies have reported that the age-related differences in force control extend to differences in the frequency profile of their force output, the pattern of regularity (based upon changes in ApEn and SampEn), and, where multiple digits are employed, changes in the coupling relations between these effectors [100, 101, 103, 105, 107, 108]. When reviewing the resultant force signals, it is interesting to compare the age-related differences in signal complexity for isometric actions with the responses generated for physiological tremor tasks. As shown in Figure 5, the force response from older adults is highlighted by an increase in complexity (increased ApEn) in comparison to younger individuals when performing more challenging isometric task (e.g., 20% MVC, sinusoidal tracking). However, during more demanding postural tremor tasks (e.g., whole arm extended, see Figure 2), the tremor output from the older adult was characterized by a decline in complexity (lower ApEn).

It would appear that, as with the discussion of the effect of aging on physiological tremor, the changes in the isometric force producing ability of older person can only in part be explained by the loss of complexity hypothesis [6, 12, 19]. While the force signal for the older adult typically exhibits increased complexity under more challenging task conditions, this pattern is not consistently prevalent across less challenging force levels or when different effectors are utilized to perform the task [57, 69, 105, 107]. This invites the interpretation that any age differences in complexity of the signal output are more a function of the interaction between extrinsic (task) and intrinsic (sacropenia, dynapenia) factors rather than biological age being the single driving factor. Consequently, the pattern of changes in the biological signal are not consistent with the view that aging is reflected by an overall loss of complexity [18]. Rather, the dynamics in the isometric force task reflect the confluence of constraints including those of the aging individual, the task constraints, and those of the environment.

8. Summary

With aging, there is a general decline in the physiological function that is often manifested by specific changes in the functional and structural properties of skeletal muscle [2–4, 51]. This decline in functional capacity of a given system has been increasingly viewed within the context of the loss of complexity hypothesis [6, 12]. While these changes alter the capacity of the individual muscle to respond, it is not clear to what degree these changes have a universal impact on an individual's behavioral movement performance in physical activity.

In the current paper, we examined the relation between aging, neuromuscular function, and physiological-behavioral complexity, specifically with reference to physiological tremor and isometric force production. These two motor outputs were selected since they both derive primarily from neuromuscular mechanisms, and the ability to control and minimize these oscillatory outputs is essential for the performance of many activities of daily living (ADL's) which contain a fine motor skill component. The examination of age-related changes in these motor processes would therefore provide greater understanding of the relation between muscle adaptations and chronological age. A central point to emerge is that there is no single pattern to the changes seen in physiological and isometric force tremor in older adults. Rather, it would appear that the specific alterations in the given motor outputs reflect a myriad of extrinsic (task related) and intrinsic (muscle weakness, loss of coordination) constraints that are unlikely to be all the direct result of the process of aging. Consequently, it is argued that any amplitude or structural changes observed in physiological and force tremor amplitude reflect the diminished ability of the older neuromuscular system to adapt to differing task demands.

Finally, the findings of this body of research do not universally support the unidirectional interpretation that aging is associated with a loss of physiological and behavioral complexity. Instead, the variable pattern of change in complexity observed across both physiological and isometric tremor forms in older adults supports the broader view

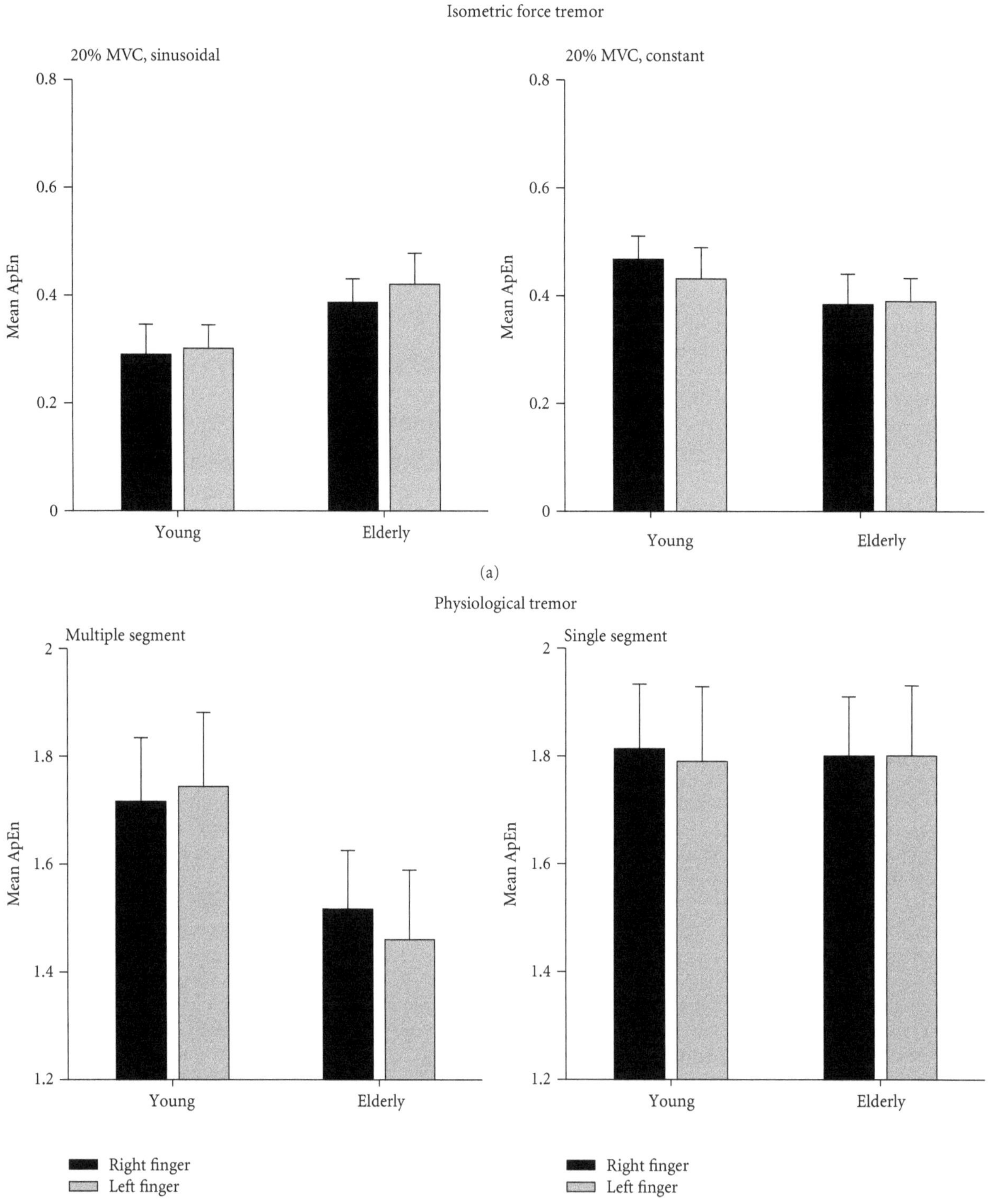

FIGURE 5: Age-related differences in approximate entropy (ApEn) measures for isometric force (a) and postural tremor (b) tasks. Changes in ApEn across the young and older individuals are shown for both the multiple segment and single-segment tremor tasks. In addition, the age-related differences during two isometric actions (20% MVC performed under sinusoidal tracking and constant force conditions) are also shown. This figure illustrates that the tremor signal tends to be less complex (lower ApEn) during multiple-segment tremor tasks and the 20% MVC constant force producing actions. However, for the 20% MVC sinusoidal funder isometric force task, the resultant signal for the older adults is more complex (higher ApEn) in comparison to the younger adults. Error bars represent one standard error of the mean.

that age-related changes in physiological complexity are bi-directional, depending to a large degree on the constraints to action. Thus, the adaptive responses of the upper limb movement dynamics studied do not simply reflect the impact aging has on motor function, in that they also depend on the task-specific requirements of the given action. Our synthesis provides further evidence that chronological age should be viewed as just an entry variable into the problem of the study of aging and not, by itself, an inevitable causal factor in neuromuscular decline and the change in physiological and behavioral complexity.

References

[1] W. W. Spirduso, *Physical Dimensions of Aging*, Human Kinetics, Champaign, Ill, USA, 1995.
[2] C. S. Klein, C. L. Rice, and G. D. Marsh, "Normalized force, activation, and coactivation in the arm muscles of young and old men," *Journal of Applied Physiology*, vol. 91, no. 3, pp. 1341–1349, 2001.
[3] J. Lexell, "Ageing and human muscle: observations from Sweden," *Canadian Journal of Applied Physiology*, vol. 18, no. 1, pp. 23–29, 1993.
[4] L. V. Thompson, "Age-related muscle dysfunction," *Experimental Gerontology*, vol. 44, no. 1-2, pp. 106–111, 2009.
[5] M. Kyriazis, "Practical applications of chaos theory to the modulation of human ageing: nature prefers chaos to regularity," *Biogerontology*, vol. 4, no. 2, pp. 75–90, 2003.
[6] L. A. Lipsitz, "Dynamics of stability: the physiologic basis of functional health and frailty," *Journals of Gerontology—Series A*, vol. 57, no. 3, pp. B115–B125, 2002.
[7] G. Deco and V. K. Jirsa, "Ongoing cortical activity at rest: criticality, multistability, and ghost attractors," *Journal of Neuroscience*, vol. 32, no. 10, pp. 3366–3375, 2012.
[8] G. Deco, V. K. Jirsa, and A. R. McIntosh, "Emerging concepts for the dynamical organization of resting-state activity in the brain," *Nature Reviews Neuroscience*, vol. 12, no. 1, pp. 43–56, 2011.
[9] A. R. McIntosh, N. Kovacevic, S. Lippe, D. Garrett, C. Grady, and V. Jirsa, "The development of a noisy brain," *Archives Italiennes de Biologie*, vol. 148, no. 3, pp. 323–337, 2010.
[10] P. J. Fadel, S. M. Barman, S. W. Phillips, and G. L. Gebber, "Fractal fluctuations in human respiration," *Journal of Applied Physiology*, vol. 97, no. 6, pp. 2056–2064, 2004.
[11] J. M. Hausdorff, "Gait dynamics, fractals and falls: finding meaning in the stride-to-stride fluctuations of human walking," *Human Movement Science*, vol. 26, no. 4, pp. 555–589, 2007.
[12] L. A. Lipsitz and A. L. Goldberger, "Loss of "complexity" and aging: potential applications of fractals and chaos theory to senescence," *Journal of the American Medical Association*, vol. 267, no. 13, pp. 1806–1809, 1992.
[13] G. E. Hicks, M. Shardell, D. E. Alley et al., "Absolute strength and loss of strength as predictors of mobility decline in older adults: The InCHIANTI study," *Journals of Gerontology—Series A*, vol. 67, no. 1, pp. 66–73, 2012.
[14] M. K. Andrew, A. Mitnitski, S. A. Kirkland, and K. Rockwood, "The impact of social vulnerability on the survival of the fittest older adults," *Age and Ageing*, vol. 41, no. 2, pp. 161–165, 2012.
[15] B. C. Clark and T. M. Manini, "Functional consequences of sarcopenia and dynapenia in the elderly," *Current Opinion in Clinical Nutrition and Metabolic Care*, vol. 13, no. 3, pp. 271–276, 2010.
[16] D. J. Clark and R. A. Fielding, "Neuromuscular contributions to age-related weakness," *Journals of Gerontology—Series A*, vol. 67, no. 1, pp. 41–47, 2012.
[17] K. M. Newell, D. E. Vaillancourt, and J. J. Sosnoff, "Aging, complexity, and motor performance," in *Handbook of the Psychology of Aging*, pp. 163–182, Academic Press, London, UK, 2006.
[18] D. E. Vaillancourt and K. M. Newell, "Changing complexity in human behavior and physiology through aging and disease," *Neurobiology of Aging*, vol. 23, no. 1, pp. 1–11, 2002.
[19] A. L. Goldberger, C. K. Peng, and L. A. Lipsitz, "What is physiologic complexity and how does it change with aging and disease?" *Neurobiology of Aging*, vol. 23, no. 1, pp. 23–26, 2002.
[20] B. J. West and W. D. Deering, *The Lure of Modern Science: Fractal Thinking*, John Wiley & Sons, New York, NY, USA, 1996.
[21] J. B. Bassingthwaighte, L. S. Liebovitch, and B. J. West, *Fractal Physiology*, Oxford University Press, New York, NY, USA, 1994.
[22] J. M. Hausdorff, Y. Ashkenazy, C. K. Peng, P. C. Ivanov, H. E. Stanley, and A. L. Goldberger, "When human walking becomes random walking: fractal analysis and modeling of gait rhythm fluctuations," *Physica A*, vol. 302, no. 1–4, pp. 138–147, 2001.
[23] G. Deuschl, M. Lauk, and J. Timmer, "Tremor classification and tremor time series analysis," *Chaos*, vol. 5, no. 1, pp. 48–51, 1995.
[24] S. Morrison and J. Sosnoff, "Age-related changes in the adaptability of neuromuscular output," *Journal of Motor Behavior*, vol. 41, no. 3, pp. 274–283, 2009.
[25] J. Timmer, S. Häussler, M. Lauk, and C. H. Lücking, "Pathological tremors: deterministic chaos or nonlinear stochastic oscillators?" *Chaos*, vol. 10, no. 1, pp. 278–288, 2000.
[26] D. E. Vaillancourt and K. M. Newell, "The dynamics of resting and postural tremor in Parkinson's disease," *Clinical Neurophysiology*, vol. 111, no. 11, pp. 2046–2056, 2000.
[27] M. M. Sturman, D. E. Vaillancourt, L. V. Metman, R. A. E. Bakay, and D. M. Corcos, "Effects of subthalamic nucleus stimulation and medication on resting and postural tremor in Parkinson's disease," *Brain*, vol. 127, no. 9, pp. 2131–2143, 2004.
[28] D. D. Garrett, N. Kovacevic, A. R. McIntosh, and C. L. Grady, "The importance of being variable," *Journal of Neuroscience*, vol. 31, no. 12, pp. 4496–4503, 2011.
[29] S. Morrison, S. R. Colberg, H. K. Parson, and A. I. Vinik, "Relation between risk of falling and postural sway complexity in diabetes," *Gait and Posture*, vol. 35, no. 4, pp. 662–668, 2012.
[30] A. Bravi, A. Longtin, and A. J. E. Seely, "Review and classification of variability analysis techniques with clinical applications," *BioMedical Engineering Online*, vol. 10, no. 1, article 90, 2011.
[31] N. Stergiou, *Innovative Analyses of Human Movement*, Human Kinetics, Champaign, Ill, USA, 2004.
[32] N. Stergiou and L. M. Decker, "Human movement variability, nonlinear dynamics, and pathology: is there a connection?" *Human Movement Science*, vol. 30, no. 5, pp. 869–888, 2011.
[33] J. B. Dingwell and J. P. Cusumano, "Nonlinear time series analysis of normal and pathological human walking," *Chaos*, vol. 10, no. 4, pp. 848–863, 2000.

[34] J. B. Dingwell, J. P. Cusumano, P. R. Cavanagh, and D. Sternad, "Local dynamic stability versus kinematic variability of continuous overground and treadmill walking," *Journal of Biomechanical Engineering*, vol. 123, no. 1, pp. 27–32, 2001.

[35] L. G. Gamero, J. Vila, and F. Palacios, "Wavelet transform analysis of heart rate variability during mycardial ischaemia," *Medical and Biological Engineering and Computing*, vol. 40, no. 1, pp. 72–78, 2002.

[36] P. C. Ivanov, L. A. Nunes Amaral, A. L. Goldberger et al., "Multifractality in human heartbeat dynamics," *Nature*, vol. 399, no. 6735, pp. 461–465, 1999.

[37] C. K. Peng, J. M. Hausdorff, S. Havlin, J. E. Mietus, H. E. Stanley, and A. L. Goldberger, "Multiple-time scales analysis of physiological time series under neural control," *Physica A*, vol. 249, no. 1–4, pp. 491–500, 1998.

[38] C. K. Peng, S. Havlin, J. M. Hausdorff, J. E. Mietus, H. E. Stanley, and A. L. Goldberger, "Fractal mechanisms and heart rate dynamics: long-range correlations and their breakdown with disease," *Journal of Electrocardiology*, vol. 28, supplement, pp. 59–64, 1995.

[39] S. M. Pincus and A. L. Goldberger, "Physiological time-series analysis: what does regularity quantify?" *American Journal of Physiology*, vol. 266, no. 4, pp. H1643–H1656, 1994.

[40] S. Pincus and B. H. Singer, "Randomness and degrees of irregularity," *Proceedings of the National Academy of Sciences of the United States of America*, vol. 93, no. 5, pp. 2083–2088, 1996.

[41] M. M. Sturman, D. E. Vaillancourt, and D. M. Corcos, "Effects of aging on the regularity of physiological tremor," *Journal of Neurophysiology*, vol. 93, no. 6, pp. 3064–3074, 2005.

[42] M. Teich, S. Lowen, and B. Jost, "Heart rate variability: measures and models," in *Nonlinear Biomedical Signal Processing—Dynamic Analysis and Modeling, Volume II*, IEEE Press, New York, NY, USA, 2001.

[43] V. K. Jirsa, O. Sporns, M. Breakspear, G. Deco, and A. R. Mcintosh, "Towards the virtual brain: network modeling of the intact and the damaged brain," *Archives Italiennes de Biologie*, vol. 148, no. 3, pp. 189–205, 2010.

[44] F. E. Yates, "Complexity of a human being: changes with age," *Neurobiology of Aging*, vol. 23, no. 1, pp. 17–19, 2002.

[45] C. Marsden, "Origins of normal and pathological tremor," in *Movement Disorders: Tremor*, L. Findley and R. Capildeo, Eds., pp. 37–84, Butterworth, London, UK, 1984.

[46] M. E. Hackel, G. A. Wolfe, S. M. Bang, and J. S. Canfield, "Changes in hand function in the aging adult as determined by the Jebsen Test of Hand Function," *Physical Therapy*, vol. 72, no. 5, pp. 373–377, 1992.

[47] V. K. Ranganathan, V. Siemionow, V. Sahgal, and G. H. Yue, "Effects of aging on hand function," *Journal of the American Geriatrics Society*, vol. 49, no. 11, pp. 1478–1484, 2001.

[48] A. T. Birmingham, H. J. Wharrad, and E. J. Williams, "The variation of finger tremor with age in man," *Journal of Neurology Neurosurgery and Psychiatry*, vol. 48, no. 8, pp. 788–798, 1985.

[49] C. D. Marsden, J. C. Meadows, G. W. Lange, and R. S. Watson, "Variations in human physiological finger tremor, with particular reference to changes with age," *Electroencephalography and Clinical Neurophysiology*, vol. 27, no. 2, pp. 169–178, 1969.

[50] J. Raethjen, F. Pawlas, M. Lindemann, R. Wenzelburger, and G. Deuschl, "Determinants of physiologic tremor in a large normal population," *Clinical Neurophysiology*, vol. 111, no. 10, pp. 1825–1837, 2000.

[51] Z. Erim, M. F. Beg, D. T. Burke, and C. J. De Luca, "Effects of aging on motor-unit control properties," *Journal of Neurophysiology*, vol. 82, no. 5, pp. 2081–2091, 1999.

[52] M. D. Grabiner and R. M. Enoka, "Changes in movement capabilities with aging," *Exercise and Sport Sciences Reviews*, vol. 23, pp. 65–104, 1995.

[53] S. V. Brooks and J. A. Faulkner, "Skeletal muscle weakness in old age: underlying mechanisms," *Medicine and Science in Sports and Exercise*, vol. 26, no. 4, pp. 432–439, 1994.

[54] M. E. Galganski, A. J. Fuglevand, and R. M. Enoka, "Reduced control of motor output in a human hand muscle of elderly subjects during submaximal contractions," *Journal of Neurophysiology*, vol. 69, no. 6, pp. 2108–2115, 1993.

[55] D. A. Keen, G. H. Yue, and R. M. Enoka, "Training-related enhancement in the control of motor output in elderly humans," *Journal of Applied Physiology*, vol. 77, no. 6, pp. 2648–2658, 1994.

[56] D. H. Laidlaw, M. Bilodeau, and R. M. Enoka, "Steadiness is reduced and motor unit discharge is more variable in old adults," *Muscle and Nerve*, vol. 23, pp. 600–612, 2000.

[57] R. M. Enoka, E. A. Christou, S. K. Hunter et al., "Mechanisms that contribute to differences in motor performance between young and old adults," *Journal of Electromyography and Kinesiology*, vol. 13, no. 1, pp. 1–12, 2003.

[58] J. G. Semmler, K. W. Kornatz, and R. M. Enoka, "Motor-unit coherence during isometric contractions is greater in a hand muscle of older adults," *Journal of Neurophysiology*, vol. 90, no. 2, pp. 1346–1349, 2003.

[59] H. Kinoshita and P. R. Francis, "A comparison of prehension force control in young and elderly individuals," *European Journal of Applied Physiology and Occupational Physiology*, vol. 74, no. 5, pp. 450–460, 1996.

[60] J. A. Faulkner, S. V. Brooks, and E. Zerba, "Skeletal muscle weakness and fatigue in old age: underlying mechanisms," *Annual Review of Gerontology & Geriatrics*, vol. 10, pp. 147–166, 1990.

[61] M. Brown, D. R. Sinacore, and H. H. Host, "The relationship of strength to function in the older adult," *Journals of Gerontology—Series A*, vol. 50, pp. 55–59, 1995.

[62] V. A. Hughes, W. R. Frontera, R. Roubenoff, W. J. Evans, and M. A. Fiatarone Singh, "Longitudinal changes in body composition in older men and women: role of body weight change and physical activity," *American Journal of Clinical Nutrition*, vol. 76, no. 2, pp. 473–481, 2002.

[63] A. J. Cruz-Jentoft, J. P. Baeyens, J. M. Bauer et al., "Sarcopenia: European consensus on definition and diagnosis," *Age and Ageing*, vol. 39, no. 4, pp. 412–423, 2010.

[64] V. Malafarina, F. Úriz-Otano, R. Iniesta, and L. Gil-Guerrero, "Sarcopenia in the elderly: diagnosis, physiopathology and treatment," *Maturitas*, vol. 71, no. 2, pp. 109–114, 2012.

[65] J. E. Morley, R. N. Baumgartner, R. Roubenoff, J. Mayer, and K. S. Nair, "Sarcopenia," *Journal of Laboratory and Clinical Medicine*, vol. 137, no. 4, pp. 231–243, 2001.

[66] B. C. Clark and T. M. Manini, "Sarcopenia $\neq$ dynapenia," *Journals of Gerontology—Series A*, vol. 63, no. 8, pp. 829–834, 2008.

[67] R. A. Fielding, B. Vellas, W. J. Evans et al., "Sarcopenia: An Undiagnosed Condition in Older Adults. Current Consensus Definition: Prevalence, Etiology, and Consequences. International Working Group on Sarcopenia," *Journal of the American Medical Directors Association*, vol. 12, no. 4, pp. 249–256, 2011.

[68] E. A. Christou and L. G. Carlton, "Old adults exhibit greater motor output variability than young adults only during rapid

discrete isometric contractions," *Journals of Gerontology—Series A*, vol. 56, no. 12, pp. B524–B532, 2001.

[69] R. M. Enoka, R. A. Burnett, A. E. Graves, K. W. Kornatz, and D. H. Laidlaw, "Task- and age-dependent variations in steadiness," *Progress in Brain Research*, vol. 123, pp. 389–395, 1999.

[70] E. Carmeli, H. Patish, and R. Coleman, "The aging hand," *Journals of Gerontology—Series A*, vol. 58, no. 2, pp. 146–152, 2003.

[71] J. Marshall, "The effect of ageing upon physiological tremor," *Journal of Neurology, Neurosurgery, and Psychiatry*, vol. 24, pp. 14–17, 1961.

[72] S. Morrison, P. M. Mills, and R. Barrett, "Differences in multiple segment tremor dynamics between young and elderly persons," *Journals of Gerontology—Series A*, vol. 61, no. 9, pp. 982–990, 2006.

[73] L. Glass and M. C. Mackay, *From Clocks to Chaos: The Rhythms of Life*, Princeton University Press, Princeton, NJ, USA, 1988.

[74] L. Glass, "Synchronization and rhythmic processes in physiology," *Nature*, vol. 410, no. 6825, pp. 277–284, 2001.

[75] F. E. Yates, "The dynamics of adaptation in living systems," in *Adaptive Control of Ill-Defined Systems*, O. G. Selfridge, E. L. Rissland, and M. A. Arbib, Eds., Plenum Press, New York, NY, USA, 1984.

[76] F. E. Yates, "The dynamics of aging and time: how physical action implies social action," in *Emergent Theories of Aging*, J. E. Birren and V. L. Bengtson, Eds., Springer, New York, NY, USA, 1988.

[77] J. H. McAuley and C. D. Marsden, "Physiological and pathological tremors and rhythmic central motor control," *Brain*, vol. 123, no. 8, pp. 1545–1567, 2000.

[78] R. J. Elble and W. C. Koller, *Tremor*, Johns Hopkins, Baltimore, Md, USA, 1990.

[79] R. J. Elble, "Tremor in ostensibly normal elderly people," *Movement Disorders*, vol. 13, no. 3, pp. 457–464, 1998.

[80] R. J. Elble, "Characteristics of physiologic tremor in young and elderly adults," *Clinical Neurophysiology*, vol. 114, no. 4, pp. 624–635, 2003.

[81] S. L. Hong, E. G. James, and K. M. Newell, "Coupling and Irregularity in the aging motor system: tremor and movement," *Neuroscience Letters*, vol. 433, no. 2, pp. 119–124, 2008.

[82] J. H. McAuley, J. C. Rothwell, and C. D. Marsden, "Frequency peaks of tremor, muscle vibration and electromyographic activity at 10 Hz, 20 Hz and 40 Hz during human finger muscle contraction may reflect rhythmicities of central neural firing," *Experimental Brain Research*, vol. 114, no. 3, pp. 525–541, 1997.

[83] P. Feys, W. F. Helsen, X. Liu, A. Lavrysen, B. Nuttin, and P. Ketelaer, "Effects of vision and arm position on amplitude of arm postural tremor in patients with multiple sclerosis," *Archives of Physical Medicine and Rehabilitation*, vol. 85, no. 6, pp. 1031–1033, 2004.

[84] J. M. Spyers-Ashby, M. J. Stokes, P. G. Bain, and S. J. Roberts, "Classification of normal and pathological tremors using a multidimensional electromagnetic system," *Medical Engineering and Physics*, vol. 21, no. 10, pp. 713–723, 1999.

[85] S. Morrison, G. Kerr, K. M. Newell, and P. A. Silburn, "Differential time- and frequency-dependent structure of postural sway and finger tremor in Parkinson's disease," *Neuroscience Letters*, vol. 443, no. 3, pp. 123–128, 2008.

[86] G. Kerr, S. Morrison, and P. Silburn, "Coupling between limb tremor and postural sway in Parkinson's disease," *Movement Disorders*, vol. 23, no. 3, pp. 386–394, 2008.

[87] I. S. Hwang, C. T. Huang, R. J. Cherng, and C. C. Huang, "Postural fluctuations during pointing from a unilateral or bilateral stance," *Human Movement Science*, vol. 25, no. 2, pp. 275–291, 2006.

[88] S. Morrison, G. Kerr, and P. Silburn, "Bilateral tremor relations in Parkinson's disease: effects of mechanical coupling and medication," *Parkinsonism and Related Disorders*, vol. 14, no. 4, pp. 298–308, 2008.

[89] I. S. Hwang, C. C. K. Lin, and P. S. Wu, "Tremor modulation in patients with Parkinson's disease compared to healthy counterparts during loaded postural holding," *Journal of Electromyography and Kinesiology*, vol. 19, no. 6, pp. e520–e528, 2009.

[90] B. Carignan, J. F. Daneault, and C. Duval, "The amplitude of physiological tremor can be voluntarily modulated," *Experimental Brain Research*, vol. 194, no. 2, pp. 309–316, 2009.

[91] S. Morrison and K. M. Newell, "Limb stiffness and postural tremor in the arm," *Motor control*, vol. 4, no. 3, pp. 293–315, 2000.

[92] S. M. Pincus, "Approximate entropy as a measure of system complexity," *Proceedings of the National Academy of Sciences of the United States of America*, vol. 88, no. 6, pp. 2297–2301, 1991.

[93] S. M. Pincus, "Greater signal regularity may indicate increased system isolation," *Mathematical Biosciences*, vol. 122, no. 2, pp. 161–181, 1994.

[94] G. Kamen and A. Roy, "Motor unit synchronization in young and elderly adults," *European Journal of Applied Physiology*, vol. 81, no. 5, pp. 403–410, 2000.

[95] J. R. Flanagan, M. K. O. Burstedt, and R. S. Johansson, "Control of fingertip forces in multidigit manipulation," *Journal of Neurophysiology*, vol. 81, no. 4, pp. 1706–1717, 1999.

[96] J. R. Flanagan and A. M. Wing, "Modulation of grip force with load force during point-to-point arm movements," *Experimental Brain Research*, vol. 95, no. 1, pp. 131–143, 1993.

[97] R. M. Enoka, "Neural strategies in the control of muscle force," *Muscle and Nerve*, vol. 20, no. 5, pp. S66–S69, 1997.

[98] J. A. C. Lazarus and J. M. Haynes, "Isometric pinch force control and learning in older adults," *Experimental Aging Research*, vol. 23, no. 2, pp. 179–199, 1997.

[99] J. K. Shim, B. S. Lay, V. M. Zatsiorsky, and M. L. Latash, "Age-related changes in finger coordination in static prehension tasks," *Journal of Applied Physiology*, vol. 97, no. 1, pp. 213–224, 2004.

[100] J. Keogh, S. Morrison, and R. Barrett, "Age-related differences in inter-digit coupling during finger pinching," *European Journal of Applied Physiology*, vol. 97, no. 1, pp. 76–88, 2006.

[101] J. W. Keogh, S. Morrison, and R. Barrett, "Strength Training Improves the Tri-Digit Finger-Pinch Force Control of Older Adults," *Archives of Physical Medicine and Rehabilitation*, vol. 88, no. 8, pp. 1055–1063, 2007.

[102] E. Christou and B. Tracy, "Aging and variability in motor output," in *Movement System Variability*, K. Davids, S. Bennet, and K. Newell, Eds., pp. 199–218, Human Kinetics, Champaign, Ill, USA, 2005.

[103] D. E. Vaillancourt, L. Larsson, and K. M. Newell, "Effects of aging on force variability, single motor unit discharge patterns, and the structure of 10, 20, and 40 Hz EMG

activity," *Neurobiology of Aging*, vol. 24, no. 1, pp. 25–35, 2003.

[104] K. Seki and M. Narusawa, "Firing rate modulation of human motor units in different muscles during isometric contraction with various forces," *Brain Research*, vol. 719, no. 1-2, pp. 1–7, 1996.

[105] J. J. Sosnoff and K. M. Newell, "Are age-related increases in force variability due to decrements in strength?" *Experimental Brain Research*, vol. 174, no. 1, pp. 86–94, 2006.

[106] J. W. L. Keogh, S. Morrison, and R. Barrett, "Strength and coordination training are both effective in reducing the postural tremor amplitude of older adults," *Journal of Aging and Physical Activity*, vol. 18, no. 1, pp. 43–60, 2010.

[107] J. J. Sosnoff and K. M. Newell, "The generalization of perceptual-motor intra-individual variability in young and old adults," *Journals of Gerontology—Series B*, vol. 61, no. 5, pp. P304–P310, 2006.

[108] D. E. Vaillancourt and K. M. Newell, "Aging and the time and frequency structure of force output variability," *Journal of Applied Physiology*, vol. 94, no. 3, pp. 903–912, 2003.

10

Use of Physical and Intellectual Activities and Socialization in the Management of Cognitive Decline of Aging and in Dementia

Myuri Ruthirakuhan, Angela C. Luedke, Angela Tam, Ankita Goel, Ayaz Kurji, and Angeles Garcia

Department of Medicine (Geriatrics) and Centre for Neuroscience, Queen's University, Kingston, ON, Canada K7L 5A2

Correspondence should be addressed to Angeles Garcia, garciaa@providencecare.ca

Academic Editor: Richard F. Gillum

Lifestyle nonpharmacological interventions can have a deep effect on cognitive aging. We have reviewed the available literature on the effectiveness of physical activity, intellectual stimulation, and socialization on the incidence of dementia and on the course of dementia itself. Even though physical activity appears to be beneficial in both delaying dementia onset and in the course of the disease, more research is needed before intellectual stimulation and socialization can be considered as treatments and prevention of the disease. Through our paper, we found that all three nonpharmacological treatments provide benefits to cognition and overall well-being in patients with age-related cognitive impairments. These interventions may be beneficial in the management of dementia.

1. Introduction

Alzheimer's disease (AD) is a neurodegenerative disorder with devastating consequences [1]. Despite being the most common cause of dementia, affecting approximately 5.4 million Americans [2] and almost 50% of people over the age 85 [3], no cure has yet been discovered. Efforts are also focusing on the development of more effective strategies to slow the progression of AD to increase the quality of life of those affected. Even a two-year delay in disease onset would reduce the prevalence of AD among Americans by two million people within fifty years [4]. If an intervention that delayed the onset of AD by five years had been applied back in 1997, we would have seen a 50% reduction in AD incidence [4]. Research on strategies to slow the development and progression of AD is arguably more important now than ever before, since the number of people with AD is expected to nearly triple over the next forty years [4], and dementia is the most important contributor to disability in the elderly [5].

Among others, three nonpharmacological interventions are particularly relevant as they might positively influence cognition, general functioning, and overall quality of life. These three strategies are *physical exercise*, *intellectual stimulation*, and *social interaction*. While there are studies that evaluate the role of individual and multimodal interventions on AD, there is a lack of literature on the combination of all three. The purpose of this paper is to review key areas of the literature that focus on the effects of physical exercise, intellectual stimulation, and socialization strategies on AD evolution, as they collectively play an important role in the management of Alzheimer's disease. Physical exercise encapsulates both aerobic exercises (e.g., walking and cycling) and nonaerobic exercises (e.g., strength and resistance training; flexibility and balance exercises). For intellectual stimulation, we examine studies that have evaluated the prognostic effects of either cognitive hobbies (e.g., reading, word puzzles, and card games) or cognitive training (e.g., computer training games/paradigms that target specific cognitive domains such as memory and attention). Social interaction is defined as the participation of an AD patient in group-related activities, such as mealtime conversations, support groups, or other forms of social engagement.

Evidence-based nonpharmacological interventions are an essential part of any management plan, especially for geriatric populations in whom the harmful effects of polypharmacy are a major concern. Nonpharmacological strategies are sometimes even more effective than pharmacological interventions and are empowering to proactive individuals who seek to gain greater personal control over their mental and physical health. We suggest that comprehensive AD management plans should include evidence-based nonpharmacological strategies.

2. Methods

Electronic databases (PubMed, Web of Science, and MEDLINE) were searched for the period from 1980 to 2012 with the combination of key words: AD, dementia, incident AD, aging, cognition, cognitive aging, exercise, aerobic exercise, resistance training, cognitive reserve, intellectual stimulation, cognitive stimulation, hobbies, cognitive training, memory training, brain games, leisure activities, socialization, loneliness, social network, support groups, quality of life, activities of daily living, nonpharmacological, and treatment. We included studies that examined the preservation of cognition in AD populations and AD incidence.

3. Physical Activity

The health benefits attributed to physical activity are numerous and well known. Exercise has been associated with a lower incidence in many chronic diseases, such as coronary heart disease [6], type 2 diabetes [7], obesity [8], cancer [9], bone loss [10], and high blood pressure [11]. We have reviewed the effects of physical exercise on cognition.

Higher cardiorespiratory fitness has been related to higher scores on tests of cognitive function [12]. A meta-analysis of randomized controlled trials examining the relationship between exercise and cognition showed modest improvements in attention, processing speed, executive function, and memory among older adults in the treatment arms [13]. This is highly relevant for the elderly population, as it suggests that physical activity can serve as a preventative measure against age-related cognitive decline [14].

Several large longitudinal studies followed older adults without cognitive impairments at baseline and measured rate of incident dementia to clarify the relationship between physical activity and incident cognitive loss. A large prospective study by Podewils et al. identified an inverse relationship between physical activity and dementia risk [15]. Compared to no exercise, physical activity has been linked with reduced risks of developing cognitive impairment and dementia [16] with the risk for dementia being further reduced with increasing levels of physical activity. Larson and colleagues found that persons who exercised three or more times per week had a reduced risk of developing dementia compared to those who exercised less, and the reduction was more marked among those with the poorest physical function at baseline [17]. These results were corroborated by Buchman et al. who found that participants in the lowest percentiles of physical activity had more than twice the risk of developing dementia than those in the highest percentiles of physical activity [18]. Furthermore, Lautenschlager et al. demonstrated that these results might be transferable to adults with mild cognitive impairment (MCI), and, thus, at high risk for dementia; participants who underwent exercise training showed modest improvements in cognition after six months [19]. Physical exercise has, therefore, been recommended as a preventative measure of mild cognitive impairment and dementia [20, 21].

There is much less research focusing on the effect of physical activity in AD patients. This may be due to the challenges of implementing an exercise regime while managing the behavioral and emotional disturbances in AD patients, particularly in the later stages of the disease. However, the results in the available literature are promising. Early research involving AD patients in nonrandomized controlled trials showed significant cognitive improvements among participants who underwent cycling training and somatic and isotonic-relaxation exercises [22, 23].

Physical exercise may have beneficial effects in AD patients beyond cognition as well. A meta-analysis on 30 randomized controlled trials that employed exercise, behavioral and environmental manipulations in patients with cognitive impairment found exercise had positive effects on strength and cardiovascular fitness in addition to improvements in behavior and cognition [24–26]. Further evidence supporting multifaceted positive effects of exercise on AD can be traced to recent randomized controlled trials of physical exercise regimes on AD patients (Table 1).

Compared to controls, patients in the intervention programs showed better physical functioning (functional reach, walking, and mobility). After treatment, these patients also showed improved performance of activities of daily living (ADLs), and less cognitive decline and cognitive improvement in some cases. Physical exercise, therefore, appears to be beneficial for AD patients. While the majority of the studies did not find any differences in depression, one study by Steinberg found increased depression and decreased quality of life in patients who underwent the exercise intervention [31]. Further research into the effect of physical exercise on mood and quality of life in AD patients is, therefore, required.

When considering the role of exercise on AD, it is important to note that any positive results may be due to a placebo effect, even in randomized controlled trials. However, due to the varied nature of the outcome measures used in these studies, it is unlikely that every intervention group demonstrated significant gains over the controls due to a placebo effect alone. Furthermore, control group members never appeared to show any improvement and often showed higher rates of functional and cognitive decline.

The majority of the reviewed studies employed aerobic exercise as a component to their therapy. Yet, two studies demonstrated that nonaerobic activity, such as strength and flexibility training, might also be beneficial to AD patients

TABLE 1: Summary of randomized controlled trials of physical exercise regimes in AD patients.

Study	Length and frequency	Type of exercise	Sample	MMSE (baseline mean)	Outcome measures	Major findings
Kemoun et al. [27]	15 wks; 1 h sessions 3x/wk	Aerobic, balance, and endurance	$n_{ex} = 16$ $n_c = 15$	12.6	Walking speed, stride length, double limb support time, and ERFC	Higher ERFC and walking parameter scores in exercise group; positive correlation between walking parameters and ERFC scores
Miu et al. [28]	3 mos; ~1 h sessions 2x/wk	Aerobic, flexibility	$n_{ex} = 36$ $n_c = 49$	20 (median)	SF-12, 6 min walk, functional reach, BBS, MMSE, ADAS-Cog, and CSDD	Improvement in walking and functional reach in exercise group
Roach et al. [29]	16 wks; 15–30 min sessions 5x/wk	Strength, flexibility, endurance, and balance	$n_{ex} = 28$ $n_{soc} = 25$ $n_{walk} = 29$	10.7	ACIF, 6 min walk, and MMSE	Improved transfer in exercise group
Rolland et al. [30]	1 yr; 1 h session 2x/wk	Aerobic, strength, flexibility, and balance	$n_{ex} = 67$ $n_c = 67$	8.8	Katz Index of ADLs, walking speed, get-up-and-go, one-leg balance, MNA, NPI, and MADRS	Less decline in overall ADLs in exercise group
Steinberg et al. [31]	12 wks; ~3x/wk	Aerobic, strength, balance, and flexibility	$n_{ex} = 14$ $n_c = 13$	20.1	YPAS, 8-ft walk, JTT, sit-to-stand, MMSE, BNT, HVLT, ADQRL, NPI, CSDD, and SCB	Improved performance in JTT and sit-to-stand, increased depression, and decreased ADQRL in exercise group
Venturelli et al. [32]	24 wks; 30 min sessions 4x/wk	Mobility, aerobic	$n_{ex} = 12$ $n_c = 12$	13	6 min walk, Barthel Index of ADLs, and MMSE	Improvements in walking and ADLs, slower decline in MMSE in exercise group
Vreugdenhil et al. [33]	4 mos; >30 mins daily	Strength, balance, and aerobic	$n_{ex} = 20$ $n_c = 20$	22.9	ADAS-Cog, MMSE, functional reach, Timed Up and Go, sit-to-stand, Barthel Index of ADLs, GDS, CIBIC-plus, and Zarit Burden Interview	Improved scores on ADAS-Cog, MMSE, CIBIC-plus, functional reach, Timed Up and Go, sit-to-stand, and ADLs in exercise group
Yàgüez et al. [34]	6 wks; 1.5 h sessions 1x/wk	Flexibility, eye-hand coordination	$n_{ex} = 15$ $n_c = 12$	22.1	CANTAB-Expedio	Improvements in attention, visual memory recognition, and working memory in exercise group

$n_{ex}, n_c, n_{soc}, n_{walk}$: number of participants in exercise program, control group, social conversation group, and walking group, respectively. ACIF: Acute Care Index of Function, ADAS-Cog: Alzheimer's Disease Assessment Scale-Cognitive Subscale, ADL: activities of daily living, ADQRL: Alzheimer's Disease Quality Related Life Scale, BBS: Berg Balance Scale, BNT: Boston Naming Test, CANTAB-Expedio: The Cambridge Neuropsychological Test Automated Battery, CIBIC-plus: Clinician's Interview-Based Impression of Change Plus Caregiver Input, CSDD: Cornell Scale for Depression in Dementia, ERFC: Rapid Evaluation of Cognitive Function, GDS: Geriatric Depression dcale, HDS: Hamilton Depression Scale, HVLT: Hopkins Verbal Learning Test, JTT: Jebsen Total Time, MADRS: Montgomery-Asberg Depression Rating Scale, MMSE: Mini-Mental State Examination, MNA: Mini-Nutritional Assessment, NPI: Neuropsychiatric Inventory, SCB: Screen for Caregiver Burden, SF-12: SF-12 Quality of Life Questionnaire, SF-36: Short-Form Health Survey, SIP: Sickness Impact Profile, and YPAS: Yale Physical Activity Survey.

[29, 34]. Studies involving cognitively normal adults and nonaerobic exercises offer insight into the potential effects of nonaerobic activity and cognitive decline. Cassilhas et al. found that participants who underwent resistance training showed significant improvements in memory measures compared to controls [35]. Liu-Ambrose and colleagues, who used a combination of resistance and balance exercises as their intervention, saw significant improvements in response inhibition in their intervention group while the control group deteriorated [36]. Resistance training may, therefore, provide protective effects for cognition. The effect of stretch exercises, such as yoga, on cognition has been briefly examined; Oken and colleagues found no cognitive differences between their control and yoga groups after treatment [37]. However, more research into stretch exercises and cognition is required to draw more definitive conclusions.

Future studies may investigate which types of exercises, or combinations of exercises, yield the greatest benefit specifically to AD patients. It is important to mention that some of the aforementioned randomized controlled trials [27, 29, 30, 32] were conducted on participants recruited from long-term care facilities, and thus were likely to be in the more moderate-advanced stages of the disease. These studies demonstrate not only the feasibility of the exercise programs in AD patients but also that patients can benefit greatly from physical exercise even in moderate-to-severe stages of the disease.

Enhanced neuroplasticity might be underlying the improvements seen. Colcombe and colleagues demonstrated that older adults without dementia who performed aerobic exercises had greater grey and white matter volumes compared to adults who engaged in stretching and toning exercises [38]. Exercise has also been associated with functional connectivity between brain networks often affected by age, such as the default mode, frontal parietal, and frontal executive networks, in older adults without dementia [39]. While randomized controlled trials in AD patients examining the relationship between neuroplasticity and exercise are underway, correlational studies examining brain volumes and cardiorespiratory fitness have been done. In AD patients, cardiorespiratory fitness has been associated with brain volume. VO_2^{peak}, peak oxygen consumption, has been positively correlated with greater whole brain volume and white matter volume [40], notably in the inferior parietal lobule, hippocampal, and parahippocampal regions [41]. Future results of randomized controlled trials will improve our knowledge in this field of research.

Overall, physical activity offers promising outcomes for cognition and physical health in the elderly population and AD patients.

4. Intellectual Activity

Engagement in intellectually stimulating activities has been linked with reduced risk of developing AD and intellectual stimulation has been widely explored as a nonpharmacological treatment option for dementia [42].

Among cognitively normal older persons, randomized control trials employing intellectual training concluded that cognitive interventions produce protective and potentially long lasting positive effects in various cognitive domains as well as activities of daily living [43]. There is also evidence that frequent engagement in hobbies, including reading, puzzles, and games, for at least six hours per week reduces the risk of incident dementia [44]. The concept of intellectual stimulation as a preventative measure for dementia in healthy older adults can be parallel to the notion of building a "compensatory mechanism" or "cognitive reserve" [45–48].

Cognitive reserve refers to the hypothesis that individual differences shaped by inherent characteristics and external sources including intelligence, years of education, occupation, and intellectual activities, may provide neural protective support against dementia [45–47]. It has been argued that these collective life experiences may contribute to building cognitive reserve and, thus, provide skills to compensate for AD pathology [45–47]. In other words, a greater cognitive reserve might delay the appearance of dementia despite the presence of neuropathology, after which a rapid progression of cognitive decline may ensue once pathology is significant enough to result in AD diagnosis. Thus, AD patients with higher education and occupation accomplishments suffer more rapid decline in cognitive abilities when compared to AD patients with less education and occupational attainment following diagnosis [49]. Another study by Helzner and colleagues [50] investigated the relationship between premorbid leisure activity and rate of cognitive decline in AD patients. Leisure activities were classified into four categories: intellectual, social, physical, and other. Higher-frequency participation in intellectual leisure activities prior to AD diagnosis was associated with delayed AD onset followed by faster cognitive decline. The study by Helzner and colleagues [50] provides evidence for the benefits of intellectual stimulation on slowing down AD development.

Besides reducing the risk of dementia, cognitive interventions later in life may affect functional decline in AD. Treiber and colleagues [51] explored the association between engaging in cognitively stimulating activities in late life and the rate of cognitive decline in incident AD. This study included a wide range of intellectual activities that required varying levels of cognitive demand, for example, completing puzzles, reading, watching television, listening to music, and cooking. The results suggested that higher-frequency participation in stimulating activities in early stages of dementia resulted in slower cognitive decline. However, as time progressed there was an overall decrease in participation in activities, which might reflect the nature of AD in terms of functional abilities.

Intellectual stimulation can be divided into several categories including cognitive stimulation, cognitive training, and cognitive rehabilitation (Table 2) [48, 52–54]. Each type of stimulation targets various cognitive domains including memory and attention, or even more generally, activities of daily living [55]. The focus of this paper is to investigate the literature on the link between intellectual stimulation and rate of cognitive decline in patients with dementia.

4.1. Cognitive Stimulation and Reality Orientation in Dementia. Cognitive stimulation therapy (CS) encompasses a variety of mentally stimulating activities and is less formal than other forms of cognitive training [53]. In addition, cognitive stimulation can be passive, such as listening to music, or active, such as playing a game [53]. The goal of CS is to enhance a wide range of functioning, including social skills, often through group discussions [48, 56]. An earlier randomized control trial included a total of 167 participants (97 in the treatment group and 70 in the control group). This study examined the relationship between CS, cognitive functioning, and quality of life [57]. The CS group participated in activities including crafts, games, and singing compared to a control group who received no intervention. The sessions ran for seven weeks and consisted of a total of 14 sessions, one 45-minute session twice a

Table 2: Summary of trials involving cognitive interventions in AD patients.

Study	Length and frequency	Type of stimulation	Sample	MMSE (baseline mean)	Outcome measures	Major findings
Buschert et al. [59]	6 months; 2 hours 1x/wk	Multicomponent intervention with focus on CS	$n_{ex} = 8$ $n_c = 7$	Experimental: 24.5 Control: 25.3	(i) MMSE (ii) ADAS-Cog (iii) TMT (iv) RBANS story memory and recall (v) QoL-AD (vi) MADRS	(i) No significant benefit
Chapman et al. [58]	8 wks; 90-minute sessions 1x/wk	Cognitive stimulation	$n_{ex} = 28$ $n_c = 26$	20.87	(i) MMSE (ii) ADAS-Cog (iii) TFLS NPI-irritability and apathy (iv) QoL-AD (v) CBIC	(i) Modest positive effects on language, global and functional abilities, and emotional wellbeing in experimental group compared to control group just treated with donepezil
Spector et al. [57]	7 wks; 45-minute sessions 2x/wk	Cognitive stimulation	$n_{ex} = 97$ $n_c = 70$	Experimental: 14.2 Control: 14.8	(i) MMSE (ii) ADAS-Cog (iii) QoL-AD (iv) HCS (v) Cornell Scale for Depression in Dementia (vi) CAPE-BRS (vii) CDR	(i) Significant improvement on the MMSE, ADAS-COG, and QoL-AD
Onder et al. [60]	25 wks; 30-minute sessions 3x/wk	Reality orientation	$n_{ex} = 70$ $n_c = 67$	Experimental: 20.2 Control: 19.9	(i) MMSE (ii) ADAS-Cog (iii) Functional status: Barthel Index, (iv) IADL (v) NPI (vi) Family caregiver outcomes: HRSD, HRSA, Caregiver Burden Inventory, SF-36	(i) Small improvement in MMSE and ADAS-COG
Loewenstein et al. [64]	12–16 weeks; 45-minute sessions 2x/wk	Cognitive rehabilitation/cognitive training	$n_{ex} = 25$ $n_c = 19$	Experimental: 23.40 Control: 24.53	(i) The face-name association task: (ii) Orientation (iii) The continuous performance test (iv) Procedural object-memory evaluation (v) Modified Making-Change-For-A-Purchase Task (vi) Balancing-A-Checkbook Task (vii) RMBPC (viii) B-ADLS (ix) CES-D (x) IQCODE	(i) Training specific improvement in orientation, face-name recall, processing speed, and making change compared to control group receiving mental stimulation

Table 2: Continued.

Study	Length and frequency	Type of stimulation	Sample	MMSE (baseline mean)	Outcome measures	Major findings
Davis et al. [65]	5 weeks; 1-hour sessions 1x/wk; home practice 30 minutes per day 6x/wk	Cognitive training	$n_{ex} = 19$ $n_c = 18$	Experimental: 21.84 Control: 22.78	(i) MMSE (ii) WMS-R logical memory (iii) WMS-R visual reproduction (iv) WAIS-R digit span (v) VSAT (vi) Controlled oral word association test (vii) Category fluency (viii) Finger taping test (ix) GDS (x) Quality of life patient	(i) Improvement in attention, recall of personal information, and face-name recall compared to mock control group (ii) Results did not extend to other neuropsychological tests or quality of life
Koltai et al. [67]	Group program: 5 wks; 1-hour sessions 1x/wk Individual program: 6 wks; 1-hour sessions 1x/wk with caregiver involvement in last 10–15 minutes	Cognitive rehabilitation/cognitive training	$n_{ex} = 14$ $n_c = 8$	Experimental: 22.9 Control: 26.6	(i) GDS and relative GDS (ii) EMQ and relative EMQ (iii) CERAD (iv) MMSE	(i) No significant differences between the experimental group and the wait-list control group (ii) Participants with insight about self-deficits perceived greater gains in memory compared to participants with no insight
Quayhagen et al. [66]	8 weeks; 1-hour sessions 5x/wk	Cognitive training	$n_{AD} = 103$ $n_c = 103$ (i) Numbers in each group (cognitive training, dyadic counseling, dual supportive seminar, and early-stage day care) not specified	Not reported	(i) Immediate memory composite: WMS-R Logical Memory 1 and visual reproduction 1, DRS (memory) (ii) Delayed memory composite: WMS logical memory 2, visual reproduction 2 (iii) Verbal fluency composite: controlled oral word association, DRS (initiation) (iv) Problem solving composite: geriatric coping schedule, DRS (conceptualization) (v) Memory and Behavior Problems Checklist (part A)	(i) Improvement in memory and communication with caregiver (ii) Other types of interventions (dual support seminar, early-stage daycare) had positive effects on communication and interactions

Table 2: Continued.

Study	Length and frequency	Type of stimulation	Sample	MMSE (baseline mean)	Outcome measures	Major findings
Cahn-Weiner et al. [71]	6 wks; 45-minute sessions 2x/wk	Memory training	$n_{ex} = 17$ $n_c = 17$	Experimental: 24.3 Control: 25.1	(i) HVLT-R (ii) BVMT-R (iii) BNT (iv) COWA (v) JLO (vi) TMT (Parts A and B) (vii) ADL questionnaire (viii) EMQ	(i) No significant effects

n_{ex}, n_c, n_{AD}: number of participants in intellectual stimulation program, control group, and group diagnosed with AD. MMSE: Mini-Mental state examination, ADAS-Cog: Alzheimer's Disease Assessment Scale-Cognitive Subscale, TMT: Trail Making Test, RBANS: Repeatable Battery for the Assessment of Neuropsychological Status Versions A (before testing) and B (after testing), QoL-AD: quality of life-Alzheimer's disease, MADRS: Montgomery-Asberg Depression Rating Scale, TFLS: Texas Functional Living Scale, NPI: Neuropsychiatric Inventory, CIBIC: Clinician's Interview-Based Impression of Change, HCS: Holden Communication Scale, CAPE-BRS: The Clifton Assessment Procedures for the Elderly-Behaviour Rating Scale, CDR: The Clinical Dementia Rating Scale, IADL: instrumental activities of daily living, HRSD: Hamilton Rating Scales for Depression, HRSA: Hamilton Rating Scales for Anxiety, SF-36: The Medical Outcomes Study 36-Item Short-Form General Health Survey, RMBPC: The Revised Memory and Behavior Problems Checklist, B-ADLS: The Bayer Activities of Daily Living Scale, CES-D: The Center for Epidemiological Studies-Depression Scale, IQCODE: the informant questionnaire of the cognitive decline in the elderly scale, WMS-R: Wechsler Memory Scale-Revised, WAIS-R: Wechsler Adult Intelligence Scale-Revised, VSAT: The Verbal Series Attention Test, GDS: Geriatric Depression Scale, EMQ: Everyday Memory Questionnaire, CERAD: Consortium to Establish a Registry for Alzheimer's Disease Test Battery, DRS: The Mattis Dementia Rating Scale, HVLT-R: Hopkins Verbal Learning Test Revised, BVMT-R: Brief Visual Spatial Memory Test Revised, BNT: Boston Naming Test, COWA: Controlled Oral Word Association Test, and JLO: Judgment of Line Orientation.

week. Assessment measures included cognitive tests and measures of quality of life, communication, behavior, global functioning, depression, and anxiety. The results indicated positive effects of CS on cognitive functioning as well as ADLs. Other studies found CS to be beneficial on measures of language [58], emotional wellbeing [58], and cognitive tests [57]. Unfortunately, not all studies found significant benefits of CS on dementia patients [59].

Reality orientation (RO) is a component of CS and focuses on orienting the individual with AD to person, place and time [52, 56]. Studies on RO in dementia indicate slight advantages on cognitive tests [60, 61]. A recent Cochrane review of fifteen randomized control trials investigated the effectiveness of RO and some CS in AD [56]. The review included 718 participants, with 407 participants in the treatment group and 311 in the control group. Intervention length varied between four weeks and 24 months, with sessions ranging from 30 to 90 minutes. Overall cognitive functioning was improved in AD patients receiving RO and CS, with some studies indicating additional positive changes to social and communicative functioning and quality of life [56].

Based on the current literature on the efficacy of CS and RO on decline in AD, it appears that both forms of intervention may provide encouraging results for slowing decline and improving quality of life [52, 56].

4.2. Cognitive Training and Cognitive Rehabilitation in Dementia. Cognitive training (CT) targets individual or multiple cognitive domains through teaching specific skills. It aims to improve functioning in the targeted area as well as the possibility of extending the improvements to more general functioning and other cognitive domains [54, 62]. Similarly, cognitive rehabilitation (CR) aims at improving daily functioning by identifying individualized strengths and weaknesses [56, 63]. Due to the significant amount of overlap between CT and CR, both interventions are sometimes combined [62].

Several reviews on CT suggest mixed outcomes in terms of effectiveness as a treatment option for AD [52, 62]. While several studies show improvement in specific cognitive domains targeted by training [64–66], others fail to report any significant changes [67] or extend results to more general functioning [65]. A Cochrane review by Clare and Woods [62] concluded that CT and CR provided no positive or negative effects on cognitive performance in AD compared to control groups. Conversely, Small and colleagues [68] found CT to have a negative impact on mood in patients with dementia and in their caregivers. A meta-analysis showed that CT had modest positive effects on various aspects of cognition, including learning, memory, executive and general functioning, and depression [55]. A randomized control trial using CR alone found that goal performance and satisfaction was improved compared to the control groups receiving relaxation therapy [63].

Another review investigated the literature on CT in preventing incident AD, preventing MCI conversion to AD, and slowing AD progression [48, 69]. The results suggested that CT may be most beneficial to healthy elderly and at risk individuals with MCI as opposed to AD treatment [48].

There is a lack of a consensus in the literature as to whether CT can ameliorate symptoms of AD [52, 62]. Although some studies show promising results for CT [55], others reveal improvement only in specific areas of cognitive training, such as learning personal information and aspects of attention [65]. CR, on the other hand, might produce more general benefits to cognitive functioning [63].

4.3. Specific Cognitive Domain Training in Dementia. Targets of intellectual stimulation can also be divided into unidomain and multidomain. While most cognitive interventions target multidomain areas of cognition and functioning, some are specific to memory training. Although some studies suggest memory rehabilitation can improve specific memory function with sufficient time and caregiver involvement [70], a randomized control study focusing on mnemonic memorization strategies found no significant difference between the treatment and control groups [71].

4.4. Comparing Interventions. Ballard and colleagues recently reviewed CT, CS, CR, and memory aids and concluded that all forms of intervention may offer modest effects, with most benefit attributed to CS [52]. In comparing CT and CS, both resulted in improvement of activities of daily living; however, only CS resulted in improvement in behavior [53, 72]. There are several reasons to explain differences in effectiveness of treatment types. There can be a significant overlap between types of intellectual stimulation, making it difficult to identify which types of interventions are most effective. The fact that some studies implementing only memory training were included in reviews of cognitive training [55] might also contribute to mixed findings in reviews of CT and cloud the effectiveness of each type of treatment. Moreover, differences in the past history and disease stages of the patients might also explain different results. Diversity in methodologies, such as sample size, variations in inclusion criteria, inconsistent outcome measures and protocols, also renders between study comparisons problematic [55]. In addition, not all studies control for medications such as cholinesterase inhibitors, which might contribute to positive effects along with stimulating activities [53].

Nonetheless, intellectual stimulation is a promising tool for slowing the progression of AD. More randomized control trials that compare generalizability of training programs, long-term effects, and rate of cognitive decline across different intervention types are needed to assess the most effective form of intellectual stimulation.

5. Socialization

AD patients' feelings of incompetence, along with societal misconceptions, may accelerate the progression of AD [73]. So far, the relevance of the social environment surrounding an individual with AD has been mostly overlooked, but the results of increased social engagement on risk of dementia open the opportunity to incorporate socialization therapies in AD.

5.1. Influence of Increased Socialization on Incident Dementia. The cognitive reserve hypothesis, as previously described [45–47], includes social engagement as an important skill set for delaying the development of AD. An increase in social engagement with the surrounding environment can be correlated with angiogenesis, synaptogenesis, and neurogenesis [74]. Fratiglioni et al. also explained the relevance of stress reduction in cognition through the stress hypothesis [74] and increased social engagement is associated with improved self-esteem [73]. The importance of social engagement in reducing the risk of AD can be further supported by the vascular hypothesis. It is important to note that vascular risk factors, which could be reduced with increased social engagement, can contribute to the pathogenesis and progression of AD [74, 75].

Table 3 showcases the importance of social engagement on the prevention of AD, there is a lack of research on the effects of social engagement on AD prognosis. Collaborative research in the fields of sociology, psychology, neuroscience, and medicine will be important in this area.

5.2. Influence of Socialization on AD Population. Many AD patients sense that their cognitive impairment isolates them from other people leading to anxiety, depression, societal withdrawal, and decreased self-confidence. Manipulating the social environment around AD patients may help them regain a sense of self-worth and a better attitude towards life. This may improve eating and exercise habits and social interactions, which may result in improved AD prognosis [73].

Shaping how cognitively normal individuals relate to AD patients can play an important role in improving patients' social environment and interactions [73]. It is extremely important that surrounding healthy individuals (friends, family members, etc.) maintain a supportive atmosphere towards AD patients to ensure that, regardless of their cognitive abilities, they have a place in society and that their identity is valued. After multiple experiences, MacRae [73] reported that married AD patients whose spouses encouraged them to live life as normally as possible, and to remain socially engaged, preserved a "positive sense of self while living with dementia." This led to healthier eating habits and increased physical exercise and participation in cognitively and socially stimulating activities, thereby improving quality of life [73].

In further support of how a positive social atmosphere can benefit individuals with AD, Keller et al. [81] analyzed how shared mealtimes can enhance social engagement. With disease progression, alterations must be made to accommodate for changes in eating conduct (difficulties with using utensils or wandering), swallowing ability, and the ability to prepare food safely. Therefore, an event that was once a traditional social occasion may become an event filled with tension, frustration, and disappointment. As a result, the social experience associated with mealtimes may become limited and possibly nonexistent. However, reports show that AD patients benefit from shared mealtimes by getting motivated through another's physical presence to improve their attentional, planning, and decision making abilities [81].

Loneliness is widely reported by patients with dementia, arising from the feeling of not having anyone to relate to, dissatisfaction with one's way of living, and social isolation. Recent studies have attempted to reduce this sense of "loneliness" and assess its effects on cognition [76]. Pitkala et al. [75] examined the effects of enhancing social stimulation on cognitive outcomes in the elderly and patients with mild dementia. Volunteers were divided into three social intervention groups, according to their preference: (1) art, inspiring activities, and discussions, (2) exercise and discussions, and (3) therapeutic writing and discussions. Within each group, they were further divided into intervention or placebo. Participants in the intervention groups improved significantly over the course of 3 months on the Alzheimer's Disease Assessment Scale (ADAS-Cog) compared to control groups. Furthermore, a health-related quality of life (HRQol) questionnaire conducted at baseline and at 12 months revealed significant improvements in quality of life in the social intervention groups [75].

Support groups are another intervention aimed to assist with the psychosocial difficulties that patients diagnosed with early-stage dementia face [82]. A clinical trial compared quality of life (QOL), depression, and family communication outcomes between an early-stage memory loss (ESML) support group and a wait-list (WL) control group [83]. The ESML condition involved 90-minute weekly sessions for 9 weeks. The WL condition did not participate in the social support groups, but received educational material from their local Alzheimer's Association group and were encouraged to contact relevant support services should any questions or concerns arise. Results showed that in comparison to control participants, ESML participants expressed better QOL and less depressive symptoms after 9 weeks. Furthermore, the improved QOL among ESML participants was associated with an improvement of cognition and family communication [83].

Results have shown that although caregivers are willing to help their loved ones; at times at a personal cost, AD caregivers have a much higher chance of being clinically depressed than age-matched controls [84, 85]. Thus, many psychosocial therapies have been explored to primarily help caregivers, which frequently lead to better care of patients. Mittelman explains that individualized counseling and involvement in caregiver support groups result in long-lasting lower caregiver distress, even at followups at one and three years later [86]. Furthermore, lower distress and depressive symptoms were observed across caregivers for patients with varying dementia severity, living conditions, and after death of the patient [86].

It appears that enhanced social interactions may decrease the risk of AD and improve patients' QOL, self-confidence, and possibly prognosis. Although it appears that socialization is important in supporting cognitive abilities in the normal elderly, further research is needed to clarify how and to what extent socialization benefits patients with AD.

Table 3: Summary of studies on the effect of socialization on incident dementia.

Study	Length and frequency	Protocol	Sample	MMSE (baseline mean)	Outcome measures	Major findings
Wilson et al. [76]	4 years; annual check up	Longitudinal clinicopathological cohort study	$n = 823$		(i) Clinical diagnosis of AD (ii) Change in measures of global cognition and specific cognitive functions	(i) Loneliness associated with cognitive decline and development of AD
Wang et al. [77]	Data collection (9 years)	Longitudinal population-based study	$n = 776$	27.3	(i) Frequency of social and leisure activities engaged 6.4 years before diagnosis (ii) Baseline MMSE (iii) MMSE of incident dementia cases	(i) Socially and mentally stimulating activity may preserve mental functioning in the elderly, reducing risk of dementia
Friedland et al. [78]		Questionnaire data collection	$n_{AD} = 193$ $n_{HC} = 358$		(i) Monthly involvement in possible 26 nonoccupational activities at early adulthood and middle adulthood	(i) AD patients are less active in midlife than HC participants
Bennet et al. [79]	6-7 years	Longitudinal, epidemiological clinicopathological cohort study	$n = 89$	25.8 (not used in analysis)	(i) Annual clinical evaluation (ii) Brain autopsy at death (iii) Social network size (number of individuals seen at least once/month)	(i) Larger social network sizes observed in participants with higher level of cognition
Fratiglioni et al. [80]	3 years	Longitudinal community-based study	$n_{HC} = 1203$	>23	(i) Social network at baseline, clinical evaluation at baseline and 3 years	(i) Limited social network ties and interaction increased risk of developing dementia

n_{HC}, n_{AD}: number of participants in healthy control group and group diagnosed with AD. MMSE: Mini-Mental State Examination.

6. Multimodal Therapy

Given that physical exercise, intellectual stimulation, and socialization have individually shown to benefit AD patients, we summarize the results of multimodal interventions, combining at least two of the three activity types.

Coelho et al. [87] found that participants who engaged in an exercise program while simultaneously completing cognitive tasks had significantly higher scores ($P < 0.001$) than the control group on the Frontal Assessment Battery, which measures frontal lobe cognitive function. Furthermore, participants in the control group demonstrated decreased executive and visuospatial abilities through lower scores on a clock drawing test. The physical exercise program consisted of aerobic, flexibility and balance exercises, and resistance training. Cognitive tasks included generating words according to specific criteria (e.g., flowers, animals) or reacting to sensory stimuli such as verbal commands. These findings suggest that there is a place for physical exercise combined with intellectual stimulation in AD management.

Arkin [88] provides further support for the use of multimodal intervention through a study of 24 AD patients engaged in exercise (aerobic and weight training), cognitive tasks (taking place before, during, and after exercise), and social activities. Compared to controls, the 4-year intervention group experienced no decline in several cognitive measures: MMSE, Clinical Dementia Rating Scale, verbal fluency, Boston Naming, and WAIS-R Comprehension. Burgener et al. [89] conducted a trial in which 24 early-AD patients received a multimodal intervention (exercise, cognitive behavioral therapy, and support group) and were compared to 19 patient control group who received attention-control educational programs. In addition to physical and behavioral outcome benefits, there was a significant difference in MMSE scores between the intervention and control groups, not present at baseline. As such, both studies suggest that multimodal intervention programs can help delay the cognitive decline characteristic of AD.

It is important to note, however, that evidence supporting multimodal intervention is not yet conclusive. A pilot study of 14 AD patients by Maci et al. [90] found that participants engaged in a multimodal program of exercise (balance, gait, and coordination), cognitive stimulation, and socialization (talking/singing with other participants) led to reduced depression and improved anxiety and quality of life. However, there were no significant between-group differences in cognition as measured by the MMSE and Frontal Assessment Battery. It is possible that behavioral improvements may have been secondary to the very small sample size. Conflicting findings such as these indicate the need for further research in this area.

While the impact of multimodal interventions (and perhaps even each intervention independently) on reducing cognitive decline in AD remains unclear, it appears that patients may benefit in other ways from physical exercise, intellectual stimulation, and socialization. More research into the effects of multimodal therapies is required.

7. Conclusions

In summary, this paper highlights key research on the effectiveness of nonpharmacological treatment options, specifically exercise, intellectual stimulation, and socialization, on the progression of AD. Based on our findings in the literature, all three intervention strategies may provide positive effects on cognition and overall wellbeing. More specifically, physical exercise appears to benefit various aspects of cognition in AD patients including stabilization of MMSE scores, and improved attention, memory and recognition, and ability to perform ADLs. It has also been demonstrated that regular exercise is helpful in reducing the risk of AD development and progression. Future studies should include a broader range of exercises to determine the most effective exercise regime for AD patients. Increased social interaction has been shown to benefit Alzheimer's patients by minimizing one's sense of loneliness, isolation, stress, and vascular factors that contribute to cognitive decline. It can also improve patients' sense of self-worth. However, limited studies exist on the benefits of socialization on cognition in the AD population. Studies focusing on these areas would help verify if a social component would provide more than simply behavioral benefits. In addition, intellectual stimulation may benefit AD patients by improving their cognition, emotional and social wellbeing as well as performance of ADLs. However, inconsistent results on the effectiveness of intellectual stimulation in delaying cognitive decline in AD patients demonstrate the need for further research.

It is necessary for future research to identify and address limitations found in the current literature. Patient recruitment can be a significant challenge in those with moderate-to-advanced AD due to the necessary comprehension levels for study completion. In addition, as dementia progresses, patients may become increasingly tired and frustrated, leading to higher attrition rates. Some of the studies do not provide adequate characterization of the enrolled population, rendering comparisons difficult. The ability to make between-study comparisons is further limited by the broad range of physical, cognitive, and social activities used in nonpharmacological therapies. Determining which nonpharmacological therapy is the most beneficial to the AD population is difficult due to the widespread and overlapping positive effects of each activity. As the goal of this paper was to provide a general overview of nonpharmacological interventions in AD, we were limited in our ability to produce statistical analysis. Therefore, a meta-analysis is suggested in order to obtain quantitative results.

Based on the literature presented in this paper, patients experience less depression and improved quality of life, ability to perform ADLs, and social relationships. Most importantly, interventions that combine physical exercise and socialization with cognitive stimulation are often highly enjoyable for patients, leading to participants expressing their approval by saying: "This has been the only thing I have found that feels like I am doing something to help myself" [89]. Thus, the aforementioned nonpharmacological therapies are recommended in AD management.

Authors' Contribution

The first three authors contributed equally to this work.

References

[1] J. L. Cummings, "Alzheimer's disease," *New England Journal of Medicine*, vol. 351, no. 1, pp. 56–67, 2004.

[2] W. Thies and L. Bleiler, "Alzheimer's disease facts and figures," *Alzheimer's and Dementia*, vol. 7, no. 2, pp. 208–244, 2011.

[3] A. L. Fitzpatrick, L. H. Kuller, D. G. Ives et al., "Incidence and prevalence of dementia in the cardiovascular health study," *Journal of the American Geriatrics Society*, vol. 52, no. 2, pp. 195–204, 2004.

[4] R. Brookmeyer, S. Gray, and C. Kawas, "Projections of Alzheimer's disease in the United States and the public health impact of delaying disease onset," *American Journal of Public Health*, vol. 88, no. 9, pp. 1337–1342, 1998.

[5] R. M. Sousa, C. P. Ferri, D. Acosta et al., "Contribution of chronic diseases to disability in elderly people in countries with low and middle incomes: a 10/66 Dementia Research Group population-based survey," *The Lancet*, vol. 374, no. 9704, pp. 1821–1830, 2009.

[6] K. E. Powell, P. D. Thompson, C. J. Caspersen, and J. S. Kendrick, "Physical activity and the incidence of coronary heart disease," *Annual Review of Public Health*, vol. 8, pp. 253–287, 1987.

[7] A. M. Kriska, S. N. Blair, and M. A. Pereira, "The potential role of physical activity in the prevention of non-insulin-dependent diabetes mellitus: the epidemiological evidence," *Exercise and Sport Sciences Reviews*, vol. 22, pp. 121–143, 1994.

[8] S. N. Blair and S. Brodney, "Effects of physical inactivity and obesity on morbidity and mortality: Current evidence and research issues," *Medicine and Science in Sports and Exercise*, vol. 31, no. 11, pp. S646–S662, 1999.

[9] I. M. Lee, "Physical activity and cancer prevention—data from epidemiologic studies," *Medicine and Science in Sports and Exercise*, vol. 35, no. 11, pp. 1823–1827, 2003.

[10] D. Bonaiuti, B. Shea, R. Iovine et al., "Exercise for preventing and treating osteoporosis in postmenopausal women," *Cochrane Database of Systematic Reviews*, no. 3, Article ID CD000333, 2002.

[11] S. N. Blair, N. N. Goodyear, L. W. Gibbons, and K. H. Cooper, "Physical fitness and incidence of hypertension in healthy normotensive men and women," *Journal of the American Medical Association*, vol. 252, no. 4, pp. 487–490, 1984.

[12] A. D. Brown, C. A. McMorris, R. S. Longman et al., "Effects of cardiorespiratory fitness and cerebral blood flow on cognitive outcomes in older women," *Neurobiology of Aging*, vol. 31, no. 12, pp. 2047–2057, 2010.

[13] P. J. Smith, J. A. Blumenthal, B. M. Hoffman et al., "Aerobic exercise and neurocognitive performance: a meta-analytic review of randomized controlled trials," *Psychosomatic Medicine*, vol. 72, no. 3, pp. 239–252, 2010.

[14] K. I. Erickson and A. F. Kramer, "Aerobic exercise effects on cognitive and neural plasticity in older adults," *British Journal of Sports Medicine*, vol. 43, no. 1, pp. 22–24, 2009.

[15] L. J. Podewils, E. Guallar, L. H. Kuller et al., "Physical activity, APOE genotype, and dementia risk: findings from the Cardiovascular Health Cognition Study," *American Journal of Epidemiology*, vol. 161, no. 7, pp. 639–651, 2005.

[16] D. Laurin, R. Verreault, J. Lindsay, K. MacPherson, and K. Rockwood, "Physical activity and risk of cognitive impairment and dementia in elderly persons," *Archives of Neurology*, vol. 58, no. 3, pp. 498–504, 2001.

[17] E. B. Larson, L. Wang, J. D. Bowen et al., "Exercise is associated with reduced risk for incident dementia among persons 65 years of age and older," *Annals of Internal Medicine*, vol. 144, no. 2, pp. 73–81, 2006.

[18] A. S. Buchman, P. A. Boyle, L. Yu, R. C. Shah, R. S. Wilson, and D. A. Bennett, "Total daily physical activity and the risk of AD and cognitive decline in older adults," *Neurology*, vol. 78, no. 17, pp. 1323–1329, 2012.

[19] N. T. Lautenschlager, K. L. Cox, L. Flicker et al., "Effect of physical activity on cognitive function in older adults at risk for Alzheimer disease: a randomized trial," *Journal of the American Medical Association*, vol. 300, no. 9, pp. 1027–1037, 2008.

[20] J. E. Ahlskog, Y. E. Geda, N. R. Graff-Radford, and R. C. Petersen, "Physical exercise as a preventive or disease-modifying treatment of dementia and brain aging," *Mayo Clinic Proceedings*, vol. 86, no. 9, pp. 876–884, 2011.

[21] M. Weih, Ü. Degirmenci, S. Kreil, and J. Kornhuber, "Physical activity and alzheimer's disease: a meta-analysis of cohort studies," *The Journal of Gerontopsychology and Geriatric Psychiatry*, vol. 23, no. 1, pp. 17–20, 2010.

[22] L. Palleschi, F. Vetta, E. De Gennaro et al., "Effect of aerobic training on the cognitive performance of elderly patients with senile dementia of Alzheimer type," *Archives of Gerontology and Geriatrics*, vol. 22, no. 1, pp. 47–50, 1996.

[23] G. F. Lindenmuth and B. Moose, "Improving cognitive abilities of elderly Alzheimer's patients with intense exercise therapy," *American Journal of Alzheimer's Care and Related Disorders and Research*, vol. 5, no. 1, pp. 31–33, 1990.

[24] P. Heyn, B. C. Abreu, and K. J. Ottenbacher, "The effects of exercise training on elderly persons with cognitive impairment and dementia: a meta-analysis," *Archives of Physical Medicine and Rehabilitation*, vol. 85, no. 10, pp. 1694–1704, 2004.

[25] C. A. Alessi, E. Yoon, J. F. Schnelle, N. R. Al-Samanai, and P. A. Cruise, "A randomized trial of a combined physical activity and environmental intervention in nursing home residents: do sleep and agitation improve?" *Journal of the American Geriatrics Society*, vol. 47, no. 7, pp. 784–791, 1999.

[26] L. Teri, L. E. Gibbons, S. M. McCurry et al., "Exercise plus behavioral management in patients with Alzheimer disease: a randomized controlled trial," *Journal of the American Medical Association*, vol. 290, no. 15, pp. 2015–2022, 2003.

[27] G. Kemoun, M. Thibaud, N. Roumagne et al., "Effects of a physical training programme on cognitive function and walking efficiency in elderly persons with dementia," *Dementia and Geriatric Cognitive Disorders*, vol. 29, no. 2, pp. 109–114, 2010.

[28] D. K. Miu, S. L. Szeto, and Y. F. Mak, "A randomised controlled trial on the effect of exercise on physical, cognitive and affective function in dementia subjects," *Asian Journal of Gerontology and Geriatrics*, vol. 3, no. 1, pp. 8–16, 2008.

[29] K. E. Roach, R. M. Tappen, N. Kirk-Sanchez, C. L. Williams, and D. Loewenstein, "A randomized controlled trial of an activity specific exercise program for individuals with Alzheimer disease in long-term care settings," *Journal of Geriatric Physical Therapy*, vol. 34, no. 2, pp. 50–56, 2011.

[30] Y. Rolland, F. Pillard, A. Klapouszczak et al., "Exercise program for nursing home residents with Alzheimer's disease: a 1-year randomized, controlled trial," *Journal of the American Geriatrics Society*, vol. 55, no. 2, pp. 158–165, 2007.

[31] M. Steinberg, J. M. Sheppard Leoutsakos, L. J. Podewills, and C. G. Lyketsos, "Evaluation of a home-based exercise program in the treatment of Alzheimer's disease: the Maximizing Independence in Dementia (MIND) study," *International Journal of Geriatric Psychiatry*, vol. 24, no. 7, pp. 680–685, 2009.

[32] M. Venturelli, R. Scarsini, and F. Schena, "Six-month walking program changes cognitive and ADL performance in patients with Alzheimer," *American Journal of Alzheimer's Disease and other Dementias*, vol. 26, no. 5, pp. 381–388, 2011.

[33] A. Vreugdenhil, J. Cannell, A. Davies, and G. Razay, "A community-based exercise programme to improve functional ability in people with Alzheimer's disease: a randomized controlled trial," *Scandinavian Journal of Caring Sciences*, vol. 26, no. 1, pp. 12–19, 2012.

[34] L. Yágüez, K. N. Shaw, R. Morris, and D. Matthews, "The effects on cognitive functions of a movement-based intervention in patients with Alzheimer's type dementia: a pilot study," *International Journal of Geriatric Psychiatry*, vol. 26, no. 2, pp. 173–181, 2011.

[35] R. C. Cassilhas, V. A. R. Viana, V. Grassmann et al., "The impact of resistance exercise on the cognitive function of the elderly," *Medicine and Science in Sports and Exercise*, vol. 39, no. 8, pp. 1401–1407, 2007.

[36] T. Liu-Ambrose, M. G. Donaldson, Y. Ahamed et al., "Otago home-based strength and balance retraining improves executive functioning in older fallers: a randomized controlled trial," *Journal of the American Geriatrics Society*, vol. 56, no. 10, pp. 1821–1830, 2008.

[37] B. S. Oken, D. Zajdel, S. Kishiyama et al., "Randomized, controlled, six-month trial of yoga in healthy seniors: effects on cognition and quality of life," *Alternative Therapies in Health and Medicine*, vol. 12, no. 1, pp. 40–47, 2006.

[38] S. J. Colcombe, K. I. Erickson, P. E. Scalf et al., "Aerobic exercise training increases brain volume in aging humans," *Journals of Gerontology*, vol. 61, no. 11, pp. 1166–1170, 2006.

[39] M. W. Voss, R. S. Prakash, K. I. Erickson et al., "Plasticity of brain networks in a randomized intervention trial of exercise training in older adults," *Froniers in Aging Neuroscience*, vol. 2, p. 32, 2010.

[40] J. M. Burns, B. B. Cronk, H. S. Anderson et al., "Cardiorespiratory fitness and brain atrophy in early Alzheimer disease," *Neurology*, vol. 71, no. 3, pp. 210–216, 2008.

[41] R. A. Honea, G. P. Thomas, A. Harsha et al., "Cardiorespiratory fitness and preserved medial temporal lobe volume in alzheimer disease," *Alzheimer Disease and Associated Disorders*, vol. 23, no. 3, pp. 188–197, 2009.

[42] R. S. Wilson, D. A. Bennett, J. L. Bienias et al., "Cognitive activity and incident AD in a population-based sample of older persons," *Neurology*, vol. 59, no. 12, pp. 1910–1914, 2002.

[43] M. Valenzuela and P. Sachdev, "Can cognitive exercise prevent the onset of dementia? systematic review of randomized clinical trials with longitudinal follow-up," *American Journal of Geriatric Psychiatry*, vol. 17, no. 3, pp. 179–187, 2009.

[44] T. F. Hughes, C. C. H. Chang, J. Vander Bilt, and M. Ganguli, "Engagement in reading and hobbies and risk of incident dementia: the MoVIES project," *American Journal of Alzheimer's Disease and other Dementias*, vol. 25, no. 5, pp. 432–438, 2010.

[45] Y. Stern, "What is cognitive reserve? Theory and research application of the reserve concept," *Journal of the International Neuropsychological Society*, vol. 8, no. 3, pp. 448–460, 2002.

[46] N. Scarmeas and Y. Stern, "Cognitive reserve and lifestyle," *Journal of Clinical and Experimental Neuropsychology*, vol. 25, no. 5, pp. 625–633, 2003.

[47] N. Scarmeas and Y. Stern, "Cognitive reserve: implications for diagnosis and prevention of Alzheimer's disease," *Current Neurology and Neuroscience Reports*, vol. 4, no. 5, pp. 374–380, 2004.

[48] L. Mowszowski, J. Batchelor, and S. L. Naismith, "Early intervention for cognitive decline: can cognitive training be used as a selective prevention technique?" *International Psychogeriatrics*, vol. 22, no. 4, pp. 537–548, 2010.

[49] Y. Stern, S. Albert, M. X. Tang, and W. Y. Tsai, "Rate of memory decline in AD is related to education and occupation: cognitive reserve?" *Neurology*, vol. 53, no. 9, pp. 1942–1947, 1999.

[50] E. P. Helzner, N. Scarmeas, S. Cosentino, F. Portet, and Y. Stern, "Leisure activity and cognitive decline in incident Alzheimer disease," *Archives of Neurology*, vol. 64, no. 12, pp. 1749–1754, 2007.

[51] K. A. Treiber, M. C. Carlson, C. Corcoran et al., "Cognitive stimulation and cognitive and functional decline in Alzheimer's disease: the Cache County Dementia Progression Study," *The Journals of Gerontology, Series B*, vol. 66, no. 4, pp. 416–425, 2011.

[52] C. Ballard, Z. Khan, H. Clack, and A. Corbett, "Nonpharmacological treatment of Alzheimer disease," *Canadian Journal of Psychiatry*, vol. 56, no. 10, pp. 589–595, 2011.

[53] F. Yu F, K. M. Rose, S. C. Burgener et al., "Cognitive training for early-stage Alzheimer's disease and dementia," *Journal of Gerontological Nursing*, vol. 35, no. 3, pp. 23–29, 2009.

[54] A. F. Kurz, S. Leucht, and N. T. Lautenschlager, "The clinical significance of cognition-focused interventions for cognitively impaired older adults: a systematic review of randomized controlled trials," *International Psychogeriatrics*, vol. 23, no. 9, pp. 1364–1375, 2011.

[55] D. I. Sitzer, E. W. Twamley, and D. V. Jeste, "Cognitive training in Alzheimer's disease: a meta-analysis of the literature," *Acta Psychiatrica Scandinavica*, vol. 114, no. 2, pp. 75–90, 2006.

[56] B. Woods, E. Aguirre, A. E. Spector, and M. Orrell, "Cognitive stimulation to improve cognitive functioning in people with dementia," *Cochrane Database of Systematic Reviews*, no. 2, Article ID CD005562, 2012.

[57] A. Spector, L. Thorgrimsen, B. Woods et al., "Efficacy of an evidence-based cognitive stimulation therapy programme for people with dementia: randomised controlled trial," *British Journal of Psychiatry*, vol. 183, pp. 248–254, 2003.

[58] S. B. Chapman, M. F. Weiner, A. Rackley, L. S. Hynan, and J. Zientz, "Effects of cognitive-communication stimulation for Alzheimer's disease patients treated with donepezil," *Journal of Speech, Language, and Hearing Research*, vol. 47, no. 5, pp. 1149–1163, 2004.

[59] V. C. Buschert, U. Friese, S. J. Teipel et al., "Effects of a newly developed cognitive intervention in amnestic mild cognitive impairment and mild Alzheimer's disease: a pilot study," *Journal of Alzheimer's Disease*, vol. 25, no. 4, pp. 679–694, 2011.

[60] G. Onder, O. Zanetti, E. Giacobini et al., "Reality orientation therapy combined with cholinesterase inhibitors in Alzheimer's disease: randomised controlled trial," *British Journal of Psychiatry*, vol. 187, pp. 450–455, 2005.

[61] A. Spector, S. Davies, B. Woods, and M. Orrell, "Reality orientation for dementia: a systematic review of the evidence of effectiveness from randomized controlled trials," *Gerontologist*, vol. 40, no. 2, pp. 206–212, 2000.

[62] L. Clare and B. Woods, "Cognitive rehabilitation and cognitive training for early-stage Alzheimer's disease and vascular dementia," *Cochrane Database of Systematic Reviews*, no. 4, Article ID CD003260, 2008.

[63] L. Clare, D. E. J. Linden, R. T. Woods et al., "Goal-oriented cognitive rehabilitation for people with early-stage alzheimer disease: a single-blind randomized controlled trial of clinical efficacy," *American Journal of Geriatric Psychiatry*, vol. 18, no. 10, pp. 928–939, 2010.

[64] D. A. Loewenstein, A. Acevedo, S. J. Czaja, and R. Duara, "Cognitive rehabilitation of mildly impaired Alzheimer disease patients on cholinesterase inhibitors," *American Journal of Geriatric Psychiatry*, vol. 12, no. 4, pp. 395–402, 2004.

[65] R. N. Davis, P. J. Massman, and R. S. Doody, "Cognitive intervention in Alzheimer disease: a randomized placebo-controlled study," *Alzheimer Disease and Associated Disorders*, vol. 15, no. 1, pp. 1–9, 2001.

[66] M. P. Quayhagen, M. Quayhagen, R. R. Corbeil et al., "Coping with dementia: evaluation of four nonpharmacologic interventions," *International Psychogeriatrics*, vol. 12, no. 2, pp. 249–265, 2000.

[67] D. C. Koltai, K. A. Welsh-Bohmer, and D. E. Schmechel, "Influence of anosognosia on treatment outcome among dementia patients," *Neuropsychological Rehabilitation*, vol. 11, no. 3-4, pp. 455–475, 2001.

[68] G. W. Small, P. V. Rabins, P. P. Barry et al., "Diagnosis and treatment of Alzheimer disease and related disorders: consensus statement of the American Association for Geriatric Psychiatry, the Alzheimer's Association, and the American Geriatrics Society," *Journal of the American Medical Association*, vol. 278, no. 16, pp. 1363–1371, 1997.

[69] L. J. Thal, "Prevention of Alzheimer disease," *Alzheimer Disease and Associated Disorders*, vol. 20, no. 2, pp. S97–S99, 2006.

[70] L. P. De Vreese, M. Neri, M. Fioravanti, L. Belloi, and O. Zanetti, "Memory rehabilitation in Alzheimer's disease: a review of progress," *International Journal of Geriatric Psychiatry*, vol. 16, no. 8, pp. 794–809, 2001.

[71] D. A. Cahn-Weiner, P. F. Malloy, G. W. Rebok, and B. R. Ott, "Results of a randomized placebo-controlled study of memory training for mildly impaired Alzheimer's disease patients," *Applied Neuropsychology*, vol. 10, no. 4, pp. 215–223, 2003.

[72] E. Farina, F. Mantovani, R. Fioravanti et al., "Evaluating two group programmes of cognitive training in mild-to-moderate AD: is there any difference between a "global" stimulation and a "cognitive-specific" one?" *Aging and Mental Health*, vol. 10, no. 3, pp. 211–218, 2006.

[73] H. MacRae, "Self and other: the importance of social interaction and social relationships in shaping the experience of early-stage Alzheimer's disease," *Journal of Aging Studies*, vol. 25, pp. 445–456, 2011.

[74] L. Fratiglioni, S. Paillard-Borg, and B. Winblad, "An active and socially integrated lifestyle in late life might protect against dementia," *The Lancet Neurology*, vol. 3, no. 6, pp. 343–353, 2004.

[75] K. H. Pitkala, P. Routasalo, H. Kautiainen, H. Sintonen, and R. S. Tilvis, "Effects of socially stimulating group intervention on lonely, older people's cognition: a randomized, controlled trial," *American Journal of Geriatric Psychiatry*, vol. 19, no. 7, pp. 654–663, 2011.

[76] R. S. Wilson, K. R. Krueger, S. E. Arnold et al., "Loneliness and risk of Alzheimer disease," *Archives of General Psychiatry*, vol. 64, no. 2, pp. 234–240, 2007.

[77] H. X. Wang, A. Karp, B. Winblad, and L. Fratiglioni, "Late-life engagement in social and leisure activities is associated with a decreased risk of dementia: a longitudinal study from the Kungsholmen Project," *American Journal of Epidemiology*, vol. 155, no. 12, pp. 1081–1087, 2002.

[78] R. P. Friedland, T. Fritsch, K. A. Smyth et al., "Patients with Alzheimer's disease have reduced activities in midlife compared with healthy control-group members," *Proceedings of the National Academy of Sciences of the United States of America*, vol. 98, no. 6, pp. 3440–3445, 2001.

[79] D. A. Bennett, J. A. Schneider, Y. Tang, S. E. Arnold, and R. S. Wilson, "The effect of social networks on the relation between Alzheimer's disease pathology and level of cognitive function in old people: a longitudinal cohort study," *The Lancet Neurology*, vol. 5, no. 5, pp. 406–412, 2006.

[80] L. Fratiglioni, H. X. Wang, K. Ericsson, M. Maytan, and B. Winblad, "Influence of social network on occurrence of dementia: a community-based longitudinal study," *The Lancet*, vol. 355, no. 9212, pp. 1315–1319, 2000.

[81] H. H. Keller, L. S. Martin, S. Dupuis, R. Genoe, H. G. Edward, and C. Cassolato, "Mealtimes and being connected in the community-based dementia context," *Dementia*, vol. 9, no. 2, pp. 191–213, 2010.

[82] R. G. Logsdon, S. M. McCurry, and L. Teri, "Evidence-based interventions to improve quality of life for individuals with dementia," *Alzheimer's Care Today*, vol. 8, no. 4, pp. 309–318, 2007.

[83] R. G. Logsdon, K. C. Pike, S. M. McCurry et al., "Early-stage memory loss support groups: outcomes from a randomized controlled clinical trial," *Journals of Gerontology*, vol. 65, no. 6, pp. 691–697, 2010.

[84] M. S. Mittelman, S. H. Ferris, E. Shulman et al., "A comprehensive support program: effect on depression in spouse-caregivers of AD patients," *Gerontologist*, vol. 35, no. 6, pp. 792–802, 1995.

[85] M. S. Mittelman, C. Epstein, and A. Pierzchala, *Counselling the Alzheimer's Caregiver: A Resource for Health Care Professionals*, American Medical Association, Chicago, Ill, USA, 2001.

[86] M. S. Mittelman, D. L. Roth, D. W. Coon, and W. E. Haley, "Sustained benefit of supportive intervention for depressive symptoms in caregivers of patients with Alzheimer's disease," *American Journal of Psychiatry*, vol. 161, no. 5, pp. 850–856, 2004.

[87] F. G. M. Coelho, L. P. Andrade, R. V. Pedroso et al., "Multimodal exercise intervention improves frontal cognitive functions and gait in Alzheimer's disease: a controlled trial," *Geriatriatrics and Gerontolology International*. In press.

[88] S. Arkin, "Language-enriched exercise plus socialization slows cognitive decline in Alzheimer's disease," *American Journal of Alzheimer's Disease and other Dementias*, vol. 22, no. 1, pp. 62–77, 2007.

[89] S. C. Burgener, Y. Yang, R. Gilbert, and S. Marsh-Yant, "The effects of a multimodal intervention on outcomes of persons with early-stage dementia," *American Journal of Alzheimer's Disease and other Dementias*, vol. 23, no. 4, pp. 382–394, 2008.

[90] T. Maci, F. Le Pira, G. Quattrocch, S. Di Nuovo, V. Percialvalle, and M. Zappia, "Physical and cognitive stimulation in Alzheimer disease. The GAIA Project: a pilot study," *American Journal of Alzheimers Disease and other Dementias*, vol. 27, no. 2, pp. 107–113, 2012.

11

Effects of Periodic Task-Specific Test Feedback on Physical Performance in Older Adults Undertaking Band-Based Resistance Exercise

Ryuichi Hasegawa,[1] Mohammod Monirul Islam,[2] Ryuji Watanabe,[3] Naoki Tomiyama,[4] and Dennis R. Taaffe[5]

[1] *Department of Occupational Therapy, College of Life and Health Sciences, Chubu University, 1200, Matsumoto, Kasugai, Aichi 487-8501, Japan*
[2] *Department of Rehabilitation, Yonaha General Hospital, 8-264-3 Izumi, Kuwana, Mie 511-0838, Japan*
[3] *Department of Rehabilitation, Tsushima City Hospital, 3-73 Tsubaki, Tsushima, Aichi 496-8537, Japan*
[4] *Division of Occupational Therapy, Faculty of Care and Rehabilitation, Seijoh University, 2-172 Fukinodai, Tokai, Aichi 476-8588, Japan*
[5] *School of Environmental and Life Sciences, The University of Newcastle, 10 Chittaway Road, Ourimbah, NSW 2258, Australia*

Correspondence should be addressed to Ryuichi Hasegawa; ryuichi@isc.chubu.ac.jp

Academic Editor: Barbara Shukitt-Hale

The purpose of this study was to determine the effects of periodic task-specific test feedback on performance improvement in older adults undertaking community- and home-based resistance exercises (CHBRE). Fifty-two older adults (65–83 years) were assigned to a muscular perfsormance feedback group (MPG, n = 32) or a functional mobility feedback group (FMG, n = 20). Both groups received exactly the same 9-week CHBRE program comprising one community-based and two home-based sessions per week. Muscle performance included arm curls and chair stands in 30 seconds, while functional mobility was determined by the timed up and go (TUG) test. MPG received fortnightly test feedback only on muscle performance and FMG received feedback only on the TUG. Following training, there was a significant ($P < 0.05$) interaction for all performance tests with MPG improving more for the arm curls (MPG 31.4%, FMG 15.9%) and chair stands (MPG 33.7%, FMG 24.9%) while FMG improved more for the TUG (MPG-3.5%, FMG-9.7%). Results from this nonrandomized study suggest that periodic test feedback during resistance training may enhance task-specific physical performance in older persons, thereby augmenting reserve capacity or potentially reducing the time required to recover functional abilities.

1. Introduction

Functional fitness not only accounts for the traditional physical fitness parameters such as muscle strength, cardiorespiratory endurance, and flexibility, but also includes balance [1]. However, it is well known that, with age, functional fitness declines [2], resulting in a reduced ability to perform activities such as rising from a chair or climbing stairs, which can be viewed as functional components of activities of daily living (ADL) performance, and may eventually compromise the ability to perform ADL [3–5]. In addition, approximately a third of community-dwelling older adults fall at least once a year, and over 30% of fallers suffer injuries requiring medical attention [6]. Strategies to prevent or attenuate the decline in physical function and balance are important for promoting independence in the elderly and thereby enhancing quality of life.

Research over the past two decades clearly shows that regular physical exercise is effective for maintaining and promoting health, physical fitness, and functional independence in older adults, especially in terms of endurance, muscular strength, flexibility, and balance [7]. Physical training programs can be undertaken in the clinic, commercial fitness centers or gymnasiums, in the community or at home. In contrast to clinic and gym-based exercise, community- and home-based exercise does not require special facilities or expensive equipment. Moreover, community- and home-based exercise is capable of reaching a broad audience and, importantly, the community setting provides an opportunity for social contact and support which may have an array of benefits, especially for those living in regional and rural settings [8]. In order to maximize compliance to community- and home-based programs, exercises should be simple, combined with appropriate equipment and personal support. Thus, community- and home-based exercises have become increasingly popular as an alternative to gym-based resistance exercise [9].

Providing feedback and prompting have been shown to be effective in increasing and maintaining physical activity as well as other positive health behaviors [10]. Moreover, feedback may also enhance the exercise response which may prove valuable in enhancing recovery of functional abilities after injury or illness [11, 12]. However, a paucity of information is currently available regarding the effects of feedback on muscular performance and functional mobility improvement in older adults undertaking resistance training in the community- and home-based setting. Hasegawa and Tomiyama have previously reported, that in middle-aged and older persons participating in a community- and home-based setting, periodic feedback enhanced muscle performance compared to those not receiving feedback [13]. Consequently, the purpose of this study was to confirm and extend these findings by examining the effects of periodic task-specific test feedback on not only muscle performance but also functional mobility in older adults undertaking resistance training with elastic bands in the community- and home-based setting.

2. Materials and Methods

2.1. Subjects. In response to a public relations magazine advertisement, 80 older adults from Tokai city, Aichi prefecture, Japan, volunteered to participate in the study. Inclusion criteria were ≥65 years of age, community residing, functionally independent, and able to perform physical exercise. Participants were excluded if they had been advised by their physician to refrain from exercise. Prior to acceptance into the study, a brief health examination was performed by an occupational therapist and questionnaires regarding medical history were completed. Current presence of disease was determined using self-reported physician-diagnosed disease information. Two persons were found medically unfit due to uncontrolled hypertension and cardiac arrhythmia. Three others were excluded from the study because they had scheduling conflicts, transportation issues, or no further interest in joining the study.

The remaining 75 participants (65 to 83 years) were included in this study. They were divided into a muscular performance feedback group (MPG) or a functional mobility feedback group (FMG) by their residential area (the two groups were from two separate communities within the same city). The two residential areas had similar living standards and socioeconomic status. Both groups participated in an identical 9-week community- and home-based resistance exercise program. All participants were asked to not alter their diet or physical activity patterns for the duration of the study. All measurements were performed before and after the 9-week program in 52 participants. Twenty-three participants did not complete follow-up measures due to travel-related reasons ($n = 18$) and medically-related problems (low back pain, $n = 2$; dizziness, $n = 1$; upper respiratory tract infection, $n = 2$). Regarding baseline characteristics, there was no difference between those who dropped out and those who completed the study within each group for age, weight or any functional fitness measure, with the only difference being in the MPG with more women than men dropping out (due to travel) and hence height of those who dropped out was lower than those who completed.

A flowchart of the study participants is provided in Figure 1. The ethics committee of Seijoh University approved the study and all participants provided written informed consent.

2.2. Exercise Program. Instruction and progression of the exercise routine occurred at a community center once per week and participants were asked to exercise an additional two times each week at home. The community-based exercise sessions consisted of 15 min of warmup, 60 min of resistance exercise, and 15 min of cooldown. The exercise sessions were supervised by experienced instructors. Pictorial guidebooks were provided to all participants in order to assist them to perform the exercises correctly. The home-based exercise program also consisted of the same resistance and stretching exercises. Participants were asked to record exercises they performed and submit a diary every week while attending the exercise classes.

2.2.1. Resistance Exercise. In order to train all major muscle groups, resistance exercises were prescribed as a combination of 3 upper body exercises, 6 lower body exercises, and 2 trunk exercises performed using an elastic resistance band (Thera-Band, Hygenic, USA). Each type of exercise was performed for 1 set of 12 repetitions per session [14]. Exertion was rated using Borg's rate of perceived exertion (RPE) scale [15, 16]. Participants were instructed to start resistance exercises at an intensity level of 13 on the RPE scale and then to progressively increase resistance to a level of 15 to 17. Participants were instructed to progressively increase resistance every two to four weeks by advancing to the next color of elastic band (lower to higher resistance of bands in order: red, green, and blue) or shortening the initial length of the band for increased resistance (Figure 2).

2.2.2. Stretching Exercise as Warmup and Cooldown. Stretching exercises consisted of eight upper body exercises and seven lower body exercises. The exercises were performed slowly and each position was held for 20 seconds. The

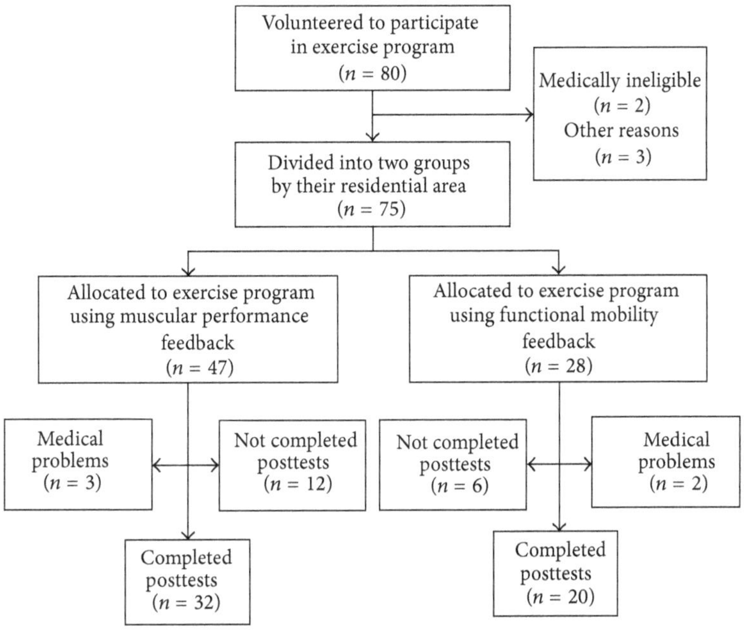

FIGURE 1: Flowchart tracking participants throughout the trial.

participants were asked to stretch to the point where they felt moderate tension without feeling pain in joints or muscles.

2.3. Feedback. Fortnightly assessments were performed by testers for three performance tests: arm curls, chair stands in 30 seconds, and the timed up and go (TUG) test. Task specific feedback, which is extrinsic or augmented information provided to a performer in regard to a specific task with the goal to enhance future performance of that task [17], was provided by the testers (not instructors) who were blinded to the participant's previous results. MPG received immediate test feedback (verbal and written) only on the arm curls and chair stand test while FMG received immediate feedback only for the TUG. Participants recorded their results on individual record sheets. In addition to the participant's results for the respective tests (muscle performance or balance), verbal feedback from the tester included statements (in front of other participants) such as "you have improved in your performance and it shows in your current score" and "keep up the exercise and you are going to improve your performance." All measurements were performed by the same tester.

2.4. Study Measures. Anthropometrics, physical symptoms by questionnaire, muscle performance, and functional mobility were evaluated at baseline and followup. Participant's height and weight were assessed and body mass index (BMI) was calculated as body weight (kg) divided by the square of height (m).

2.4.1. Measurement of Muscular Performance. Upper body muscle performance was assessed using the 30-second arm curl test (arm curl) [18, 19]. On a signal, participants were instructed to flex and extend the elbow of the dominant hand, lifting a weight dumbbell (men: 8-lbs [3.6 kg], women: 5-lbs [2.3 kg]) through the complete range of motion, as many times as possible in 30 seconds. A practice trial of one or two repetitions was given, followed by two test trials. The score was the number of repetitions completed with the best performance used for analysis.

Lower body muscle performance was assessed using the 30-second chair stand test [18, 19]. The participant's arms were crossed at the wrists and held against the chest. On a signal, participants rose to a standing position from a chair and then returned to a seated position and continued to complete as many full stands as possible in 30 seconds. A practice trial of one or two repetitions was given, followed by two test trials. The score was the total number of stands executed correctly with the best performance used for analysis.

2.4.2. Measurement of Functional Mobility. Functional mobility was assessed using the 8-foot timed up and go (TUG) test [18–20]. Participants sat in a chair with their hands on their thighs and feet flat on the floor. On a signal, participants stood from the chair without pushing off with the arms, walked as quickly as possible around a cone placed 8-feet (2.44 m) ahead of the chair, and returned to a fully seated position in the chair. Participants were instructed to walk as quickly as possible without running. Participants walked through the test one time as a practice and then were given two test trials with the best performance time used for analysis.

2.5. Statistical Analysis. Data were analyzed using the PASW statistics 18 software package (SPSS Inc., Chicago, IL, USA). Comparisons between MPG and FMG at baseline were performed using an independent Student's t-test or Chi-square test as appropriate. The effect of the intervention was determined using a repeated measures analysis of covariance

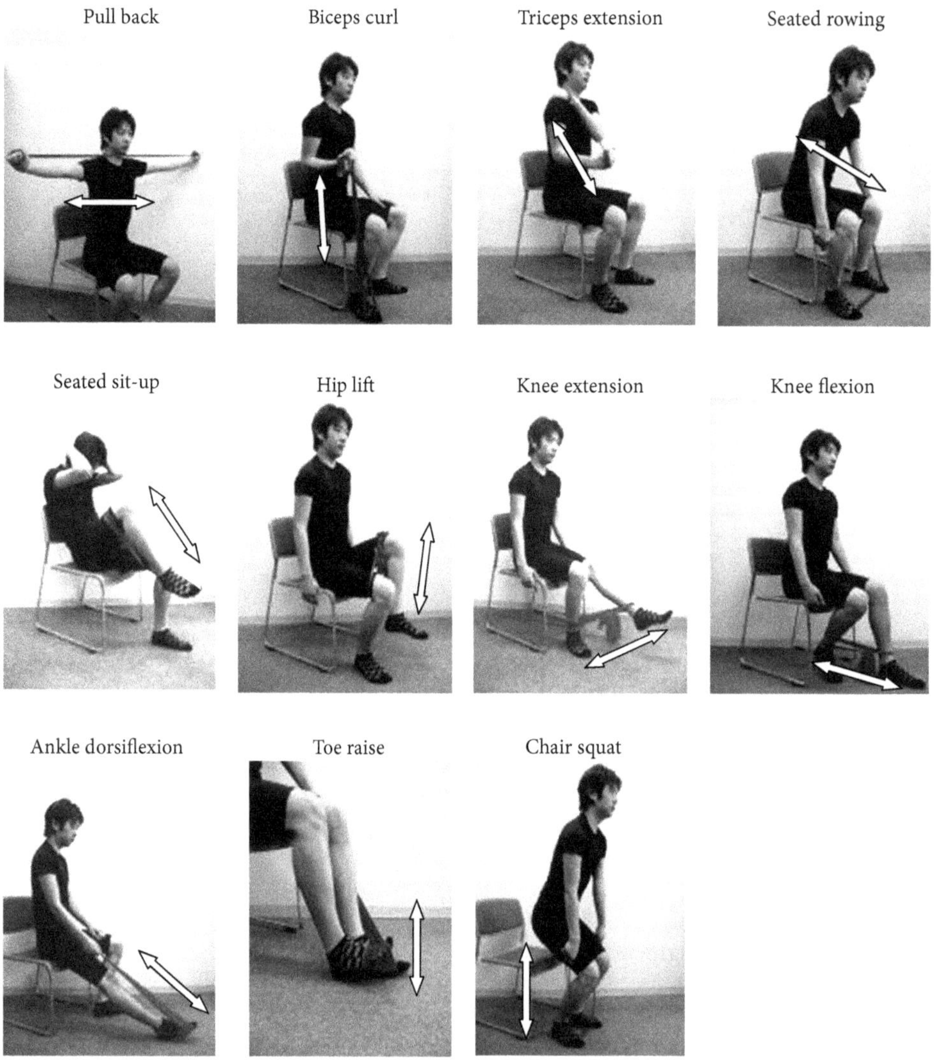

FIGURE 2: Resistance exercises undertaken in the community- and home-based setting. The resistance training program consisted of exercises that used an elastic resistance band (Thera-Band, Hygenic, USA). Each type of exercise was performed for 12 repetitions/session. Exertion was rated using Borg's rate of perceived exertion (RPE) scale.

(ANCOVA) adjusted for gender and within group changes by a paired t-test. All tests were two tailed and a P value of less than 0.05 was considered statistically significant. Values reported are the mean ± SD.

3. Results

3.1. Pretraining Data. There were no differences between groups at baseline for age, height, weight, and prevalent disease (Table 1) or muscle performance and functional mobility (Table 2).

3.2. Training Data. The average adherence rates in the exercise class at the community center were 92 ± 13% for MPG and 87 ± 12% for FMG. Both groups performed home-based exercises in addition to community-based classes for a total of 2.7 ± 1.3 days/week in MPG and 2.1 ± 1.0 days/week in FMG. No differences were observed between the two groups in adherence or home-based training frequency (Table 1). There were no accidents or injuries during the exercise classes at the community center or at home.

There was a significant group × time interaction for the arm curl (F = 15.2) and chair stand test (F = 5.2) with MPG improving more than FMG, while FMG improved more than MPG for the TUG (F = 4.1) (Table 2). In the MPG, the muscle performance measures for the arm curl and chair stand test increased by 31.4% (P = 0.001) and 33.7% ($P < 0.001$), respectively, while TUG performance time was reduced by 3.5% ($P < 0.001$). In the FMG, arm curl and chair stand test significantly increased by 15.9% ($P < 0.001$) and 24.9% ($P < 0.001$), respectively, while time to perform the TUG was reduced by 9.7% ($P = 0.049$).

4. Discussion

Maintaining or enhancing muscle performance and functional mobility in older persons is critical for undertaking

TABLE 1: Participant characteristics (mean ± SD).

Variables	Muscle performance feedback group	Functional mobility feedback group	P values
No. of participants	32	20	
Demographic			
Gender (men/women)†	16/16	5/15	0.09
Age (years)‡	71.4 ± 4.3	73.7 ± 5.5	0.10
Anthropometrics			
Height (cm)‡	155.4 ± 6.8	152.1 ± 7.5	0.11
Weight (kg)‡	56.7 ± 9.0	55.5 ± 8.5	0.63
BMI (kg/m^2)‡	23.4 ± 3.0	24.0 ± 3.2	0.53
Prevalent disease [number (%)]			
Hypertension†	8 (25%)	9 (45%)	0.14
Knee osteoarthritis†	8 (25%)	5 (25%)	1.00
Diabetes mellitus†	4 (13%)	3 (15%)	0.55
Heart disease†	4 (13%)	3 (15%)	0.55
Osteoporosis†	2 (6%)	1 (5%)	0.67
Compliance of exercise			
Adherence at community center (%)‡	92.0 ± 13.0	87.2 ± 12.1	0.11
Frequency (days/week)‡	2.7 ± 1.3	2.1 ± 1.0	0.19

Note: BMI: body mass index.
No significant differences at baseline were present between groups for all indexes.
†χ^2 test was used to evaluate differences between the groups.
‡Student's t-test was used to evaluate the difference between the groups.

daily activities and for sustaining an appropriate quality of life. In the current study, we found significant improvements in muscle performance and functional mobility following a 9-week community- and home-based exercise regimen undertaken with elastic bands. Importantly, gains were partly dependent on fortnightly test feedback suggesting that this is an important component of the training session in order to maximize gains resulting from the program.

The muscular performance results are in agreement with other studies that have used elastic bands in a community setting. Bohlken et al. reported significant increases of 16% in arm curl and 18% in chair stand performance in older women who participated in a 12-week exercise program (3 d/wk) using elastic bands [21]. Similarly, a 23% and 19% increase in arm curl and chair stand performance, respectively, was reported by Rogers et al. who enrolled older women in a 4-week (3 d/wk) elastic band resistance exercise program [22]. However, gains resulting from home-based programs may not be of the same magnitude as that of supervised gym- or community-based programs with Yamauchi et al. reporting improvements of 18% in the arm curl test and only 6% in the chair stand test for older adults following 12 weeks of a home-based exercise program [9].

In the current study, the FMG had an average improvement for the arm curl test of 16%, which is comparable to other studies with a similar training period. However, the MPG improvement on this task was double that of the FMG with gains of 31%. These results suggest that task-specific feedback of serial testing may be an effective strategy to enhance performance in older persons. For the chair stand test, there was also a significant difference between the two feedback groups with the task-specific group enhancing their performance by ~34% while the FMG increased by ~25%. Moreover, the results in MPG were higher than previous studies with comparable training programs [9, 21, 22]. The improvements in the chair stand test are particularly important given the role that lower body muscle performance, as does balance, plays in maintaining physical function.

Similarly, for the timed up and go test, which was used to assess functional mobility in our cohort, improvement was greater for the FMG who decreased their performance time by ~10% whereas the MPG experienced a reduction of only 3.5%. This suggests that improvements in functional mobility are also associated with the use of feedback in older persons.

These results indicate that the magnitude of improvement in muscular function and functional mobility are associated with the feedback provided and would be beneficial to older persons in order to maximize program-related gains. The importance of data feedback has been previously described by Mihalko et al. who reported that individual fitness feedback influences exercise attendance [23]. Positive feedback is effective in intensifying competence [24]. In addition, it is suggested that relatedness is intensified in group work and exercise programs in which the participant's interaction is increased [25]. Moreover, Bourbonnais et al. reported that treatment of the lower limb in stroke patients based on muscle force-feedback produced an improvement in gait velocity [26], while feedback has also been found to improve pelvic floor muscle training in those with urinary incontinence [27]. In athletes, providing verbal feedback has been associated with a modest enhancement in muscle performance [28] and tuck-jump performance [29], although not in time trial cycling [30]. Our results reinforce the importance of providing feedback if serial performance assessments are undertaken.

Feedback can be classified as either "intrinsic" or "extrinsic" with task-specific feedback categorized as knowledge of results [16]. Indeed, the observations of Leventthal have documented the importance of providing relevant information in order to encourage an action [31]. It may well be that awareness of muscular performance or functional mobility improvement and the encouragement provided by the tester (in delivering the feedback in a face-to-face situation) enhanced the participant's self-efficacy [32] for these respective tasks and their intrinsic motivation [33, 34] and this contributed to task-specific performance differences in the MPG and FMG. In addition, the feedback may have reinforced or enhanced the participant's goal-setting which in turn enhanced their intrinsic motivation [35]. The finding that feedback of performance may have increased motivation is consistent with previous literature and cognitive evaluation theory [36] which proposes that, when feelings of competence are enhanced, motivation increases.

Table 2: Improvements in muscle performance and functional mobility.

	Muscle performance feedback group			Functional mobility feedback group			Interaction (F ratio)
	Pre	Post	% Change	Pre	Post	% Change	
Muscle performance							
Arm curl (reps/30 sec.)	21.6 ± 2.7	28.4 ± 3.6	31.4%$^{\$}$	20.7 ± 3.0	24.0 ± 3.7	15.9%$^{\$}$	15.2*
Chair stand (reps/30 sec.)	20.2 ± 2.4	27.0 ± 4.2	33.7%$^{\$}$	18.9 ± 5.1	23.6 ± 5.1	24.9%$^{\$}$	5.2*
Functional mobility							
Timed up & go (sec)#	4.87 ± 0.57	4.70 ± 0.50	−3.5%$^{\$}$	5.18 ± 1.00	4.68 ± 0.78	−9.7%$^{\$}$	4.1*

Note: Values are mean ± SD.
Pre: baseline; post: after the 9-week exercise program.
No significant differences at baseline were present between groups for all indexes.
#Improvement on test results in a negative value.
*Analysis of covariance (ANCOVA) significant group by time interaction, $P < 0.05$.
$^{\$}$Paired t-test, $P < 0.05$.

Motivating older adults to perform exercises on a regular basis is an important factor in maintaining the effects of exercise [9]. In the current study, we held community-based exercise classes once a week in addition to the home-based exercise program 2 days per week. The adherence to the community-based classes was over 85% and the frequency of the community- and home-based exercise was over 2 days per week. This finding of frequency meets the current guidelines for resistance exercise [12]. Most participants mentioned that they were glad to make new friends and enjoyed exercising as a group in the community setting. This supports previous findings [37] that community-based exercise classes have positive psychological effects as well as physical effects on community-dwelling older adults. After completion of this 9-week program, participants continued to exercise and currently attend exercise classes twice a month. Enhanced self-efficacy resulting from participation may be one factor that contributed to the participation rates during the study period as well as with the participation postintervention [32].

There are several limitations of the study which are worthy of comment. Given the homogeneity of participants in the study (age, socioeconomic status, and geographical location), caution should be taken when extrapolating our results to all older community-dwelling persons. Moreover, the participants were not randomized to the treatment conditions as it was not possible to blind participants to the exercise program, leaving them vulnerable to a variety of tester and subject effects that may influence test results and introduce bias in our findings. Our program was also of a relatively short-term nature and it is unclear if differences based on feedback would exist with a longer program, such as 6 or 12 months. Nevertheless, our results show, even within a relatively short training period, that task-specific test feedback appears to have a beneficial effect in enhancing physical performance, and, regardless of the underlying mechanism for the improvement, this is an important practical outcome for those involved in the exercise training of older persons. A future direction would be in determining if task-specific feedback is a valuable strategy to enhance performance in those disabled or recovering from illness/disease or injury. In addition, a more extensive test battery could be employed to measure additional aspects of functional and ambulatory ability. Lastly, it would be of interest to determine if performance was enhanced by motivation, whether it was motivation to train harder or to perform the tests or to the combination.

5. Conclusion

This study was designed to determine the efficacy of test performance feedback to improve muscle performance and functional mobility in older adults. Following the 9-week community- and home-based intervention, a significant interaction was noted for the muscle performance and functional mobility tests suggesting that periodic test feedback during resistance training may enhance task-specific physical performance in older persons. Providing regular feedback on test performance in the community and, if possible, the home exercise setting may facilitate gains in muscle and balance performance resulting in enhanced physical function and a greater safety margin for functional thresholds.

Conflict of Interests

The authors declare that there is no conflict of interests regarding the publication of this paper.

Acknowledgments

The authors wish to thank the participants for their involvement in this study. This work was supported by grants from Seijoh University in Japan.

References

[1] R. E. Rikli and C. J. Jones, "Functional fitness normative scores for community-residing older adults, ages 60–94," *Journal of Aging and Physical Activity*, vol. 7, no. 2, pp. 162–181, 1999.

[2] V. A. Freedman, L. G. Martin, and R. F. Schoeni, "Recent trends in disability and functioning among older adults in the United States: a systematic review," *Journal of the American Medical Association*, vol. 288, no. 24, pp. 3137–3146, 2002.

[3] K. Y. Z. Forrest, J. M. Zmuda, and J. A. Cauley, "Correlates of decline in lower extremity performance in older women: a 10-year follow-up study," *Journals of Gerontology A*, vol. 61, no. 11, pp. 1194–1200, 2006.

[4] R. S. Lindle, E. J. Metter, N. A. Lynch et al., "Age and gender comparisons of muscle strength in 654 women and men aged 20–93 yr," *Journal of Applied Physiology*, vol. 83, no. 5, pp. 1581–1587, 1997.

[5] T. Rantanen, K. Avlund, H. Suominen, M. Schroll, K. Frändin, and E. Pertti, "Muscle strength as a predictor of onset of ADL dependence in people aged 75 years," *Aging Clinical and Experimental Research*, vol. 14, no. 3, pp. 10–15, 2002.

[6] R. Orr, "Contribution of muscle weakness to postural instability in the elderly. A systematic review," *European Journal of Physical and Rehabilitation Medicine*, vol. 46, no. 2, pp. 183–220, 2010.

[7] M. E. Nelson, W. J. Rejeski, S. N. Blair et al., "Physical activity and public health in older adults: recommendation from the American College of Sports Medicine and the American Heart Association," *Medicine and Science in Sports and Exercise*, vol. 39, no. 8, pp. 1435–1445, 2007.

[8] D. E. Gillis, M. D. Grossman, B. Y. McLellan, A. C. King, and A. L. Stewart, "Participants' evaluations of components of a physical-activity-promotion program for seniors (CHAMPS II)," *Journal of Aging and Physical Activity*, vol. 10, no. 3, pp. 336–353, 2002.

[9] T. Yamauchi, M. M. Islam, D. Koizumi, M. E. Rogers, N. L. Rogers, and N. Takeshima, "Effect of home-based well-rounded exercise in community-dwelling older adults," *Journal of Sports Science and Medicine*, vol. 4, no. 4, pp. 563–571, 2005.

[10] B. Rooney, T. Hooks, K. Baciak, S. Havens, and H. Gilles, "Minutes in motion: motivating a community to move," *Wisconsin Medical Journal*, vol. 107, no. 3, pp. 118–123, 2008.

[11] B. H. Marcus and L. H. Forsyth, *Motivating People to Be Physically Active*, Human Kinetics, Champaign, Ill, USA, 2003.

[12] American College of Sports Medicine, *ACSM's Guidelines for Exercise Testing and Prescription*, Lippincott Williams and Wilkins, Philadelphia, Pa, USA, 8th edition, 2009.

[13] R. Hasegawa and N. Tomiyama, "Data feedback to participants strengthen the efficacy of resistance exercise in community-dwelling older adults," *The Journal of Japanese Association of Occupational Therapist*, vol. 29, no. 4, pp. 488–498, 2010 (Japanese).

[14] M. S. Feigenbaum and M. L. Pollock, "Strength training: rationale for current guidelines for adult fitness programs," *The Physician and Sportsmedicine*, vol. 25, no. 2, pp. 44–63, 1997.

[15] G. A. V. Borg, "Psychophysical bases of perceived exertion," *Medicine and Science in Sports and Exercise*, vol. 14, no. 5, pp. 377–381, 1982.

[16] B. S. Row, K. M. Knutzen, and N. J. Skogsberg, "Regulating explosive resistance training intensity using the rating of perceived exertion," *Journal of Strength and Conditioning Research*, vol. 26, no. 3, pp. 664–671, 2012.

[17] A. W. Salmoni, R. A. Schmidt, and C. B. Walter, "Knowledge of results and motor learning: a review and critical reappraisal," *Psychological Bulletin*, vol. 95, no. 3, pp. 355–386, 1984.

[18] R. E. Rikli and C. J. Jones, "Development and validation of a functional fitness test for community-residing older adults," *Journal of Aging and Physical Activity*, vol. 7, no. 2, pp. 129–161, 1999.

[19] N. Takeshima, N. L. Rogers, M. E. Rogers, M. M. Islam, D. Koizumi, and S. Lee, "Functional fitness gain varies in older adults depending on exercise mode," *Medicine and Science in Sports and Exercise*, vol. 39, no. 11, pp. 2036–2043, 2007.

[20] D. Podsiadlo and S. Richardson, "The timed "Up and Go": a test of basic functional mobility for frail elderly persons," *Journal of the American Geriatrics Society*, vol. 39, no. 2, pp. 142–148, 1991.

[21] R. M. Bohlken, M. E. Rogers, J. D. F. Shores, N. L. Rogers, and L. R. Sporleder, "Effects of a community-based intervention using elastic bands on strength in older adults," *Medicine & Science in Sports & Exercise*, vol. 34, no. 5, p. S75, 2002.

[22] M. E. Rogers, H. S. Sherwood, N. L. Rogers, and R. M. Bohlken, "Effects of dumbbell and elastic band training on physical function in older inner-city African-American women," *Women and Health*, vol. 36, no. 4, pp. 33–41, 2002.

[23] S. L. Mihalko, K. L. Wickley, and B. L. Sharpe, "Promoting activity in independent living communities," *Medicine and Science in Sports and Exercise*, vol. 38, no. 1, pp. 112–115, 2006.

[24] J. B. Allen and B. L. Howe, "Player ability, coach feedback, and female adolescent athletes' perceived competence and satisfaction," *Journal of Sport and Exercise Psychology*, vol. 20, no. 3, pp. 280–299, 1998.

[25] H. Matsumoto and K. Takenaka, "Motivational profiles and stages of exercise behavior change," *International Journal of Sport and Health Science*, vol. 2, pp. 89–96, 2004.

[26] D. Bourbonnais, S. Bilodeau, Y. Lepage, N. Beaudoin, D. Gravel, and R. Forget, "Effect of force-feedback treatments in patients with chronic motor deficits after a stroke," *The American Journal of Physical Medicine and Rehabilitation*, vol. 81, no. 12, pp. 890–897, 2002.

[27] R. Herderschee, E. J. C. Hay-Smith, G. P. Herbison, J. P. Roovers, and M. J. Heineman, "Feedback or biofeedback to augment pelvic floor muscle training for urinary incontinence in women," *Cochrane Database of Systematic Reviews*, no. 7, Article ID CD009252, 2011.

[28] C. K. Argus, N. D. Gill, J. W. L. Keogh, and W. G. Hopkins, "Acute effects of verbal feedback on upper-body performance in elite athletes," *Journal of Strength and Conditioning Research*, vol. 25, no. 12, pp. 3282–3287, 2011.

[29] B. W. Stroube, G. D. Myer, J. L. Brent, K. R. Ford, R. S. Jr. Heidt, and T. E. Hewett, "Effects of task-specific augmented feedback on deficit modification during performance of the tuck-jump exercise," *Journal of Sport Rehabilitation*, vol. 22, no. 1, pp. 7–18, 2013.

[30] C. A. Williams, S. D. Bailey, and A. R. Mauger, "External exercise information provides no immediate additional performance benefit to untrained individuals in time trial cycling," *British Journal of Sports Medicine*, vol. 46, no. 1, pp. 49–53, 2012.

[31] H. Leventhal, "Fear communications in the acceptance of preventive health practices," *Bulletin of the New York Academy of Medicine*, vol. 41, no. 11, pp. 1144–1168, 1965.

[32] A. Bandura, "Self-efficacy: the foundation of agency," in *Control of Human Behavior, Mental Processes and Consciousness*, W. J. Perrig and A. Grob, Eds., Erlbaum, Mahwah, NJ, USA, 2000.

[33] R. J. Vallerand, "The effect of differential amounts of positive verbal feedback on the intrinsic motivation of male hockey players," *Journal of Sport Psychology*, vol. 5, no. 1, pp. 100–107, 1983.

[34] A. Mouratidis, M. Vansteenkiste, W. Lens, and G. Sideridis, "The motivating role of positive feedback in sport and physical education: evidence for a motivational model," *Journal of Sport and Exercise Psychology*, vol. 30, no. 2, pp. 240–258, 2008.

[35] R. S. Weinberg and D. Gould, *Foundations of Sport and Exercise Psychology*, Human Kinetics, Champaign, Ill, USA, 5th edition, 2011.

[36] E. L. Deci and R. M. Ryan, *Intrinsic Motivation and Self-Determination in Human Behavior*, Springer, New York, NY, USA, 1985.

[37] T. Yamauchi, T. Yamada, M. M. Islam, A. Okada, T. Takahashi, and N. Takeshima, "Effects of well-rounded exercise program on overall fitness in older outpatients," *Japanese Journal of Physical Fitness and Sports Medicine*, vol. 52, no. 5, pp. 513–523, 2003.

12

Effects of Resistance Training on Immunoinflammatory Response, TNF-Alpha Gene Expression, and Body Composition in Elderly Women

Luís Ângelo Macêdo Santiago,[1] Lídio Gonçalves Lima Neto,[2] Guilherme Borges Pereira,[3] Richard Diego Leite,[4] Cristiano Texeira Mostarda,[5] Janaina de Oliveira Brito Monzani,[5] Wandson Rodrigues Sousa,[6] Aruanã Joaquim Matheus Rodrigues Pinheiro,[2] and Francisco Navarro[5]

[1]*Department of Medicine, Federal University of Maranhão (UFMA), Pinheiro, MA, Brazil*
[2]*Laboratory of Immunology and Microbiology of Respiratory Infections, LAMIR, Universidade CEUMA, São Luis, MA, Brazil*
[3]*Undergraduate Program in Physical Education at the Catholic University of Brasilia, Brasília, Brazil*
[4]*Department of Physical Education, Federal University of Espírito Santo (UFES), Vitória, ES, Brazil*
[5]*Department of Physical Education, Federal University of Maranhão (UFMA), São Luis, MA, Brazil*
[6]*Postgraduate Program in Adult and Child Health, PPGSAC, UFMA, São Luis, MA, Brazil*

Correspondence should be addressed to Luís Ângelo Macêdo Santiago; luisangelomacedo@gmail.com

Academic Editor: Jean-Francois Grosset

The aim of this study was to determine the effects of resistance training on the immunologic response, body composition, tumor necrosis factor-alpha (TNF-alpha) gene expression obtained from blood leukocytes, and the cytokines interleukin-6, TNF-alpha, and C-reactive protein (CRP), in the elderly women (mean age 63 ± 2 y). A randomized controlled trial was performed using a bi-set training method for eight weeks in nineteen elderly women. Peripheral blood samples were collected by puncture in pre-training (Pre) and posttraining (Post) moments. In the resistance training group, there was a statistically significant decrease from 38.43 ± 9.48 pg/mL to 11.76 ± 5.19 pg/mL ($p = 0.01$) in the serum levels of interleukin-6. Considering serum levels of TNF-alpha, there was a statistically significant difference, comparing the resistance training group at Pre (66.27 ± 10.31 pg/mL) and Post (37.85 ± 9.05 pg/mL) moments ($p = 0.01$). In molecular analysis of TNF-alpha gene expression, there was a statistically significant decrease ($p = 0.007$) between Pre (0.010 ± 0.01 ng/ml) and Post (0.0002 ± 0.0001 ng/ml) moments. Among CRP data, in the resistance training group, there was a statistically significant reduction, between Pre (2.04 ± 0.32 mg/L) and Post (0.90 ± 0.22 mg/L) moments ($p = 0.001$). In the Control group, there was no statistical significance between these two moments. Therefore, the resistance training demonstrated changes in the TNF-alpha gene expression in elderly women, as well as decreased serum levels of interleukin-6, TNF-alpha, and CRP. Such conditions may be related to immune modulation and anti-inflammatory effects, since resistance training releases cytokines, especially interleukin-6, which acts as a TNF-alpha antagonist during exercise.

1. Introduction

In recent years, life expectancy has grown considerably. Nowadays, there are 14.3 million Brazilians over 60 years. Until the year 2025, Brazil will become the sixth country in the number of elderly people [1]. Due to this increase in life expectancy and aging, many researchers have investigated several aspects about this theme [2].

Human aging is a process characterized by biological and physiological changes with repercussion on body composition and onset of chronic systemic inflammation, pointed by the increase of inflammatory markers such as interleukin-6 (IL-6), tumor necrosis factor-alpha (TNF-α), and C-reactive protein (CRP) [2, 4]. According to Silva and Mura [5], several diseases in this life stage result in changes in the immune system with consequent disturbance in cytokine homeostasis.

Cytokines are proteins that respond to pathogens with cells of innate and adaptive immunity and also act on inflammatory processes [6]. Among cytokines, TNF-α is the main mediator of acute inflammatory response whose physiological function is stimulation of leukocytes, signaling to sites of inflammation and activating them in order to eradicate microorganisms and reduce inflammation [3, 7].

Another important cytokine in the inflammatory process is IL-6. It is synthesized from mononuclear phagocytes, vascular endothelial cells, fibroblasts, and adipose and muscle tissues. Its function is stimulation of neutrophil production by bone marrow progenitors, promoting synthesis of proinflammatory cytokines and inhibiting TNF-α. Thus, the body returns to its resting state as the inflammatory process is eradicated [6].

C-reactive protein is a risk marker for cardiovascular disease, which also features an important function in the inflammatory process, especially in the acute phase, when CRP can increase up to 1000 times its normal serum level. This protein is produced and released into the bloodstream by hepatocytes, but it can also be produced by arterial walls. Its synthesis is stimulated by IL-1 and IL-6, which are released by macrophages [5]. Among several functions attributed to CRP, perhaps the most important is the synthesis of phagocytic components, which remove structures from blood circulation and induce an anti-inflammatory effect. These events promote tissue repair [8–10].

Several systemic, tissue, cellular, and molecular changes happen in the aging process, featured by progressive dysfunction of the immune system, with an imbalance in the concentrations of pro- and anti-inflammatory cytokines and other inflammatory markers associated with the development of cardiovascular diseases, and the increase in morbidity and mortality, in the elderly [11, 12]. Resistance training is a modality of exercise to prevent diseases, especially cardiovascular diseases and type 2 diabetes mellitus [13]. Thus, some studies suggest that the resistance training is effective in decreasing serum concentrations of proinflammatory cytokines (TNF-α, IL-1β, and IL-8), being also recommended for health promotion in the elderly [13–16].

Therefore, the role of immunological and inflammatory markers such as TNF-α, IL-6, and CRP in the face of chronic resistance training in the elderly can be a good tool for several health professionals and, especially, for the general population, because of the beneficial effects of exercise in this senile age. Thus, this study is mainly aimed at analyzing the immunological response, gene expression, inflammatory markers through cytokines such as TNF-α, IL-6, and CRP, and body composition, in a group of elderly women, so as to better understand these events.

Therefore, the role of immunological and inflammatory markers such as TNF-α, IL-6, and CRP in relation to resistance training in the elderly can be a good appliance for several health professionals, and especially for the general population, as these effects will be beneficial in this age by reducing proinflammatory cytokines and thereby reducing various types of chronic degenerative diseases due to aging. Thus, this study is aimed at analyzing the behavior of the immune system, through gene expression, inflammatory markers of TNF-α, IL-6, and CRP, and body composition in a group of elderly women to better understand these events.

2. Materials and Methods

2.1. Study Characteristics. It is an experimental and controlled study. The Ethics and Research Committee of the CEUMA University, through the Brazil Platform Ministry of Health, National Health Council, National Commission of Ethics in Research-Division of Experimental Research Involving Human Beings, approved this study under CAEE permit number 10863313.2.1001.5084 (protocol no. 372453/2013). All participants signed an individual consent form, so their identification is included in this article. All procedures performed in this study were in accordance with the Ethical Standards of the Institutional and/or National Research Committee and with the Helsinki Declaration of 1975 and its later amendments or comparable ethical standards.

2.2. Sample Selection. This is a nonprobabilistic sample. A list with names and telephone contacts of women aged between 60 and 70 was initially requested from the Integrated Seniors University (UNITI/UFMA). From the telephone contacts available, subjects were invited to take part in the study, and those who had not entered any other structured RT program in the last six months were selected. A meeting was held for explanation about project logistics, for delivering the schedule of activities to all participants, and for the consent form to be signed by them. Also, there were scheduled days, times, and locations for anthropometric evaluation and blood collection. For inclusion criteria, participants should be between 60 and 70 years; not be enrolled in structured RT programs in the last six months; be nonsmokers; have no degree of obesity according to the World Health Organization [17], using body mass index (BMI) and waist-to-hip ratio (WHR) as parameters ($BMI \leq 30\ kg/m^2$ and $WHR \leq 1.00$); and voluntarily sign the consent term. For exclusion criteria, participants should not have untreated hypertension or diabetes mellitus (these criteria were controlled through directed anamnesis and measurement of changes in total leukocyte numbers, which could indicate acute infectious processes). The total initial sample consisted of 23 elderly women. After eight weeks of RT, the final sample was 19 participants. Two people from the initial sample presented leukocyte values above the reference for inclusion criteria, and the other two attended less than 85% of the training sessions.

2.3. Design of the Experiment. A pretest/posttest with a control group design was adopted for the study. Both groups were pretested and posttested at eight weeks. The participants were randomly (http://www.randomization.com, Protocol no. 2538 08/2014, available on 08/18/2014) divided into the control group (Control) and experimental group (RT). The Control received no intervention, and the RT performed resistive training. It happened this way: first, the entire sample (n = 19) was submitted to anthropometric assessment and blood collection; then, the entire sample was randomly assigned. One group (n = 9) performed RT, while the other (n = 10) received no intervention. After 24 hours, corresponding to eight weeks, all participants returned for a new anthropometric evaluation and blood collection. Then, the Control group started the intervention (n = 10), performing RT for eight weeks as well. Afterwards, they were again submitted to anthropometric evaluation and blood collection. Then, the groups that performed RT were paired, forming the RT group (n = 19) and the Control group (n = 10) (Figure 1).

2.4. Resistive Training Program. The RT protocol was based on a critical analysis of the databases in [13, 18–20]. Thus, the training sessions were performed on fitness equipment for eight weeks. The type of training was the bi-set method, which consists of two exercises without time intervals for different muscle groups: lower limbs (LL) and upper limbs (UL).

For the protocol procedure, before and after all training sessions, participants rested for 5 minutes and then blood pressure was measured. The RT was supervised by one physiotherapist and two physical education professionals. The model of resistance training was by means of 8–12 maximal repetitions (MRs), aiming at muscular hypertrophy. In relation to the weekly frequency, the training protocol was performed three times per week, where eight exercises were performed in LL and UL: sitting leg press, sitting supine, knee extension, pulley (back), lying down knee flexion, low pulley elbow flexion, seated leg press, and pulley elbow extension. As for the increase in intensity (load (kg)), two criteria were adopted: (1) exercise intensity and load increase were obtained using the BORG scale; in other words, participants were instructed to mention any number from this scale, provided that the number actually corresponded to their perceived effort after each exercise series was performed. (2) After that, all participants performed their RT program within a maximum repetition (MR) zone of 8 to 12 repetitions; thus, whenever the participants exceeded the limits of this zone, a new increase of load occurred which would remain within the established zone, corresponding to 15% of the initial load. The time interval between the repetitions was one minute for each series, and the duration of the training protocol sessions lasted on average 50 minutes. In relation to the speed of execution of the exercise preestablished in four seconds for each movement, the repetition rate was performed with a concentric action of 2 seconds and an eccentric action of 2 seconds, controlled by visual and verbal commands to standardize angles of movement. The intervention of resistance training was very intense, and the participants were elderly and had not trained for at least six months, so in order to avoid possible side effects and possible withdrawal of the participants in the research, we chose to do a one-week adaptation training in the participants performed two sets of 15 submaximal repetitions with low loads, aiming at neuromuscular adaptation avoiding late-onset muscular pain.

2.5. Procedures and Data Collection

2.5.1. Anthropometry and Body Composition. All participants were submitted to anthropometric assessment in pretest and posttest (eight weeks later). Body mass was measured using a digital scale (Welmy® W300, Brazil) with a maximum capacity of 300 kg. Height was measured using an anthropometric scale between 1.00 and 2.00 m. These measurements were used to calculate the body mass index (BMI). Also, waist and hip circumference was measured using the metric tape (Waist Fit®, Brazil) to calculate the waist-to-hip ratio. Prior to the measurements of body composition, participants were instructed to not eat 2-3 hours before, not drink alcohol, not perform any physical exercise for 24 hours, monitor fluid intake, and urinate 30 minutes prior to assessment. To begin the assessment, the participants were asked to lie down on the hammock, and then electrodes were put at predetermined points which were sanitized using 70% alcohol.

The emitter electrodes were placed at the dorsal surface of the right hand, near the metacarpophalangeal joint, and at the transverse arch of the upper surface of the right foot. The detector electrodes were placed between the distal prominences of the radius and ulna of the right wrist, and another one was placed between the medial malleolus and lateral malleolus of the right ankle [21]. This procedure was performed using a four-pole electrical bioimpedance (Maltron BF-906 Body Fat Analyzer®, England), whose technique is based on the fact that tissues with high water and electrolyte contents have high electrical conduction capacity and tissues with low water concentration show lower electrical conduction capacity; thus, this difference creates a good predictor for body parameters [5, 22]. All these procedures were performed at LAFIPEMA-UFMA at pretest (Pre) and posttest (Post), eight weeks after pretest.

2.5.2. Blood Collection. Blood samples were collected by a trained pharmaceutical and in accordance with the biosafety standards recommended by NR32. The blood collection was performed at Pre (fasting) and Post (24 hours after the last day of RT) moments. At the moment Pre, all participants were instructed to go to the Laboratory of Physiology and Exercise Prescription (LAFIPEMA-UFMA), at 6 am, fasted for 8–12 hours. At the time Post, participants in the Control group made blood collections after a time period of 8 weeks. Already, the participants who performed RT made blood collections 24 hours after the last day of training. A total volume of 14 ml, approximately, was collected at vacuum and then distributed into a 4 ml EDTA tube (Vacuette) and two dry tubes containing 5 ml separating gel (Vacuette). The samples collected proceeded with the

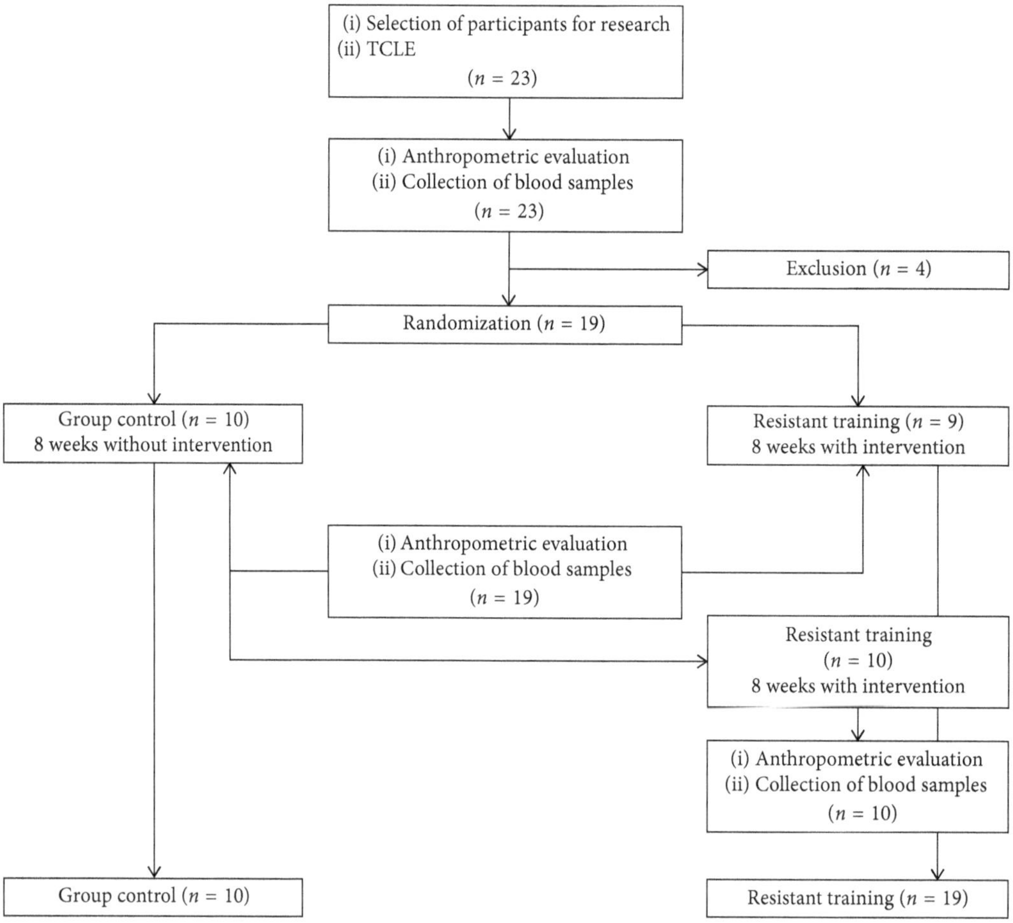

FIGURE 1: Study design flowchart.

following usage: (a) the tube containing the EDTA anticoagulant was used to perform the complete blood count and the analysis of TNF-α gene expression and (b) the tubes containing the separating gel were used to perform the biochemical analysis of the high-sensitivity CRP and the ELISA immunoassays for cytokines IL-6 and TNF-α.

2.6. Analysis of Biochemical Parameters of High-Sensitivity CRP. This was analyzed to measure the CRP serum levels and feature the degree of risk for cardiovascular diseases. Therefore, biochemical analysis was performed by immunoturbidimetry.

2.7. Analysis of Cytokines IL-6 and TNF-α

2.7.1. Serum Concentrations of IL-6 and TNF-α. The analysis of the blood concentrations of IL-6 and TNF-α was performed through ELISA tests at the Laboratory of Immunology and Microbiology of Respiratory Infections (LAMIR), CEUMA University. To process the immunoassay, serum aliquots and the IL-6 ELISA kits (SIGMA-ALDRICH 3050™, USA) and TNF-α ELISA kits (EIA-4641-DRG®, USA) were used, according to the manufacturer's instructions. This technique was performed using IL-6 and TNF-α monoclonal antibodies (MAbs), marked with enzymes, for chromogenic reactions. The quantification of IL-6 and TNF-α concentrations was performed by calorimetry, measuring the absorbance proportional to the concentration of each cytokine studied. A calibration curve was drawn, and the concentrations of both cytokines (IL-6 and TNF-α) were determined by interpolation from the curve.

All concentrations of IL-6 and TNF-α were determined by an enzyme immunoassay, using a microplate reader device with an 8-channel optical photometric system to measure the optical density of vertical light (Thermoplate® model TP Reader Basic, Brazil).

2.8. Analysis of TNF-α Gene Expression

2.8.1. Total RNA Extraction and cDNA and TNF-α Preparation. The RNA isolation was performed from blood leukocytes collected in a vacuum tube containing the EDTA anticoagulant. A sample volume of 20 μL was used for RNA extraction, according to the protocol using the GeneJET RNA Purification Kit (Thermo Scientific®, USA), in line with the manufacturer's recommendations. The total RNA was resuspended in 20 μL of RNase-free water and quantified using a GeneQuant 100 spectrophotometer (GE Healthcare, Wisconsin, USA); after that, cDNA was synthesized from 200 μg of total RNA, using the RevertAid First Strand cDNA

Synthesis Kit (Thermo Scientific®, USA), according to the manufacturer's recommendations. In short, approximately 200 μg of total RNA was reverse transcribed in a final volume of 20 μL of reaction. The resulting cDNA was stored at −30°C until real-time PCR analysis.

2.8.2. Real-Time Quantitative PCR Assay for TNF-α. Real-time quantitative PCR assays were performed for TNF-α gene analysis from blood leukocytes. A pair of primers presenting the following sequences were synthesized: TNF-α-5′-GTAGGACCCTGGAGGCTGAAC-3′ (sense) and 5′-CCCAAAAGAAATGGAGGCAAT-3′ (antisense), and GAPDH 5′-GGAAGGTGAAGGTCGGAGTCA-3′ (sense) and 5′-CTGGAAGATGGTGATGGGATTTC-3′ (antisense). Their construction was based on the gene sequences described by Schattner et al. [23]. GAPDH mRNA was used as the endogenous reference gene. Relative expression was calculated using the 2-ΔCt method. The real-time PCR was performed using the QuantStudio™ 6 Flex Real-Time PCR System (Thermo Fisher Scientific, USA). The reaction mix contained 2 μL of the cDNA sample, 1.0 μL of forward and reverse primers (200 nM), 10 μL of Supermix, and 7.0 μL of nuclease-free water. The oligonucleotides used in PCR were selected using the Primer Premier 6.1 Program (Premier Biosoft International®, USA). The amplicons were generated under the following thermocycling conditions: 1 cycle at 50°C for 2 min (UNG activation), 1 cycle at 95°C for 10 min (UNG inactivation), and 40 cycles at 95°C for 15 s and 60°C for 1 min.

2.9. Statistical Data Analysis. The statistical analysis was performed using the software GraphPad Prism 6.0. First, the Shapiro–Wilk normality test was performed, considering parametric tests ($p > 0.05$). The descriptive analysis of the variables, between the groups, was presented as mean and standard deviation, followed by Student's T-test for independent samples. To compare the anthropometric variables, body composition and lipid profile, at Pre and Post moments, the paired Student's T-test was performed. A one-way ANOVA test—paired for repeated measures and followed by Tukey's post hoc test—was performed to compare dependent samples of the load increase in the RT group. A two-way ANOVA test was performed to compare outcome variables between intra- and intergroups. The significance level was set at $p < 0.05$.

3. Results

3.1. Sample Characterization. Both groups presented similar variables, except for height ($p = 0.01$) and body weight ($p = 0.04$) (Table 1).

Comparing Pre and Post moments for RT and Control groups, there was a statistically significant difference in the RT group for the variables: decreased fat mass ($p = 0.02$), body fat percentage ($p = 0.01$), and WHR and increased lean mass ($p = 0.02$), lean mass percentage ($p = 0.01$), and body weight (Table 2).

Table 1: Characteristics of study participants.

Variable	Control ($n = 10$)	RT ($n = 19$)	p value
Age (years)	63.0 ± 1.0	63.0 ± 2.0	0.08
Height (m)	1.4 ± 0.0	1.5 ± 0.0	0.01*
Body mass (kg)	58.5 ± 3.8	63.7 ± 2.4	0.04*
Fat percentage (%)	39.1 ± 2.6	39.3 ± 1.4	0.60
Lean mass percentage (%)	60.8 ± 2.6	60.7 ± 1.4	0.60

Data are presented as mean ± standard deviation. Student's T-test for independent samples: *statistically significant difference ($p < 0.05$) between RT and Control groups.

Following the load evolution at the 1st, 4th, and 8th training weeks, there was a load increase in their respective exercises with a significant difference between the weeks ($p = 0.0001$) (Table 3).

With respect to serum concentration of IL-6, a statistically significant interaction ($p = 0.05$) between the groups (Control vs RT) and their respective moments (Pre vs Post) was noted, as well as a significant reduction ($p = 0.01$) in the RT group between their respective moments (Pre vs Post) (Figure 2).

With respect to serum concentration of TNF-α, there was a statistically significant interaction ($p = 0.05$) between the groups (Control vs RT) and their respective moments (Pre vs Post), as well as a significant reduction ($p = 0.01$) in the RT group between their respective moments (Pre vs Post) (Figure 3).

The molecular analysis of TNF-α gene expression between groups (Control vs RT), showed that although Pre values in the RT group were higher than the Pre values in the Control group, these values did not interfere in the statistically significant decrease observed in the RT group ($p = 0.007$) (Figure 4).

With respect to serum concentration of CRP, there was a statistically significant interaction ($p = 0.01$) between the groups (Control vs TR) and their respective moments (Pre vs Post), as well as a significant reduction ($p = 0.001$) in the RT group between their respective moments (Pre vs Post) (Figure 5).

4. Discussion

This study aimed to evaluate the effects of eight weeks of RT on the immune response of IL-6 and TNF-α, the inflammatory marker of high-sensitivity CRP, and the TNF-α gene expression, as well as to analyze body composition in elderly women. Thereby, the initial hypothesis was confirmed, and there were observed a decrease in the serum concentrations of IL-6, TNF-α, and CRP after eight weeks of TR and a decrease in cellular activation, translated into the TNF-α gene expression. In addition, we observed a decrease in fat mass and an increase in lean mass and training load.

The objective of this study was to evaluate the behavior of the immune system of IL-6 and TNF-α and inflammatory marker of high-sensitivity PCR, as well as the gene expression of TNF-α in elderly women after eight weeks of intervention through the resistance training protocol. Thus,

Table 2: Anthropometric characteristics, body composition and lipid profile, in RT and Control groups at Pre and Post (8 weeks) moments.

Variables	Control (n = 10)		p value	RT (n = 19)		p value
	Pre	Post		Pre	Post	
Body mass (kg)	58.5 ± 3.8	58.1 ± 3.8	0.9	63.7 ± 2.4	65.0 ± 2.5	0.1
Fat mass (kg)	22.8 ± 2.9	22.2 ± 3.0	0.2	25.0 ± 1.7	23.5 ± 1.7*	0.02
Lean mass (kg)	35.6 ± 1.1	35.7 ± 1.0	0.8	38.6 ± 3.6	41.4 ± 4.1*	0.02
Fat percentage (%)	39.1 ± 2.6	38.2 ± 2.7	0.9	39.3 ± 1.4	36.2 ± 1.5*	0.01
Lean mass percentage (%)	60.8 ± 2.6	61.7 ± 2.7	0.5	60.7 ± 1.4	63.7 ± 1.5*	0.01
BMI (kg/m^2)	26.8 ± 1.7	26.0 ± 1.7	0.1	27.7 ± 0.9	27.5 ± 1.0	0.7
WHR (cm)	0.8 ± 0.0	0.8 ± 0.0	0.3	0.8 ± 0.0	0.8 ± 0.0	0.1

Data are presented as mean ± standard deviation. Student's T-test: *statistically significant difference ($p < 0.05$) compared to Pre moment. BMI: body mass index; WHR: waist-to-hip ratio.

Table 3: Evolution of training load in first, fourth, and 8th weeks of RT.

Exercises	RT (n = 19)			Effect size (Δ)	p value
	1st week	4th week	8th week		
Seated leg press (kg)	20.7 ± 3.8	33.6 ± 1.1*	45.48 ± 1.4*†	6.3	0.0001
Elbow flexion (low pulley) (kg)	9.0 ± 1.8	13.8 ± 0.3*	17.83 ± 0.4*†	4.8	0.0001
Knee extension (kg)	9.9 ± 0.5	18.4 ± 0.6*	25.90 ± 0.8*†	28.0	0.0001
Supine seated (kg)	7.1 ± 0.3	13.8 ± 0.4*	17.96 ± 0.7*†	29.2	0.0001
Lying knee flexion (kg)	7.9 ± 0.4	15.5 ± 2.0*	17.09 ± 0.5*	22.1	0.0001
Pulley (back) (kg)	13.2 ± 0.5	21.9 ± 0.4*	27.03 ± 0.5*†	26.4	0.0001
Plantar flexion (seated leg press) (kg)	20.0 ± 0.7	33.38 ± 0.9*	43.56 ± 1.2*†	30.9	0.0001
Elbow extension (pulley) (kg)	8.6 ± 0.6	16.42 ± 0.4*	20.20 ± 0.4*†	19.0	0.0001

Data are presented as mean ± standard deviation. One-way ANOVA test followed by Tukey's post hoc test: *statistically significant difference ($p < 0.05$) compared to the first week; †statistically significant difference ($p < 0.05$) compared to the fourth week. Δ: effect size measures on the evolution of training load among the analyzed weeks. RT: resistance training.

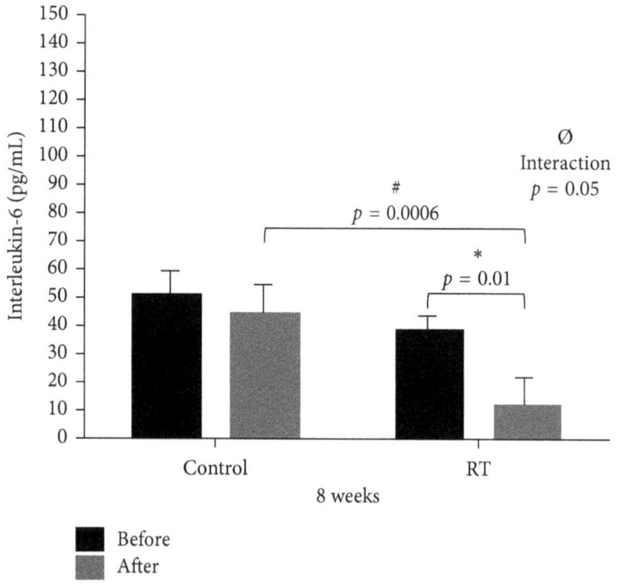

Figure 2: Dispersion measurements of interleukin-6 between Control (n = 10) and RT (n = 19) groups at Pre and Post moments. Two-way ANOVA test: *statistically significant difference (p = 0.01) between Pre and Post moments in the RT group; #statistically significant difference (p = 0.0006) between Post moments in the RT vs Control groups; Øsstatistically significant interaction (p = 0.05).

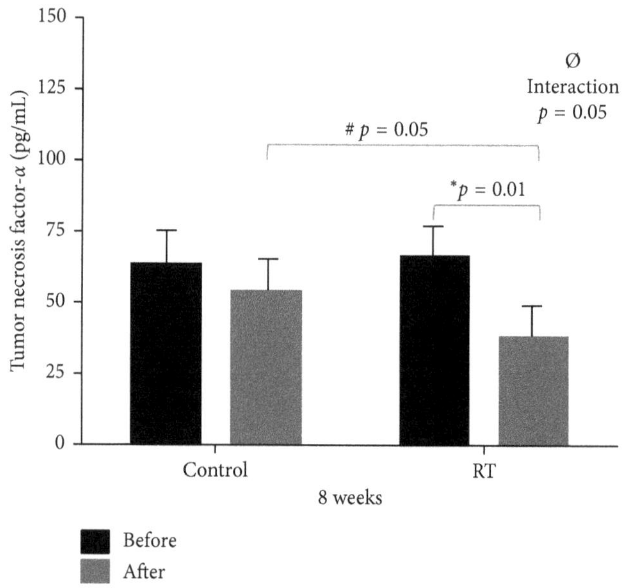

Figure 3: Dispersion measurements of tumor necrosis factor-α between Control (n = 10) and RT (n = 19) groups at Pre and Post moments. Two-way ANOVA test: *statistically significant difference (p = 0.01) between Pre and Post moments in the RT group; #statistically significant difference (p = 0.05) between Post moments in the RT vs Control groups; Østatistically significant interaction (p = 0.05).

the initial hypothesis was confirmed, and a decrease in the serum concentrations of IL-6, TNF-α, and CRP after eight weeks of RT and a decrease in the cellular activation, translated into expression of the TNF-α gene, were observed. In addition, we observed a decrease in fat mass and an increase in lean mass, along with an increase in strength

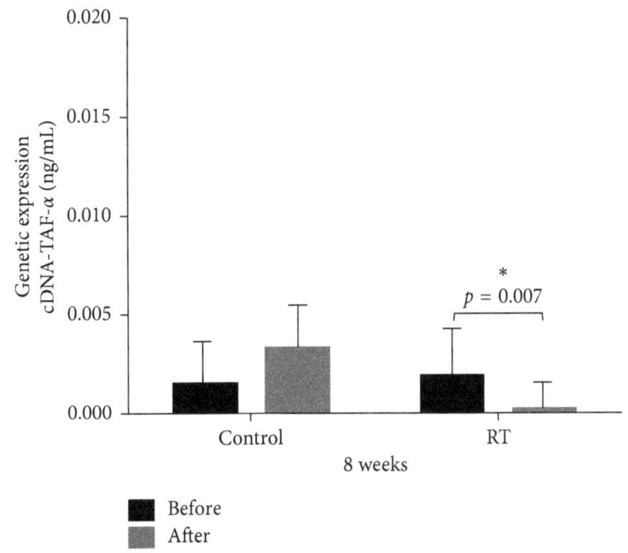

FIGURE 4: Measurements of tumor necrosis factor-α gene expression between Control ($n = 4$) and RT ($n = 5$) groups at Pre and Post moments. Two-way ANOVA test: *statistically significant difference ($p = 0.007$) between Pre and Post moments in the RT group.

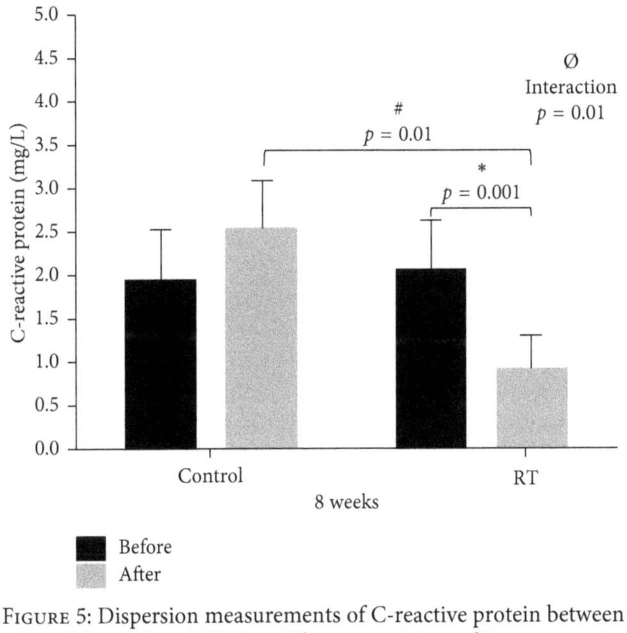

FIGURE 5: Dispersion measurements of C-reactive protein between Control ($n = 10$) and RT ($n = 19$) groups at Pre and Post moments. Two-way ANOVA test: *statistically significant difference ($p = 0.001$) between Pre and Post moments in the RT group; #statistically significant difference ($p = 0.01$) between Post moments in the RT vs Control groups; Østatistically significant interaction ($p = 0.01$).

represented by the evolution of load along the resistance training.

In this study, eight weeks of RT significantly decreased the serum concentrations of IL-6, TNF-α, and CRP in the elderly women. TNF-α and IL-6 are cytokines produced by immune, endothelial, adipose, and smooth and skeletal muscle cells [24, 25]. Their main functions are to modulate innate and acquired immunity and regulate the response of the body during inflammatory processes [6]. These cytokines (IL-6 and TNF-α) have receptors on several cell types, including hepatocytes, and signal the synthesis of acute-phase proteins, such as CRP [5]. The TNF-α also stimulates the process of phagocytosis to repair and regenerate tissue [10, 24, 27]. For Abramson and Vaccarino [28], Costa and Vaisberg [29], Petersen and Pedersen [25], and Rossetti et al. [30], physical exercise is associated with muscle cell injury and, hence, the synthesis of anti-inflammatory cytokines (IL-6 and IL-10), from the bone marrow into the bloodstream, in balance with proinflammatory cytokines (TNF-α and IL-1Ra). The IL-6 has an important function in this muscle repair, since it increases soon after the beginning of the exercise and promotes anti-inflammatory actions and also inhibitory effects on the production and secretion of TNF-α (mainly), which cause a chronic adaptation to exercise [14].

Therefore, to analyze the chronic effects of physical exercise on inflammatory markers, it is essential to understand the acute effects of exercise on cytokine concentrations. Pereira et al. [31] investigated the effects of a single RT session on the serum concentrations of cytokines (TNF-α, IL-1a, IL-1b, IL-12, IL-6, and IL-10) in women with metabolic syndrome. No statistical difference was observed; however, there was a trend to decrease TNF-α concentration and to increase IL-1b and IL-6 concentrations 60 minutes after the training. This result indicates that a single RT session can modulate and reduce proinflammatory cytokines and shows that periodized and systematized training programs have a positive effect on cytokine concentrations. Rossetti et al. [30] explain that RT releases myokines (cytokines produced in active muscles), particularly IL-6, stimulating the production of anti-inflammatory cytokines (IL-6 and IL-10), which in turn inhibit the production of the proinflammatory cytokine (TNF-α). This process occurs in acute and consecutive training sessions and supports the systemic decrease in serum concentrations of total cytokines and, hence, in the acute inflammatory marker (CRP) [32, 33].

This was observed by Córdova et al. [14], who investigated the association between eight weeks of RT and serum concentrations of IL-6, TNF-α, and IFN-γ in elderly women. The study demonstrated that RT in elderly women is associated with low serum concentrations of proinflammatory cytokines, evidenced the impact of RT on these markers, and showed that sedentary lifestyle is a risk factor for diseases related to the aging process. Ho et al. [34] observed the effects of 12 weeks of training on inflammatory markers TNF-α, IL-6, and CRP in overweight and obese individuals and reinforced that idea because all studied variables decreased in the training group compared with the control.

Searching evidence about the molecular mechanisms behind these findings, it was verified that RT produces modulatory effects on TNF-α gene expression, influencing this proinflammatory mediator production. The results of the present study showed a significant decrease in TNF-α

gene expression after 8 weeks of training, and this may be related to immunomodulation mediated by IL-6, since this cytokine acts as a natural TNF-α antagonist during long-term physical exercise and also promotes stimulation of anti-inflammatory cytokines production, like IL-1 antagonist receptor (IL-1Ra) and interleukin-10 (IL-10) [5, 6, 25].

In order to understand the control of TNF-α gene expression in terms of molecular mechanisms, Keller et al. [35] used an experimental model of induction of physical activity with *knockout* mice for the two main signaling pathways: TNF-α receptor 1 (p55) and TNF-α receptor 2 (p75). After training, TNF-α gene expression levels decreased in both *knockout* models, thus indicating that the activation of TNF-α receptors is one of the main mechanisms by which physical exercise regulates the TNF-α gene expression, although it is believed that other pathways may also be involved in this regulation.

As well, it is important to point out that the RT group presented significant gains in lean mass and loss of fat mass. These findings may also have contributed to the suppression of TNF-α gene expression, since, in obesity, adipose tissue produces a low-grade systemic inflammatory state, characterized by an increase in transcription and elevated levels of circulating TNF-α mRNA [25, 35].

Based on these data, adipose tissue contributes to the increase in TNF-α and CRP concentrations, which reverberates in their increased serum concentrations [25, 36]. Physical exercise induces a reduction in fat mass, by the mobilization of lipids and stimulation of lipolysis, which is regulated by lipase and activated by beta-oxidative stimulation. Thus, it increases the uptake and oxidation of fatty acids by the skeletal muscle and serves as an energetic substrate by the glucose fatty acid cycle mechanism, which directly reflects on the reduction of adipose tissue and, hence, on the reduction in serum concentrations of inflammatory markers (IL-6, TNF-α, and CRP). This is beneficial because it has a protective effect against cardiovascular diseases [25, 37]. The research conducted by Willis et al. [16] corroborates the findings of this study once it evaluated the effects of eight months of aerobic, resistance, and concurrent training on the body composition in overweight and obese adults and showed that aerobic and concurrent training reduced fat mass. Another similar study was conducted by Ho et al. [34], in which they investigated the effects of those three training modalities (aerobic, resistance, and concurrent training), for 12 weeks, in participants aged 40–66 years, and noted a decrease in fat mass and an increase in lean mass. Lee et al. [15] followed the effects on body composition, CRP, IL-6, and TNF-α, caused by two training modalities (aerobic and concurrent training), for eight weeks, in elderly women, and they observed a reduction in fat mass and an increase in lean mass, especially in aerobic training. Considering inflammatory markers, concurrent training decreased serum concentrations of CRP, IL-6, and TNF-α, compared to aerobic training. Based on the previously presented studies, it is possible to speculate that the decrease in fat mass and the increase in lean mass, verified in this study, were determinant for the decrease in serum concentrations of TNF-α, IL-6, and CRP, in the elderly women.

In this research, an increase in muscle strength was also observed, evidenced by the progressive increase in training load and in muscle volume, over the eight weeks of training. According to Prestes et al. [38], an adjustment of the body to training overload induces physiological and structural changes (neural and muscular factors, respectively), which results in an increase in muscle strength. The increase in muscle volume and strength may directly influence the decrease in serum concentrations of inflammatory markers (IL-6, TNFα, and CRP), as these variables have a strong relationship with each other [32]. For Rossetti et al. [30] and Petersen and Pedersen [25], this relationship is due to the fact that resistance training has an important neuro-immunoendocrine function; among them, myokines are cytokines produced in active muscles. The IL-6 has its wide action in other areas of the body, by means of important effects of the physical exercise in the adaptive process, since the muscular fibers seem to produce it through an independent way, stimulating in the circulation the appearance of other anti-inflammatory cytokines, as to IL-10, which in turn inhibits the production of the inflammatory cytokine TNF-α, via TNF-α receptor, TNF-R.

Mavros et al. [39] and Santiago et al. [40] studied the effects of 12 months of RT on the CRP in the elderly and associated its reduction with changes in body composition. They concluded that RT reduced serum concentrations of CRP and associated it with increased skeletal muscle mass ($p = 0.01$). Thereby, they corroborate the findings of the present study. Moreover, Lera et al. [42] observed the importance of 16 weeks of RT on body composition, blood glucose, and CRP in menopausal, sedentary, and overweight elderly women. Their results indicated that RT increased muscle strength and muscle mass and prevented increased glucose and CRP.

The systematized and progressive RT program is developed through appropriate and specific training purposes. Among several protocols available, the bi-set method shows an efficient proposal for a well-structured and individualized RT program, which follows the RT prescription recommendations for the elderly. In view of this, it was decided to determine the training intensity by means of an RM range between 8 and 12 [13, 18–20, 43]. The results of this study suggest that chronic RT reduces serum concentrations of cytokines (IL-6 and TNF-α) and CRP and also induces molecular changes in TNF-α gene expression, in elderly women.

A possible limitation of this study may be related to the representativeness of the sample, since it is a limited group of women who are available to participate in institutional care research. Another limitation of the study was in relation to the elderly women who have passed th0065 menopause period, and it is known that the hormonal changes that occur in the postmenopausal period can influence the responses to the cytokines through body composition, mainly in the fat weight. In this way, we controlled this limitation with the decrease of the fat weight with the resistance training in relation to the basal values.

In summary, the results of the present study showed that eight weeks of RT caused molecular changes in TNF-α gene expression, in the elderly women, as well as a decrease in serum levels of IL-6, TNF-α, and CRP. This may be related to an immunomodulation and anti-inflammatory effect, since RT releases myokines (cytokines produced in active muscles), particularly IL-6, thus acting as a TNF-α antagonist during exercise. Therefore, the performance and adaptation to chronic RT controlled inflammatory conditions, which resulted in a balanced action between pro- and anti-inflammatory effectors in different tissues, especially in the striated skeletal muscle.

Conflicts of Interest

The authors declare that they have no conflicts of interest.

Authors' Contributions

LÂMS organized and designed the experiments. LÂMS, LGLN, WRS, and AJMCRP performed the experiments. GBP, RDL, and CTM wrote the manuscript. LÂMS, LGLN, and JOBM reviewed the manuscript. LÂMS, LGLN, and FN gave approval of the final manuscript version.

Acknowledgments

This project was funded by the Federal University of Maranhão (UFMA) and Foundation for Research Support of the State of Maranhão (FAPEMA-BM-01486/13). Luís Ângelo Macêdo Santiago was an FAPEMA productivity scholarship student.

References

[1] N. M. Papaléo and J. R. Ponte, *Aging: Challenge in the Transition of the Century*, Atheneu, São Paulo, SP, Brazil, 2002.

[2] O. T. Nóbrega, V. P. Faleiros, and J. L. Telles, "Gerontology in the developing Brazil: achievements and challenges in public policies," *Geriatrics & Gerontology International*, vol. 9, no. 2, pp. 135–139, 2009.

[3] T. C. Adam, "The TNF and TNF receptor super families: integration mammalian biology," *Cell*, vol. 104, pp. 487–501, 2001.

[4] P. N. Amaral, D. M. Pomatti, and V. L. F. Fortes, "Physical Activities in human aging: a creative sensitive reading," *Brazilian Journal of the Sciences of the Aging Human*, vol. 4, no. 1, pp. 18–27, 2007.

[5] S. M. C. S. Silva and J. D. P. Mura, *Food, Nutrition and Diet Therapy Treaty*, Roca, São Paulo, SP, Brazil, 2007.

[6] F. O. C. Silva and D. V. Macedo, "Physical exercise, inflammatory process and adaptation: an overview," *Brazilian Journal of Cineanthropometry and Human Performance*, vol. 13, pp. 320–328, 2011.

[7] G. Opdenakker, W. E. Fibbe, and J. Van Damme, "The molecular basis of leukocytosis," *Immunology Today*, vol. 19, no. 4, pp. 182–187, 1998.

[8] L. Mosca, "C-reactive protein—to screen or not to screen?," *New England Journal of Medicine*, vol. 347, no. 20, pp. 1615–1617, 2002.

[9] J. Cermak, N. S. Key, R. R. Bach, J. Balla, H. S. Jacob, and G. M. Vercellotti, "C-reactive protein induces human peripheral blood monocytes to synthesize tissue factor," *Blood Journal*, vol. 82, no. 2, pp. 513–520, 1993.

[10] M. G. Santos, M. Pegoraro, F. Sandrini, and E. C. Macuco, "Risk factors in the development of atherosclerosis in childhood and adolescence," *Arquivos Brasileiros de Cardiologi*, vol. 90, no. 4, 2008.

[11] G. Pawelec and A Larbi, "Immunity and ageing in man: annual review, 2006/2007," *Experimental Gerontology*, vol. 43, pp. 34–38, 2008.

[12] A. C. Tonet and O. T. Nóbrega, "Immunossenescence: the relationship between leukocytes, cytokines and chronic diseases," *Brazilian Journal of Geriatrics and Gerontology*, vol. 2, no. 11, 2008.

[13] C. E. Garber, B. Blissmer, M. R. Deschenes et al., "Quantity and quality of exercise for developing and maintaining cardiorespiratory, musculoskeletal, and neuromotor fitness in apparently healthy adults," *Medicine & Science in Sports & Exercise*, vol. 43, no. 7, pp. 1334–1359, 2011.

[14] C. Córdova, F. Lopes-e-Silva Jr., A. S. Pires et al., "Long-term resistance training is associated with reduced circulating levels of IL-6, IFN-gamma and TNF-alpha in elderly women," *Neuroimmunomodulation*, vol. 18, no. 3, pp. 165–170, 2011.

[15] J. S. Lee, C. G. Kim, T. B. Seo, H. G. Kim, and S. J. Yoon, "Effects of 8-week combined training on body composition, isokinetic strength, and cardiovascular disease risk factors in older women," *Aging Clinical and Experimental Research*, vol. 27, no. 2, pp. 179–186, 2014.

[16] L. Willis, C. A. Slentz, L. A. Bateman et al., "Effects of aerobic training and/or endurance on body mass and fat mass in overweight or obese adults," *Journal of Applied Physiology*, vol. 113, no. 12, pp. 1831–1837, 2012.

[17] WHO, World Health Organization, "Preventing and managing the global epidemic," Report of a WHO Consultation on Obesity, vol. 3, WHO, Geneva, Switzerland, 1998.

[18] AHA-American Heart Association, "Cardiology and council on nutrition, physical activity, and metabolism update: a scientific statement from the american heart association council on clinical resistance exercise in individuals with and without cardiovascular disease," *Circulation: Journal of the American Heart Association*, vol. 116, no. 5, pp. 572–584, 2007.

[19] H.-S. Kim and D.-G. Kim, "Effect of long-term resistance exercise on body composition, blood lipid factors, and vascular compliance in the hypertensive elderly men," *Journal of Exercise Rehabilitation*, vol. 9, no. 2, pp. 271–277, 2013.

[20] R. Tibana and S. Balsamo, "Manipulation of the order of the exercises in the prescription of resistance training," *Brazilian Journal of Exercise Physiology*, vol. 10, no. 1, pp. 41–45, 2011.

[21] K. R. Segal, M. Van Loan, P. I. Fitzgerald, J. A. Hodgdon, and T. B. Van Itallie, "Lean body mass estimation by bioelectrical impedance analysis: a four-site cross validation study," *American Journal of Clinical Nutrition*, vol. 47, no. 1, pp. 7–14, 1998.

[22] W. D. Mcardle, I. K. Frank, and L. K. Victor, *Fisiologia do Exercício Energia, Nutrição e Desempenho Humano*, Guanabara-Koogan, Rio de Janeiro, RJ, Brazil, 2003.

[23] E. J. Schattner, D.-H. Yoo, M. K. Crow, and S. M. Friedman, "Superantigen-dependent TH cell/B cell interaction: a model for TH cell-mediated B cell activation and apoptosis," in

Human B Cell Superantigens, M. Zouali, Ed., R.G. Landes, Austin, TX, USA, 1996.

[24] A. K. Abbas, A. H. Lichtman, and S. Pillai, *Imunologia Celular e Molecular*, Elsevier Editora Ltda., Rio de Janeiro, Brazil, 7th edition, 2012.

[25] A. M. W. Petersen and B. K. Pedersen, "The anti-inflammatory effect of exercise," *Journal Applied Physiology*, vol. 98, no. 4, pp. 1154–1162, 2005.

[26] G. R. Person, T. Pettersson, O. Ohlsson, and S. Renvert, "High-sensitivity sérum C-reactive protein levels in subjects with or without myocardial infarction or periodontitis," *Journal of Clinical Periodontology*, vol. 32, no. 3, pp. 219–224, 2005.

[27] W. B. Santos, M. Pegoraro, F. Sandrini, and E. C. Macuco, "C-reactive protein and cardiovascular disease. The basis of scientific evidence," *Brazilian Archives of Cardiology*, vol. 80, no. 4, pp. 452–458, 2003.

[28] J. L. Abramson and V. Vaccarino, "Relationship between physical activity and inflammation among apparently healthy middle-aged and older US adults," *Archives of Internal Medicine*, vol. 162, no. 11, pp. 1286–1292, 2002.

[29] R. L. Costa and M. W. Vaisberg, "Influences of exercise on the immune response," *Brazilian Journal of Sports Medicine*, vol. 8, pp. 167–172, 2002.

[30] M. B. Rossetti, R. R. Britto, and R. C. Norton, "Primary prevention of cardiovascular diseases in childhood and juvenile obesity: anti-inflammatory effect of physical exercise," *Brazilian Journal of Sports Medicine*, vol. 15, no. 6, pp. 472–475, 2009.

[31] G. B. Pereira, R. A. Tibana, J. Navalta et al., "Acute effects of resistance training on cytokines and osteoprotegerin in women with metabolic syndrome," *Clinical Physiology and Functional Imaging*, vol. 33, no. 2, pp. 122–130, 2012.

[32] C. J. Brito, P. A. C. Volp, O. T. Nóbrega et al., "Physical exercise as a factor preventing the inflammatory processes due to aging," *Motriz: Revista de Educação Física*, vol. 17, no. 3, pp. 544–555, 2011.

[33] B. K. Pedersen and C. P. Fischer, "Beneficial health effects of exercise—the role of IL-6 as a myokine," *Trends in Pharmacological Sciences*, vol. 28, no. 4, pp. 152–156, 2007.

[34] S. S. Ho, S. S. Dhaliwal, A. P. Hills, and S Pal, "Effects of chronic exercise training on inflammatory markers in australian overweight and obese individuals in a randomized controlled trial," *Inflammation*, vol. 36, no. 3, pp. 625–632, 2013.

[35] C. Keller, P. Keller, M. Giralt, J. Hidalgo, and B. K. Pedersen, "Exercise normalises overexpression of TNF-α in knockout mice," *Biochemical and Biophysical Research Communications*, vol. 321, no. 1, pp. 179–182, 2004.

[36] S. Akira, T. Taga, and T. Kishimoto, "Interleukin-6 in biology and medicine," *Advances in Immunology*, vol. 54, pp. 1–78, 1993.

[37] L. Silveira, C. H. J. Pinheiro, C. C. Zoppi et al., "Regulation of glucose and fatty acid metabolism in the musculoskeletal during exercise," *Brazilian Archive of Endocrinology and Metabolism*, vol. 55, no. 5, pp. 303–313, 2011.

[38] J. Prestes, D. Foschin, P. Maarchetti, M. Charro, and R. Tibana, *Prescrição e Periodização do Treinamento de Força em Academias*, Editora Manole Ltda., Barueri, SP, Brazil, 2010.

[39] Y. Mavros, S. Kay, K. A. Simpson et al., "Reductions in C-reactive protein in older adults with type 2 diabetes are related to improvements in body composition following a randomized controlled trial of resistance training," *Journal Cachexia, Sarcopenia and Muscle*, vol. 5, no. 2, pp. 111–120, 2014.

[40] L. A. M. Santiago, L. G. L. Neto, P. V. A. Santana, P. C. Mendes, W. K. R. Lima, and F. Navarro, "Resisted training reduces cardiovascular risk in elderly women," *Brazilian Journal of Sports Medicine*, vol. 21, no. 4, pp. 261–265, 2015.

[41] M. Toigo and U. Boutellier, "New fundamental resistance exercise determinants of molecular and cellular muscle adaptations," *European Journal Applied Physiology*, vol. 97, no. 6, pp. 643–663, 2006.

[42] O. Lera, E. A. Nahas, N. Maestá et al., "Effects of resistance training frequency on body composition and metabolics and inflammatory markers inoverweight postmenopausal women," *Journal of Sports Medicine and Fitness*, vol. 3, no. 54, pp. 317–325, 2014.

[43] R. Tibana, G. B. Pereira, J. W. Navalta, M. Bottaro, and J. Prestes, "Acute effects of resistance exercise on 24-h blood pressure in middle aged overweight and obese women," *International Journal Sports Medicine*, vol. 34, no. 5, pp. 460–464, 2013.

13

10-Hydroxy-2-decenoic Acid, the Major Lipid Component of Royal Jelly, Extends the Lifespan of *Caenorhabditis elegans* through Dietary Restriction and Target of Rapamycin Signaling

Yoko Honda,[1] Yoko Araki,[2] Taketoshi Hata,[2] Kenji Ichihara,[2] Masafumi Ito,[3] Masashi Tanaka,[1] and Shuji Honda[1]

[1]*Department of Genomics for Longevity and Health, Tokyo Metropolitan Institute of Gerontology, Sakaecho, Itabashiku, Tokyo 173-0015, Japan*
[2]*Nagaragawa Research Center, Api Company Limited, Nagara, Gifu 502-0071, Japan*
[3]*Research Team for Mechanism of Aging, Tokyo Metropolitan Institute of Gerontology, Sakaecho, Itabashiku, Tokyo 173-0015, Japan*

Correspondence should be addressed to Shuji Honda; hondas@center.tmig.or.jp

Academic Editor: F. R. Ferraro

Royal jelly (RJ) produced by honeybees has been reported to possess diverse health-beneficial properties and has been implicated to have a function in longevity across diverse species as well as honeybees. 10-Hydroxy-2-decenoic acid (10-HDA), the major lipid component of RJ produced by honeybees, was previously shown to increase the lifespan of *Caenorhabditis elegans*. The objective of this study is to elucidate signaling pathways that are involved in the lifespan extension by 10-HDA. 10-HDA further extended the lifespan of the *daf-2* mutants, which exhibit long lifespan through reducing insulin-like signaling (ILS), indicating that 10-HDA extended lifespan independently of ILS. On the other hand, 10-HDA did not extend the lifespan of the *eat-2* mutants, which show long lifespan through dietary restriction caused by a food-intake defect. This finding indicates that 10-HDA extends lifespan through dietary restriction signaling. We further found that 10-HDA did not extend the lifespan of the long-lived mutants in *daf-15*, which encodes Raptor, a target of rapamycin (TOR) components, indicating that 10-HDA shared some longevity control mechanisms with TOR signaling. Additionally, 10-HDA was found to confer tolerance against thermal and oxidative stress. 10-HDA increases longevity not through ILS but through dietary restriction and TOR signaling in *C. elegans*.

1. Introduction

One of the most important challenges in the study of aging is the discovery of compounds with longevity-promoting activities and the elucidation of their underlying mechanisms. Such compounds could provide potential nutraceutical or pharmaceutical approaches to slow aging and the onset of age-related diseases in humans [1]. Royal jelly (RJ) is produced by the hypopharyngeal, postcerebral, and mandibular glands of the worker bees and has been implicated to be involved in the longer lifespan of queens in contrast with workers in the honeybee *Apis mellifera* L., because queens are fed throughout their lives with RJ, whereas workers are fed RJ for only a short period of time during their larval stage [2–5]. RJ has been also reported to extend the lifespan of nematodes [6, 7], flies [8, 9], and mice [10] indicating that RJ has a common role in longevity across phyla. RJ comprises proteins, sugars, lipids, vitamins, and free amino acids, together with a variety of bioactive substances [11]. The identities of the components that play critical roles in longevity are not fully understood. A single protein, termed royalactin contained in RJ, was reported to extend the lifespan of *D. melanogaster* and *C. elegans* [9, 12]. We previously found 10-hydroxy-2-decenoic acid (10-HDA), which is the major lipid component of RJ [13] and has several health-beneficial effects in mammals [14], such as antitumor activity [15], anti-inflammatory activity [16], and antiangiogenic activity [17]. It also extends the lifespan of *C. elegans* [6]. However, how 10-HDA extends lifespan is not well elucidated.

It has been reported that lifespan is regulated mainly through insulin-like signaling (ILS) and dietary restriction signaling in *C. elegans* as well as *Drosophila melanogaster* and other experimental animals [18]. In the present study, we found that 10-HDA extended the lifespan of *C. elegans* not through ILS but through dietary restriction signaling. Dietary restriction signaling has been reported to mediate lifespan extension through various downstream signaling pathways including target of rapamycin (TOR) signaling [19]. We suggest in this report that 10-HDA extends the lifespan via the TOR signaling.

2. Methods

2.1. Culture and Strains of C. elegans. C. elegans strains were maintained at 20°C on nematode growth medium agar with *Escherichia coli* OP50 as a food source, as previously described [20]. The N2 Bristol strain was used as the wild type *C. elegans*. The mutant strains used in this study were CB1370: *daf-2(e1370)* III; DA465: *eat-2(ad465)* II; CB138: *unc-24(e138)* IV; DR412: *unc-24(e138)/daf-15(m81)* IV; and LG344: *geIs8[gpa-4p::skn-1b::gfp + rol-6(su1006)]*.

2.2. Treatment with 10-HAD. 10-HDA was purchased from Alfresa Pharma Co., Ltd., Osaka, Japan. 10-HDA was added to liquid NGM that had been autoclaved and cooled to 50°C, using DMSO as a solvent at a final concentration of 0.03%. The media were immediately dispensed into Petri dishes. 10-HDA was provided at 20°C from adult 0-day to death in the lifespan assay and from hatched L1 stage in the progeny production assay. Experiments involving 10-HDA were conducted in parallel with those involving a control group treated with an equivalent volume of DMSO.

2.3. Lifespan Determination. Lifespan was determined as previously described [6]. UV-killed *E. coli* strain OP50 was used as a food source in the experiment to avoid any effects of live *E. coli* on 10-HDA and any effects of 10-HDA on growth and metabolism of live *E. coli*. Lifespan under UV-killed *E. coli* is longer compared to that under live *E. coli* probably because of the diminished toxicity of growing bacteria [21]. Worms were raised until the L4 molt and were then transferred onto a new plate containing 40 μM 5-fluoro-2′-deoxyuridine (Sigma Aldrich, St. Louis, MO, USA) to prevent self-fertilization [22, 23]. The day of transfer at the L4 molt was counted as adult 0-day. Worms were judged to be dead when they did not respond to a mechanical stimulus. To focus on aging, worms that had become desiccated on the side of the plate after crawling off or those that displayed extruded internal organs were excluded from our analysis. The results of the survival assays were analyzed using the Kaplan-Meier method, and significance was measured with the log-rank test using the statistical analysis package StatMate III (ATMS, Tokyo, Japan).

2.4. Measurement of Progeny Production. Single newly hatched N2 worm was placed on a plate containing UV-killed OP50. Worms were transferred every day or every other day to fresh plates. The resulting progenies were left to develop for 2 days for measurement of progeny number.

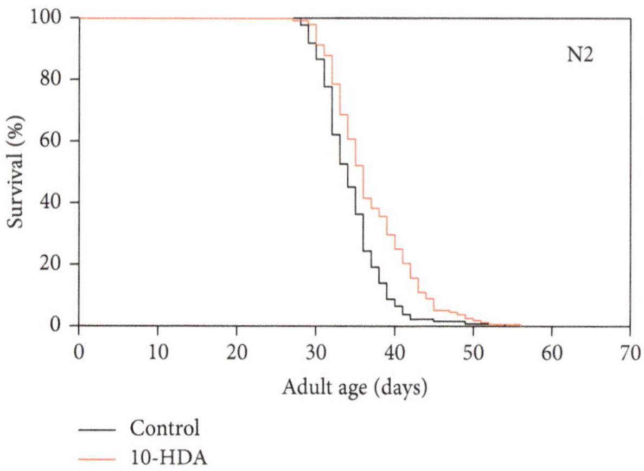

Figure 1: The effect of 10-HDA on the lifespan of N2 wild type *C. elegans*. The curves shown in Figures 1, 2, 3, and 5 represent pooled data from three to four experiments (Table 1).

2.5. Assays of Stress Resistance. To assess thermotolerance, young adult hermaphrodites were placed on NGM plates at 35°C and scored for viability. To assess oxidative stress, young adult hermaphrodites were placed on NGM plates, which included 50 mM paraquat (Sigma Aldrich) at 20°C and were scored for viability.

3. Results

3.1. 10-HDA Extends Lifespan Independently of ILS. As shown in Figure 1 and Table 1, 10-HDA extended the lifespan of N2, a wild type strain of *C. elegans* as previously described [6]. To investigate whether this lifespan extension effect of 10-HDA was due to ILS, we evaluated the effect of 10-HDA on the lifespan of the insulin-like receptor *daf-2* mutants, which reduce ILS and show long lifespan [18]. We found that 10-HDA further extended the lifespan of *daf-2* (Figure 2 and Table 1) indicating that 10-HDA affected lifespan independently of ILS. The previous finding that 10-HDA extended the lifespan of the mutants in *daf-16*, which encodes the FOXO transcription factor, the downstream target of ILS [6], also supports this notion. Alternatively, 10-HDA appeared to extend the lifespan of the *daf-2* mutants to a greater extent than that of the wild type (Figure 2 and Table 1) suggesting some interaction between 10-HDA and ILS.

3.2. 10-HDA Extends Lifespan through Dietary Restriction Signaling. To determine whether the lifespan extension by 10-HDA is mediated through dietary restriction signaling, we examined the effect of 10-HDA on the lifespan of the *eat-2* mutants, which display the extended lifespan through the feeding impairment-based dietary restriction [24]. As shown in Figure 3 and Table 1, 10-HDA did not further extend the lifespan of the *eat-2* mutants, suggesting that 10-HDA shared common lifespan control mechanisms with dietary restriction signaling. We wondered if 10-HDA directly exerts

TABLE 1: The effects of 10-HDA on the lifespan of various mutants.

Exp.	Genotype	Treatment	Mean life span ± SEM (days)	% change	Maximum life span (days)	% change	*N* (animal)	Significance
1	N2	Control	34.8 ± 0.8	+11	54	−4	34	$P < 0.01$
	N2	10-HDA 25 μM	38.7 ± 1.0		52		26	
2	N2	Control	34.4 ± 0.6	+10	49	+14	45	$P < 0.01$
	N2	10-HDA 25 μM	37.7 ± 0.8		56		29	
3	N2	Control	34.3 ± 0.5	+6	45	+11	56	$P < 0.01$
	N2	10-HDA 25 μM	36.2 ± 0.5		50		95	
1	*daf-2*	Control	61.3 ± 12.3	+10	82	+20	31	$P < 0.01$
	daf-2	10-HDA 25 μM	67.2 ± 11.7		98		34	
2	*daf-2*	Control	63.7 ± 10.5	+24	87	+46	49	$P < 0.01$
	daf-2	10-HDA 25 μM	79.2 ± 17.5		127		41	
3	*daf-2*	Control	63.0 ± 11.9	+14	83	+18	53	$P < 0.01$
	daf-2	10-HDA 25 μM	71.8 ± 13.9		98		61	
1	*eat-2*	Control	32.5 ± 2.8	+6	39	+25	23	
	eat-2	10-HDA 25 μM	34.5 ± 4.4		49		21	
2	*eat-2*	Control	39.8 ± 4.8	−13	56	−14	30	
	eat-2	10-HDA 25 μM	34.8 ± 5.1		48		11	
3	*eat-2*	Control	37.0 ± 5.3	−7	54	−4	71	
	eat-2	10-HDA 25 μM	34.4 ± 4.4		52		83	
1	*unc-24/+*	Control	37.8 ± 0.8	+4	46	+9	58	
	unc-24/+	10-HDA 25 μM	40.2 ± 1.1		50		61	
	unc-24/daf-15	Control	39.6 ± 1.3	−5	49	−14	71	
	unc-24/daf-15	10-HDA 25 μM	36.4 ± 0.6		42		65	
2	*unc-24/+*	Control	36.6 ± 0.5	+4	46	+9	58	$P < 0.01$
	unc-24/+	10-HDA 25 μM	38.1 ± 0.6		50		61	
	unc-24/daf-15	Control	37.7 ± 0.5	−5	49	−14	71	
	unc-24/daf-15	10-HDA 25 μM	35.8 ± 0.4		42		65	
3	*unc-24/+*	Control	37.7 ± 0.6	+6	47	+13	43	$P < 0.01$
	unc-24/+	10-HDA 25 μM	39.8 ± 0.7		53		47	
	unc-24/daf-15	Control	39.1 ± 0.6	−5	53	−11	85	
	unc-24/daf-15	10-HDA 25 μM	37.2 ± 0.4		47		83	
4	*unc-24/+*	Control	36.5 ± 4.6	+7	46	+11	38	$P < 0.01$
	unc-24/+	10-HDA 25 μM	39.0 ± 5.8		51		41	
	unc-24/daf-15	Control	37.8 ± 5.3	−3	50	−10	37	
	unc-24/daf-15	10-HDA 25 μM	36.5 ± 4.1		45		39	

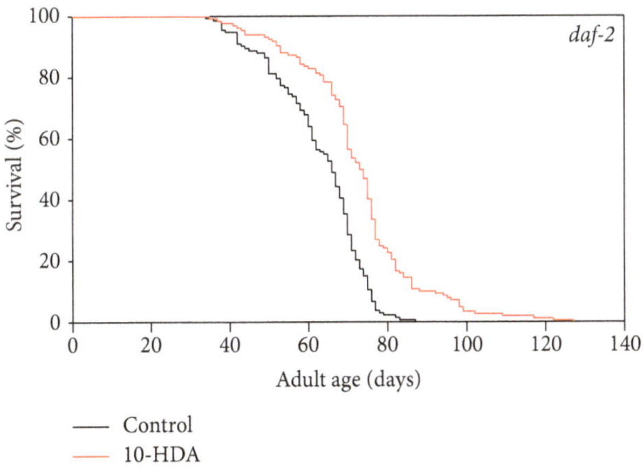

FIGURE 2: The effect of 10-HDA on the lifespan of the *daf-2* mutants.

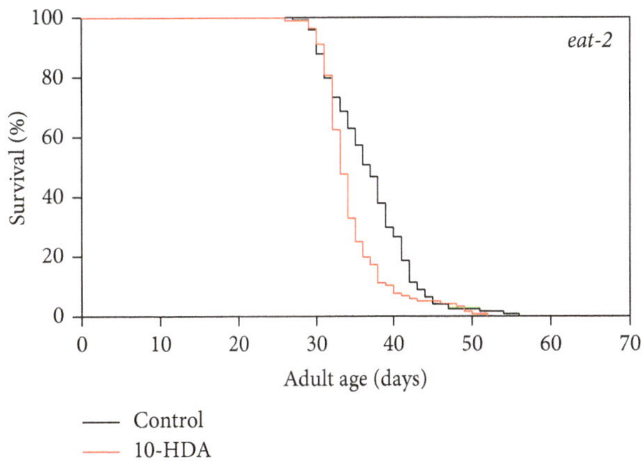

FIGURE 3: The effect of 10-HDA on the lifespan of the *eat-2* mutants.

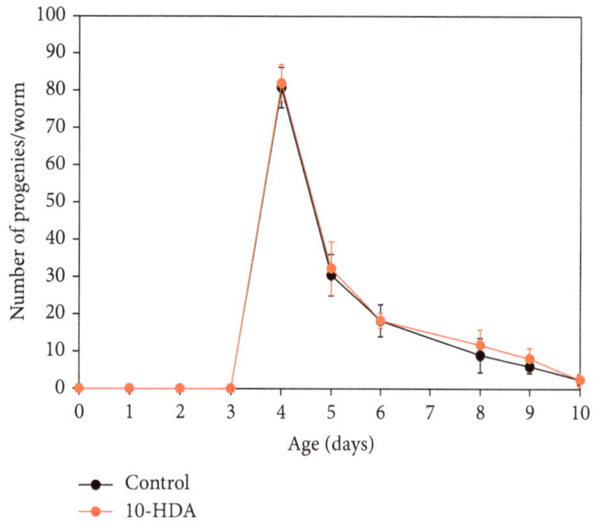

FIGURE 4: The effect of 10-HDA on the progeny production of wild type *C. elegans*. The progeny production is plotted against age at transfer. Mean values and SD are shown ($n = 6$). Day 0 corresponds to the hatched L1 stage.

dietary restriction. Dietary-restricted worms are known to produce progeny in a delayed manner [17]. 10-HDA-treated worms produced progeny in a similar manner to untreated ones (Figure 4), suggesting that 10-HDA is unlikely to directly restrict diet. Taken together, these findings suggest that 10-HDA extended lifespan by affecting the downstream process of the dietary restriction signaling.

3.3. 10-HDA Extends Lifespan through TOR Signaling. Dietary restriction has been reported to extend lifespan through various downstream signalings including TOR signaling [15]. To determine whether 10-HDA extended lifespan via the TOR signaling, we evaluated the effect of 10-HDA on the lifespan of mutants in *daf-15*, which encodes Raptor (the regulatory associated protein of mTOR), a component of the TOR complex [25]. The *daf-15* homozygous mutants show larval arrest and heterozygotes display lifespan extension [22]. As shown in Figure 5(b) and Table 1, 10-OHDA did not further extend the lifespan of the *daf-15* heterozygous mutants; 10-HDA extended the lifespan of the control *unc-24/+* mutants (Figure 5(a) and Table 1). This finding suggests that lifespan extension by 10-HDA is mediated through TOR signaling.

3.4. 10-HDA Confers Tolerance against Thermal and Oxidative Stresses. To assess whether 10-HDA confers tolerance against thermal and oxidative stresses, we examined the effects of 10-HDA treatment on survival during heat exposure and paraquat exposure. As shown in Figures 6(a) and 6(b), 10-HDA increased survival during both heat exposure and paraquat exposure.

4. Discussion

The findings we have presented here suggest that 10-HDA, the major lipid component of RJ, extends the lifespan of *C. elegans* through dietary restriction and TOR signaling. RJ is believed to have several components with lifespan-extending activity, including peptides (6), royalactin (9, 12), and 10-HDA, which work through a variety of signaling pathways, such as ILS, EGF, or TOR. This seems to indicate that RJ originally has diverse functions in honeybees, such as cast differentiation, queen longevity, and nourishment.

A variety of compounds have been shown to extend the lifespan of *C. elegans* [1]. Among them, anticonvulsants like ethosuximide [26], valproic acid [27], icariin [28], and caffeic acid phenethyl ester [29] extend lifespan via ILS. The present study showed that 10-HDA further extended the lifespan of *daf-2* mutants that showed long lifespan via ILS, indicating that 10-HDA extends lifespan independently of ILS.

On the other hand, dietary restriction mimetics including 2-deoxyglucose extend lifespan like direct dietary restriction [30]. Further, several compounds that target downstream of dietary restriction signaling also extend lifespan: α-ketoglutarate via the TOR signaling [31]; diallyl trisulfide [32] via SKN-1 pathway; metformin via AMP-activated protein kinase (AMPK); and SKN-1 pathways [33]. The SKN-1 transcription factor is the ortholog of mammalian Nrf2 and known to control stress protection. 10-HDA was found to confer tolerance against thermal and oxidative stresses (Figures 6(a) and 6(b)). However, we failed to find the induction of *skn-1* by 10-HDA treatment using the reporter of *skn-1*: *geIs8[gpa-4p::skn-1b::gfp]* (unpublished observation), suggesting that 10-HDA may not be involved in the SKN-1 pathway. Metformin has also been reported to retard aging by directly affecting metabolism of folate and methionine in *E. coli*, the worm's food [34]. Resveratrol extended lifespan via Sir2 [35] and AMPK pathways [19]. However, resveratrol has also been reported not to extend the lifespan of worms or flies [36] or mice [37]. Furthermore, oxaloacetate extended worm lifespan via both IIS and dietary restriction [38] but was reported not to extend mouse lifespan [37].

In the present study, we found that 10-HDA extended *C. elegans* lifespan via dietary restriction and the TOR pathway. RJ, whose major lipid component is 10-HDA, plays an important role in an epigenetic fate determination between worker and long-lived queen honeybees with identical genome composition [2–5, 39]. TOR has been reported to participate in the caste fate determination in honeybees [40–42]. Although it is unknown whether 10-HDA is involved in the caste fate determination, it may be relevant that 10-HDA functions as an inhibitor of histone deacetylase, which is known to play a main role in epigenesis [43] and that 10-HDA affects the expression of histone deacetylase 3 and DNA methyltransferase 3, both of which also play a role in epigenesis in honeybees [44].

TOR is known to be a nutrient sensor and controls lifespan as well as protein synthesis and degradation, cell growth, and autophagy [45–48]. Rapamycin, which inhibits TOR, extends the lifespan of yeasts [49], nematodes [50], flies [51], and mice [52]. However, chronic administration of rapamycin in rodents has several side effects such as glucose intolerance, insulin tolerance, and cataracts [53–57]. It may be possible that 10-HDA contained in RJ which is widely taken as a health food could be used as nutraceutical intervention

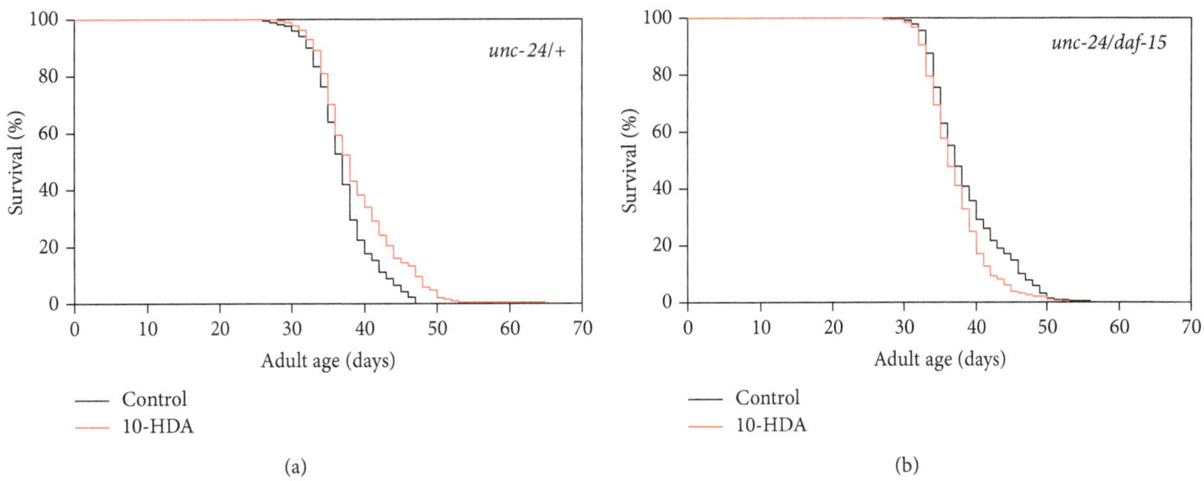

FIGURE 5: The effect of 10-HDA on the lifespan of the *daf-15* mutants. (a) *unc-24/+* and (b) *unc-24/daf-15*.

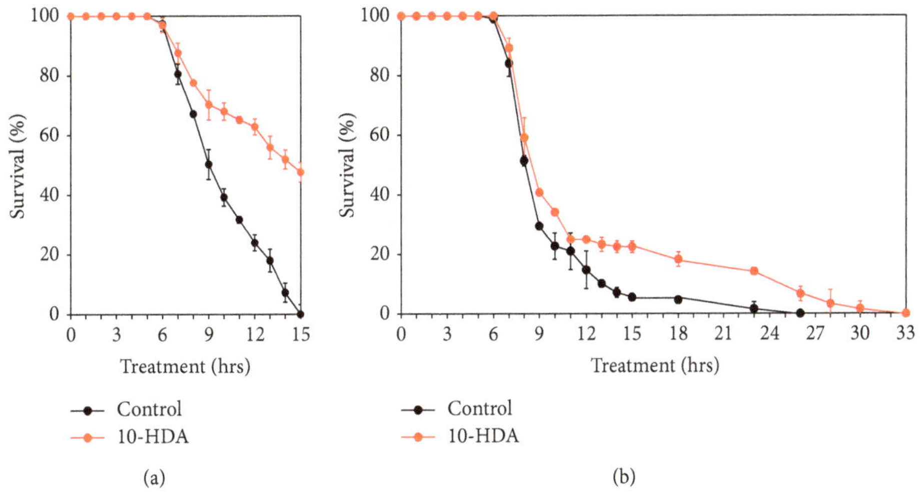

FIGURE 6: (a) Thermal stress. (b) Oxidative stress. Treatment with or without 25 μM 10-HDA began at the egg stage. Mean values and SD of triplicate samples are plotted.

aimed at mammalian TOR (mTOR) inhibition to delay aging and the onset of age-related diseases.

5. Conclusions

The present study indicates that 10-HDA extends lifespan of *C. elegans* not via ILS but via dietary restriction and the TOR signaling. It may be possible that 10-HDA contained in RJ which is widely taken by human as a health food could be used as nutraceutical intervention aimed at mTOR inhibition to delay aging and the onset of age-related diseases.

Conflict of Interests

This work was essentially supported by the Tokyo Metropolitan Institute of Gerontology financially and was partially funded by Api Company Limited, which engages in the manufacture and sale of royal jelly products and of which Yoko Araki, Taketoshi Hata, and Kenji Ichihara are employees. The authors confirm that this declaration does not alter their adherence to all the Journal of Aging Research policies on sharing data.

Acknowledgments

Some strains were provided by the CGC, which is funded by NIH Office of Research Infrastructure Programs (P40 OD010440).

References

[1] M. Lucanic, G. J. Lithgow, and S. Alavez, "Pharmacological lifespan extension of invertebrates," *Ageing Research Reviews*, vol. 12, no. 1, pp. 445–458, 2013.

[2] M. L. Winston, *The Biology of the Honey Bee*, Harvard University Press, Cambridge, Mass, USA, 1991.

[3] S. C. Remolina and K. A. Hughes, "Evolution and mechanisms of long life and high fertility in queen honey bees," *Age*, vol. 30, no. 2-3, pp. 177–185, 2008.

[4] A. Chittka and L. Chittka, "Epigenetics of royalty," *PLoS Biology*, vol. 8, no. 11, Article ID e1000532, 2010.

[5] R. E. Page Jr. and C. Y. S. Peng, "Aging and development in social insects with emphasis on the honey bee, *Apis mellifera* L," *Experimental Gerontology*, vol. 36, no. 4–6, pp. 695–711, 2001.

[6] Y. Honda, Y. Fujita, H. Maruyama et al., "Lifespan-extending effects of royal jelly and its related substances on the nematode *Caenorhabditis elegans*," *PLoS ONE*, vol. 6, no. 8, Article ID e23527, 2011.

[7] X. Wang, L. F. Cook, L. M. Grasso, M. Cao, and Y. Dong, "Royal jelly-mediated prolongevity and stress resistance in *Caenorhabditis elegans* is possibly modulated by the interplays of DAF-16, SIR-2.1, HCF-1, and 14-3-3 proteins," *The Journal of Gerontology, A Biological Science and Medical Science*, 2014.

[8] T. S. Gardner, "The use of *Drosophila melanogaster* as a screening agent for longevity factors; pantothenic acid as a longevity factor in royal jelly," *The Journals of Gerontology*, vol. 3, no. 1, pp. 1–8, 1948.

[9] M. Kamakura, "Royalactin induces queen differentiation in honeybees," *Nature*, vol. 473, no. 7348, pp. 478–483, 2011.

[10] S. I. Inoue, S. Koya-Miyata, S. Ushio, K. Iwaki, M. Ikeda, and M. Kurimoto, "Royal Jelly prolongs the life span of C3H/HeJ mice: correlation with reduced DNA damage," *Experimental Gerontology*, vol. 38, no. 9, pp. 965–969, 2003.

[11] T. Takenaka, "Chemical composition of royal jelly," *Honeybee Science*, vol. 3, no. 2, pp. 69–74, 1982.

[12] G. Detienne, W. de Haes, U. R. Ernst, L. Schoofs, and L. Temmerman, "Royalactin extends lifespan of *Caenorhabditis elegans* through epidermal growth factor signaling," *Experimental Gerontology*, vol. 60, pp. 129–135, 2014.

[13] A. Butenandt and H. Rembold, "Royal jelly of the honeybee. I. Isolation, constitution analysis, and incidence of 10-hydroxy-delta 2-decenoic acid," *Hoppe-Seyler's Zeitschrift für Physiologische Chemie*, vol. 203, no. 5-6, pp. 284–289, 1957.

[14] X. Li, C. Huang, and Y. Xue, "Contribution of lipids in honeybee (*Apis mellifera*) royal jelly to health," *Journal of Medicinal Food*, vol. 16, no. 2, pp. 96–102, 2013.

[15] G. F. Townsend, J. F. Morgan, S. Tolnai, B. Hazlett, H. J. Morton, and R. W. Shuel, "Studies on the in vitro antitumor activity of fatty acids. I. 10-Hydroxy-2-decenoic acid from royal jelly," *Cancer Research*, vol. 20, no. 4, pp. 503–510, 1960.

[16] X. Y. Yang, D. S. Yang, J. M. Wang et al., "10-Hydroxy-2-decenoic acid from Royal jelly: a potential medicine for RA," *Journal of Ethnopharmacology*, vol. 128, no. 2, pp. 314–321, 2010.

[17] H. Izuta, Y. Chikaraishi, M. Shimazawa, S. Mishima, and H. Hara, "10-Hydroxy-2-decenoic acid, a major fatty acid from royal jelly, inhibits VEGF-induced angiogenesis in human umbilical vein endothelial cells," *Evidence-Based Complementary and Alternative Medicine*, vol. 6, no. 4, pp. 489–494, 2009.

[18] C. J. Kenyon, "The genetics of ageing," *Nature*, vol. 464, no. 7288, pp. 504–512, 2010.

[19] E. L. Greer and A. Brunet, "Different dietary restriction regimens extend lifespan by both independent and overlapping genetic pathways in *C. elegans*," *Aging Cell*, vol. 8, no. 2, pp. 113–127, 2009.

[20] S. Brenner, "The genetics of *Caenorhabditis elegans*," *Genetics*, vol. 77, no. 1, pp. 71–94, 1974.

[21] D. Garigan, A.-L. Hsu, A. G. Fraser, R. S. Kamath, J. Abringet, and C. Kenyon, "Genetic analysis of tissue aging in *Caenorhabditis elegans*: a role for heat-shock factor and bacterial proliferation," *Genetics*, vol. 161, no. 3, pp. 1101–1112, 2002.

[22] R. Hosono, "Sterilization and growth inhibition of *Caenorhabditis elegans* by 5-fluorodeoxyuridine," *Experimental Gerontology*, vol. 13, no. 5, pp. 369–374, 1978.

[23] D. H. Mitchell, J. W. Stiles, J. Santelli, and D. R. Sanadi, "Synchronous growth and aging of *Caenorhabditis elegans* in the presence of fluorodeoxyuridine," *The Journals of Gerontology*, vol. 34, no. 1, pp. 28–36, 1979.

[24] B. Lakowski and S. Hekimi, "The genetics of caloric restriction in *Caenorhabditis elegans*," *Proceedings of the National Academy of Sciences of the United States of America*, vol. 95, no. 22, pp. 13091–13096, 1998.

[25] D.-H. Kim, D. D. Sarbassov, S. M. Ali et al., "mTOR interacts with raptor to form a nutrient-sensitive complex that signals to the cell growth machinery," *Cell*, vol. 110, no. 2, pp. 163–175, 2002.

[26] K. Evason, C. Huang, I. Yamben, D. F. Covey, and K. Kornfeld, "Anticonvulsant medications extend worm life-span," *Science*, vol. 307, no. 5707, pp. 258–262, 2005.

[27] K. Evason, J. J. Collins, C. Huang, S. Hughes, and K. Kornfeld, "Valproic acid extends *Caenorhabditis elegans* lifespan," *Aging Cell*, vol. 7, no. 3, pp. 305–317, 2008.

[28] W.-J. Cai, J.-H. Huang, S.-Q. Zhang et al., "Icariin and its derivative icariside II extend healthspan via insulin/IGF-1 pathway in *C. elegans*," *PLoS ONE*, vol. 6, no. 12, Article ID e28835, 2011.

[29] S. Havermann, Y. Chovolou, H. U. Humpf, W. Wätjen, and J. Sadoshima, "Caffeic acid phenethylester increases stress resistance and enhances lifespan in *Caenorhabditis elegans* by modulation of the insulin-like DAF-16 signalling pathway," *PLoS ONE*, vol. 9, no. 6, Article ID e100256, 2014.

[30] T. J. Schulz, K. Zarse, A. Voigt, N. Urban, M. Birringer, and M. Ristow, "Glucose restriction extends *Caenorhabditis elegans* life span by inducing mitochondrial respiration and increasing oxidative stress," *Cell Metabolism*, vol. 6, no. 4, pp. 280–293, 2007.

[31] R. M. Chin, X. Fu, M. Y. Pai et al., "The metabolite α-ketoglutarate extends lifespan by inhibiting ATP synthase and TOR," *Nature*, vol. 510, no. 7505, pp. 397–401, 2014.

[32] A. A. Powolny, S. V. Singh, S. Melov, A. Hubbard, and A. L. Fisher, "The garlic constituent diallyl trisulfide increases the lifespan of *C. elegans* via skn-1 activation," *Experimental Gerontology*, vol. 46, no. 6, pp. 441–452, 2011.

[33] B. Onken and M. Driscoll, "Metformin induces a dietary restriction-like state and the oxidative stress response to extend *C. elegans* healthspan via AMPK, LKB1, and SKN-1," *PLoS ONE*, vol. 5, no. 1, Article ID e8758, 2010.

[34] F. Cabreiro, C. Au, K.-Y. Leung et al., "Metformin retards aging in *C. elegans* by altering microbial folate and methionine metabolism," *Cell*, vol. 153, no. 1, pp. 228–239, 2013.

[35] M. Viswanathan, S. K. Kim, A. Berdichevsky, and L. Guarente, "A role for SIR-2.1 regulation of ER stress response genes in determining *C. elegans* life span," *Developmental Cell*, vol. 9, no. 5, pp. 605–615, 2005.

[36] T. M. Bass, D. Weinkove, K. Houthoofd, D. Gems, and L. Partridge, "Effects of resveratrol on lifespan in *Drosophila melanogaster* and *Caenorhabditis elegans*," *Mechanisms of Ageing and Development*, vol. 128, no. 10, pp. 546–552, 2007.

[37] R. Strong, R. A. Miller, C. M. Astle et al., "Evaluation of resveratrol, green tea extract, curcumin, oxaloacetic acid, and medium-chain triglyceride oil on life span of genetically heterogeneous mice," *The Journals of Gerontology Series A: Biological Sciences and Medical Sciences*, vol. 68, no. 1, pp. 6–16, 2013.

[38] D. S. Williams, A. Cash, L. Hamadani, and T. Diemer, "Oxaloacetate supplementation increases lifespan in *Caenorhabditis elegans* through an AMPK/FOXO-dependent pathway," *Aging Cell*, vol. 8, no. 6, pp. 765–768, 2009.

[39] R. Kucharski, J. Maleszka, S. Foret, and R. Maleszka, "Nutritional control of reproductive status in honeybees via DNA methylation," *Science*, vol. 319, no. 5871, pp. 1827–1830, 2008.

[40] A. Patel, M. K. Fondrk, O. Kaftanoglu et al., "The making of a queen: TOR pathway is a key player in diphenic caste development," *PLoS ONE*, vol. 2, no. 6, article e509, 2007.

[41] N. S. Mutti, A. G. Dolezal, F. Wolschin, J. S. Mutti, K. S. Gill, and G. V. Amdam, "IRS and tor nutrient-signaling pathways act via juvenile hormone to influence honey bee caste fate," *The Journal of Experimental Biology*, vol. 214, no. 23, pp. 3977–3984, 2011.

[42] D. E. Wheeler, N. A. Buck, and J. D. Evans, "Expression of insulin/insulin-like signalling and TOR pathway genes in honey bee caste determination," *Insect Molecular Biology*, vol. 23, no. 1, pp. 113–121, 2014.

[43] A. Spannhoff, Y. K. Kim, N. J.-M. Raynal et al., "Histone deacetylase inhibitor activity in royal jelly might facilitate caste switching in bees," *EMBO Reports*, vol. 12, no. 3, pp. 238–243, 2011.

[44] W. X. Wang, L. Q. Tian, Q. Huang, X. B. Wu, and Z. J. Zeng, "Effects of 10-Hydroxy-2-decenoic acid on the development of honey bee (*Apis mellifera*) larvae," *Journal of Apicultural Research*, vol. 53, no. 1, pp. 171–176, 2014.

[45] T. Vellai, K. Takacs-Vellai, Y. Zhang, A. L. Kovacs, L. Orosz, and F. Müller, "Influence of TOR kinase on lifespan in *C. elegans*," *Nature*, vol. 426, no. 6967, p. 620, 2003.

[46] P. Kapahi, B. M. Zid, T. Harper, D. Koslover, V. Sapin, and S. Benzer, "Regulation of lifespan in *Drosophila* by modulation of genes in the TOR signaling pathway," *Current Biology*, vol. 14, no. 10, pp. 885–890, 2004.

[47] P. Kapahi, D. Chen, A. N. Rogers et al., "With TOR, less is more: a key role for the conserved nutrient-sensing TOR pathway in aging," *Cell Metabolism*, vol. 11, no. 6, pp. 453–465, 2010.

[48] J. J. Wu, J. Liu, E. B. Chen et al., "Increased mammalian lifespan and a segmental and tissue-specific slowing of aging after genetic reduction of mTOR expression," *Cell Reports*, vol. 4, no. 5, pp. 913–920, 2013.

[49] A. L. Alvers, M. S. Wood, D. Hu, A. C. Kaywell, W. A. Dunn Jr., and J. P. Aris, "Autophagy is required for extension of yeast chronological life span by rapamycin," *Autophagy*, vol. 5, no. 6, pp. 847–849, 2009.

[50] S. Robida-Stubbs, K. Glover-Cutter, D. W. Lamming et al., "TOR signaling and rapamycin influence longevity by regulating SKN-1/Nrf and DAF-16/FoxO," *Cell Metabolism*, vol. 15, no. 5, pp. 713–724, 2012.

[51] I. Bjedov, J. M. Toivonen, F. Kerr et al., "Mechanisms of life span extension by rapamycin in the fruit fly *Drosophila melanogaster*," *Cell Metabolism*, vol. 11, no. 1, pp. 35–46, 2010.

[52] D. E. Harrison, R. Strong, Z. D. Sharp et al., "Rapamycin fed late in life extends lifespan in genetically heterogeneous mice," *Nature*, vol. 460, no. 7253, pp. 392–395, 2009.

[53] V. P. Houde, S. Brûlé, W. T. Festuccia et al., "Chronic rapamycin treatment causes glucose intolerance and hyperlipidemia by upregulating hepatic gluconeogenesis and impairing lipid deposition in adipose tissue," *Diabetes*, vol. 59, no. 6, pp. 1338–1348, 2010.

[54] N. Deblon, L. Bourgoin, C. Veyrat-Durebex et al., "Chronic mTOR inhibition by rapamycin induces muscle insulin resistance despite weight loss in rats," *British Journal of Pharmacology*, vol. 165, no. 7, pp. 2325–2340, 2012.

[55] D. W. Lamming, L. Ye, P. Katajisto et al., "Rapamycin-induced insulin resistance is mediated by mTORC2 loss and uncoupled from longevity," *Science*, vol. 335, no. 6076, pp. 1638–1643, 2012.

[56] J. E. Wilkinson, L. Burmeister, S. V. Brooks et al., "Rapamycin slows aging in mice," *Aging Cell*, vol. 11, no. 4, pp. 675–682, 2012.

[57] F. Neff, D. Flores-Dominguez, D. P. Ryan et al., "Rapamycin extends murine lifespan but has limited effects on aging," *The Journal of Clinical Investigation*, vol. 123, no. 8, pp. 3272–3291, 2013.

14

Older Adults with Hoarding Behaviour Aging in Place: Looking to a Collaborative Community-Based Planning Approach for Solutions

Kyle Y. Whitfield,[1] Jason S. Daniels,[1] Keri Flesaker,[2] and Doneka Simmons[3]

[1] *Faculty of Extension, University of Alberta, Enterprise Square, Room 2-215, 10230 Jasper Avenue, Edmonton, Alberta, Canada T5J 4P6*
[2] *Department of Educational Psychology, University of Alberta, 6-102 Education North, Edmonton, Alberta, Canada T6G 2G5*
[3] *Senior Association of Greater Edmonton, 15 Sir Winston Churchill Square, Edmonton, Alberta, Canada T5J 2E5*

Correspondence should be addressed to Kyle Y. Whitfield, kyle.whitfield@ualberta.ca

Academic Editor: Frank Oswald

This paper reports on and synthesizes new research that examines how a collaborative community response can promote successful aging in place for older adults with hoarding behaviour. Through interviews with older adults with hoarding behaviour, who used a particular community support and a focus group interview with members of the community collaborative that directed supports for this population, our findings suggest that there were valuable outcomes for both groups. These older adults with hoarding behaviour were able to remain in their own homes, their safety was enhanced, their sense of isolation was minimized, empowerment was fostered, and they gained valuable insight into their behaviour. The members of the community collaborative were able to access the expertise of other professionals, maximize their own expertise, and they generated an enhanced understanding of the experience of older adults living with hoarding behaviour in Edmonton. This study is a significant addition to the much too sparse literature about the community planning needs of older adults with hoarding behaviour. It offers knowledge that is integral to theories and principles of better aging in place but attempts to translate this into practice.

1. Introduction

Older adults with hoarding behaviour are often at a high risk of being homeless making aging in place extremely complex. This paper reports on a study that examines the value of a community-based planning approach that responds to the needs of this population, a population that is both increasing in number and that is very seldom studied [1]. It synthesizes new research about the complexities associated with remaining in one's own home when he/she is over 55 and has compulsive hoarding behaviour. And it examines how a collaborative community response promotes successful aging in place for this population. Not only are community-based services necessary to better understand because they are central to all health sectors [2], but also current research surrounding those with hoarding behaviour is mostly focussed on methods addressing individual-level behavioural characteristics of hoarding through cognitive behavioural therapy (cf., the extensive work of Frost and Steketee). Missing are descriptions of community-based planning approaches for health and social service sectors working hard to make aging in place a possibility.

For older individuals with hoarding behaviour, aging in place is complex because hoarding behaviour is multifaceted; it touches on social, environmental, familial, and personal issues [3]. Aging in place is also not simple for those with hoarding behavior because they want to remain living in their own homes, neighbourhoods and communities which seem to require that a collection of agencies, often representing different sectors, understand their needs in order to help them stay in the community and age in place. In this paper, aging in place refers to an ideal where people can age in the familiarity of their homes, neighbourhoods, and communities where their quality of life is maximized by the availability and accessibility of supports and services that respond to their needs and capacities [4, 5]. Aging in place, in addition, is about belonging to a community that supports one's many needs, for example, physically, socially, mentally, environmentally, and so forth [6]. To understand the varying aspects of aging in place in late life, older individuals with hoarding behaviour need to be further understood so their aging journey is successful; collaborative approaches by community support agencies can help to make that possible.

In our case, social and health related organizations from different sectors, that in some way supported people with hoarding behaviour in Edmonton, AB, Canada, were brought together in 2007 through the leadership of the social worker of a seniors support agency called SAGE (Seniors Association of Greater Edmonton). After having visited a number of individuals with hoarding behaviour (age 55+) in her professional role, she noticed, as did those members of the imminent community collaborative, that those with hoarding behaviour were at a high risk for being evicted from their homes, and they experienced shame associated with their hoarding resulting in isolation, as well as depression; they were at risk of falling in their own homes, and generally, they were living in unsanitary conditions. To approach this highly vulnerable population, to respond to some of their needs, especially to prevent their potential eviction, a concerted effort by a broad representation of social, health, and other agencies was necessary. The collaborative met together regularly (e.g., once every 2 months over the years and as of June 2011, it continues to meet) to continually plan for and improve the support of older adults with hoarding behaviour in the Edmonton area.

Although little is still known about the effects of one's neighbourhood on the mental health of older adults, positive mental health in later life may be influenced by the way in which older people feel about their neighbourhood [7]. It is fair to conclude, therefore, that for older adults with hoarding behaviour, place matters and the role of place as locality is key when making meaning at both the individual and the collective levels. In particular, local place is an important factor in identity, in ones sense of community, and attachment; this is crucial to the determinants of attachment, satisfaction, and behaviour [8]. Also important is place and the person-place relationship are very much grounded in a context of fear over loss of place [9] and the obliteration of locality [10]. Aging and compulsive hoarding behaviour need to be examined in concert with one another.

As our aging population rapidly increases, the number of older adults with hoarding behaviour will also quickly increase. Although hoarding behaviour usually begins in early adolescents, its severity increases with age [11]. Results from the Hopkins Epidemiology of Personality Disorder Study found that the odds of hoarding were over two times as great in the oldest compared with the youngest age group [12], and in a study of hoarding-related complaints to public health departments in Massachusetts, 40% of individuals that hoarded were involved with elder service agencies [13].

Referring to Frost and Hartl [14] when defining hoarding behaviour, there are key characteristics: the acquisition of and failure to discard a large number of possessions that seem to be of little use or limited value; cluttered living spaces that cannot be used as intended; significant distress and/or impairment associated with the clutter. Hoarded possessions clutter living spaces until rooms are difficult or impossible to use for their designed purpose, causing significant stress to the individuals themselves. Possessions may be purchased through compulsive buying [15] and/or through acquiring things like newspapers or discarded items from dumpsters [16]. Some individuals may even steal new possessions. After acquiring possessions, discarding these items is extremely difficult [17]. In serious instances, household clutter may interfere with and prevent daily activities, like food preparation, moving freely in one's home, and using the bathroom [11, 17]. And as clutter increases, falling, fire, sanitation issues, depression, and isolation are possible, creating significant risk for a number of outcomes but especially eviction and thus homelessness [18].

Community collaboration is one way to respond to social and health needs of a population. In fact, genuine collaborate is say to be the very thing that successfully reforms health systems [14]. Although there are many ways to define collaboration, most definitions emphasize the importance of shared responsibility and a team approach [20], and using a collaborative approach can significantly increase the available pool of resources from which team members can draw [21]. A response to the multiple challenges of older adults with hoarding behaviour requires a comprehensive and far-reaching approach, more than one single agency can provide alone [22, 23]. Philosophically, collaboration is rooted in systems theory which says that entities in a system are dependent on one another [24] and ecological theory in particular proposes that causes and solutions of health and/or social problems are beyond the individual and are associated with such determinants as the health and social services that we receive [25]. Service recipients can benefit from a collaborative approach to the provision of community health services as can the agencies participating in the collaborative [26–28]. Using a collective made up of representative agencies to support this vulnerable population creates potential for an approach that builds on the strengths of all those involved.

2. Methods

Between January 2007 and January 2010, approximately 75 older adults (ages 55+) with hoarding behaviour in Edmonton, AB, Canada, were provided with community supports to prevent them from being evicted from their homes [29]. The Seniors Association of Greater Edmonton (SAGE) offers support through a program referred to as *This Full House*. And *This Full House* is a direct outcome of the work of the community collaborative. The aim of *This Full House* for older individuals with hoarding behaviour is to prevent eviction from their home, improve their health and well-being, maintain positive social contacts, and contribute to the building of a healthy community [29]. As the population of potential participants with hoarding behaviour in Edmonton is not particularly large, a small-n approach was used in an attempt to create heuristic generalizations which Tsoukas [30] defines as opportunities to refine analytic understanding and to make more incisive distinctions than were previously possible. Small-n studies are not designed to support or refute a theory, but rather, to further refine it. As such, the purpose of this study is to further examine the role of a collaborative planning approach in a community setting when seeking to help those over 55 years with issues relevant to having compulsive hoarding behaviour and wanting to age well in one's community.

To further understand the value of collaboration and, in particular, its role and value in this community support, interviews and a focus group were conducted with seniors with hoarding issues involved with *This Full House* and with the community collaborative. All interviews were semi-structured and conducted by a third party researcher (i.e., Research Assistant). Ethics approval for this research was received from the University of Alberta, Research Ethics Board.

2.1. Interviews with Individuals with Hoarding Behaviour. Individual interviews were conducted with five ($N = 5$) individuals with hoarding behaviour involved with *This Full House*, all of whom were over the age of 55. The semistructured, face to face interviews took place at a location expressed as being most comfortable to the interviewee, for example, at their homes, at a university office, at a nearby coffee shop. These study participants were first contacted by the social worker from SAGE who directs *This Full House*. The individuals with hoarding behaviour had either referred themselves to *This Full House* or had been referred to it by one of their health care practitioners or family members. At an appointment with the individuals, the social worker informed them about the study asking if they might be interested in being interviewed by a researcher about their experience with *This Full House*. If they agreed (which all five did), she gave them a one-page written description of the study. She then went through the summary of the study ensuring they understood what was being requested from them. With their agreement, their telephone numbers were provided to the researcher (i.e., Research Assistant) who contacted them and established a location and time to meet for the interview. The aim of the one-hour interviews was to gather information regarding their experience with *This Full House*. In particular, the interview was used to understand their perceptions of the impact of or value of their association with *This Full House*, that is, the aspects of the program they benefitted from most.

2.2. Focus Group with the Community Collaborative Members. A community collaborative made up of social and health related agency representatives providing insights into the ongoing development of *This Full House* was formed. The focus group interview included ten members ($N = 10$) (of the possible 11 members in total) and was conducted in a face-to-face manner for approximately 1.5 hours. Members of this collaborative represented a number of expert groups: social workers, home care nurses, geriatric neuropsychologists, geriatric nurses, fire and safety investigators, public health practitioners, and environmental health and safety officers. The focus group questions centered on the nature of the working relationship between and amongst the members and their observations about the value and impact their work may have had on the service users, that is, those with hoarding behaviour. The questions guiding the semistructured interview were generated from key themes highlighted in the literature (i.e., health services, collaboration, community support, etc.) that aligned with the purpose of the study.

3. Results

Use of a grounded theory framework was quite valuable for our data analysis. Grounded theory means that the data analysis essentially, is "grounded" in the data [31]. Therefore, the concepts and themes we describe in our results have evolved from and are embedded in the data collected and have been mined through a process of conceptual ordering. Grounded theories are said to provide further insight, to enhance understanding, and to be used as a guide to inform action (i.e., acting on the results). As Strauss and Corbin [31] describe in more detail, our interview data, in the form of pages of the exact words from the interview, was organized into categories that were not predetermined but that evolved after reading and rereading this data many times. And that, mainly described ideas and offered explanations from interviewees that had commonalities to each other. The themes described here are those that were mentioned frequently and carried the same meaning.

Because our aim in this study was to further our understanding of how older adults with hoarding behaviour were supported by a particular community-based planning approach, grounded theory provided the most effective means of organizing, reducing, and understanding the data. Suggested below is a picture that describes how the work of the community collaborative, because of its high level of collaboration, resulted in many important benefits for older people with hoarding behaviour that align well with and facilitate the goals and ideals associated with an aging in place model. The picture also describes how the community collaborative members valued their experience on the team.

3.1. The Work of the Community Collaborative Benefitted People with Hoarding Behaviour. As a result of this group working together to respond to the needs of older adults with hoarding behaviour, several themes evolved from the data demonstrating direct benefits for these individuals: being able to remain in their own homes; reducing their potential for harm, and minimizing their isolation all which allowed them to experience a feeling of empowerment which also helped them to generate insight into issues surrounding their hoarding behaviour.

3.1.1. Remaining in Own Home. There are considerable challenges associated with aging in one place for older individuals with hoarding behaviour. They can be at significant risk of being evicted from their homes and their behaviour can be a major public health concern leading to eviction as a result of violating building, fire, or property maintenance codes. It may not be until a particular emergency occurs (i.e., water leakage, fire, and pest infestation) that a landlord is notified [32]. One focus group member describes their role, as a member of the community collaborative, in minimizing evictions for this population:

> *"Our legislation says that we do have the right to go into any public or private place if we believe there may be a public health nuisance... and if that means we have to order their suite cleaned out, we'll do it. Um, because you can't get control of bedbugs and cockroaches unless you treat all the suites and if somebody's hoarding, you can't get rid of them... so, so they have to clean up."*

The five interviewees in this study were all in a situation where eviction from their homes was a potential, but they were able to remain at home as a result of a community-based approach that addressed some of their needs. Prior to the existence of this community collective, one focus group member describes how the health inspector had to play all roles and visit clients once a week and "nag people into cleaning up, which was mostly unsuccessful." For example, when there is a potential home eviction for individuals with hoarding behaviour, the social worker and a public health worker, together with the client and other members of the collaborative, that is, where necessary such as a fire and safety representative, provide input into the problem-solving process. A professional organizer usually assists with the practical aspects associated with cleaning up including heavy lifting, removing garbage, and reorganizing resulting in "[these clients being able to] stay living at home without being on the street and [being] homeless." Being able to age in one's own home, one's neighbourhood, and community fosters independence significantly impacts a more positive relationship in the person-place relationship [33].

The five people with hoarding behaviour that we interviewed spoke about the value of being able to remain living in their own homes. One person found it motivating to have someone help him/her to clean up his/her apartment, "it's the motivation of having someone there plus... the helper doing the heavy lifting and heavy carrying... making... 76 thousand trips to the garbage bin... its stressful but helpful [and] I certainly would not have been able to hire a company on my own [...] if the program had not been in effect [and] I would be in deep do-do with Capital Health." For another individual, what helped him remain in his own home was having the home care worker put him in touch with the social worker and the cleaning person who helped him find ways to deal with issues of parting with his stuff. And for this gentleman, the social worker supported him by suggesting options: "she made life more convenient for me by offering me options." And for another person, the social worker and the cleaner reminded her that the condition of her house, the bugs, the mouse droppings, the make up from years ago, the shiny covered magazines all over, and the infestation that she had, was not her fault and she could probably face organizing and cleaning it with encouragement and the help of a plan.

3.1.2. Reducing Harm and Promoting Safety. Hoarding behaviour creates a significant safety risk for the individual him/her self and for the community [32]. Harm reduction is a core principle that is essential to address the needs of those with compulsive hoarding behaviour because promoting safety is foremost [13]. In this case, focusing on harm reduction by the community collective ensured that safety was embedded within all the actions, initiatives, and supports they provided. One focus group member talks about the value of taking on this strategic focus: "We subsequently learned the value of focusing on a harm reduction approach wherein we address issues of harm first so that the person [with hoarding behaviour], at least, will be safe. Even though they may be living with a significant amount of stuff every day of their lives, but at least they are safe." A harm reduction philosophy considers behaviour change to be incremental and assumes that people will maintain their behaviour change when they have decision-making power to influence their goals and put them into action [34].

This focus on safety and reducing harm or the potential for harm helped the individuals with hoarding behaviour buy into the larger process at hand, that is, to contribute to the building of healthy neighbourhoods, supporting their well-being, and helping them stay in their homes as long as possible. Instead of suddenly or immediately removing the person from a potentially unsafe environment or situation, the aim instead is first to reduce the potential for harm and create a safe place to live. In the case of these five individuals, it meant such things as: hiring a person to help them remove and reorganize their excessive items, getting help to fumigate their apartments, openly talking about their hoarding situation to help them reflect upon it, receiving nonjudgemental support, and establishing a plan to minimize household items. One interviewee describes the value of setting goals and generating a plan, "we set a plan and the social worker would come back and generally we would accomplish that goal whatever it was." It also meant helping the person at risk of potential eviction, for example, to respond to requests made by the Public Health Inspector. One person with hoarding behaviour describes the role of this service (i.e., *This Full House*): "they sort of mediate [between varying agencies] and rub off the sharp corners." Reducing harm by promoting safety enables an aging in place philosophy and model as both can facilitate positive and long-term aging in one location.

3.1.3. Minimizing Loneliness. The community collaborative, used in this study as a planning approach helped to address the problem of isolation for these older adults. Several of the representative organizations of the community collaborative, that is, a social worker, public health nurse, geriatric nurse, and so forth, offer home visitation to many of their clients and observe their living environment. As observed by one community collaborative member, "a lot of these seniors are very lonely, very isolated, and so the fact that they have someone that's coming to their home often, helps." Another member talked about the impact of the support group (which is provided for people with hoarding behaviour on a monthly basis as part of *This Full House* services) on minimizing their sense of loneliness and connecting with people that have similar experiences: "[there is] value of that coming together, meeting with other people and seeing and hearing that you're not alone." Two interviewees with hoarding behaviour confirmed this same sentiment, about the importance of feeling connected to a group: "the group has helped me" and "[I realized] you are not the odd one out." As a result of not feeling alone and part of a group, interviewees with hoarding behaviour said that they felt empowered.

3.1.4. Fostering Empowerment. Empowerment can be an outcome of collaborative relationships; it offers a catalyst for new community programs and other supports, changes in policies, and advancing health practices [35, 36]. The members of the community collaborative intentionally aimed to facilitate empowerment using it as a principle to guide their work that addressed the needs of older individuals with hoarding behaviour in the greater Edmonton area. During the focus group interview, one member describes how empowerment as a guiding principle was translated into action benefitting a particular individual with hoarding behaviour:

> *"We [the community collaborative] have entertained some really creative approaches in terms of dealing with management [i.e., housing manager] and having the client lead those interventions [...] as opposed to, we [the service providers] meet[ing] with management, then... meet[ing] with the client... we really include the client in those interventions, so that the client really is aware of everyone that's involved, what's being discussed and then they are really empowered to be part of the action plan."*

When individuals with hoarding behaviour are more involved in directing their own support, they may experience greater control in such decision making which can lead to empowerment [13]. As observed by another community collaborative member, "[empowerment provides] a sense of control in a situation that they may feel a lack of control."

3.1.5. Communicating Insight into Their Hoarding Behaviour. The most successful reported treatment for those with compulsive hoarding behaviour is the use of behavioural treatment, in other words, a cognitive behavioural model [37]. To be motivated to discard their possessions, insight into their hoarding behaviour is significant [14, 38]. Members of the community collaborative said that individuals with hoarding behaviour seemed to gain insight into their behaviour as a result of the support provided by this collaborative. This observation was expressed during the focus group interview by the social worker:

> *"... the insights that come out as a part of the intervention, as you go along, then they [clients with hoarding behaviour] start to reveal some insight as to "how did I ever get to this place? and, "I can't believe this happened to me" and "I can't believe that I'm actually, I'm making some decisions now that I was not able to before"."*

During an individual interview, one individual with hoarding behaviour reflected on the changes in her own behaviour of accumulating things: "I would still be walking down one little path between the bathroom, bedroom and one side of the kitchen and that would have been it." Another interviewee with hoarding behavior expresses insight into her hoarding behavior: "they [the social worker] finally were able to get me to accept... this condition... that it probably was not my fault and that I could probably face it... it's been a great support... eye opening." And another person said something similar: "when I think how far I came from the first day.... it [my behavior] improved." She also said "I need to continue both thinking about and maybe following up [...] with counseling [...] is there an answer why I have become a person who allows clutter around myself [...]?". In the one-on-one interviews, individuals reported an improved feeling of independence and a sense of empowerment. This occurred because the collaborative team joined forces, they were united by a common goal of supporting, to the best of their ability, the needs of this population who they noticed to be struggling more and more and who they were being called upon more frequently to try to assist.

3.2. Participating in the Community Collaborative Benefitted the Group Members, Individually and Collectively. On individual and collective levels, the members of the community collaborative experienced three significant benefits as a consequence of participating in this group. For example, members of the collaborative were able to access the expertise of other professionals, they maximized the use of their own skills and knowledge and significantly enhanced their understanding of hoarding behaviour.

3.2.1. Accessing Expertise from the Other Group Members. Working on the collaborative team allowed the individual members an opportunity to access a broader range of skills and knowledge than those who were found solely in their own area of expertise or their own organization. In one instance, a professional social worker described how she could now present the risks associated with hoarding behaviour more objectively to a client with greater confidence as she could make reference to and more easily call on the authoritative role of the local fire department. Because the firefighter and social worker were both members of the collaborative, a close working partnership was facilitated. This benefit was expressed in this way: "when I mention to her [the client with compulsive hoarding behavior] the possibility of having someone from [the fire department] come and just do an assessment to let her know what her risk level is [i.e., of eviction from her home], she was suddenly open to that." As a result of working collaboratively, members also got to know more about the professional resources available to them in the community through their ongoing communication together. As one health professional of the community collaborative said: "it is a professional benefit to see and use the expertise around this table for the benefit of the individual clients."

Evaluating collaborative planning practices must consider not just the purpose of the collaboration but the value of its relational interactions [28]. For example, asking how social relations are changed can reveal how certain conditions are impacted for the group. Access to new areas of expertise is one descriptor of the quality of social relations. The sharing of expertise between and amongst the members was said to directly benefit the older people with hoarding behaviour using the services of *This Full House*. In the words of one member of the community collaborative, "a benefit of the collaborative process was working with everybody, to partner, to ensure that we're getting our clients the best support."

3.2.2. Maximizing their Own Expertise. Participating in this group allowed team members to maximize the use of their own expertise. One member, a public health inspector, recounted a time when such a collaborative approach was not used to support older adults with hoarding behaviour illustrating the tremendous limitations of working in isolation:

> *"Before... [the community collaborative existed] it was [up to]... the health inspector to try and play all roles and just sort of go and visit once a week and try and nag people into cleaning up. Which was mostly unsuccessful and wasn't really our job. I mean we are not social workers, we're not mental health workers, we are public health inspectors."*

Functioning alone, the health inspector had to operate as the only contact for this client group. Working in isolation took away time from the job he/she was actually trained and hired to do forcing them to work beyond their professional scope of practice. As further evidence of the value of being able to maximize one's own expertise, the professional organizer, who provides hands-on assistance with the cleanup of client homes, can now maximize her cleaning and organizational skills while directing clients' emotional issues to a trained professional. As described by the social worker during the focus group interview: "A big portion of her [the professional organizer's] time was addressing the [clients] emotional issues. So we've now learned that when those issues come up, it's a direct link back to me."

3.2.3. Enhancing Their Knowledge of Hoarding Behaviour. Members of the community collaborative described how their partnering with one another as professionals helped to enhance their knowledge and understanding of compulsive hoarding behaviour. Gaining new knowledge and a more "enlightened understanding" of compulsive hoarding behaviour was said to be the result of participating in this ongoing process. One member of the collaborative described the value of the increase of his knowledge stating "another professional benefit [of being a member of the community collaborative] is deepening my personal understanding of what hoarding is and what the dynamics are. Certainly, it's helped me in recognizing that it's multi-faceted." Group members said they were then able to take their learning back to their representative organizations: "I think working with [the collaborative] has really helped to educate me and hopefully the rest of [name of organization]." Successful aging in place requires that support by community-based organizations exists that it is available and accessible and responsive to a variety of their needs; therefore, knowledge about aging and its long list of associated issues, such as compulsive hoarding behaviour, is imperative.

4. Discussion

The aim of our discussion is to explain several matters that underpin the major themes of our results. Explaining why such themes evolved and their relationship to the broader phenomenon being studied is what Strauss and Corbin refer to as the process of theorizing [31]. At the heart of this study is community-based planning as a phenomenon of which a number of related concepts are embedded: aging in place, social support, collaboration, vulnerable populations, and community services. Overall, our research attempted to discover how a collaborative approach to planning for and addressing the needs of older adults with hoarding behaviour, living in the community, provided value. For these vulnerable adults living in Edmonton, Alberta, Canada, a collaborative planning approach that involved multiple agencies (representing varying sectors) that worked continuously to improve their quality of life made a difference. And, the members of this community collaborative also benefitted. From this approach they were able to access the professional expertise of the other group members, maximize the use of their own skills and knowledge, overall, giving them an opportunity to generate new insights into hoarding behaviour which they described as helping them provide the best possible care and support to this population. It is feasible; therefore, to use such results to inform the many ways to age in place more successfully in late life.

Currently there is no systemic, long-term process to support older people living in the community that have compulsive hoarding behavior. Nor in Canada, is there an overall strategy to plan for our aging population, therefore aging in place, at a national, political scale, is not yet a priority. But, because people with this behavior will increase in numbers, and the complexities associated with their need to live safely in their own communities, a national strategy must also address their specific and unique needs. As emphasized by The Canadian Health Services Research Foundation [39], our study also finds a need for enhanced integration, cooperation, and coordination at the system and at the service delivery levels. That is, integration and collaboration between health and social services, between ranges of sectors, between disciplines of front line workers, and between government ministries. Collaboration and integration need to be part of the foundation upon which aging in one's own home and community can be realized. In addition, our study supports the findings of Keonig et al. [3] who found that when having to facilitate ethical dilemmas for this population, older adults with hoarding behavior benefit from the use of teams whose members have a variety of disciplines.

Well evidenced in the health services planning literature, applied to an aging population, is the need for improved collaboration, both at a principle and a practice-based level [35]. Our study also confirms and emphasizes this important need. Not only do our findings align with the literature but it provides further insight into the challenges associated with older individuals that want and deserve to remain in their own homes. Our particular case is specific to older individuals that have hoarding behaviour that were supported through the efforts of a community collaborative planning approach. Our study adds to the current aging in place literature and extends it. The current literature supports collaboration and integration at varying levels of the health and social support system. But studies that examine community planning approaches grounded in collaboration are uncommon. This population will increase in numbers over time and they deserve to remain in their own communities with the support of surrounding agencies and organizations that work togather to best support older individuals with hoarding behaviour to age well in their own homes.

5. Conclusions

At the heart of several concepts and themes arising from interviews with older people with compulsive hoarding behavior and members of a community collaborative working to support this population is an approach founded on collaboration between and amongst service providers. Results demonstrated that when a highly collaborative approach to planning is used, there were quite direct benefits for older adults with hoarding behavior and, at the same time, there were benefits for the members of the community collaborative. This approach to planning for the health and social needs of this population resulted in people with hoarding behavior being able to remain in their own homes when eviction was a potential, enhancing their safety, helping to minimize their isolation, and creating opportunities to increase control in their own decision making. The members of the community collaborative could now access the expertise of other professionals, maximize their own expertise, and they generated new insight and understanding of the experience of older adults living with hoarding behaviour in Edmonton. Our study needs to be viewed within certain boundaries. Although our data conveys that this approach to planning has quite positive outcomes, our data is short term and situational. Our use of a single, one-time only interview method only allows us to draw insights and observations about that moment in time and not over an extended trajectory. As well, our study is grounded in five interviews with older adults with compulsive hoarding behavior. And although a collaborative approach to addressing the needs of older people with hoarding behaviour conveyed comprehensive benefits, collaboration as a planning approach is rarely the complete answer or solution to people's social and health needs. Health Integrated Delivery systems, for example, are far more comprehensive but do view collaborative planning as a core principle [2]. Viewed in this light, aging in place may not always be possible, but it must be realized that community-level social and health related supports maximize the quality of later life while aging at home [5]. And further building on that is the need for a well-coordinated model of care [5, 35] where supports are comprehensive, easily accessible, and well connected [5].

Acknowledgments

The authors are grateful to the Seniors Association for Greater Edmonton for helping to facilitate this study. As well, they very much appreciate the individuals with hoarding behaviour and professionals that agreed to participate in an interview. This research was made possible through a University of Alberta, Faculty of Extension Research Grant.

References

[1] S. A. Luchian, R. J. McNally, and J. M. Hooley, "Cognitive aspects of nonclinical obsessive-compulsive hoarding," *Behaviour Research and Therapy*, vol. 45, no. 7, pp. 1657–1662, 2007.

[2] F. Lega, "Organisational design for health integrated delivery systems: theory and practice," *Health Policy*, vol. 81, no. 2-3, pp. 258–279, 2007.

[3] T. Koenig, R. Chapin, and R. Spano, "Using multi-disciplinary teams to address ethical dilemmas with older adults who hoard," *Journal of Gerontological Social Work*, vol. 53, no. 2, pp. 137–147, 2010.

[4] C. Dye, D. Willoughby, and D. Battisto, "Advice from rural elders: what it takes to age in place," *Educational Gerontology*, vol. 37, no. 1, pp. 74–93, 2011.

[5] Institute for Life Course and Aging, *Mapping Aging in Place in a Changing Neighborhood*, University of Toronto, Toronto, Canada, 2008.

[6] A. Bookman, "Innovative models of aging in place: transforming our communities for an aging population," *Community Work and Family*, vol. 11, no. 4, pp. 419–438, 2008.

[7] C. Gale, E Dennison, C. Cooper, and A. Sayer, "Neighbourhood environment and positive mental health in older people: the Hertfordshire Cohort Study," *Health and Place*, vol. 17, no. 4, pp. 867–874, 2011.

[8] R. Stedman, "Toward a social psychology of place: predicting behavior from place-based cognitions, attitude, and identity," *Environment and Behavior*, vol. 34, no. 5, pp. 561–581, 2002.

[9] E. Relph, "Geographical experiences and being-in-the-world: the phenomenological origins of geography," in *Dwelling, Place and Environment*, D. Seamon and R. Mugerauer, Eds., pp. 15–32, Columbia University, New York, NY, USA, 1985.

[10] D. Massey, "The conceptualization of place," in *A Place in the World?* D. Massey and P. Jess, Eds., pp. 45–86, Open University Press, Milton Keynes, UK, 1995.

[11] J. Grisham, R. O. Frost, G. Steketee, H. J. Kim, and S. Hood, "Age of onset of compulsive hoarding," *Journal of Anxiety Disorders*, vol. 20, no. 5, pp. 675–686, 2006.

[12] J. F. Samuels, O. J. Bienvenu, M. A. Grados et al., "Prevalence and correlates of hoarding behaviour in a community-based sample," *Behaviour Research and Therapy*, vol. 46, no. 7, pp. 836–844, 2008.

[13] R. O. Frost, G. Steketee, and L. Williams, "Hoarding: a community health problem," *Health and Social Care in the Community*, vol. 8, no. 4, pp. 229–234, 2000.

[14] R. O. Frost and T. L. Hartl, "A cognitive-behavioral model of compulsive hoarding," *Behaviour Research and Therapy*, vol. 34, no. 4, pp. 341–350, 1996.

[15] R. O. Frost and G. Steketee, *Stuff: Compulsive Hoarding and the Meaning of Things*, Houghton Mifflin Harcourt, Boston, Mass, USA, 2009.

[16] R. O. Frost, H. J. Kim, C. Morris, C. Bloss, M. Murray-Close, and G. Steketee, "Hoarding, compulsive buying and reasons for saving," *Behaviour Research and Therapy*, vol. 36, no. 7-8, pp. 657–664, 1998.

[17] G. Steketee and R. O. Frost, *Compulsive Hoarding and Acquiring: Therapist Guide*, Oxford University Press, New York, NY, USA, 2006.

[18] C. L. Damecour and M. Charron, "Hoarding: a symptom, not a syndrome," *Journal of Clinical Psychiatry*, vol. 59, no. 5, pp. 267–272, 1998.

[19] R. Lindstrom, S. M. MacLeod, and A. Levy, "Twisting the lion's tail: collaborative health policy making in British Columbia," *Healthcare Papers*, vol. 11, no. 2, 2011.

[20] E. A. Henneman, J. L. Lee, and J. I. Cohen, "Collaboration: a concept analysis," *Journal of Advanced Nursing*, vol. 21, no. 1, pp. 103–109, 1995.

[21] M. M. Friend and L. Cook, *Interactions: Collaboration Skills for School Professionals*, Allyn and Bacon, Boston, Mass, USA, 5th edition, 2007.

[22] J. G. Emshoff, A. J. Darnell, D. A. Darnell, S. W. Erickson, S. Schneider, and R. Hudgins, "Systems change as an outcome and a process in the work of community collaboratives for health," *American Journal of Community Psychology*, vol. 39, no. 3-4, pp. 255–267, 2007.

[23] C. A. McAiney, L. M. Hillier, M. Ringland, and N. Cooper, "Getting a bigger bang for your buck: a collaborative approach to enhancing dementia education planning in long-term care homes," *Healthcare Policy*, vol. 5, no. 2, pp. e125–e140, 2009.

[24] F. Capra, *The Web of Life: A New Understanding of Living Systems*, Anchor Books, New York, NY, USA, 1996.

[25] J. Mikkonen and D. Raphael, *Social Determinants of Health: The Canadian Facts*, York University School of Health Policy and Management, Toronto, Canada, 2010.

[26] S. Dieleman, K. Farris, D. Feeny, J. A. Johnson, R. T. Tsuyuki, and S. Brilliant, "Primary health care teams: team members' perceptions of the collaborative process," *Journal of Interprofessional Care*, vol. 18, no. 1, pp. 75–78, 2004.

[27] P. Drew, B. Jones, and D. Norton, "Team effectiveness in primary care networks in Alberta," *Healthcare Quarterly*, vol. 13, no. 3, pp. 33–38, 2010.

[28] P. Healey, "Collaborative planning in perspective," *Planning Theory*, vol. 2, no. 2, pp. 101–123, 2003.

[29] D. Simmons, "This full house: an intervention program to assist elderly compulsive hoarders," 2009, http://www.seniorscouncil.net/uploads/files/This%20Full%20House.pdf.

[30] H. Tsoukas, "Craving for generality and small-N studies: a Wittgensteinian approach towards the epistemology of the particular in organization and management studies," in *The Sage Handbook of Organizational Research Methods*, D. A. Buchanan and A. Bryman, Eds., pp. 285–301, Sage, London, UK, 2009.

[31] A. Strauss and J. Corbin, *Basics of Qualitative Research*, Sage, London, UK, 1998.

[32] C. Rodriguez, L. Panero, and A. Tannen, "Personalized intervention for hoarders at risk of eviction," *Frontline Reports*, vol. 61, no. 2, p. 205, 2010.

[33] K. Johansson, S. Josephsson, and M. Lilja, "Creating possibilities for action in the presence of environmental barriers in the process of 'ageing in place'," *Ageing & Society*, vol. 29, no. 1, pp. 49–70, 2009.

[34] S. J. Rogers and T. Ruefli, "Does harm reduction programming make a difference in the lives of highly marginalized, at-risk drug users?" *Harm Reduction Journal*, vol. 1, pp. 1–7, 2004.

[35] R. Hebert, P. Durand, A. Tournigy, and PRISMA Group, "PRISMA: a new model of integrated service delivery for the frail older people in Canada," *International Journal of Integrated Care*, vol. 3, 2003, http://www.ijic.org/.

[36] S. Fawcett, A. Paine-Andrews, V. T. Francisco et al., "Using empowerment theory in collaborative partnerships for community health and development," *American Journal of Community Psychology*, vol. 23, no. 5, pp. 677–697, 1995.

[37] J. A. Cermele, L. Melendez-Pallitto, and G. J. Pandina, "Intervention in compulsive hoarding: a case study," *Behavior Modification*, vol. 25, no. 2, pp. 214–232, 2001.

[38] T. L. Hartl and R. O. Frost, "Cognitive-behavioral treatment of compulsive hoarding: a multiple baseline experimental case study," *Behaviour Research and Therapy*, vol. 37, no. 5, pp. 451–461, 1999.

[39] Canadian Health Services Research Foundation, "Better with age: health systems planning for the aging population," 2011, http://www.chsrf.ca/.

15

Physical Activity Improves Verbal and Spatial Memory in Older Adults with Probable Mild Cognitive Impairment

Lindsay S. Nagamatsu,[1] Alison Chan,[2] Jennifer C. Davis,[2] B. Lynn Beattie,[3,4] Peter Graf,[1] Michelle W. Voss,[5] Devika Sharma,[2] and Teresa Liu-Ambrose[2,4]

[1] *Department of Psychology, University of British Columbia (UBC), 2136 West Mall, Vancouver, BC, Canada V6T 1Z4*
[2] *Department of Physical Therapy, University of British Columbia (UBC), 212-2177 Wesbrook Mall, Vancouver, BC, Canada V6T 1Z3*
[3] *Alzheimer Clinic, G37 Purdy Pavilion, UBC Hospital, University of British Columbia (UBC), 2211 Wesbrook Mall, Vancouver, BC, Canada V6T 2B5*
[4] *Brain Research Centre, University of British Columbia (UBC), 2211 Wesbrook Mall, Vancouver, BC, Canada V6T 2B5*
[5] *Department of Psychology, The University of Iowa, E11 Seashore Hall, Iowa City, IA 52242-1409, USA*

Correspondence should be addressed to Teresa Liu-Ambrose; tlambrose@exchange.ubc.ca

Academic Editor: Louis Bherer

We report secondary findings from a randomized controlled trial on the effects of exercise on memory in older adults with probable MCI. We randomized 86 women aged 70–80 years with subjective memory complaints into one of three groups: resistance training, aerobic training, or balance and tone (control). All participants exercised twice per week for six months. We measured verbal memory and learning using the Rey Auditory Verbal Learning Test (RAVLT) and spatial memory using a computerized test, before and after trial completion. We found that the aerobic training group remembered significantly more items in the loss after interference condition of the RAVLT compared with the control group after six months of training. In addition, both experimental groups showed improved spatial memory performance in the most difficult condition where they were required to memorize the spatial location of three items, compared with the control group. Lastly, we found a significant correlation between spatial memory performance and overall physical capacity after intervention in the aerobic training group. Taken together, our results provide support for the prevailing notion that exercise can positively impact cognitive functioning and may represent an effective strategy to improve memory in those who have begun to experience cognitive decline.

1. Introduction

Cognitive decline is one of the most pressing health care issues of the 21st century. Currently worldwide, one new case of dementia is detected every seven seconds [1] and the number of people affected is projected to be over 80 million by 2040 [1]. Thus, the societal value of developing effective intervention strategies cannot be overstated [2]. To date, pharmacological interventions for dementia have remained medically challenging at best. As a result, there has been growing interest in exercise training as an alternative intervention strategy.

The primary aim of our current study was to investigate the efficacy of exercise as an intervention strategy to improve memory performance in older adults who have already begun to experience cognitive decline—namely, those with mild cognitive impairment (MCI). MCI is characterized by cognitive decline that is greater than expected for an individual's age and education level, but does not significantly interfere with everyday function (i.e., instrumental activities of daily living) [3]. Importantly, MCI is a well-recognized risk factor for dementia; longitudinal studies report that seniors with MCI develop Alzheimer's disease at a rate of 10–30% annually [4, 5], compared to 1-2% of seniors without MCI [5]. Thus, MCI represents a critical window of opportunity to intervene and alter the trajectory of both cognitive and functional decline in seniors.

Exercise is a promising strategy for improving cognitive functions. Previous research has found that both resistance training [6, 7] and aerobic training [8] positively impact cognitive functioning and result in functional plasticity in healthy older adults. Furthermore, emerging evidence also suggests that exercise training has cognitive benefits for seniors with MCI. For example, a 24-week home-based physical activity program improved performance on the Alzheimer Disease Assessment Scale-Cognitive Subscale in seniors with probable MCI [9]. Additionally, a six-month aerobic training program improved selective attention and conflict resolution, processing speed, and verbal fluency in senior women with amnestic MCI [10].

Expanding upon the existing body of knowledge on exercise and cognitive functions, we found that twice-weekly progressive resistance training in our six-month intervention improved associative memory—or the memorization of two items in conjunction—in senior women with probable MCI [11]. These findings were further corroborated by our neuroimaging results, where resistance training was associated with increased activation over time in key cortical regions that subserve associative memory. Importantly, other research groups have found complementary evidence for a relationship between physical activity and memory in seniors with MCI [12]. However, a comparison has not been conducted between resistance and aerobic training for their propensity to improve various forms of memory in older adults who are showing signs of memory decline.

For our study reported here, we analyzed the secondary outcome measures of our randomized controlled trial that was previously published [11]. Our current analysis was primarily designed to examine the efficacy of both resistance training and aerobic training to improve memory performance in senior women with probable MCI. To this end, we examined the impact of exercise on two distinct forms of memory: (1) verbal memory and learning and (2) spatial memory. The second aim of our study was to determine whether memory performance at the end of the trial might be associated with physical performance measures. While research on the effects of resistance training on cognitive function has been limited, preliminary evidence does suggest that different forms of exercise (e.g., aerobic versus resistance training) alter distinct cognitive processes [6, 11]. Consistent with this idea, Cassilhas and colleagues [13] recently reported differences in underlying molecular mechanisms between the two types of exercise for how they may improve cognitive function; whereas resistance training appeared to increase levels of serum IFG-1, aerobic training increased levels of brain-derived neurotrophic factors (BDNF) in the hippocampus. Therefore, we hypothesized that both types of exercise training would yield beneficial—although potentially divergent—impacts on memory.

2. Methods

2.1. Study Design. We conducted a 26-week, single-blinded, randomized trial of exercise (NCT00958867) with assessments at baseline, mid-point, and trial completion. Details of the trial have been reported elsewhere [11].

2.2. Participants. Our study only included women due to sex differences in cognitive response to exercise [14]. From April 2009 to August 2009, we recruited participants using advertisements in local media and a memory clinic. Individuals were screened by a standardized telephone interview and by a 30-minute in-person assessment. Women who lived in Vancouver, Canada, were eligible for study entry if they (1) were aged 70 to 80 years; (2) were living independently in their own home; (3) scored ≥24/30 on the Mini-Mental State Examination (MMSE); (4) scored <26/30 on the Montreal Cognitive Assessment (MoCA) [15]; (5) answered "yes" to the question "do you have any difficulty with your memory?" [9]; (6) scored ≥6/8 on the Lawton and Brody [16] Instrumental Activities of Daily Living; (7) had a visual acuity of at least 20/40, with or without corrective lenses; and (8) obtained their physician's clearance to start a supervised exercise program. We excluded those who (1) had a current medical condition for which exercise is contraindicated; (2) had participated regularly in resistance training or aerobic training in the last six months; (3) had a neurodegenerative disease and/or stroke; (4) had a diagnosed psychiatric condition (e.g., depression); (5) had a diagnosis of dementia of any type; (6) did not speak and understand English fluently; or (7) were on oestrogen replacement therapy.

In Figure 1, the CONSORT (Consolidated Standards of Reporting Trial) flowchart shows the number and distribution of participants. Ethical approval was obtained from the Vancouver Coastal Health Research Institute and the University of British Columbia's Clinical Research Ethics Board. All participants provided written informed consent.

2.3. Descriptive Variables. Current level of physical activity was determined by the Physical Activities Scale for the Elderly (PASE) self-report questionnaire [17]. The 15-item Geriatric Depression Scale [18] screened for depression. The Functional Comorbidity Index was calculated to estimate the degree of comorbidity associated with physical functioning [19]. We used the Lawton and Brody [16] Instrumental Activities of Daily Living Scale to subjectively assess ability to perform daily activities.

2.4. Verbal Memory and Learning. The Rey Auditory Verbal Learning Test (RAVLT) [20] assessed verbal memory and learning. Participants were read a list of 15 common words five times. Immediately after each time, they were required to recall as many words as possible. After the fifth trial, an interference list was presented, after which participants had to spontaneously recall the original words. Finally, participants were required to spontaneously recall the original words after a 20 minute delay. Scores were calculated as the total number of words recalled (1) across the five trials

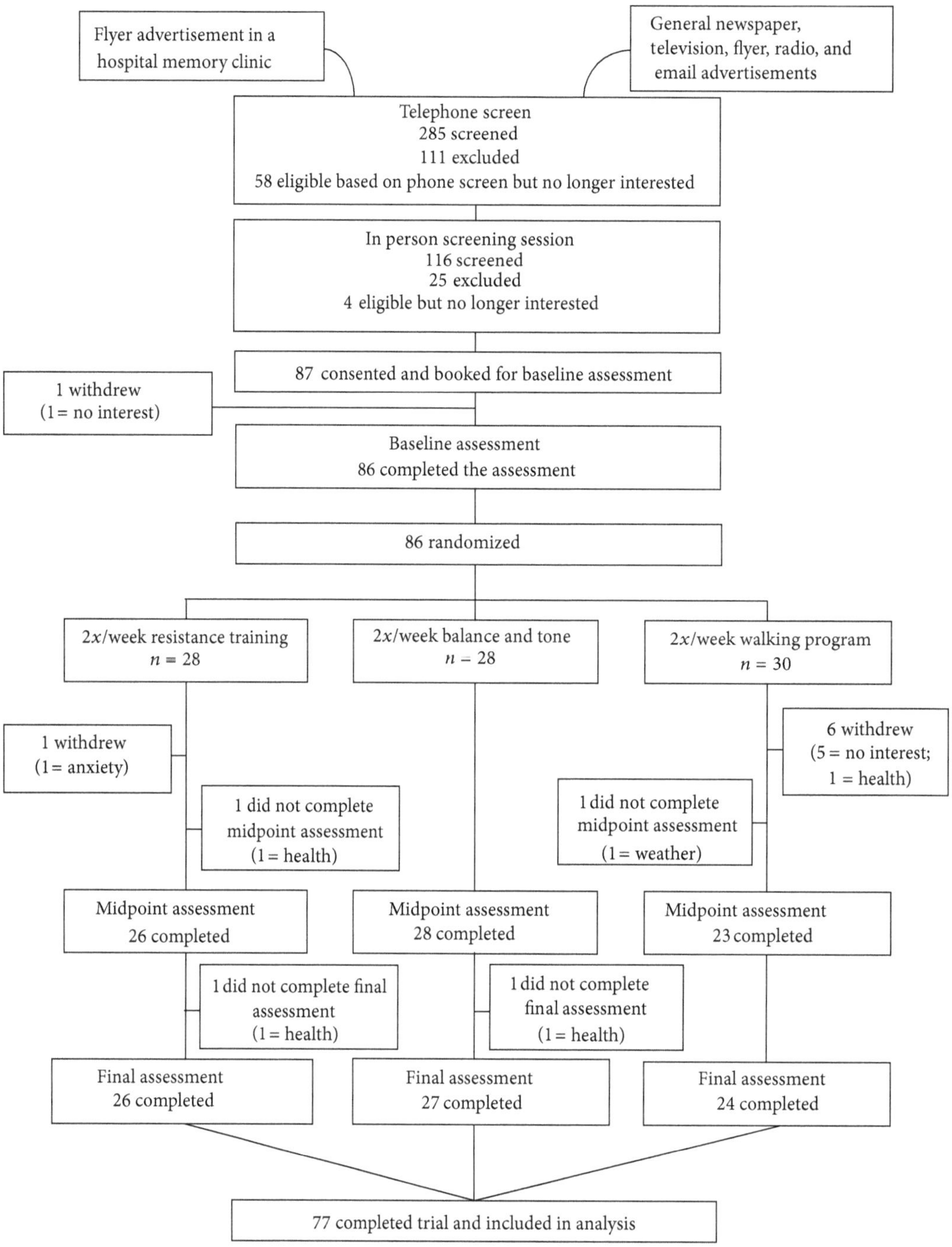

FIGURE 1: The CONSORT (Consolidated Standards of Reporting Trials) flowchart.

(total acquisition); (2) after the interference list (recall after interference); (3) on the fifth trial minus after the interference (loss after interference); and (4) after the delay (long delay free recall).

2.5. Spatial Memory. Spatial memory was assessed using a computerized task developed in-house by one of our co-authors along with her collaborators. This task was chosen because it has previously been found to modulate with physical activity [21–23] and allows for the collection of reaction times and accuracy—rather than just working memory span which other spatial memory tasks provide. Our spatial memory task required participants to recall the spatial location of dots presented on a screen. Specifically, one, two, or three dots appeared at randomly selected locations on the screen for 500 ms. Next, a fixation-cross appeared for 3 s. At the end of the delay, a single red test dot was presented on the screen, either at the same location as one of the previous black dots (match), or at a new location (nonmatch). Subjects

Table 1

Variable[a]	BAT (n = 28) Mean (SD)	AT (n = 30) Mean (SD)	RT (n = 28) Mean (SD)	Total N = 86 Mean (SD)
Age, years	75.1 (3.6)	75.6 (3.6)	73.9 (3.4)	74.9 (3.5)
Height, cm	158.2 (7.3)	159.2 (5.9)	158.7 (7.0)	158.7 (6.7)
Weight, kg	66.4 (14.0)	64.8 (12.8)	65.2 (10.7)	65.4 (12.4)
Physical activity scale for the elderly	133.2 (78.1)	121.6 (52.9)	151.8 (74.9)	135.2 (69.52)
Education, No (%)				
Less than grade 9	0 (0)	2 (2.3)	0 (00	2 (2.3)
Grade 9 to 12 without certificate or diploma	5 (5.8)	3 (3.5)	2 (2.3)	10 (11.6)
High school certificate or diploma	7 (8.1)	7 (8.1)	7 (8.1)	21 (24.4)
Trades or professional certificate or diploma	5 (5.8)	2 (2.3)	3 (3.5)	10 (11.6)
University certificate or diploma	8 (9.3)	8 (9.3)	8 (9.3)	24 (27.9)
University degree	3 (3.5)	8 (9.3)	8 (9.3)	19 (22.1)
Geriatric depression scale[b]	1.0 (1.8)	1.1 (1.8)	1.4 (2.0)	1.2 (1.8)
Functional comorbidities index[c]	2.6 (2.2)	2.9 (1.5)	3.0 (1.9)	2.8 (1.8)
Instrumental activities of daily living[d]	7.8 (0.5)	7.8 (0.5)	7.7 (0.8)	7.8 (0.6)
Montreal cognitive assessment[e]	22.5 (2.8)	22.2 (2.8)	21.4 (3.4)	22.1 (3.0)
Minimental state examination[f]	27.1 (1.7)	27.4 (1.5)	27.0 (1.8)	27.2 (1.6)
Exercise class compliance, %	59 (14.8)	60 (18.7)	54 (14.7)	57 (16.1)

Abbreviations: BAT: balance and tone; AT: aerobic training; RT: resistance training.
[a] Unless otherwise indicated, data are expressed as mean (SD). Percentages (%) have been rounded and may not total 100.
[b] Maximum was 15 points.
[c] Maximum was 18 points.
[d] Maximum was 8 points.
[e] Maximum was 30 points.
[f] Maximum was 30 points.

were required to indicate whether the red test dot was a match or a nonmatch to any of the previously presented black dots by pressing the designated key on a computer keyboard ("x" = nonmatch; "m" = match). Participants were instructed to respond as quickly and accurately as possible. The entire task consisted of 120 trials (40 trials for each set size, divided into 20 match and 20 nonmatch conditions). Participants were provided with practice trials prior to beginning the test to ensure they understood the task instructions. Reaction times and accuracy were recorded.

2.6. Choice Reaction Time. Choice reaction times were collected to use as a covariate in our statistical analyses for computerized tasks measuring reaction times to account for differences in basic processing speed secondary to memory performance [24]. Participants were required to indicate whether a number (1, 2, 3, 4, 6, 7, 8, 9) presented on a computer screen was higher or lower than the number "5". Numbers were presented individually for 1500 ms in the centre of the screen, and the same number did not repeat twice in a row. Using one hand, they were required to press one button with their index finger if the correct answer was "higher" than five and another button with their middle finger if the number was "lower" than five. Participants were instructed to respond as quickly and accurately as possible.

2.7. Physical Performance. General balance and mobility was assessed using the Short Physical Performance Battery, which is a composite score of the following tasks: (1) tandem standing; (2) four-metre walk (gait speed); and (3) chair stands. General cardiovascular capacity was assessed using the Six-Minute Walk Test, where the total distance walked at participants' usual pace in six minutes was measured in metres.

2.8. Randomization. The randomization sequence was generated by (http://www.randomization.com) and was concealed until interventions were assigned. This sequence was held independently and remotely by the Research Coordinator. Participants were enrolled and randomized by the Research Coordinator to the twice-weekly exercise groups: resistance training (RT), aerobic training (AT), or balance and tone (BAT).

2.9. Exercise Intervention. The exercise protocol has been reported elsewhere [11]. Briefly, classes began one month after baseline assessments and were held at a fully equipped gym in a research centre. Classes were led by certified fitness instructors who received additional training from the study investigators. The classes were 60 minutes in duration (10-minute warm-up, 40 minutes of core content, and 10-minute cool-down). Attendance was recorded daily, which was used to calculate compliance (i.e., percentage of total classes attended). Strategies were implemented to promote participant engagement [6, 25].

2.9.1. Resistance Training. For the RT program, both a Keiser Pressurized Air system and free weights were used [6]. The Keiser-based exercises consisted of biceps curls, triceps extension, seated row, latissimus dorsi pull downs, leg press, hamstring curls, and calf raises. The intensity of the training stimulus was at a work range of six to eight repetitions (two sets). The training stimulus was subsequently increased using the 7RM method—when two sets of six to eight repetitions were completed with proper form and without discomfort. Other key strength exercises included minisquats, minilunges, and lunge walks.

2.9.2. Aerobic Training. The AT program was an outdoor walking program. The intensity of the training stimulus was at approximately 40% of one's age specific target heart rate (i.e., heart rate reserve; HRR) and progressed over the first 12 weeks to the range of 70% to 80% of HRR. Exercise intensity was monitored through heart rate monitors. Participants also monitored the intensity of their workouts by the Borg's Rating of Perceived Exertion [26] and the "talk" test [27, 28].

2.9.3. Balance and Tone. The BAT program consisted of stretching exercises, range of motion exercises, balance exercises, functional sand relaxation techniques [6]. Other than bodyweight, no additional loading (e.g., hand weights, etc.) was applied. This group served to control for confounding variables such as physical training received by traveling to the training centres, social interaction, and changes in lifestyle secondary to study participation.

2.10. Adverse Effects. Participants were questioned about the presence of any adverse effects, such as musculoskeletal pain or discomfort, at each exercise session. Instructors monitored participants for symptoms of angina and shortness of breath during the exercise classes.

2.11. Statistical Analysis. All analyses were "full analysis set" [29] (defined as the analysis set which is as complete and as close as possible to the intention-to-treat ideal of including all randomized participants). Data were analyzed using IBM SPSS STATISTICS (Version 20).

Performance on the RAVLT was measured using univariate ANOVAs for each outcome measure, with two planned simple contrasts to assess differences between (1) RT versus BAT and (2) AT versus BAT. Baseline scores were entered as covariates. For the spatial memory task, repeated measures ANOVAs were performed to examine changes over the course of the trial in both reaction time and accuracy, with number of items (one, two, or three) as the within-subjects factor and group as the between-subjects factor. The reaction time analysis included choice reaction time as a covariate to account for differences in processing speed [24]. Bivariate Pearson correlations were calculated to examine the relationship between memory and physical performance

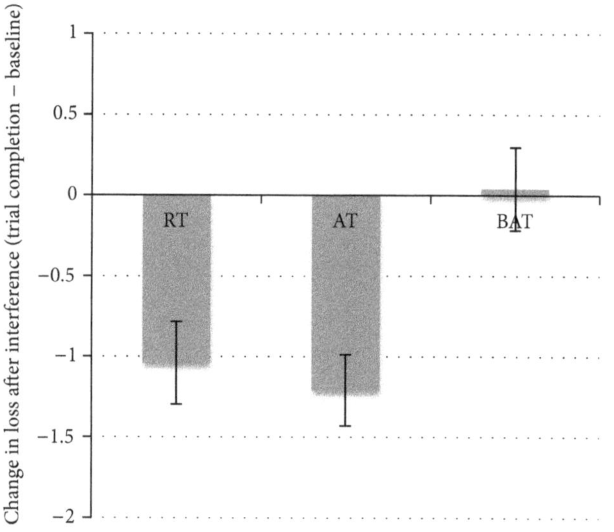

FIGURE 2: Change between baseline and trial completion in loss after interference on the RAVLT as a function of exercise group. The AT group showed significantly more change compared to the BAT group. Error bars represent standard error of the mean.

at trial completion within each group. For all analyses the overall alpha was set at $P \leq 0.05$.

3. Results

3.1. Descriptive Variables, Physical Activity, and Participants. In this trial, 86 participants were recruited and randomized (Figure 1). Baseline demographic and characteristics of the 86 participants are shown in Table 1. Physical activity levels (PASE scores) did not differ significantly between the groups at midpoint ($P = 0.93$) or trial completion ($P = 0.67$). Of the 86 participants, 77 completed the 26-week trial. The number of dropouts was the greatest in the AT group (Figure 1).

3.2. Verbal Memory and Learning. Table 2 shows the baseline, mid-point, and trial completion results for verbal memory and learning performance. For the RAVLT, there were no significant between-group differences at trial completion in total acquisition, recall after interference, and long delay free recall (all P's > 0.15). However, there was a significant difference in loss after interference at trial completion between the AT and BAT groups, $P = 0.04$ (Figure 2). Conversely, the RT and BAT contrast for loss after interference was nonsignificant, $P = 0.20$. Overall, loss after interference was reduced by 43.4% and 32.5% in the AT group and the RT group, respectively. In contrast, the BAT group demonstrated a 1.45% increase in loss after interference. The improvement observed in the AT group was not present at mid-point, $P = 0.71$.

3.3. Spatial Memory. Table 3 shows the baseline, mid-point, and trial completion results for reaction time and accuracy

TABLE 2: Mean values (SDs) for RAVLT performance.

Variable	Baseline Mean (SD)	Midpoint Mean (SD)	Final Mean (SD)
RT	$n = 25$	$n = 24$	$n = 25$
Total acquisition	40.88 (8.36)	46.79 (12.68)	44.36 (11.29)
Recall after interference	7.48 (2.50)	8.58 (3.89)	8.52 (3.50)
Loss after interference	3.2 (1.85)	3.38 (2.63)	2.16 (1.80)
Long delay free recall	7.52 (2.76)	8.83 (4.10)	7.79 (4.23)
AT	$n = 24$	$n = 23$	$n = 24$
Total acquisition	39.58 (9.04)	47.22 (11.01)	43.38 (10.95)
Recall after interference	7.83 (3.21)	8.83 (3.73)	9.29 (3.21)
Loss after interference	2.79 (1.79)	2.87 (2.32)	1.58 (1.86)
Long delay free recall	7.46 (3.08)	8.91 (4.28)	8.13 (3.70)
BAT	$n = 25$	$n = 24$	$n = 25$
Total acquisition	41.00 (8.63)	43.75 (9.55)	43.00 (9.61)
Recall after interference	7.60 (2.81)	8.54 (3.22)	8.12 (3.52)
Loss after interference	2.76 (1.92)	2.71 (2.05)	2.80 (2.58)
Long delay free recall	7.84 (3.33)	8.26 (3.68)	8.04 (3.36)

Abbreviations: BAT: balance and tone; AT: aerobic training; RT: resistance training.

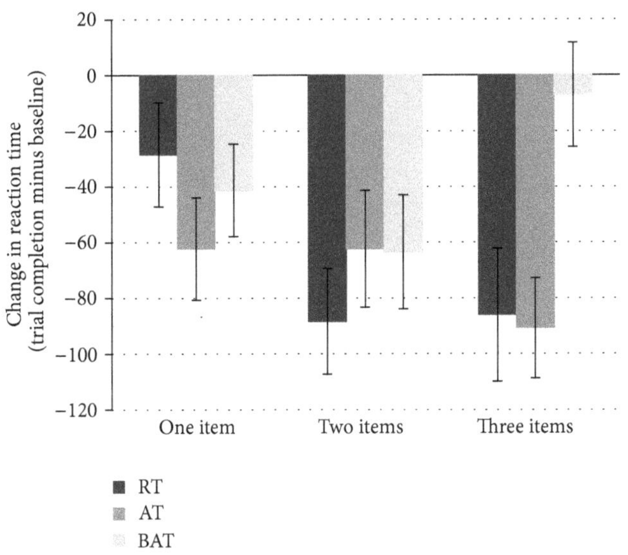

FIGURE 3: Change between baseline and trial completion on the spatial memory task as a function of number of items presented and exercise group. Both the RT and AT groups showed improved performance compared to the BAT group for the memorization of three items. Error bars represent standard error of the mean.

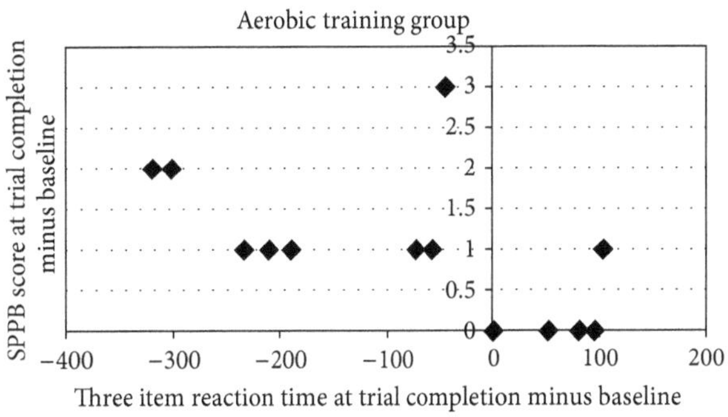

FIGURE 4: Significant correlations between change in reaction time performance on the spatial memory task and change in performance on the SPPB for the AT group. SPPB performance was negatively correlated with spatial memory reaction time, where better balance and mobility were associated with faster reaction times.

on the spatial memory task. The exercise groups differed in reaction time changes after completion of the trial as a function of number of items to be remembered. This was evidenced by a significant item by group interaction, $F(4,100) = 2.41$, $P = 0.05$. Examining the plots (Figure 3), the RT and AT groups appear to have improved their reaction times for memorizing the spatial location of three items more than the BAT group. Notably, this between-groups difference was not present at mid-point, $P = 0.18$. There were no significant differences between the exercise groups in accuracy for spatial memory for either mid-point or trial completion ($P = 0.83$ and 0.14, resp.).

3.4. Correlations between Memory and Physical Performance. Changes in physical performance as a function of exercise group have been previously reported [11]. In this study, faster reaction times at trial completion compared to baseline during the three-item condition on the spatial memory task were associated with better performance on the SPPB in the AT group (Figure 4). This was confirmed via a significant negative correlation between the two variables, $r(13) = -0.57$, $P = 0.04$. Spatial memory reaction times and SPPB were not significantly correlated in the RT or BAT groups ($P = 0.20$ and 0.79, resp.). Furthermore, reaction times were not associated with performance on the Six-Minute Walk Test (all P's > 0.17). There were no significant correlations between

TABLE 3: Mean values (SDs) for spatial memory performance.

Variable	Baseline Mean (SD)	Midpoint Mean (SD)	Final Mean (SD)
RT	$n = 19$	$n = 18$	$n = 19$
Reaction time, ms			
One item	981.02 (141.18)	941.05 (167.40)	952.57 (193.75)
Two items	1036.40 (176.36)	997.00 (196.59)	948.09 (219.19)
Three items	1092.71 (148.86)	1072.64 (189.75)	1006.69 (189.75)
Accuracy[a]			
One item	0.76 (0.17)	0.82 (0.14)	0.74 (0.17)
Two items	0.81 (0.16)	0.81 (0.13)	0.75 (0.19)
Three items	0.72 (0.15)	0.78 (0.13)	0.73 (0.17)
Choice reaction time, ms	895.26 (158.07)	880.42 (149.10)	889.41 (163.19)
AT	$n = 17$	$n = 16$	$n = 17$
Reaction time, ms			
One item	958.77 (161.91)	927.12 (179.21)	896.51 (172.92)
Two items	1013.56 (198.95)	982.32 (146.48)	951.22 (165.06)
Three items	1093.65 (186.34)	1039.24 (172.98)	1002.91 (195.64)
Accuracy			
One item	0.73 (0.11)	0.79 (0.13)	0.77 (0.12)
Two items	0.75 (0.15)	0.84 (0.10)	0.84 (0.09)
Three items	0.71 (0.11)	0.78 (0.10)	0.74 (0.09)
Choice reaction time, ms	877.82 (128.62)	894.49 (130.15)	910.08 (164.62)
BAT	$n = 19$	$n = 19$	$n = 19$
Reaction time, ms			
One item	993.26 (155.19)	968.55 (179.74)	952.00 (178.40)
Two items	1070.66 (210.78)	1010.36 (198.28)	1007.27 (187.55)
Three items	1084.62 (215.32)	1061.94 (190.76)	1077.48 (223.07)
Accuracy			
One item	0.73 (0.14)	0.74 (0.14)	0.79 (0.12)
Two items	0.76 (0.13)	0.76 (0.15)	0.79 (0.12)
Three items	0.71 (0.14)	0.68 (0.15)	0.74 (0.10)
Choice reaction time, ms	864.91 (111.95)	885.06 (169.32)	838.30 (101.36)

Abbreviations: BAT: balance and tone; AT: aerobic training; RT: resistance training.
[a]Maximum was 1.00.

RAVLT performance and either of the physical performance measures (all P's > 0.37).

3.5. Adverse Events. Adverse effects included episodes of shortness of breath that resolved with rest ($n = 2$) and noninjurous falls ($n = 4$). Results of the Chi Square test indicated no significant between-group differences ($P = 0.54$) in the proportion of participants reporting adverse events.

4. Discussion

We analyzed our secondary data from a six-month intervention to examine the effects of aerobic training and resistance training on two distinct forms of memory. Our specific aims were to evaluate whether either type of exercise would improve verbal memory and learning and/or spatial memory and to determine whether an association might exist between postintervention memory performance and physical measures. In this regard, we report three key findings. First, we found that twice-weekly aerobic training for six months remembered significantly more items in the loss after interference condition on the verbal memory test. Second, our results suggest that both types of exercise improved reaction times during the spatial memory test compared to the control group. Last, spatial memory performance appears to be positively associated with physical performance in the aerobic training group after the intervention. The results of our present study extend those from our previous work [11], where we found that resistance training significantly improved associative memory. Within this context, several noteworthy points of discussion follow.

To begin with, our finding that aerobic exercise significantly improved verbal memory and learning is consistent with previous reports. Specifically, Pereira and colleagues

[30] found that three months of aerobic exercise improved performance on the RAVLT. While the benefits of aerobic activity on verbal memory and learning in our study were only observed after six months—compared to three months in the study by Pereira et al. [30], differences in study design may account for this apparent discrepancy. For example, participants in the study by Pereira et al. [30] were young, healthy adults who engaged in aerobic activity four times per week; this is contrasted with older adults in our study who were already experiencing cognitive decline and exercised twice per week. This suggests that a higher dose of exercise may result in observable changes in memory more quickly. It is worth mentioning that in our study, the resistance training group also showed a greater reduction in loss after interference after the trial compared with the control group, although this change was not significant. Nevertheless, future studies with larger sample sizes may discover that resistance training does yield similar benefits to aerobic training for verbal memory performance.

Second, we found that both of our experimental exercise groups showed improved reaction time performance for recalling the spatial location of three items, as compared to the balance and tone group. Task performance on the spatial memory test has been shown to systematically decline as a function of load [31]. That the between-group difference was solely observed for three items—the most difficult condition for the spatial memory task—suggests that exercise distinctively improves higher-level cognitive processing required for more complicated tasks. These findings directly support those from previous studies, where both resistance and aerobic training improved executive functioning—such as selective attention and conflict resolution, as measured by the Stroop task [6, 8, 11].

Third, in light of our initial findings regarding improved associative memory performance after six months of twice-weekly resistance training, the results of our present study suggest that different types of exercise may selectively target distinct cognitive processes—and their underlying neural correlates. To recapitulate, we previously reported that resistance training resulted in improved associative memory performance and increased functional activation in three key regions of the cortex: the right lingual and occipital-fusiform gyri and the right frontal pole [11]. In contrast, here we found that *both* types of exercise training led to improved spatial memory. Importantly, spatial memory has neural underpinnings in the hippocampus [21, 32], thus suggesting that both forms of exercise training may impact hippocampal structure and/or function. Indeed, it has been established that the hippocampus is the structure most sensitive to exercise-induced change via neurogenesis and cell proliferation. For example, aerobic exercise has been found to increase hippocampal volume and levels of BDNF—a neurotrophic factor involved in cell growth and survival and memory promotion [21]. Thus, while there are multiple potential mechanisms to account for the relationship between cognitive functions and physical activity, such as increased cerebral blood flow [33], reduced neuroinflammation [34], and contribution of white matter hyperintensities [35], we can speculate that underlying changes in hippocampal structure and/or function may be a mediating observed relationship between spatial memory and physical performance.

Finally, the link between physical activity and cognitive functioning is further supported by the significant correlation we have reported between our measure of overall physical performance and spatial memory in the aerobic training group. Notably, these results correspond to our previous findings that improvements in conflict resolution and selective attention, as measured by Stroop performance, were significantly correlated to improved gait speed after 12 months of resistance training [6]. That these two studies found relationships between different types of exercise (aerobic versus resistance training) and two different measures of cognitive function further supports the notion presented above that the two types of exercise may target distinct molecular pathways [13]—and thus, modify different subtypes of cognitive function. However, in combination, evidence from these two studies demonstrate that higher levels of physical performance are associated with better cognitive performance. Given that there are multiple ways to improve general physical performance levels, our results therefore suggest that individuals may gain cognitive benefits from a wide variety of exercise options. Future work is needed to explore this possibility.

The conclusions of our study are tempered by our exclusion of men and those older or younger than 70–80 years old. Additionally, our study was only powered to compare the resistance training versus the control group and the aerobic training versus the control group; therefore, we were unable to directly compare changes in performance between our two exercise groups. Hence, future research on how our results may apply to the broader population with larger sample sizes is warranted.

In sum, our study provides preliminary evidence that multiple benefits for memory can be observed after six months of exercise training. However, the mechanisms behind how resistance training and aerobic training may differentially impact cognition remain unclear; thus future work should be aimed at further understanding the contribution of each type of exercise to cognitive functioning, functional plasticity, and brain structure. Furthermore, while our study did find performance improvements after six months, we did not see comparable changes after only three months using a twice-weekly exercise protocol. Therefore, the dose-response relationship of exercise needs to be elucidated so that future recommendations for the most effective program can be translated to health care practitioners and the public.

Conflict of Interest

All authors have no conflict of interests to declare.

Acknowledgments

The Pacific Alzheimer's Research Foundation provided funding for this study (to T. L. Ambrose). The authors thank the instructors for their commitment to the participants' health and safety. T. L. Ambrose is a Michael Smith Foundation for Health Research Scholar and a Canada Research Chair in Physical Activity, Mobility, and Cognitive Neuroscience. L. Nagamatsu is a Michael Smith Foundation for Health Research Senior Graduate trainee and a Natural Sciences and Engineering Research Council of Canada Doctoral trainee.

References

[1] C. P. Ferri, M. Prince, C. Brayne et al., "Global prevalence of dementia: a Delphi consensus study," *The Lancet*, vol. 366, no. 9503, pp. 2112–2117, 2005.

[2] R. Brookmeyer, E. Johnson, K. Ziegler-Graham, and H. M. Arrighi, "Forecasting the global burden of Alzheimer's disease," *Alzheimer's and Dementia*, vol. 3, no. 3, pp. 186–191, 2007.

[3] R. C. Petersen, R. Doody, A. Kurz et al., "Current concepts in mild cognitive impairment," *Archives of Neurology*, vol. 58, no. 12, pp. 1985–1992, 2001.

[4] A. Busse, J. Bischkopf, S. G. Riedel-Heller, and M. C. Angermeyer, "Mild cognitive impairment: prevalence and incidence according to different diagnostic criteria. Results of the Leipzig Longitudinal Study of the Aged (LEILA75+)," *British Journal of Psychiatry*, vol. 182, pp. 449–454, 2003.

[5] R. C. Petersen, G. E. Smith, S. C. Waring, R. J. Ivnik, and E. Kokmen, "Mild cognitive impairment: clinical characterization and outcome," *Archives of Neurology*, vol. 56, no. 3, pp. 303–308, 1999.

[6] T. Liu-Ambrose, L. S. Nagamatsu, P. Graf, B. L. Beattie, M. C. Ashe, and T. C. Handy, "Resistance training and executive functions: a 12-month randomized controlled trial," *Archives of Internal Medicine*, vol. 170, no. 2, pp. 170–178, 2010.

[7] T. Liu-Ambrose, L. S. Nagamatsu, M. W. Voss, K. M. Khan, and T. C. Handy, "Resistance training and functional plasticity of the aging brain: a 12-month randomized controlled trial," *Neurobiology of Aging*, vol. 33, no. 8, pp. 1690–1698, 2011.

[8] S. J. Colcombe, A. F. Kramer, K. I. Erickson et al., "Cardiovascular fitness, cortical plasticity, and aging," *Proceedings of the National Academy of Sciences of the United States of America*, vol. 101, no. 9, pp. 3316–3321, 2004.

[9] N. T. Lautenschlager, K. L. Cox, L. Flicker et al., "Effect of physical activity on cognitive function in older adults at risk for Alzheimer disease: a randomized trial," *Journal of the American Medical Association*, vol. 300, no. 9, pp. 1027–1037, 2008.

[10] L. D. Baker, L. L. Frank, K. Foster-Schubert et al., "Effects of aerobic exercise on mild cognitive impairment: a controlled trial," *Archives of Neurology*, vol. 67, no. 1, pp. 71–79, 2010.

[11] L. S. Nagamatsu, T. C. Handy, C. L. Hsu, and T. Liu-Ambrose, "Resistance training promotes cognitive and functional brain plasticity in seniors with probable mild cognitive impairment," *Archives of Internal Medicine*, vol. 172, no. 8, pp. 666–668, 2012.

[12] J. C. Smith, K. A. Nielson, J. L. Woodard et al., "Does physical activity influence semantic memory activation in amnestic mild cognitive impairment?" *Psychiatry Research*, vol. 193, no. 1, pp. 60–62, 2011. *Neuroscience*, vol. 202, pp. 309–317,

[13] R. C. Cassilhas, K. S. Lee, J. Fernandes et al., "Spatial memory is improved by aerobic and resistance exercise through divergent molecular mechanisms," 2012.

[14] S. Colcombe and A. F. Kramer, "Fitness effects on the cognitive function of older adults: a meta-analytic study," *Psychological Science*, vol. 14, no. 2, pp. 125–130, 2003.

[15] Z. S. Nasreddine, N. A. Phillips, V. Bédirian et al., "The Montreal Cognitive Assessment, MoCA: a brief screening tool for mild cognitive impairment," *Journal of the American Geriatrics Society*, vol. 53, no. 4, pp. 695–699, 2005.

[16] M. P. Lawton and E. M. Brody, "Assessment of older people: self-maintaining and instrumental activities of daily living," *Gerontologist*, vol. 9, no. 3, pp. 179–186, 1969.

[17] R. A. Washburn, E. McAuley, J. Katula, S. L. Mihalko, and R. A. Boileau, "The Physical Activity Scale for the Elderly (PASE): evidence for validity," *Journal of Clinical Epidemiology*, vol. 52, no. 7, pp. 643–651, 1999.

[18] J. A. Yesavage, "Geriatric depression scale," *Psychopharmacology Bulletin*, vol. 24, no. 4, pp. 709–710, 1988.

[19] D. L. Groll, T. To, C. Bombardier, and J. G. Wright, "The development of a comorbidity index with physical function as the outcome," *Journal of Clinical Epidemiology*, vol. 58, no. 6, pp. 595–602, 2005.

[20] M. D. Lezak, *Neuropsychological Assessment*, Oxford University Press, New York, NY, USA, 3rd edition, 1995.

[21] K. I. Erickson, M. W. Voss, R. S. Prakash et al., "Exercise training increases size of hippocampus and improves memory," *Proceedings of the National Academy of Sciences of the United States of America*, vol. 108, no. 7, pp. 3017–3022, 2011.

[22] M. W. Voss, K. I. Erickson, R. S. Prakash et al., "Functional connectivity: a source of variance in the association between cardiorespiratory fitness and cognition?" *Neuropsychologia*, vol. 48, no. 5, pp. 1394–1406, 2010.

[23] K. I. Erickson, R. S. Prakash, M. W. Voss et al., "Aerobic fitness is associated with hippocampal volume in elderly humans," *Hippocampus*, vol. 19, no. 10, pp. 1030–1039, 2009.

[24] S. Heo, R. S. Prakash, M. W. Voss et al., "Resting hippocampal blood flow, spatial memory and aging," *Brain Research*, vol. 1315, pp. 119–127, 2010.

[25] T. Liu-Ambrose, K. M. Khan, J. J. Eng, P. A. Janssen, S. R. Lord, and H. A. McKay, "Resistance and agility training reduce fall risk in women aged 75 to 85 with low bone mass: a 6-month randomized, controlled trial," *Journal of the American Geriatrics Society*, vol. 52, no. 5, pp. 657–665, 2004.

[26] G. Borg, "Ratings of perceived exertion and heart rates during short-term cycle exercise and their use in a new cycling srength test," *International Journal of Sports Medicine*, vol. 3, no. 3, pp. 153–158, 1982.

[27] R. Persinger, C. Foster, M. Gibson, D. C. W. Fater, and J. P. Porcari, "Consistency of the Talk Test for exercise prescription," *Medicine and Science in Sports and Exercise*, vol. 36, no. 9, pp. 1632–1636, 2004.

[28] C. Foster, J. P. Porcari, J. Anderson et al., "The talk test as a marker of exercise training intensity," *Journal of Cardiopulmonary Rehabilitation and Prevention*, vol. 28, no. 1, pp. 24–30, 2008.

[29] ICH Expert Working Group, "ICH Harmonised Tripartite Guideline: statistical principals in clinical trials," *Statistics in Medicine*, vol. 18, pp. 1905–1942, 1999.

[30] A. C. Pereira, D. E. Huddleston, A. M. Brickman et al., "An in vivo correlate of exercise-induced neurogenesis in the adult dentate gyrus," *Proceedings of the National Academy of Sciences of the United States of America*, vol. 104, no. 13, pp. 5638–5643, 2007.

[31] P. M. Greenwood, T. Sunderland, C. Lambert, and R. Parasuraman, "Effects of apolipoprotein E genotype on spatial attention, working memory, and their interaction in healthy, middle-aged

adults: results from the National Institute of Mental Health's BIOCARD study," *Neuropsychology*, vol. 19, no. 2, pp. 199–211, 2005.

[32] M. L. Smith and B. Milner, "The role of the right hippocampus in the recall of spatial location," *Neuropsychologia*, vol. 19, no. 6, pp. 781–793, 1981.

[33] I. J. Rhyu, J. A. Bytheway, S. J. Kohler et al., "Effects of aerobic exercise training on cognitive function and cortical vascularity in monkeys," *Neuroscience*, vol. 167, no. 4, pp. 1239–1248, 2010.

[34] A. Parachikova, K. E. Nichol, and C. W. Cotman, "Short-term exercise in aged Tg2576 mice alters neuroinflammation and improves cognition," *Neurobiology of Disease*, vol. 30, no. 1, pp. 121–129, 2008.

[35] E. V. Cyarto, N. T. Lautenschlager, P. M. Desmond et al., "Protocol for a randomized controlled trial evaluating the effect of physical activity on delaying the progression of white matter changes on MRI in older adults with memory complaints and mild cognitive impairment: the AIBL Active trial," *BMC Psychiatry*, vol. 12, article 167, 2012.

16

Health-Related Social Control over Physical Activity: Interactions with Age and Sex

Kelly A. Cotter

Department of Psychology, Sacramento State University, 6000 J Street, Sacramento, CA 95819, USA

Correspondence should be addressed to Kelly A. Cotter, cotterk@csus.edu

Academic Editor: Iris Reuter

Despite the disease prevention benefits of engaging in life-long regular physical activity, many adults remain sedentary. The social environment provides an important context for health and health behavior across the lifespan, as well as a potential point of intervention for increasing physical activity. Self-reports of perceived social support, social strain, positive social control, and negative social control were examined for their cross-sectional relationships to physical activity frequency in purposive samples of younger and older adults ($N = 371$, ages from 18 to 97, 68% women). Hierarchical regression analyses revealed that perceived support and perceived strain were not correlated with physical activity. However, age and sex interacted with social control, such that more positive social control was associated with more frequent physical activity for younger men. Furthermore, more positive and negative social control were significantly associated with less frequent physical activity for older men, while social control was not associated with physical activity among women. While younger men may be encouraged toward healthier behaviors by positive social control messages, social control attempts may backfire when targeting older men. Implications for physical activity promotion are discussed.

1. Introduction

Engaging in regular physical activity is a powerful tool for maintaining health and reducing disability across the lifespan [1]. The Centers for Disease Control and Prevention (CDC, [2]) recommend that all adults, including older adults, should accumulate *at least* 150 minutes of moderate-intensity aerobic activity (e.g., brisk walking) or 75 minutes of vigorous-intensity aerobic activity (e.g., running) on most days of the week. An equivalent combination of moderate and vigorous aerobic activity is also acceptable. In addition to strengthening the cardiovascular system through aerobic activity, the CDC also recommends that adults participate in strength-building activity on at least two days per week. Importantly, these activity bouts can be broken into 10-minute sessions and spread throughout the week. Furthermore, these activity bouts do not have to be planned, structured exercise sessions; Leisure activities like gardening or bowling also "count" toward the accumulation of health-enhancing activity minutes, as long as the individual participating in the activity perceives it to be moderately or vigorously intense.

The CDC's physical activity recommendations are based on research demonstrating that physical activity effectively reduces risk for age-related diseases including diabetes, heart disease, cerebrovascular disease, osteoarthritis, and some cancers [3]. In addition, greater physical activity is associated with more strength and balance, relief of many disease symptoms, and increased longevity [3]. Due to its profound health effects, it is imperative to understand how to promote physical activity behavior across the lifespan. The social landscape provides one important context for physical activity behavior [1], and it also changes in meaningful ways for men and women as they age [4]. Thus, in the present study, I examined the direct and moderated relationships of physical activity to perceived social support, perceived social strain, positive social control, and negative social control.

Perceived social support, defined by Walen and Lachman as "one's perceived notion of the caring and understanding exhibited by the [social] network" [5, page 7], has a consistent positive influence on health and health behaviors [6].

On the other hand, perceived strain, defined as "individuals' general perception of the critical, irritating, and unreliable nature of their network" [5, page 7], typically has negative implications for health and health behaviors [7].

The structure of the social network, and thus the availability of support and strain, changes in meaningful ways as people age. The social network narrows in later life, such that older adults maintain or increase contact with intimates (including spouses and close friends) but reduce contact with acquaintances [8]. This pattern is consistent with socioemotional selectivity theory [4], which states that people are motivated by emotional goals when they perceive time as limited. Applying the sense of time-sensitivity to the lifespan, older adults (relative to younger adults) are more motivated to maintain bonds with sources of support and sever ties with sources of strain because older adults are closer to the end of the lifespan and thus more motivated to induce positive emotional states [8]. Therefore, older adults should report more support and less strain from their social partners than do younger adults. Consistent with this assertion, Walen and Lachman [5] found that older adults (age 60–75) reported more family support and less family strain than younger adults (age 25–39) in a sample of married or cohabitating adults. Furthermore, older men reported more support from their spouse than younger men [5].

In addition to predicting health directly, perceived support is also linked to greater physical activity participation [1]. Furthermore, although perceived strain is associated with poor health outcomes, it has a positive relationship with physical activity. For example, in a large national survey of adults aged 35 to 84 years, participants who reported more perceived strain also reported more frequent physical activity [1]. The relationship between perceived strain and physical activity was moderated by age, such that it was stronger for older adults. To explain the counterintuitive relationship between strain and physical activity, some authors have suggested that people may use social sanctions to elicit desired behavior in social partners [9]. These interactions, while potentially well intended and effective, may be perceived as straining and controlling. Indeed, health-related social control, broadly defined as the efforts of network members to change a target's health behavior [10], provides a potential pathway to health.

At the most basic level, health-related social control is theorized to act as the mechanism by which network members influence health, such that someone in the social network exerts social control, which causes the recipient to change his or her targeted health behavior, which in turn affects the recipient's health [11]. These control attempts can be perceived as positive (e.g., encouragement) or negative (e.g., criticism) [12]. For example, a person who wants to support a friend by including her in activities might invite her to a water aerobics class. This friend may interpret such support as encouragement for healthy behaviors (positive social control), or she might feel nagged to exercise (negative social control). Thus, social control may explain the relationship of perceived support to health behaviors, such that social control provides one of many strategies to offer support [1]. In fact, social control and general perceived support are moderately correlated [13].

It is important to point out that general perceived support is not the same concept as domain-specific social support [13]: general support refers to a person's global perceptions about his or her available supports, while domain-specific support refers to a person's perceptions of available support or actual support received given specific circumstances. Domain-specific support has received a lot of attention in the physical activity literature. Studies show that greater exercise-support or physical activity-support predict greater exercise or physical activity participation [14]. Domain-specific support is the same concept as positive social control (i.e., encouragement for physical activity participation), but the terms used to describe the concept have differed in the literature. I use the social control terminology in this paper.

An overwhelming majority of research has found that positive social control is linked to health behavior change [15], including physical activity [16], while negative social control is associated with resistance to behavior change [17]. However, the influence of social control may change across the life course. For example, Tucker et al. found that older adults reported fewer people in their networks who provided social control than younger adults [18]. Additionally, older adults who reported more positive affect from social control attempts were more likely to hide unhealthy behaviors from the social network [19]. Tucker et al. argue that older adults want to maintain harmony with the social network but may be unwilling to give up negative health behaviors, so instead they hide these behaviors [19]. This explanation is consistent with socioemotional selectivity theory, which states that older adults are more motivated than younger adults to satisfy emotional goals, like maintaining harmony with the social network [4]. Tucker and colleagues' results suggest that positive social control may not necessarily promote health behavior among older adults, particularly if they enjoy high-quality relationships [19].

In addition to being less effective for older adults than for younger adults, social control attempts may also be less effective for women than for men. Men are more likely than women to be the targets of social control in marriages [20], and wives are more successful social control agents than husbands [21]. Even outside of the marital relationship, social control attempts from the partner, family, and friends were effective at reducing men's smoking behavior over four months but had no effect on women's smoking [22]. Taken together, previous research suggests that social control may not be an effective strategy for changing the health behaviors of older adults or women. However, social control may be successful when targeting the health behaviors of younger men. Because younger men might react differently to social control than older men or women react, the potential interaction between age, sex, and social control was explored in the present study.

The present study was designed to examine the links between physical activity behavior, perceived support and strain, and health-related social control. As argued above, positive social control shares conceptual similarities to social support and may even act as a method of providing emotional, informational, and instrumental support [13]. While research has demonstrated the independence of social control from social support [13], social control has not yet been examined for its independence from social strain, despite conceptual similarities. In fact, Cotter and Lachman have argued that social partners may intend to be supportive with their health-related messages, but that recipients of those messages may perceive such interactions as straining [1]. Therefore, from the perspective of the target, strain may share an even stronger relationship to social control than support does. Examining all four forms of social influence together is imperative for informing health behavior interventions because this will identify which type has the strongest relationship to health behavior, and thus the most appropriate target for intervention.

Based on the results of previous studies, I predicted that more frequent physical activity would be associated with more perceived support and strain, and that the positive relationship of strain to physical activity would be stronger among older adults than among younger adults [1]. I also explored a potential interaction between age and sex in the context of health-related social control. Based on previous research revealing that social control was ineffective when targeting older adults [19] and women [22], I predicted that age and sex would moderate the relationship of social control to physical activity in the present study, such that more positive and less negative social control would be associated with more frequent physical activity for younger men, but that social control would not be related to physical activity for older adults and for women.

2. Method

2.1. Procedure. Data for the present study were simultaneously collected from two different sources: undergraduate psychology majors at a northern California university and community-dwelling older adults (who were recruited through flyers and presentations at local senior centers). Upon volunteering, participants were guided through an informed consent procedure. Next, participants completed the survey. A research assistant was available to answer questions as the participants completed the survey. Finally, participants were debriefed and given information about psychological and fitness resources. Undergraduates received course research credit for their participation, and older adults were entered into a raffle for one of fifteen \$25 gift cards. The protocol received institutional approval for the ethical treatment of participants.

2.2. Participants. Participants were 371 noninstitutionalized, English-speaking adults ages from 18 to 97 (M = 45.28, SD = 26.93), who volunteered to participate in a paper-and-pencil survey. The sample recruited through the university ranged between 18 and 52 years old (M = 22.02, SD = 4.46), while the sample recruited through senior centers ranged between 46 and 97 years old (M = 73.71, SD = 10.72). Information regarding the demographic characteristics of race/ethnicity, marital status, education, and income was also collected (see Table 1), and each of these variables was dichotomized for analyses.

For the race/ethnicity variable, White participants comprised one group (51.3%) and all other races were combined to create the non-White group (48.7%). Marital status was recoded with one category of participants who were currently married (17%) and the second category with participants who were separated, divorced, widowed, or never married (83%). Education was dichotomized with one group of participants who had earned up to a high school diploma or GED (22.9%) and the other group who attended some college or higher education (77.1%). Finally, annual household income was recoded such that participants earning \$20,000 or less comprised one group (50%) and participants earning \$20,001 or more comprised the other group (50%).

The undergraduate sample reflects an accurate representation of the age and ethnicity of the undergraduate population of the university. However, women are overrepresented [23]. Older women, African Americans, and people of multiethnic heritage are overrepresented in the older adult sample compared to the population of American older adults [24, 25]. Furthermore, it should be presumed that the older adults sampled for the present study represent a relatively healthy and active segment of the older adult population. While participants were not asked specific questions regarding health conditions or pain; all were healthy enough to either attend classes at a university or to attend functions and activities at a community center.

2.3. Measures

2.3.1. Perceived Support and Strain. Responses to questions reflecting perceived social support (e.g., "How much do your friends really care about you?") and perceived social strain (e.g., "How often does your family criticize you?") from the spouse/partner, family, and friends were averaged across source [5], with higher scores reflecting more support (M = 3.45, SD = .48, α = .84) or strain (M = 1.92, SD = .58, α = .85). Although only 17% of the sample reported being married, most participants (54%) had a significant other to which they referred on items regarding partner support and strain. The range of scores in the present sample reflects the possible range (1 = Not at all to 4 = A lot) and published reliability (α range from .79 to .91) [5].

2.3.2. Social Control over Physical Activity. Social control over physical activity was measured as positive and negative social control from the spouse/partner, family, and friends. The positive social control scale (e.g., "How much does your partner encourage you to exercise?") was adapted from Sallis et al. [26], who reported high test-retest and internal consistency reliability for the measure. Responses to items were averaged, with higher scores reflecting more positive social control (M = 2.39, SD = .99, α = .97). The range of scores in the present sample reflects the possible range (1 = Never to 5 = Very Often).

Table 1: Summary of participant characteristics.

Variable	Total Sample (N = 371) N	%	Younger Adults (N = 205) N	%	Older Adults (N = 166) N	%
Sex						
Male	171	31.7	56	27.9	60	36.1
Female	252	68.3	145	72.1	106	63.9
Race/Ethnicity						
White	183	51.3	81	41.5	101	63.1
African American	41	11.5	17	8.7	24	15.0
Mexican American	43	12.0	31	15.9	11	6.9
Native American	7	2.0	4	2.1	3	1.9
Asian or Pacific Islander	46	12.9	42	21.2	4	2.5
Other	14	3.9	10	5.1	4	2.5
Multiracial	23	6.4	10	5.1	13	8.1
Marital Status						
Married	61	17.0	12	6.0	49	31.4
Separated	6	1.7	0	0	6	3.8
Divorced	42	11.7	0	0	42	26.9
Widowed	45	12.5	1	.5	43	27.6
Never Married	205	57.1	188	93.5	16	10.3
Education						
No school/some grade school	2	.6	0	0	2	1.3
Junior high school	7	2.0	0	0	7	4.6
Some high school	11	3.1	0	0	11	7.2
GED	4	1.1	0	0	4	2.6
High school diploma	26	7.3	0	0	26	17.1
1-2 years of college	130	36.7	109	54.2	20	13.2
3 or more years of college	64	18.1	54	26.9	10	6.6
Associate's degree	49	13.8	32	15.9	17	11.2
Bachelor's degree	27	7.6	6	3.0	21	13.8
Some graduate school	11	3.1	0	0	11	7.2
Master's degree	19	5.4	0	0	19	12.5
Professional degree	4	1.1	0	0	4	2.6
Annual Income						
Less than $10,000	91	27.2	57	29.1	34	24.8
$10,001–$20,000	77	23.0	35	17.9	40	29.2
$20,001–$50,000	81	24.2	42	21.4	39	28.5
$50,001–$75,000	33	9.9	23	11.7	10	7.3
$75,000 or more	53	15.8	39	19.9	14	10.2

Note: Age ranged from 18 to 42 ($M = 21.76$, SD = 3.56) for younger adults and from 46 to 97 ($M = 73.44$, SD = 11.02) for older adults.

The negative social control measure was created for the present study to measure negative social control from the spouse/partner, family, and friends aimed at promoting exercise behavior. Modeled after the positive social control measure [26], respondents were asked to report how often their spouse/partner, family members not including the spouse or partner, or friends did each of the following in the past month: nag you about exercise, demand that you exercise on recreational outings, demand that you discuss exercise, tell you ideas on how you can get more exercise, make negative comments about your physical appearance, pressure you to exercise, and make remarks about how much you should be exercising. Participants responded on a five-point scale (1 = Never, 2 = Rarely, 3 = Sometimes, 4 = Often, 5 = Very Often).

A principal components factor analysis was conducted on each subscale, and each subscale had an eigenvalue above 2. The factor solution for the partner domain included one factor that accounted for 53.74% of the variance with an eigenvalue of 3.76 ($\alpha = .84$). The factor solution for the family domain included one factor that accounted for 55.56% of the variance with an eigenvalue of 3.89 ($\alpha = .86$). The factor solution for the friend domain included one factor that accounted for 45.97% of the variance with an eigenvalue of 3.22 (α = .77). Responses were averaged across social partner for the present study, with possible scores ranging from 1 to 5. Higher scores reflect more negative social control (range = 1–5, M = 1.53, SD = .56, α = .89).

2.3.3. Physical Activity. Physical activity was measured with 9 items assessing participants' frequency of vigorous and moderate physical activity on a six-point scale ranging from 0 (Never) to 5 (Several times a week). Participants' scores reflected the possible range in the present sample. Based on Cotter and Lachman's measure [1], the setting in which the participant was most active (work, home, or leisure) comprised the participants' vigorous and moderate scores. In other words, the highest "moderate" score of the three settings was used as the indicator of frequency of moderate physical activity, and the highest "vigorous" score of the three settings was used as the indicator of frequency of vigorous physical activity. In this manner, if the participant performed regular activity in the home but not at work or for leisure, the respondent was still classified as regularly active. Next, the higher of the moderate versus vigorous scores was used as the indicator of total physical activity frequency (M = 3.89, SD = 1.59). Moderate (M = 3.77, SD = 1.63) and vigorous (M = 3.10, SD = 1.88) activity were highly correlated with each other in the present study: r = .66, P < .001. Cotter and Lachman [1] reported that calculating the physical activity score in this manner yields the best approximation possible to data from the Centers for Disease Control and Prevention [2], which recommends that adults accumulate at least 30 minutes of moderate aerobic activity on most days of the week or 20 minutes of vigorous aerobic activity three days per week.

3. Results

First, analyses were conducted on all variables to ensure normality of the distribution and reliability of measures. The negative social control measure was positively skewed and was transformed using a log 10 transformation. Next, exploratory analyses were conducted to determine whether there were different patterns of results based on different sources of influence (partner, family, and friends). Patterns were consistent between the partner, family, and friend domains. Thus, social influence variable scores were averaged across the domains, as described above in the measures section. All continuous independent variables were centered, and 2- and 3-way interaction terms were calculated by multiplying the centered support, strain, positive social control, or negative social control score by sex (0 = male, 1 = female) and age (0 = younger, 1 = older). Age was dichotomized at the mean of 45 years because the sampling technique led to a very bimodal distribution (n = 205 for younger adults, n = 166 for older adults, see Table 1).

Zero-order correlations between all variables were calculated and examined (see Table 2). Next, the direct and moderated cross-sectional relationships with physical activity frequency were examined in Hierarchical Multiple Regression (HMR) analyses using pairwise deletion and the MODPROBE procedure for SPSS developed by Hayes and Matthes [27]. Interactions with positive social control and negative social control were each examined in separate analyses in order to reduce problems associated with multicollinearity. Thus, age, sex, perceived support, perceived strain, positive social control, and negative social control were entered on Step 1 of both HMR analyses. Two-way age, sex, and *positive* social control interaction terms were entered on Step 2 of Model 1 (presented in the top half of Table 3), and two-way age, sex, and *negative* social control interaction terms were entered on Step 2 of Model 2 (presented in the bottom half of Table 3). The three-way interaction term age-by-sex-positive social control was entered on Step 3 of Model 1, and the three-way interaction term age-by-sex-by-negative social control was entered on Step 3 of Model 2. The Johnson-Neyman technique was used in follow-up analyses to examine regions of significance for the interactions [27].

Regression analyses revealed that none of the demographic characteristics had a significant relationship to physical activity when age and sex were in the models, so demographic characteristics were trimmed from the analyses to conserve statistical power. Furthermore, consistent with the bivariate relationships presented in Table 2, regression analyses revealed no statistically significant direct or moderated relationships between perceived social support and perceived social strain with physical activity. Thus, the three-way interaction terms of age-by-sex-by-perceived support and age-by-sex-by-perceived strain were also trimmed from the reported models to conserve power, but are available upon request. The results of the regression analyses are shown in Table 3, with interactions involving positive social control presented in the top half of the table and interactions involving negative social control presented in the bottom half of the table.

3.1. Positive Social Control. Variables in the model examining positive social control explained 20.1% of the total variance in physical activity frequency, F (10, 262) = 6.60, P < .001, and revealed a significant 3-way interaction between age, sex, and positive social control (β = .27, P = .05, see top half of Table 3) even after controlling for the relationships of perceived support, perceived strain, and negative social control. To plot the interaction, the data were split by sex and the 2-way interactions of age and positive social control were examined separately for men and women. The figures show predicted regression lines for younger and older adults at one standard deviation below (low) and one standard deviation above (high) the mean of positive social control. As shown in Figure 1, the 2-way age-by-positive social control interaction was significant among men, ΔR^2 = .10, F (1, 73) = 9.85, P < .001. Follow-up analyses used the Johnson-Neyman technique to determine regions of significance within the interactive effect [27]. Specifically, the effect of positive social control at each level of age (younger versus older) was examined among men and women. The follow-up analyses revealed that more positive social control was associated with more frequent physical activity for younger men (t = 1.67,

Table 2: Correlations between all variables.

		1	2	3	4	5	6	7	8	9	10	11
1	Age	—	−.09	**−.22**	**.34**	**−.21**	−.07	−.05	**−.18**	−.09	−.10	**−.38**
2	Sex		—	−.00	*−.10*	.01	−.07	**.17**	*−.13*	.07	−.08	−.03
3	Race			—	−.08	−.05	−.06	−.08	**.25**	−.03	.08	.03
4	Marital status				—	.00	**.19**	.07	.09	*.12*	−.01	**−.16**
5	Education					—	*.13*	.05	−.04	*.11*	.00	**.18**
6	Income						—	*.12*	−.05	−.01	**−.17**	.01
7	Support							—	−.08	**.34**	.04	.11
8	Strain								—	**.17**	**.52**	.03
9	PSC									—	**.28**	.12
10	NSC										—	−.01
11	Physical activity											—

Note: $P \leq .05$, $P < .01$. Age was dichotomized such that 0 = younger than 45 and 1 = older than 45, sex was dichotomized such that 0 = male and 1 = female, race/ethnicity was dichotomized such that 0 = White and 1 = all other races, marital status was dichotomized such that 0 = separated, divorced, widowed, or never married, and 1 = currently married, education was dichotomized such that 0 = up to a high school diploma or GED and 1 = attended some college or higher education, and annual household income was dichotomized such that 0 = \$20,000 or less and 1 = \$20,001 or more. PSC refers to positive social control and NSC refers to negative social control.

Table 3: Summary of two HMR analyses predicting physical activity frequency.

	Step 1			Step 2			Step 3		
	B	SE	β	B	SE	β	B	SE	β
Age	−1.25	.18	−.39**	−1.20	.32	−.38**	−1.24	.32	−.39**
Sex	−.30	.20	−.09	−.29	.27	−.09	−.30	.27	−.09
Support	.26	.20	.08	.34	.20	.10*	.34	.20	.11
Strain	−.07	.18	−.02	−.05	.19	−.02	−.00	.19	-.00
PSC	.13	.10	.08	.37	.21	.23	.74	.28	.46**
NSC	−.80	.80	−.07	−.59	.80	−.05	−.55	.80	−.05
PSC *Age				−.46	.19	−.20*	−1.03	.35	−.45**
PSC *Sex				−.04	.21	−.02	−.52	.32	−.26
Age *Sex				−.07	.39	−.02	−.01	.39	−.00
PSC *Age *Sex							.82	.42	.27*
Change stats	$\Delta R^2 = .17$, $F(6, 266) = 9.16^{**}$			$\Delta R^2 = .02$, $F(3, 263) = 1.99^{+}$			$\Delta R^2 = .01$, $F(1, 262) = 3.87^{*}$		
Age	−1.25	18	−.39**	−1.15	.32	−.36**	−1.05	.32	−.33**
Sex	−.30	.20	−.09	−.25	.27	−.07	−.15	.27	−.05
Support	.26	.20	.08	.30	.20	.09	.33	.20	.10
Strain	−.07	.18	−.02	−.00	.19	−.00	.10	.19	.04
PSC	.13	.10	.08	.15	.10	.09	.15	.10	.09
NSC	−.80	.80	−.07	−.21	1.57	−.02	4.04	1.99	.34*
NSC *Age				−2.01	1.45	−.13	−8.14	2.32	−.52**
NSC *Sex				.72	1.49	.04	−5.33	2.33	−.33*
Age* Sex				−.12	.40	−.04	−.13	.39	−.04
NSC* Age* Sex							9.91	2.97	.41**
Change stats	$\Delta R^2 = .17$, $F(6, 265) = 9.12^{**}$			$\Delta R^2 = .01$, $F(3, 262) = .93^{+}$			$\Delta R^2 = .03$, $F(1, 261) = 11.16^{**}$		

Note: $^{+}P < .10$, $^{*}P < .05$, $^{**}P < .01$. PSC refers to positive social control, NSC refers to negative social control, *age refers to the interaction with age, and *sex refers to the interaction with sex.

$P = .10$), while more positive social control was associated with significantly less frequent physical activity for older men ($t = -2.30$, $P = .03$). The interaction was not significant for women, $\Delta R^2 = .001$, $F(1, 174) = .31$, $P = .58$. Instead, only the direct relationship of age and physical activity was statistically significant, such that younger age was related to more frequent physical activity ($\beta = -.37$, $P < .001$).

3.2. Negative Social Control. Variables in the model examining negative social control explained 18.3% of the total

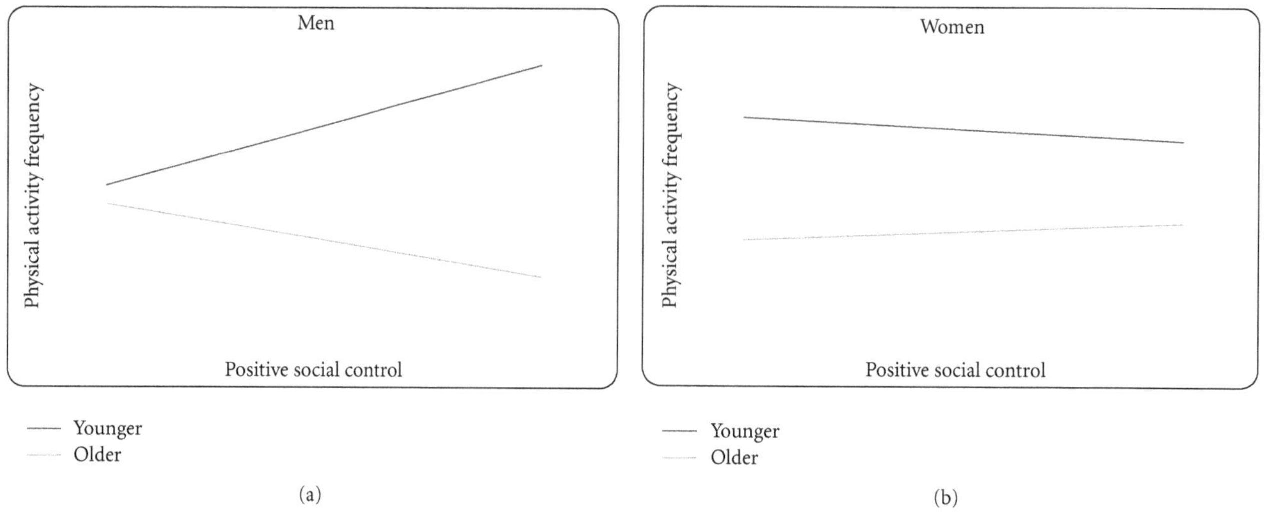

Figure 1: (a) The interaction of age and positive social control on physical activity for men. (b) The interaction of age and positive social control on physical activity for women. *Note:* the figures show predicted regression lines for one standard deviation above (high) and one standard deviation below (low) the mean of positive social control. The simple slope is statistically significant for older men.

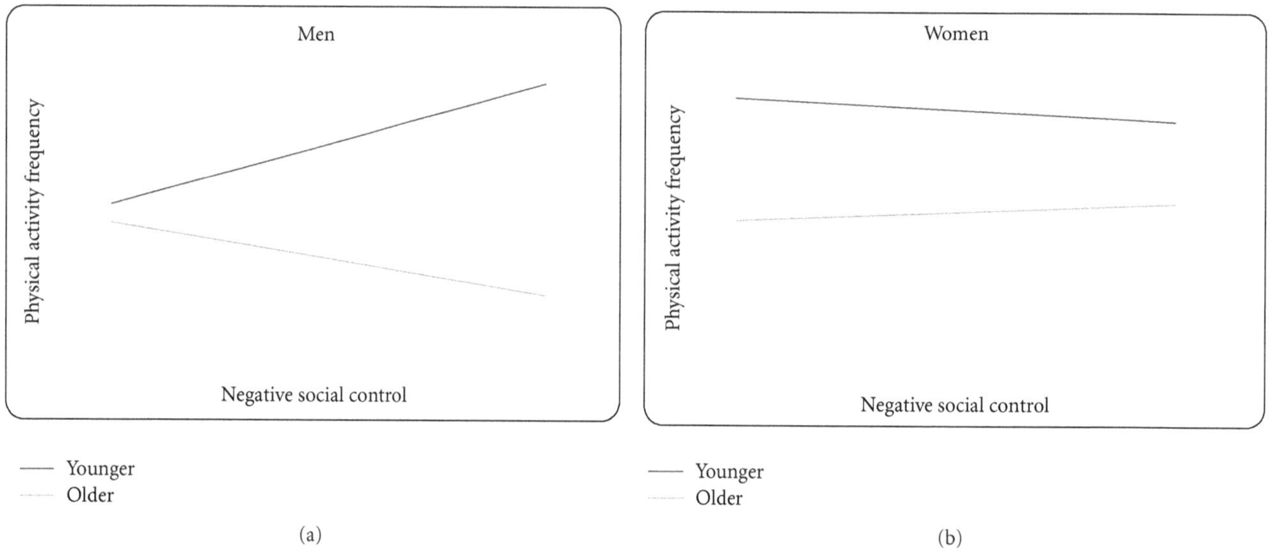

Figure 2: (a) The interaction of age and negative social control on physical activity for men. (b) The interaction of age and negative social control on physical activity for women. *Note:* the figures show predicted regression lines for one standard deviation above (high) and one standard deviation below (low) the mean of negative social control. The simple slope is statistically significant for older men.

variance in physical activity frequency, $F(10, 261) = 7.09$, $P < .001$, and revealed a significant 3-way interaction between age, sex, and negative social control ($\beta = .41$, $P = .001$, see bottom half of Table 3) even after controlling for the relationships of perceived support, perceived strain, and positive social control. The interaction was plotted following the same method described above (see Figure 2), and further analysis using the Johnson Neyman technique [27] revealed that the 2-way age-by-negative social control interaction was significant among men, $\Delta R^2 = .09$, $F(1, 73) = 8.57$, $P = .005$, such that more negative social control was associated with less frequent physical activity for older men ($t = -2.52$, $P = .01$), while negative social control was not significantly associated with physical activity for younger men ($t = .90$, $P = .37$). Again here, the interaction was not significant for women, $\Delta R^2 = .003$, $F(1, 174) = .66$, $P = .42$. Instead, only the direct relationship of younger age and more frequent physical activity was statistically significant for women ($\beta = -.38$, $P < .001$).

4. Discussion

Younger age was associated with more frequent physical activity in all analyses. This is consistent with a large body of research demonstrating younger adults as more active than older adults [28]. Younger adults are less likely than older adults to suffer from disabling conditions [29] and are more aware of the benefits of exercise [30]. Thus, younger adults may have more opportunity to be active.

While the main effect of age on physical activity is important for public health intervention, the present study is among the first to examine the interactive effect of age, sex, and social control on physical activity. As predicted, age and sex moderated the relationship of social control to physical activity, such that more positive social control was associated with more frequent physical activity for younger men (albeit at trend-level statistical significance). These results are consistent with results from a sample of men living with HIV, demonstrating that positive social control from friends, family members, and romantic partners was associated with behavior change [17]. Because the current data are cross-sectional, we cannot determine if young men engage in health behaviors in response to social control attempts or, alternatively, if they receive social control in response to health behaviors. However, based on previous experimental research where social control predicted health behavior change [31], the social control to behavior direction seems more likely than the opposite.

In contrast to younger men, older men in the present study reported significantly less physical activity when they perceived more social control. These results do not support my hypothesis that social control would not affect older men. This hypothesis was based on a study from Tucker and colleagues, who found that older adults who reported more positive affect from social control attempts were more likely to hide unhealthy behaviors from the social network [19]. Consistent with socioemotional selectivity theory [4], Tucker et al. argued that older adults want to maintain harmony with the social network, but may be unwilling to give up negative health behaviors, so instead they hide these behaviors from their loved ones.

Alternatively, older men may suffer from more health conditions that benefit from engaging in physical activity. For example, older men are more likely than younger men to suffer from heart disease [32], a chronic illness that can be controlled through regular physical activity [33]. Social partners may engage in health-related social control in an attempt to encourage illness-management [13], but heart disease also makes physical activity more difficult to complete [33]. Thus older men may actively refrain from engaging in this health behavior, despite the social control attempts of their network members, because they are unable or unwilling to begin or maintain a physical activity regimen. In addition to health, response bias provides another potential explanation for the negative relationship between physical activity and social control: older men may perceive more social control from their social partner, or they may be more willing to report social control than younger men [20].

Consistent with previous research [22] and with hypotheses, social control had no relationship to physical activity among women in the present study. Westmaas et al. suggest that receiving social control may undermine women's perceptions of themselves as the health-keepers of their families and as positive role models for health behaviors [22]. Westmaas et al. explain that this psychological burden may interfere with women's ability to change their health behavior. Thus, women may need to bolster their cognitive and emotional resources (i.e., self-efficacy) before attempting a physical activity behavior change. Because older adults have low confidence in their ability to adopt and maintain a physically active lifestyle [34], they may also need to strengthen their self-efficacy before becoming active. Once they are confident in their physical abilities, positive social control may further enhance self-efficacy and promote activity [35].

While the relationship between social control and self-efficacy still needs to be examined empirically, there is evidence for a relationship between exercise self-efficacy and *exercise-specific* social support (which I have argued is the same concept as positive social control for exercise) [14], as well as exercise self-efficacy and *general* social support [36] among older adults. Furthermore, positive and negative aspects of social relations may have different relationships to outcomes depending on whether they are examined cross-sectionally or longitudinally [37]. Therefore, future research should examine physical activity's longitudinal relationship to both positive and negative social control, as well as social control's cross-sectional and longitudinal relationship to exercise self-efficacy.

Contrary to predictions, general perceived support and strain were not associated with physical activity in the current investigation. These results are inconsistent with a study demonstrating that more perceived support and strain were associated with more frequent physical activity among adults [1]. The discrepancy here may be attributed to study design and statistical power. Cotter and Lachman examined data from over 3,000 participants, whereas I examined data from approximately 300 participants in the current investigation. It is possible that with more statistical power the relationships found in the current investigation would have reached statistical significance. In fact, effect sizes for the relationships in the present study, while not statistically significant, are similar to the effect sizes reported by Cotter and Lachman.

Perceived support was moderately related to positive social control in bivariate analyses in the present study, consistent with results reported by Helgeson et al. [13] and McAuley et al. [14]. Additionally, perceived strain was moderately related to both negative social control and positive social control. These results are consistent with assertions that strain may share a stronger relationship to social control than support does, particularly from the perspective of the recipient of social influence [1]. Social partners, then, should be encouraged to be careful to remain positive in their interactions with social control targets. Positive social control is more likely to elicit positive affect, which leads to behavior change without also eliciting negative affect [16]. Thus, positive social control attempts have greater potential for success with fewer negative repercussions.

When evaluating suggestions based on the present results, it is important to consider the study's strengths and limitations. Regarding the limitations, variables were all examined using a self-report method. Thus, some of the shared variance can be accounted for by the method of data collection. Second, the present study may have lacked sufficient power to corroborate the statistical significance of relationships that have been found using larger samples [1]. Most importantly, the present investigation is based on cross-sectional data. Thus, conclusions regarding causal relationships cannot be made. Furthermore, age differences may be attributed to cohort effects rather than developmental effects. For example, the older adults sampled, particularly the older women, may have approached physical activity differently than the younger adults due to generational differences in attitudes, beliefs, and normative behaviors. While care was taken when collecting the present data to describe physical activity in detail at the outset, older and younger adults may have responded to questions regarding physical activity according to preconceived definitions and thus the results must be interpreted with caution.

The current study also had a number of strengths. First, perceived support and strain and positive and negative social control were all examined simultaneously, making comparisons between different types of social interaction possible. Indeed, this was the first study to examine perceived strain's relationship to social control. Results from the present investigation suggest that social control may be a more efficacious avenue to explore for physical activity promotion than general support and strain. Second, the use of younger and older adult samples allowed for age comparisons, which revealed different patterns of relationships between variables for younger and older cohorts. Finally, the present sample contained a high percentage of minority participants who are typically underrepresented in research. Thus, the results of the present study are generalizable to a broad population of healthy younger and older adults.

The results of the current investigation demonstrate how and for whom social control is associated with physical activity. However, longitudinal work must be completed in order to determine the causal direction of these relationships. This is especially important given that previous research shows that social influence variables have different cross-sectional and longitudinal relationships to outcomes [36]. Furthermore, experience time sampling designs, such as daily diary studies, would be useful to determine how daily interactions influence physical activity on that day or in a given week. Daily diary designs would be particularly informative for understanding how, when, and from whom social control might promote physical activity [38]. Finally, self-efficacy plays an important role in behavior adoption [39] and is influenced by the social environment [40]. Therefore, future work should examine the relationship of social control to self-efficacy.

In conclusion, health professionals and intimate social partners should be discouraged from using negative social control strategies because of the potential to induce negative affect, because these strategies may be ineffective for women and younger men, and because these strategies may be counterproductive for older men. Instead, it might be more appropriate to use positive social control strategies, particularly for younger male targets, in order to maintain feelings of support and positive affect while encouraging health behavior change. On the other hand, alternative strategies should be pursued for improving the health and fitness of women and older adults. For example, bolstering self-efficacy may provide an efficacious strategy within these populations.

Acknowledgments

Special thanks are due to the Active Aging Lab for their support with data collection. This paper was partially supported by the Sacramento State University 2009-2010. Research and Creative Activity Award Program Summer Fellowship Grant.

References

[1] K. A. Cotter and M. E. Lachman, "No strain, No Gain: psychosocial predictors of physical activity across the adult lifespan," *Journal of Physical Activity and Health*, vol. 7, no. 5, pp. 584–594, 2010.

[2] Centers for Disease Control and Prevention, "Physical activity for everyone," 2011, http://www.cdc.gov/nccdphp/dnpa/physical/everyone/recommendations/.

[3] American College of Sports Medicine, *ACSM's Guidelines for Exercise Testing and Prescription*, Lippincott, Williams, and Wilkins, Philadelphia, Pa, USA, 2000.

[4] L. L. Carstensen, D. M. Isaacowitz, and S. T. Charles, "Taking time seriously: a theory of socioemotional selectivity," *American Psychologist*, vol. 54, no. 3, pp. 165–181, 1999.

[5] H. R. Walen and M. E. Lachman, "Social support and strain from partner, family, and friends: costs and benefits for men and women in adulthood," *Journal of Social and Personal Relationships*, vol. 17, no. 1, pp. 5–30, 2000.

[6] S. Cohen, "Social relationships and health," *American Psychologist*, vol. 59, no. 8, pp. 676–684, 2004.

[7] T. C. Antonucci, H. Akiyama, and J. E. Lansford, "Negative effects of close social relations," *Family Relations*, vol. 47, no. 4, pp. 379–384, 1998.

[8] L. L. Carstensen, "Social and emotional patterns in adulthood: support for socioemotional selectivity theory," *Psychology and Aging*, vol. 7, no. 3, pp. 331–338, 1992.

[9] N. Krause, L. Goldenhar, J. Liang, I. G. Jay, and D. Maeda, "Stress and exercise among the Japanese elderly," *Social Science and Medicine*, vol. 36, no. 11, pp. 1429–1441, 1993.

[10] K. S. Rook, "Support, companionship, and control in older adults' social networks: implications for well-being," in *Handbook of Communication and Aging Research*, J. F. Nussbaum and J. Coupland, Eds., pp. 437–463, Lawrence Erlbaum Associates, Inc, Hillsdale, NJ, USA, 1995.

[11] D. Umberson, "Family status and health behaviors: social control as a dimension of social integration," *Journal of Health and Social Behavior*, vol. 28, no. 3, pp. 306–319, 1987.

[12] M. A. Lewis and R. M. Butterfield, "Social control in marital relationships: effect of one's partner on health behaviors," *Journal of Applied Social Psychology*, vol. 37, no. 2, pp. 298–319, 2007.

[13] V. S. Helgeson, S. A. Novak, S. J. Lepore, and D. T. Eton, "Spouse social control efforts: relations to health behavior and well-being among men with prostate cancer," *Journal of Social and Personal Relationships*, vol. 21, no. 1, pp. 53–68, 2004.

[14] E. McAuley, G. J. Jerome, S. Elavsky, D. X. Marquez, and S. N. Ramsey, "Predicting long-term maintenance of physical

activity in older adults," *Preventive Medicine*, vol. 37, no. 2, pp. 110–118, 2003.

[15] M. Logic, M. A. Okun, and J. A. Pugliese, "Expanding the mediational model of the effects of health-related social control," *Journal of Applied Social Psychology*, vol. 39, no. 6, pp. 1373–1396, 2009.

[16] M. M. Franks, M. A. P. Stephens, K. S. Rook, B. A. Franklin, S. J. Keteyian, and N. T. Artinian, "Spouses' provision of health-related support and control to patients participating in cardiac rehabilitation," *Journal of Family Psychology*, vol. 20, no. 2, pp. 311–318, 2006.

[17] E. Fekete, T. R. Geaghan, and J. A. Druley, "Affective and behavioural reactions to positive and negative health-related social control in HIV+ men," *Psychology and Health*, vol. 24, no. 5, pp. 501–515, 2009.

[18] J. S. Tucker, D. J. Klein, and M. N. Elliott, "Social control of health behaviors: a comparison of young, middle-aged, and older adults," *Journals of Gerontology—Series B*, vol. 59, no. 4, pp. P147–P150, 2004.

[19] J. S. Tucker, M. Orlando, M. N. Elliott, and D. J. Klein, "Affective and behavioral responses to health-related social control," *Health Psychology*, vol. 25, no. 6, pp. 715–722, 2006.

[20] D. Umberson, "Gender, marital status and the social control of health behavior," *Social Science and Medicine*, vol. 34, no. 8, pp. 907–917, 1992.

[21] M. A. Lewis, R. M. Butterfield, L. A. Darbes, and C. Johnston-Brooks, "The conceptualization and assessment of health-related social control," *Journal of Social and Personal Relationships*, vol. 21, no. 5, pp. 669–687, 2004.

[22] J. L. Westmaas, T. C. Wild, and R. Ferrence, "Effects of gender in social control of smoking cessation," *Health Psychology*, vol. 21, no. 4, pp. 368–376, 2002.

[23] Voluntary System of Accountability Program College Portrait, "California State University, Sacramento college portrait," 2011, http://wwwcollegeportraits.org/CA/CSUS/characteristics.

[24] L. M. Howden and J. A. Meyer, "Age and sex composition: 2010," Census Briefs, 2010, http://www.census.gov/prod/cen2010/briefs/c2010br-03.pdf.

[25] J. J. Pirkl, "The demographics of aging...," 2011, http://www.transgenerational.org/aging/demographics.htm#Characteristics.

[26] J. F. Sallis, R. M. Grossman, R. B. Pinski, T. L. Patterson, and P. R. Nader, "The development of scales to measure social support for diet and exercise behaviors," *Preventive Medicine*, vol. 16, no. 6, pp. 825–836, 1987.

[27] A. F. Hayes and J. Matthes, "Computational procedures for probing interactions in OLS and logistic regression: SPSS and SAS implementations," *Behavior Research Methods*, vol. 41, no. 3, pp. 924–936, 2009.

[28] Centers for Disease Control and Prevention, "Public health and aging: trends in aging—United States and worldwide," *Morbidity & Mortality Weekly Report*, vol. 52, no. 6, pp. 101–106, 2003.

[29] J. Cohen-Mansfield, M. S. Marx, and J. M. Guralnik, "Motivators and barriers to exercise in an older community-dwelling population," *Journal of Aging and Physical Activity*, vol. 11, no. 2, pp. 242–253, 2003.

[30] A. C. King, S. N. Blair, D. E. Bild et al., "Determinants of physical activity and interventions in adults," *Medicine and Science in Sports and Exercise*, vol. 24, no. 6, pp. S221–S236, 1992.

[31] M. A. Lewis and R. M. Butterfield, "Antecedents and reactions to health-related social control," *Personality and Social Psychology Bulletin*, vol. 31, no. 3, pp. 416–427, 2005.

[32] Federal Interagency Forum on Aging-Related Statistics, *Older Americans 2010: Key Indicators of Well-Being*, Federal Interagency Forum on Aging-Related Statistics, Washington DC, USA, 2010.

[33] Centers for Disease Control and Prevention, "Know the facts about heart disease," 2012, http://www.cdc.gov/heartdisease/docs/ConsumerEd_HeartDisease.pdf.

[34] F. D. Lees, P. G. Clark, C. R. Nigg, and P. Newman, "Barriers to exercise behavior among older adults: a focus-group study," *Journal of Aging and Physical Activity*, vol. 13, no. 1, pp. 23–33, 2005.

[35] J. S. Tucker and S. L. Anders, "Social control of health behaviors in marriage," *Journal of Applied Social Psychology*, vol. 31, no. 3, pp. 467–485, 2001.

[36] K. A. Cotter and A. M. Sherman, "Love hurts: the influence of social relations on exercise self-efficacy for older adults with osteoarthritis," *Journal of Aging and Physical Activity*, vol. 16, no. 4, pp. 465–483, 2008.

[37] K. S. Rook, "The negative side of social interaction: impact on psychological well-being," *Journal of Personality and Social Psychology*, vol. 46, no. 5, pp. 1097–1108, 1984.

[38] M. R. Mehl and T. S. Conner, *Handbook of Research Methods for Studying Daily Life*, The Guilford Press, New York, NY, USA, 2012.

[39] A. Bandura, *Self-Efficacy: the Exercise of Control*, W. H. Freeman, New York, NY, USA, 1997.

[40] E. McAuley, G. J. Jerome, D. X. Marquez, S. Elavsky, and B. Blissmer, "Exercise self-efficacy in older adults: social, affective, and behavioral influences," *Annals of Behavioral Medicine*, vol. 25, no. 1, pp. 1–7, 2003.

The Impact of Quality of Life on the Health of Older People from a Multidimensional Perspective

Luis Miguel Rondón García[1] **and Jose Manuel Ramírez Navarrro**[2]

[1]*Faculty of Social Work, University of Granada, Granada, Spain*
[2]*Faculty of Social Studies, University of Málaga, Málaga, Spain*

Correspondence should be addressed to Luis Miguel Rondón García; madgrana1@gmail.com

Academic Editor: Antonello Lorenzini

Background. This research analyzes the impact of quality of life as a metavariable that conditions the health and social welfare of the elderly. The sample of this study is composed of 500 people, randomly selected from the major day centers for the elderly in the province of Granada (Spain). *Method.* For the inferential analysis, we used the CUBRECAVI questionnaire, which is a multidimensional scale of health and quality of life, along with the Katz and García measure questionnaires, which are also applied to quality of life. Through the technique of the interview, we have distributed the participants into two groups: experimental and control. *Results and Conclusions.* Once the tests have been completed, we have concluded from the meta-analysis and validation tests that the participants have a good perception of their quality of life, considering health, leisure, environmental quality, functional capacity, level of satisfaction, social support, social networks, and positive social interactions as the determinants of their well-being, although social contact reduces as the age advances. We conclude that multidimensional evaluation is an effective tool to evaluate the quality of life and the objective and subjective health of the elderly. These variables can be related to the improvement of health and well-being.

1. Introduction

The World Health Organization [1] defined quality of life as an "individual perception of his or her living situation, understood in a cultural context, value system and in relation to the objectives, expectations and standards of a given society" (p. 2). From this perspective, health-related quality of life includes areas such as physical health, psychological state, level of independence of the person, personal relationships, beliefs in a particular context or the natural environment, social support, and perceived social support [2–6].

The different discursive approaches have recognized the importance of implementing health measures from a multidimensional perspective. This means that while analyzing the quality of life, factors such as the various social conditions and social, cultural, and psychological networks that exist within the different study groups should be considered [7–13]. We add social networks, which are a fundamental element to understand this analysis, as they are an important vector of the quality of life.

However, for a general approach to the state of health from the quality of life perspective, it is necessary to consider more precise questions, and it is, therefore, important to distinguish health from life satisfaction, which involves complacency with the life of the present and past experiences. In this sense, many gerontologists claim that older people who successfully age are those who feel happy and satisfied with their past and present and enjoy positive social relationships and contacts. This concept also refers to a subjective dimension of welfare, to an adequate capacity to adapt to, accept, and recognize the environment, in order to have a better perception of health and welfare. It is about explaining how people experience their lives, their cognitive assessment, their emotional reactions, and their adaptation to life.

As we have already mentioned, quality of life and life satisfaction are different concepts, but at the same time, they are complementary. Life satisfaction represents an indicator of quality of life, a specific part of it, since it focuses on moral, cognitive, and affective aspects, on the tasks carried out independently, and on satisfaction with social support received and, in general, is related to life expectancy [14, 15]. On the contrary, quality of life is more closely linked to factors strictly related to health [16]. To put it more accurately and pragmatically, many older people relate quality of life to the ability to be independent in their daily activities. This is the reason why it is so important to take into account the improving self-esteem, satisfaction with functioning, a sense of independence in daily life tasks, and a sense of participation, which are important components of the whole structure that makes up the standards of quality of life of the elderly.

From this perspective, it is common in professional practice to measure the quality of life according to signs of satisfactory living. More recently, the cultural context, the meaning of life for a person from a quality of life perspective, has been introduced. This shows that quality of life, in addition to being multidimensional, must take into account the person's life experience and how they feel and interpret their life in relation to other people involved. This idea becomes more relevant in people who suffer from dementia, who need to foster their empowerment, so that they can express how they feel and their needs, when more specific stimulation is required for them.

It is worth mentioning that, in recent decades, research is related to health, quality of life, and gerontology as linked subjective health with psychological welfare beyond the absence of disease [17–19]. The Gwozdz and Sousa-Poza study [20] shows that happy people can live longer, and this idea envisions interesting research prospects for the future. Previous research has already highlighted the relationship between the age evolution and happiness in the elderly [21–24]. In this sense, and in line with our main research objective, professionals must look beyond the aspects related to the health of older people, that is, how to restore psychological and social crisis, as this leads to acceptance of the ageing process. Results of White's study assessed "life experiences, describing personality, past traumas, social support, and level of activity, along with physical and psychological health, influencing levels of happiness and satisfaction in the elderly" (p. 54). These findings explain the need to review the variables involved in success or satisfaction with life, such as psychological and physical health, level of activity, and social support. The combination of these factors can give a sense of usefulness and a positive feeling in the review or balance of life in the elderly.

Other specific factors should also be considered when analyzing life satisfaction in people with reduced capacity or dependency. In these specific cases, social, physical, and economic aspects interact with each other as a combination that determines the optimal quality of life [25]. Especially the feeling of loneliness, the degree of self-care capacity, the feeling of concern, the scarcity of financial resources to manage personal independence, and the basic activities of daily life in relation to real needs are the factors that condition health [26].

To finish with, we conclude that no clear consensus exists over the definition of quality of life in elderly to develop the concept based on all its extent for further evaluation from a psychological, cultural, or social point of view. In fact, instead, there is a wide variety of terminology that includes a satisfying life, subjective and psychological welfare, personal development, and other elements that many authors consider synonymous with a satisfying life and welfare. These authors found some approaches to the three dimensions of the concept proposed by Borthwick-Duffy [27] by adding a fourth dimension that seems key to our study: the satisfaction experienced by people in their living conditions, the combination of subjective and objective elements along with the sensations they experience, according to their scale of values, personal expectations, and aspirations held by all elderly people.

From the above analysis, it is evident that the quality of life, in addition to being multidimensional, must take into account the person's life experience, how they feel, and how they interpret their lives [28]. These factors, along with good habits, social support, and relationships, significantly affect health.

Finally, and as a synthesis, the ability to evaluate and learn about these elements allows us to manage health and disease and to identify those factors that can affect. It also improves the quality of life of older people from an integral point of view, that is, from a medical, psychological, and social perspective. It is a multifaceted, interdisciplinary, holistic approach, focused on the person searching for new support strategies for the care and improvement of the health of the elderly, from an interdisciplinary point of view. This approach is beginning to be implemented in clinical practice in some projects of care for dependent and independent elderly people. In summary, the main objective of this research is to analyze the quality of life and the perception of health of the elderly from a multidimensional perspective. The following objectives are pursued:

(i) To assess health in general, from a subjective and objective point of view
(ii) To assess functional, recreational, and leisure skills
(iii) To analyze life satisfaction, taking into account the social contacts and networks, and other social variables
(iv) To determine the relationship between the variables described above and how they complement each other

2. Materials and Methods

According to data from the National Institute of Statistics [29] for the year 2017, the total population over 65 years of age in Granada in 2017 is 47,257 (20.48%). Based on these data, the sample group is made up of 510 people, selected at random from the municipal population census, from five social centers for the elderly in the province of Granada

(Spain). This type of random sampling is suitable for this type of research, since all people in the universe have the same probability of being chosen, discarding those who, due to their dementia or disability, could not collaborate in the survey.

The selection of participants was coordinated with the help of a technical team. Each of the interviewers chose a center to conduct the random questionnaires, selected from the available list of the Health and Social Services. The surveys have been thorough and were conducted from January to May 2017. In order to improve effectiveness, four months elapsed between the first evaluation and second evaluation, with the time needed for a rigorous analysis of the results obtained in the two groups studied. Before starting, a pilot study was carried out to adapt the items or questions to the characteristics of this sector of the population. In both cases, the sample had sociodemographic and health characteristics similar to those of social center users, with representative quotas by sex and age, and an age range of 60 to 85 years for both genders. The experimental group was composed of 250 people, and the control group was composed of 260 people.

The applied research design has been a longitudinal panel design. In the first part of the empirical research, the statistical tool SPSS version 22 was used for the inferential analysis, based on the data obtained from the validated questionnaire CUBRECAVI [30], which is a reliable and valid scale for multidimensional measurement of health and quality of life. It is a validated questionnaire that has the psychometric guarantees of reliability and internal consistency and is very appropriate to our research objectives. It is easy to complete, of short duration (approximately 20 minutes), and measures the following areas related to quality of life: health (subjective, objective, and psychic), social integration, functional capacities, activity and leisure, environmental quality, life satisfaction, education, income, and social and health services. By means of individual and group interviews, we have arranged the participants into two groups: experimental and control. In order to analyze the reliability of the CUBRECAVI scale, the Cronbach alpha index was applied to the main variables that made up the questionnaire: health, integration, activity and leisure, functional capacities, and environmental quality. Subsequently, a regression analysis was conducted, based on the responses to the CUBRECAVI questionnaire, in the experimental and control groups. This was followed by a comprehensive statistical analysis of the most significant variables related to social relations, health, and quality of life. This analysis involved social contacts, frequency, social networking, and cohabitation with family members. The questionnaires included sociodemographic data, social support OARS, daily activities, health-related quality of life scales (QL-Index), and the Garcia scale [31, 32]. These scales were designed to assess the frequency and degree of satisfaction with the social contact received from different sources in relation to quality of life. This study also tested the reliability of the questionnaire, its criteria, and its structural validity, already demonstrated by the authors who validated the tool. The correlative analysis showed significant positive associations between the scores obtained and measures of the explanatory or independent variables, as explained below. Finally, a multivariate descriptive analysis was carried out with the sample studied.

Table 1: Internal consistency of the CUBRECAVI tool.

Variable	*N*	Alpha
Health	857	0.61
Social integration	341	0.22
Leisure and activities	862	0.66
Functional capacities	509	0.81
Environmental quality	893	0.73

For the analysis of inferential statistics, descriptive results and sociodemographic variables were initially analyzed. Later, we studied both the magnitude and the significance of the association between the dependent variables and each of the independent variables (Mantel–Haenszel chi square) in both the experimental and control groups. The magnitude of the associations is expressed with odds ratios and the differences in percentages, as well as their reliable intervals. In contrast to the hypotheses of the quantitative variables, techniques such as Student's and analysis of variance were used if the necessary conditions were met. In order to identify independent risk factors, multivariate analysis techniques and nonconditional logistic regression with binary dependent variables and Cox regression were performed. All these, as indicated, are performed with the SPSS statistical tool.

3. Results

In the descriptive results of the sociodemographic variables, we found that the percentage of men is slightly higher than that of women, which represents 43.6%. In terms of age, all of them are older adults aged between 60 and 70, with 43% of the sample being between 60 and 70 years old, compared to 57% between 70 and 87 years old. The socioeconomic level of the participants is medium low, with an average income ranging from 500 to 600€ per month, although they are within the national average. No significant differences have been found in gender dimensions or educational levels, although age is significant. Hence, the older the person, the greater the deterioration in the quality of life.

As soon as the sociodemographic data were identified, we examined the specific components of quality of life which are most relevant for the older participants in the study of both groups. First, in Table 1, we began to analyze the internal consistency of each of the scales indicated by CUBRECAVI to measure the reliability of this tool. For this purpose, the Cronbach alpha index has been calculated for the subvariables: health, social integration, leisure and activities, functional capacities, and environmental quality. As the scales have only one item, an index of the five scales indicated above has been calculated.

The previous results indicate that the scale used in our research (CUBRECAVI) allows us to predict a subjective criterion of quality of life, that is, whether the subject is satisfied with life. As explained at the beginning of this

TABLE 2: Regression analysis of experimental and control groups.

Variable	Environmental group			Control group		
	Beta	T	Signification	Beta	T	Signification
Health	0.32	5.25	0.001	0.39	2.79	0.001
Functional capacities	0.02	0.11	0.0021	0.19	2.07	0.031
Leisure and activities	0.15	2.89	0.002	0.19	2.09	0.033
Environmental quality	0.9	2.08	0.0026	0.9	0.91	0.02
Income	−0.9	1.45	NS	−0.02	−0.29	NS

Note: variance explained of the experimental group: 25%; variance explained of the control group: 25%; NS = no significance.

document, satisfaction with life is related to quality of life, although specific aspects of each of these concepts are measured. According to the data in Table 1, the internal consistency indices are moderate (between 0.81 and 0.61) in all the subvariables (health, leisure and activities, environmental quality, and functional capacities), with the exception of the social integration that it is low (0.22).

Once the reliability of the scale has been verified, in Table 2, we proceed to apply the regression analysis with the five variables indicated by CUBRECAVI and analyzed in our questionnaires already indicated in the table.

In the multiple regression process, the aim is to describe the impact of the quantitative factors applied on the CUBRECAVI scale on the dependent variable proposed in our study on quality of life, which in turn is related to the health of older people, which, as we have explained in the initial introduction, usually have multiple causes. In this specific case, health and quality of life phenomena relate to several independent factors or variables that influence a priori, such as health, functional capacities, leisure and activities, environmental quality, and income. For this reason, multivariate analysis analyzes the five variables simultaneously, relating them to the impact on the quality of life of the elderly, in order to know how they can affect. It is a question of finding out from a statistical research whether they are in any way related to each other, so it is possible that they can be mathematically related. In order to achieve this purpose, we calculate the regression line in Table 2, where we represent the results of this parametric test with the two groups studied:

Once the regression analysis was carried out, as shown in Table 2, which differentiates the results of the experimental and control groups, we concluded that health, leisure, activity, and environmental quality are the significant variables with the greatest influence on older people in both groups. In detail, in the experimental group, four of the five variables established by CUBRECAVI have been validated as determinants, with the exception of income. These values represent 25% of the total variance in the experimental group. In the control group, the same thing happens as in the previous case, and only the income variable is not significant, where the variance represents 31% of the total.

The results of the two groups have in common the importance given to leisure, spare time, health, and the influence of these factors on the quality of life. However, the participants in the control group attach more importance to functional skills and leisure activities. In contrast, in the experimental group, they value environmental conditions more. These differences, nevertheless, are minimal.

Therefore, we understand that the elderly consider transcendental, for their lives, having the capacity to carry out the basic activities of daily life, but also having sufficient physical capacities to allow them access to leisure and spare time, in an suitable environmental context. In simple terms, this is interpreted as the need to be able to carry out their personal autonomy and community participation in the environment, or the natural environment, close to their reference nuclei, taking into account the limitations of age. After all, being well, being able to do the basics for oneself, and enjoying spare time are priority aspects in this stage of life because they make it possible to feel more empowered and better. For obvious reasons, the connotations of these elements are direct with the state of health because they influence the fact of feeling better and, consequently, of being better, of the perception one has of one's health and quality of life.

To complement the results of the previous analysis obtained in the factors determined by the scale CUBRECAVI, a new element has been introduced, which in our opinion may be of interest for the purpose of this study. We are referring to the effects that social contacts and social relations have on the quality of life of the elderly and, of course, also on their health situation. To this end, we have taken into account what has been published in the latest research and articles in the area of geriatrics and gerontology that places contact, its duration, frequency, and interactions as a crucial axis in the health and illness binomial. Thus, in Table 3, we show the multivariate analysis of nonconditional logistic regression in the same subjects, with both models, in relation to the independent variable called social contact. Three specific aspects or dimensions are calculated: the association between the duration of visits, weekly contacts, and cohabitation as explanatory subvariables. The data are intended to determine whether or not the probability of these variables occurring will influence the quality of life and health of the elderly and whether they are a complement to the variables studied in the table above. The strength of association is expressed in odds ratios.

If we compare the variables set out in Table 3 in the results of both groups, we find some differences in the scores obtained. First, in the control group, we find negative associations in the coexistence subvariable, when contact with children occurs (HR 0.99), and positive association when it is with other family members (HR 1.28). HR stands for the hazard ratio. Also, as reflected in the odds ratio data, they are negative when the number of visits per week is increased. Specifically, the association is more negative when the visits

TABLE 3: Logistic regression analysis of the association size of the network and social contacts in both groups.

Variable	Environmental group (model 1)				Control group (model 2)			
	P	Hazard ratio	95% CI of HR		*P*	Hazard ratio	95% CI of HR	
			Lower limit	Upper limit			Lower limit	Upper limit
Coexistence								
Alone (basal)	1				1			
Spouse	0.211	1.068	0.806	1.434	0.325	1.089	0.794	1.387
Son/daughter	0.019	1.289	0.989	1.68	0.389	0.995	0.791	1.335
Siblings	0.003	1.335	1.119	1.988	0.169	1.1	0.833	1.469
Other people	0.008	1.499	1.108	1.995	0.048	1.285	0.886	1.893
Contacts and weekly visits								
>5 (basal)	1				1			
2–4 per week	0.499	1.401	0.799	1.132	0.428	0.824	0.659	1.089
1-2 per week	0.599	1.048	0.795	1.244	0.11	1.08	0.88	1.386
0	0.24	1.22	0.78	1.249	0.229	0.795	0.495	1.081
Times to visit the social network								
>1-2 day (basal)	1				1			
2–5 per week	0.699	1.024	0.842	1.203	0.504	1.079	0.765	1.109
1-2 per week	0.297	1.097	0.865	1.259	0.069	1.182	0.895	1.34
0	0.1	1.123	0.889	1.295	0.897	0.924	0.828	1.829

Note: model 1 was adjusted by sociodemographic variables in the experimental group; model 2 was adjusted by sociodemographic variables in the control group; 95% CI of HR = confidence interval for *b*.

are more frequent than two per week (HR 0.82) but also when there are no visits at all (HR 0.79). On the contrary, 1 or 2 contacts with people per week are positive for this group (HO 1.08). We can conclude from these data that the ideal is to have visitors, but not too many, given that elderly value quality more than quantity.

Secondly, in the experimental group, there is a positive association with the quality of life and health of the elderly, in the variables called coexistence and contacts, but also with divergences from the previous group. In the case of contacts, both the length of time they last and the frequency or number of times they occur influence this model. That is to say, the longer and more frequent the visits, the better the association or dependency. Hence, we can consider that the experimental group does value the frequency and number of social interactions and not so much their quality as the other group does.

Specifically, by analyzing each of the three dimensions of contact in experimental and control duality, the differences in scores are minimal. It is interesting to observe results in common, in the variable related to coexistence. In particular, this relationship is more positive, with second-degree relatives and other persons outside the primary group, than with those closest to them, such as the spouse or children. That is to say, other members than the direct family provide a more positive relationship in the elderly of both groups, with an even greater incidence in the control group. We can conclude, then, that in this study, the incidence of the contact subvariable is clearly a determinant of the quality of life of the experimental group with an HR between 1.04 and 1.40, and a 95% confidence Interval, compared to the control group with an HR between 0.79 and 1.08. In any case, in both groups, it is closer to the value 1 when the contacts range from 1 to 2 per week. This means that older people who have social contacts are more likely to improve their quality of life when they have weekly contacts with others, regardless of kinship.

As for the variable related to the contacts made with different people during the week, although they are valued as important in general, it seems that they are more positive when they are of a medium frequency but not intense. The ideal is between 2 and 4 contacts per week in the experimental group (HR 1.401). In this respect, the two groups do not agree on this point, and the number of contacts per week is more important for the experimental group. The common point, or coincidence, occurs when considering two average contacts per week as the average of positive contacts for quality of life.

We insist once again that social relationships depend on several factors as determinants of quality of life. For this reason, in addition to coexistence and contacts, the length of time these contacts last is also important. According to these results, as for the number of visits, the opposite occurs when the visits decrease to none per week, which is a negative association in the experimental group. When they increase, that is, between 2 and 5 visits per week (control group HR 1.024), it is considered a positive element in the perception of quality of life. In the control group, the scores are slightly lower, peaking at 1.182 in 1 to 2 visits per week. Consequently, the higher the number of visits, the better the quality of life. That is, having visitors or contacts is an important predictor as well, with a clear positive association with the dependent variables.

4. Discussion

Data from multivariate analysis show that the determinants indicated in the variables analyzed above, if added together, are considered as a metavariable measure of health and quality of life. If we take into account the regression analysis, they influence according to their number or frequency and the relationship that social contact has with the elderly person; in fact, living with close relatives is less valued than living with other people. In addition, contacts are influenced not only by how long they last but also by their influence or importance. It is not important to have contact with many different people, but it is important to have contact with those who provide a sense of comfort, who are chosen by the older person, who are not imposed, and, above all, who last long enough to be able to interact, talk, and share common topics of conversation.

As a final summary, we conclude that there is a positive and significant association between the variables described. Therefore, the validity of these scales is confirmed as a proven element for assessing the quality of life in older adults. Multivariable analysis shows that family support or cohabitation is as important for health as social contacts, which are a true welfare factor, and that, by influencing both their number and frequency, they can be considered an estimate of quality of life. Therefore, they are also social factors that generate or predict health in the elderly. At the same time, the deterioration of health in old age requires more participation, more social contacts that act as protectors of health.

Nowadays, due to the higher rate of longevity and the increase in health expenditure, the need to study the psychological, social, and health-related aspects is becoming more and more necessary. The appropriate approach to the aspects mentioned in our study, such as social contact and the main elements of quality of life from a multidimensional perspective, allows us to act as a preventive factor and mitigate the impact of age on health and illness. From this perspective, the psychological and social variables that we have found to be related to the quality of life of older adults are environmental quality, the use of spare time and community facilities, the capacity for personal autonomy and for carrying out basic activities of daily living, and the quantity and quality of social contacts. The combination of all of them makes up a metavariable that acts as a complementary axis to the important medical dimension, which can be understood as an explanatory health factor from an integral, social, and psychic point of view, beyond the absence or presence of illness.

Finally, multidimensional assessment is an effective tool for assessing the quality of life and the objective and subjective health of the elderly. These variables may be related to improving health.

5. Conclusions

The biopsychosocial approach is fundamental in the work of professionals dealing with the elderly, as the constant interaction of the different areas of functioning described can explain the causality between them. This is what happens in this case with the relationship between functional skills, leisure, health, and quality of life: when there is greater involvement with others, and more satisfaction in social contacts, there is a better performance of instrumental or daily activities. This can lead to greater autonomy and better control of certain pathologies and physical limitations. However, it is important to mention that the older adult's concept of health, which in this case has been optimal, is a predictor of physical fitness, which is associated with psychological conditions such as life satisfaction, self-esteem, functional skills, activities, participation, and social interaction.

Conflicts of Interest

The authors declare that they have no conflicts of interest.

References

[1] World Health Organization (WHO), *World Health Day 2012: Ageing and Health: Toolkit for Event Organizer. Instruments WHOQOL-SRPB Field-Test Instrument*, 2012, http://apps.who.int/iris/bitstream/10665/77777/1/WHO_MSD_MER_Rev.2012.04_eng.pdf?ua=1.

[2] J. H. Kahn, R. M. Hessling, and D. W. Russell, "Social support, health, and well-being among the elderly: what is the role of negative affectivity?," *Personality and Individual Differences*, vol. 35, no. 1, pp. 5–17, 2003.

[3] L. Odell, M. Troutman-Jordan, and A. Newman, "Social support and successful aging in assisted living residents," *Educational Gerontology*, vol. 40, no. 1, pp. 61–70, 2013.

[4] A. M. White, G. S. Philogene, L. Fine, and S. Sinha, "Social support and self-reported health status of older adults in the United States," *American Journal of Public Health*, vol. 99, no. 10, pp. 1872–1878, 2009.

[5] T. M. Lyyra and R. L. Heikkinen, "Perceived social support and mortality in older people," *Journal of Gerontology B: Psychological Science*, vol. 61, no. 3, pp. S147–S152, 2006.

[6] K. L. Siedlecki, T. A. Salthouse, S. Oishi, and S. Jeswani, "The relationship between social support and subjective well-being across age," *Social Indicators Research*, vol. 117, no. 2, pp. 581–576, 2014.

[7] A. Walker, *Understanding Quality of Life in Old Age*, Open University Press, Berkshire, UK, 2005.

[8] A. Walker, "A European perspective on quality of life in old age," *European Journal of Ageing*, vol. 2, no. 1, pp. 2–12, 2005.

[9] M. P. Walker, "A refined model of sleep and the time course of memory formation," *Behavioral and Brain Sciences*, vol. 28, no. 1, pp. 51–64, 2005.

[10] A. Walker and C. H. Hennessy, *Growing Older: Quality of Life in Old Age*, Open University Press, Berkshire, UK, 2004.

[11] A. Walker and H. Mollenkopf, "International and multi-disciplinary perspectives on quality of life in old age," in *Quality of Life in Old Age*, H. Mollenkopf and A. Walker, Eds., Springer, Dordrecht, Netherlands, 2007.

[12] G. A. Good, S. LaGrow, and F. Alpass, "An age-cohort study of older adults with and without visual impairments: activity, independence and life satisfaction," *Journal of Visual Impairment and Blindness*, vol. 102, no. 9, pp. 517–527, 2008.

[13] G. Good and A. Kabel, "An exploration of relationships between social comparisons, disability and life satisfaction association for the association for the education and rehabilitation of the blind and visually impaired, AER," *Research and Practice in Visual Impairment and Blindness*, vol. 2, no. 1, 2009.

[14] R. C. Mannel and S. Dupuis, "Life satisfaction," in *Encyclopedia of Gerontology Age, Aging, and the Aged*, J. E. Birren, Ed., pp. 59–64, Academic Press, San Diego, CA, USA, 1996.

[15] P. B. Baltes and J. Smith, "New frontiers in the future of aging: from successful aging of the young old to the dilemmas of the fourth age," *Gerontology*, vol. 49, no. 2, pp. 123–135, 2003.

[16] J. G. Beaumont and P. M. Kenealy, "Quality of life perceptions and social comparisons in healthy old age," *Ageing and Society*, vol. 24, no. 5, pp. 755–769, 2004.
[17] D. J. H. Deeg, R. J. Bosscher, M. I. Broese van Groenou, L. M. Horn, and C. Jonker, *Ouder Worden in Nederland*, Thela Thesis, Amsterdam, Netherlands, 2000.
[18] S. Degges-White and K. Stoltz, "Archetypal identity development, meaning in life, and life satisfaction: differences among clinical mental health counselors, school counselors, and counselor educators," *Adultspam Journal*, vol. 14, no. 1, pp. 49–61, 2015.
[19] J. Smith, "Well-being and health from age 70 to 100: findings from the Berlin Aging Study," *European Review*, vol. 9, no. 4, pp. 461–477, 2001.
[20] W. Gwozdz and A. Sousa-Poza, "Ageing, health and life satisfaction of the oldest old: an analysis for Germany," *Social Indicators Research*, vol. 97, no. 3, pp. 397–417, 2009.
[21] C. Chen, "Aging and life satisfaction," *Social Indicators Research*, vol. 54, no. 1, pp. 57–79, 2001.
[22] D. K. Mroczek and A. Spiro, "Change in life satisfaction during adulthood: findings from the veterans affairs normative aging study," *Journal of Personality and Social Psychology*, vol. 88, no. 1, pp. 189–202, 2005.
[23] A. Steptoe, P. Demakakos, and C. De Oliveira, *The Psychological Well-Being, Health and Functioning of Older People in England, ELSA Wave 6 Report*, English Longitudinal Study of Ageing, St Helens, UK, 2012.
[24] M. Kolosnitsyna, N. Khorkina, and N. Khongor, "What happens to happiness when people get older? Socio-economic determinants of life satisfaction," in *Later Life. HSE Working Papers*, National Research University Higher School of Economics, Moscow, Russia, 2014.
[25] C. Borg, I. R. Hallberg, and K. Blomqvist, "Life satisfaction among older people (65+) with reduced self-care capacity: the relationship to social, health and financial aspects," *Journal of Clinical Nursing*, vol. 15, no. 5, pp. 519–656, 2006.
[26] J. B. Morganti, M. F. Nehrke, I. M. Hulicka, and J. F. Cataldo, "Life-span differences in life satisfaction, self-concept, and locus of control," *International Journal of Aging*, vol. 26, no. 1, pp. 45–56, 1988.
[27] S. A. Borthwick-Duffy, "Quality of life and quality of care in mental retardation," in *Mental Retardation in the Year 2000*, L. Rowitz, Ed., pp. 52–56, Springer-Verlag, Berlin, Germany, 1992.
[28] R. Fernández-Ballesteros, "Quality of life: the differential conditions," *Psychology in Spain*, vol. 2, pp. 57–65, 1998.
[29] *National Institute of Statistics, INE*, 2016, http://www.ine.es/jaxiT3/Tabla.htm?t=2871.
[30] R. Fernández-Ballesteros and M. D. Zamarron, *CUBRECA VI. Short Questionnaire on Quality of Life*, Tea Ediciones, Madrid, Spain, 2007.
[31] S. Katz, A. B. Ford, R. W. Moskowiz, B. A. Jackson, and M. W. Jaffe, "Studies of illness in the age. The index of ADL: a standardized measure of biological and psychosocial function," *JAMA*, vol. 185, no. 12, pp. 914–919, 1963.
[32] F. J. García García, M. I. Garcia Garcia, and A. Sanchez Ayala, "The prevalence of dementia and its main subtypes in subjects older than 65 years: impact of occupation and education. The Toledo Study," *Clinical Medicine*, vol. 116, no. 11, pp. 401–407, 2001.

18

Associations between ACE-Inhibitors, Angiotensin Receptor Blockers, and Lean Body Mass in Community Dwelling Older Women

Jennifer W. Bea,[1] **Sylvia Wassertheil-Smoller**,[2] **Betsy C. Wertheim**,[1] **Yann Klimentidis**,[3] **Zhao Chen**,[3] **Oleg Zaslavsky**,[4] **Todd M. Manini**,[5] **Catherine R. Womack**,[6] **Candyce H. Kroenke**,[7] **Andrea Z. LaCroix**,[8] **and Cynthia A. Thomson**[9]

[1]*University of Arizona Cancer Center, 1515 N. Campbell Ave, P.O. Box 245024, Tucson, AZ 85724-0524, USA*
[2]*Department of Epidemiology and Population Health, Albert Einstein College of Medicine of Yeshiva University, 1300 Morris Park Avenue, Belfer Building, Room 1308B, Bronx, NY 10461, USA*
[3]*Department of Epidemiology and Biostatistics, Mel and Enid Zuckerman College of Public Health, University of Arizona, 1295 N. Martin, P.O. Box 245211, Drachman Hall A238, Tucson, AZ 85724, USA*
[4]*Department of Biobehavioral Nursing and Health Systems, University of Washington, P.O Box 357266, 1959 NE Pacific Ave., Seattle, WA 98195-7266, USA*
[5]*Department of Aging and Geriatric Research, University of Florida, P.O. Box 100107, Gainesville, FL 32610, USA*
[6]*Department of Medicine, University of Tennessee, 956 Court Avenue, Memphis, TN 38163, USA*
[7]*Kaiser Permanente Northern California, Division of Research, 2000 Broadway, Oakland, CA 94612, USA*
[8]*Department of Family Medicine and Public Health, University of California, 9500 Gilman Drive No. 0725, San Diego, La Jolla, CA 92093, USA*
[9]*Department of Health Promotion Sciences, Mel and Enid Zuckerman College of Public Health, University of Arizona, 1295 N. Martin, P.O. Box 245209, Drachman Hall A260, Tucson, AZ 85724, USA*

Correspondence should be addressed to Jennifer W. Bea; jbea@uacc.arizona.edu

Academic Editor: Adam B. Salmon

Studies suggest that ACE-inhibitors (ACE-I) and angiotensin receptor blockers (ARBs) may preserve skeletal muscle with aging. We evaluated longitudinal differences in lean body mass (LBM) among women diagnosed with hypertension and classified as ACE-I/ARB users and nonusers among Women's Health Initiative participants that received dual energy X-ray absorptiometry scans to estimate body composition ($n = 10,635$) at baseline and at years 3 and 6 of follow-up. Of those, 2642 were treated for hypertension at baseline. Multivariate linear regression models, adjusted for relevant demographics, behaviors, and medications, assessed ACE-I/ARB use/nonuse and LBM associations at baseline, as well as change in LBM over 3 and 6 years. Although BMI did not differ by ACE-I/ARB use, LBM (%) was significantly higher in ACE-I/ARB users versus nonusers at baseline (52.2% versus 51.3%, resp., $p = 0.001$). There was no association between ACE-I/ARB usage and change in LBM over time. Reasons for higher LBM with ACE-I/ARB use cross sectionally, but not longitundinally, are unclear and may reflect a threshold effect of these medications on LBM that is attenuated over time. Nevertheless, ACE-I/ARB use does not appear to negatively impact LBM in the long term.

1. Introduction

Sarcopenia, defined as a progressive loss of skeletal muscle mass, is a significant public health concern linked to diminished quality of life, disability, and even mortality in older adults [1, 2]. Investigating strategies to increase muscle mass or minimize losses in older adults is important and a bourgeoning area of research [1, 2]. Correspondingly, within older populations, antihypertensive medications, such as ACE-inhibitors (ACE-I) and angiotensin receptor blockers (ARBs), are regularly prescribed to those at risk for or diagnosed with hypertension and cardiovascular diseases (CVDs) [3]. Interestingly, these medications target angiotensin II, a protein upregulated in hypertension and CVD, which has been associated with a phenomenon called cardiac cachexia, in which the skeletal muscle mass is lost more rapidly than would be expected under normal aging conditions [4]. Thus, ACE-I and ARBs, respectively, may help to preserve lean body mass (LBM) among older adults. Studies suggest that these medications not only target smooth muscle relaxation, aiding in blood pressure control, but also have a direct positive effect on skeletal muscle [2, 4, 5].

The extent of ACE-I and ARB mechanisms of action on muscle is not fully understood; the potential favorable effects of these medications on muscle mass and function could inform on the best options for blood pressure control, particularly for older individuals [5]. In fact, the Health ABC study, including >2400 elderly males and females, found that larger lower extremity muscle mass was associated with ACE-I use [6]. Meanwhile, functional studies related to skeletal muscle performance have yielded mixed results. For example, the Women's Health Initiative (WHI) found no associations between ACE-Is and frailty, physical performance, and strength with 3 and 6 years follow-up, respectively [7, 8]. Similarly, Health ABC found no association between ACE-I and risk of mobility limitations over 6.5 years [9]. In contrast, the Women's Healthy Aging Study found positive associations between ACE-I, muscle strength, and walking speed at 3 years, even after adjusting for cardiovascular events [10]. Unfortunately, these prior analyses were limited to those over the age of 65 years, and none of them directly evaluated LBM prospectively. However, hypertension, commonly treated with ACE-I/ARBs, is present in 34% of US adults aged 45–64 years [11].

Fortunately, a subset of WHI participants ($n = 10,635$) completed repeated body composition over six years. Of those with DXA scans, 2642 self-reported being currently treated for hypertension. The aim of the present analysis was to evaluate baseline differences in LBM among ACE-I/ARB users and nonusers and to determine if longitudinal changes in LBM are associated with ACE-I/ARB use among postmenopausal women. We hypothesized that taking antihypertensive medications, specifically ACE-I and ARBs, would be associated with higher LBM and preservation of LBM with aging.

2. Methods

2.1. Study Population. Between 1993 and 1998, healthy postmenopausal women aged between 50 and 79 years were enrolled in the WHI clinical trials and observational study at 40 clinical centers across the U.S. ($n = 161,808$) [12, 13]. A subcohort consented to complete body composition measurements at the WHI clinical centers in Pittsburgh, PA; Birmingham, AL; and Tucson-Phoenix, AZ ($n = 11,020$) [14]. All participants with body composition at baseline and for whom medication information could be ascertained were included in the analysis ($n = 10,635$); of those, 2642 were treated for hypertension at baseline. The protocol and consent forms were approved by the institutional review board at each site, and all participants provided written informed consent. Study design and participant characteristics have been described in detail elsewhere [12, 13, 15].

2.2. Body Composition. Total and regional body composition was determined by performing total body dual energy X-ray absorptiometry (DXA) scans (QDR2000, 2000+, or 4500W; Hologic Inc, Bedford, MA) at baseline and at years 3 and 6. Percent total body fat [%TBF = TBF (kg)/weight (kg)], LBM [%LBM = LBM (kg)/weight (kg)], and appendicular lean mass [aLM% = $LBM_{arms} + LBM_{legs}$ (kg)/$weight_{arms} + weight_{legs}$ (kg)] were computed. DXA-derived fat and lean mass have been validated against gold standard, magnetic resonance imaging, within a subset of this study population ($n = 101$; WHI MRI precision error < 1%; fat, Pearson rho = 0.99; lean, Pearson rho = 0.94, $p < 0.001$) [16].

The WHI DXA quality assurance program has been well described previously. It included standard positioning and analysis protocols; certification of technicians; local daily and weekly phantom scans; circulating Hologic calibration phantoms; and machine and technician performance monitoring by review of phantom and problematic scans, as well as random sampling [17].

2.3. Medications. Participants brought all current medications to their baseline and year 3 visit at the local WHI clinics. All medications were assigned drug codes in the Medi-Span software database (First DataBank, Inc., San Bruno, CA). The antihypertensive medications of interest in this analysis, ACE-I and ARBs, were coded according to therapeutic classes as follows: ACE Inhibitors; Angiotensin II Receptor Antagonist; ACE Inhibitors and Calcium Blockers; ACE Inhibitors and Thiazide/Thiazide-Like; and Angiotensin II Receptor Antagonist and Thiazides. For baseline analyses, binary categorization of users and nonusers of ACE-I or ARB was used. For follow-up analyses, the following categories were created: nonuse, no use at baseline or year 3; intermediate use, use at either time point; use, use at both time points.

2.4. Covariates. Potential covariates were initially identified from published literature evaluating body composition and medications. Self-report questionnaires were used to determine demographic characteristics, health history, and lifestyle behaviors, such as age, neighborhood socioeconomic status (NSES) [18], race/ethnicity, dietary energy consumption (kcal/day) [19] and quality (Healthy Eating Index, HEI 2005) [20], physical activity (MET-hr/wk) [21], physical function [22], smoking (pack-years), and alcohol use. Polypharmacy categories (0–4 or ≥5 medications) were created utilizing all reported medications. Weight (kg) and height (cm) were measured during clinic visits on a balance-beam scale and wall-mounted stadiometer, respectively. Body mass index (BMI) was calculated as weight (kg)/height $(m)^2$.

2.5. Statistical Analysis. Baseline characteristics were compared between ACE-I/ARB users and nonusers by *t*-test for continuous variables and chi-square tests for categorical variables. Within the full DXA cohort ($n = 10,635$), key potential confounding variables were found to be clinically and statistically significantly different between ACE-I/ARB users ($n = 944$) and nonusers ($n = 9691$). ACE-I/ARB users were significantly older (2 years), physically larger (2.0 kg/m^2), and more racially/ethnically diverse and reported less education, poorer health, lower alcohol consumption, lower hormone therapy use, lower physical activity, lower energy intake, and greater use of other CVD-related medications than nonusers ($p \leq 0.005$; *data not presented*). Therefore, the present analysis is primarily focused on those reporting being treated for hypertension at baseline ($n = 2642$), to better evaluate the differences between ACE-I/ARB users ($n = 782$) and nonusers ($n = 1860$) rather than the differences between those treated for hypertension and those without hypertension. All analyses were repeated in the full cohort for comparison.

The cross-sectional association between ACE-I/ARB use and LBM at baseline was assessed by linear regression. Absolute and relative *changes* in LBM from baseline to year 3 or year 6 based on exposure to ACE-I/ARB during the first three years of the study period were evaluated using multivariate-adjusted linear regression models and the ACE-I/ARB use classifications above. Covariates were scanner serial number; clinical trial arm; self-reported age, race/ethnicity, smoking, physical activity, history of diabetes treatment, history of arthritis, cancer, CVD, depressive symptoms, HRT use (never, past, and current), general health (excellent, very good, good, or fair/poor), physical function (dichotomized as <90 or ≥90 points), dietary energy, dietary protein, and HEI; polypharmacy; SES; and clinic measured systolic and diastolic blood pressure and height at baseline. Models evaluating change in LBM were further adjusted for baseline lean mass measure and year 3 physical activity. The effects of *new* use of either drug at year 3 on change in LBM and aLM between years 3 and 6 were explored in similar models. New users were defined by ACE-I/ARB use reported at year 3 but not at baseline ($n = 174$), which was compared to no ACE-I/ARB use reported at baseline nor year 3 (non-users, $n = 837$). Due to the high levels of missing data among covariates, multiple imputation with chained equations was employed to fill in the gaps [23]. The imputation model used all variables listed above as covariates. Twenty complete datasets were created, analyzed, and combined. All statistical analyses were conducted using Stata 15.1 (StataCorp, College Station, TX), and significance was set at $p < 0.05$.

3. Results

Among those being treated for hypertension ($n = 2642$), there were significant differences between ACE-I/ARB users ($n = 782$) and nonusers ($n = 1860$) in terms of age, SES, race/ethnicity, smoking status, or hormone therapy use (Table 1). Users had slightly higher systolic, but not diastolic, blood pressure and were more likely to be treated for diabetes, prescribed a greater number of medications (polypharmacy), and reported lower general health. Diet quality was higher among users. Absolute body size and composition were not significantly different at baseline between users and nonusers; however, TBF (%) was 0.8% higher and LBM (%) was correspondingly lower among nonusers at baseline.

Total body lean mass (kg) was significantly greater among ACE-I/ARB users compared to nonusers in fully adjusted models at baseline (Table 2; lean mass, kg: β: 0.42; standard error (SE): 0.20; $p < 0.04$). The absolute lean mass association with ACE-I/ARB use stratified by BMI (normal weight (18.5–24.9 kg/m^2), overweight (25.0–29.9 kg/m^2), and obese (≥30 kg/m^2)) remained significant for normal weight (0.77 (0.28); $p = 0.007$) and overweight (0.67 (0.22); $p = 0.002$) categories, but not for obese women (0.14 (0.28); $p = 0.621$). Percent LBM and aLM were also significantly greater among ACE-I/ARB users than nonusers (β: 0.76, SE: 0.26 and β: 1.08, SE: 0.28, resp.; both $p < 0.01$).

Baseline ACE-I/ARB use was not significantly associated with total LBM or aLM change in between baseline and the year 3 visit. However, a substantial proportion (21%) of participants did not have data available at year 3, and these women were different from those with follow-up data with regard to several baseline characteristics. Women lacking follow-up data were significantly older with lower NSES, lower physical activity, higher systolic blood pressure, higher BMI, and lower HEI than women with follow-up data. Additionally, those without follow-up were more likely than those with follow-up data to be black or Hispanic, smoke currently or previously, take 5+ prescription medications, and have diabetes, arthritis, or depressive symptoms. Furthermore, women lacking follow-up data had significantly worse physical functioning and general health than women with follow-up data. There were no significant differences between these two groups of women with regard to personal history of cancer or cardiovascular disease or dietary energy or protein (data not shown).

Similarly, change in total LBM or aLM was not different between ACE-I/ARB use categories over 3 years and 6 years (Table 3). All analyses related to *change* in lean mass comparing ACE-I/ARB users to nonusers, regardless of hypertensive status, were repeated using the full DXA cohort ($n = 10,635$), and results remained null (*data not presented*).

4. Discussion

Within the largest and most diverse prospective study of postmenopausal women with body composition information, we found ACE-I/ARB use to be significantly associated with higher LBM in cross-sectional analyses. However, ACE-I/ARB use among hypertensives was not associated with change in LBM or aLM longitudinally. The higher lean mass with ACE-I/ARB use that was demonstrated cross sectionally, but not longitudinally, herein could reflect a threshold effect of these medications on LBM that is attenuated over time. The fact that ACE-I/ARB use did not negatively impact LBM long term is important clinically in that it does not deter clinicians from prescribing these medications long term.

TABLE 1: Baseline characteristics of hypertensive women in the Women's Health Initiative DXA Cohort by ACE-I/ARB use*†.

Characteristic: mean ± SD or n%	Total n = 2642	Nonusers n = 1860	Users n = 782	p
Age (years)	65.1 ± 7.2	65.0 ± 7.2	65.1 ± 7.2	0.666
NSES	69.2 ± 10.3	69.0 ± 10.5	69.5 ± 9.8	0.283
Race/ethnicity				0.112
Non-Hispanic white	1736 (65.7)	1205 (64.8)	646 (68.4)	
Black	737 (27.9)	543 (29.2)	194 (24.8)	
Hispanic	116 (4.39)	77 (4.14)	39 (4.99)	
Other or unknown	53 (2.01)	35 (1.88)	18 (2.30)	
Smoking status				0.744
Never	1471 (56.6)	1029 (56.4)	442 (57.0)	
Former	961 (37.0)	673 (36.9)	288 (37.1)	
Current	169 (6.50)	123 (6.74)	46 (5.93)	
Physical activity (MET-hr/wk)	9.44 ± 12.3	9.36 ± 11.8	9.64 ± 13.5	0.593
Blood pressure				
Systolic (mmHg)	138.2 ± 18.4	137.7 ± 18.1	139.5 ± 19.2	0.021
Diastolic (mmHg)	77.0 ± 9.7	77.1 ± 9.7	76.8 ± 9.7	0.390
Body size				
Height (cm)	161.2 ± 6.5	161.3 ± 6.6	160.8 ± 6.3	0.080
Weight (kg)	78.8 ± 17.7	79.1 ± 18.3	78.0 ± 16.2	0.138
BMI (kg/m^2)	30.2 ± 6.3	30.2 ± 6.4	30.1 ± 5.9	0.668
Lean mass (kg)	39.1 ± 6.0	39.0 ± 6.1	39.3 ± 5.9	0.316
Lean mass (%)	51.5 ± 6.6	51.3 ± 6.7	52.1 ± 6.5	0.005
Fat mass (%)	45.7 ± 6.9	45.9 ± 7.0	45.1 ± 6.7	0.009
Appendicular lean mass (%)	45.7 ± 6.8	45.3 ± 6.9	46.5 ± 6.7	<0.001
Medical history				
Diabetes treatment	327 (12.4)	189 (10.2)	138 (17.7)	<0.001
Polypharmacy (≥5)	980 (37.1)	623 (33.5)	357 (45.7)	<0.001
Depressive symptoms	375 (14.6)	271 (15.0)	104 (13.7)	0.399
Arthritis	1653 (62.9)	1163 (62.8)	490 (62.9)	0.973
Cancer	216 (8.22)	151 (8.15)	65 (8.37)	0.857
Cardiovascular disease	726 (27.9)	527 (28.8)	199 (25.7)	0.112
General health				0.001
Excellent	132 (5.02)	105 (5.66)	27 (3.48)	
Very good	661 (25.1)	480 (25.9)	181 (23.4)	
Good	1231 (46.8)	876 (47.3)	355 (45.8)	
Fair/poor	605 (23.0)	393 (21.2)	212 (27.4)	
Physical function construct <90	1808 (70.1)	1276 (70.2)	532 (69.9)	0.888
Hormone replacement therapy				0.686
Never used	1288 (48.8)	914 (49.2)	374 (47.8)	
Past use	465 (17.6)	320 (17.2)	145 (18.5)	
Current use	888 (33.6)	625 (33.6)	263 (33.6)	
Diet				
Energy intake (kcal/d)	1656 ± 724	1681 ± 735	1595 ± 694	0.006
Protein intake (%)	16.6 ± 3.3	16.5 ± 3.3	16.8 ± 3.3	0.035
Healthy Eating Index	65.4 ± 11.3	65.1 ± 11.4	66.2 ± 11.0	0.023

*ACE-inhibitor, ACE-I; angiotensin receptor blocker, ARB; cardiovascular disease, body mass index, BMI; Healthy Eating Index, HEI; hormone replacement therapy, HRT; neighborhood socioeconomic status, NSES; standard deviation, SD; †missing data: NSES 42; smoking 41; physical activity 9; blood pressure (systolic/diastolic) 2/3; height 15; weight 4; BMI 19; diabetes 6; depression 72; arthritis 12; cancer 13; CVD 36; general health 13; physical function 63; HRT 1; diet (energy, protein, HEI) 125.

TABLE 2: Association between baseline ACE-I/ARB use and measures of lean mass using linear regression in hypertensive women from the Women's Health Initiative*.

Outcome	Baseline lean mass β (SE) $n = 2642$		Change in lean mass (baseline to year 3) β (SE) $n = 2095$	
	Model 1†	Model 2‡	Model 1†	Model 2‡
Lean mass (kg)				
Nonuser	Ref.	Ref.	Ref.	Ref.
User	0.31 (0.25)	0.42 (0.20)	0.06 (0.09)	0.14 (0.09)
p value	0.212	0.038	0.481	0.137
Lean mass (%)				
Nonuser	Ref.	Ref.	Ref.	Ref.
User	0.73 (0.28)	0.76 (0.26)	−0.28 (0.14)	−0.21 (0.15)
p value	0.009	0.004	0.055	0.141
Appendicular lean mass (%)				
Nonuser	Ref.	Ref.	Ref.	Ref.
User	1.16 (0.29)	1.08 (0.28)	−0.14 (0.15)	−0.12 (0.16)
p value	<0.001	<0.001	0.358	0.452

*ACE-inhibitor, ACE-I; angiotensin receptor blocker, ARB; †Model 1 adjusted for scanner serial number. The change model is also adjusted for the baseline lean mass measure; ‡Model 2 further adjusted for age, neighborhood socioeconomic status, race/ethnicity, smoking, physical activity, systolic blood pressure, diastolic blood pressure, height, diabetes, polypharmacy, depressive symptoms, arthritis, cancer, cardiovascular disease, hormone replacement therapy use, general health, physical function, dietary energy, dietary protein, and healthy eating index. The change model is also adjusted for physical activity at year 3 and clinical trial arm(s). Multiple imputation was used to fill in missing values for baseline covariates (see Methods for details and Table 1 footnote for missing data frequencies); however, participants missing medication use at year 3 were excluded from this analysis ($n = 35$).

TABLE 3: Association between ACE-I/ARB use over time and change in lean mass in hypertensive women from the Women's Health Initiative*.

	Baseline to year 3 β (SE); p $n = 2060$		Baseline to year 6 β (SE); p $n = 1687$	
	Model 1†	Model 2‡	Model 1†	Model 2‡
Lean mass (kg)				
Nonuser	Ref.	Ref.	Ref.	Ref.
Intermediate user	0.06 (0.10); 0.54	0.10 (0.10); 0.34	0.08 (0.15); 0.59	0.08 (0.15); 0.58
User	0.07 (0.11); 0.52	0.18 (0.11); 0.12	0.23 (0.16); 0.16	0.29 (0.16); 0.08
Lean mass (%)				
Nonuser	Ref.	Ref.	Ref.	Ref.
Intermediate user	−0.14 (0.16); 0.40	−0.15 (0.16); 0.34	−0.14 (0.22); 0.53	−0.28 (0.22); 0.21
User	−0.33 (0.18); 0.07	−0.31 (0.18); 0.09	−0.04 (0.25); 0.87	−0.05 (0.25); 0.85
Appendicular lean mass (%)				
Nonuser	Ref.	Ref.	Ref.	Ref.
Intermediate user	−0.06 (0.17); 0.71	−0.08 (0.17); 0.65	−0.04 (0.23); 0.85	−0.18 (0.23); 0.43
User	−0.23 (0.19); 0.23	−0.22 (0.20); 0.27	0.17 (0.25); 0.49	0.17 (0.25); 0.51

*ACE-inhibitor, ACE-I; angiotensin receptor blocker, ARB; †Model 1 adjusted for scanner serial number and baseline lean mass measure; ‡Model 2 further adjusted for age, neighborhood socioeconomic status, race/ethnicity, smoking, physical activity (baseline and year 3), systolic blood pressure, diastolic blood pressure, height, diabetes, polypharmacy, depressive symptoms, arthritis, cancer, cardiovascular disease, hormone replacement therapy use, general health, physical function, dietary energy, dietary protein, healthy eating index, and clinical trial arm(s). Multiple imputation was used to fill in missing values for covariates (see Methods for details and Table 1 footnote for missing data frequencies).

Reducing angiotenin II or its activity via ACE-I and ARBs, respectively, was hypothesized to preserve LBM in postmenopausal women, a population that losses significant LBM annually through the end of life [24]. Health ABC findings of greater lower extremity LBM in older persons using ACE-I cross sectionally, similar to the cross-sectional differences in ACE-I/ARB users versus nonusers herein, suggest LBM as a possible explanation of the benefits of ACE/ARB use in wasting syndromes [6]. However, no longitudinal effects on LBM were demonstrated within the WHI. Results from a previous analysis of 25% random sample of WHI clinical trial participants aged ≥65 demonstrated no difference in mean annual change in function over time among hypertensives taking ACE-I compared to nonusers [8]. Similar null effects on grip strength were reported for the Hertfordshire Cohort Study ($n = 639$, 50% female, aged 65 yrs) for ACE-I use [25].

The robust measure of body composition, detailed characterization of the cohort, broader age range, diversity, and large sample size were strengths of the present analysis. Similar results across LBM and aLM indicate that health conditions that may influence LBM measures by DXA, such as organ enlargement with serious health conditions, did not significantly influence results.

Accounting for body size was important, with height being a major confounder, significantly increasing the point estimate. Limiting to hypertensive individuals in the primary analyses and separately evaluating results by BMI strata further minimized the potential for cross-sectional associations between LBM and ACE-I/ARB to be due to larger body sizes typically associated with hypertension and CVD. Lifestyle factors (e.g., diet and physical activity) were included in the models to minimize behavioral confounding. It is important to note that we adjusted for other important covariates such as race/ethnicity, blood pressure, diabetes treatment, and polypharmacy given that clinical guidelines have begun to differentiate treatment strategies based on various characteristics such as hypertensive stage at presentation, race, diabetes, and other comorbidities [26].

4.1. Limitations. The present analysis cannot be applied to men or younger women. Minimal overlap between DXA and physical function subcohorts precluded concomitant evaluation. Comparisons between drug classes and monotherapy versus combination therapy (i.e., ACE-I combined with thiazide) were limited by power and prescribing patterns of the time [27], similar to other large studies [6]. Patients prescribed an ACE-I commonly switch to an ARB and vice versa depending on side effects and may do so several times during the course of treatment. Therefore, although we recognize that the medications may have different effects, beyond the hemodynamic effects for which they are prescribed, we could not adequately account for crossovers given the periodicity of medication monitoring within WHI, and we examined both antihypertensive medications in combination. In addition, we did not have information on the doses prescribed or taken, prohibiting examination between dose and LBM. Though multiple imputation was employed to account for missing covariates, differences between participants lost to follow-up and those remaining in the analysis may have introduced some bias.

Nevertheless, ACE-I and ARB medications continue to be routinely prescribed early in the medical management of CVD, heart failure, and hypertension, particularly if the patient presents with stage 2 hypertension [26, 28–30]. We expect that new medications, including those that affect the Renin–angiotensin–aldosterone system (e.g., angiotensin II receptor blocker neprilysin inhibitors) [31] will be increasingly incorporated in the management of hypertension. We could not examine these newer medications. Comparisons between medications in relation to their effects on body composition should continue and will be facilitated by the advent of an ICD-10 Code specific to sarcopenia (M62.84, as of Oct. 1, 2016).

In conclusion, our results support the use of ACE-I/ARB use without concern for deleterious changes in LBM among hypertensives. New cohorts are needed to determine if there are differences in the effects on LBM between the two common antihypertensive medications examined here, as well as newer medications.

Conflicts of Interest

The authors declare that they have no conflicts of interest.

Acknowledgments

The WHI program is funded by the National Heart, Lung, and Blood Institute, National Institutes of Health, and U.S. Department of Health and Human Services through contracts HHSN268201600018C, HHSN268201600001C, HHSN268201600002C, HHSN268201600003C, and HHSN268201600004C. The authors are thankful for the contribution of the WHI Investigators and staff at the clinical centers, clinical coordinating center, and project office. A short list of WHI investigators is as follows. *Program Office*: (National Heart, Lung, and Blood Institute, Bethesda, Maryland) Jacques Rossouw, Shari Ludlam, Joan McGowan, Leslie Ford, and Nancy Geller. *Clinical Coordinating Center: Clinical Coordinating Center*: (Fred Hutchinson Cancer Research Center, Seattle, WA) Garnet Anderson, Ross Prentice, Andrea LaCroix, and Charles Kooperberg. *Investigators and Academic Centers*: (Brigham and Women's Hospital, Harvard Medical School, Boston, MA) JoAnn E. Manson; (MedStar Health Research Institute/ Howard University, Washington, DC) Barbara V. Howard; (Stanford Prevention Research Center, Stanford, CA) Marcia L. Stefanick; (The Ohio State University, Columbus, OH) Rebecca Jackson; (University of Arizona, Tucson/ Phoenix, AZ) Cynthia A. Thomson; (University at Buffalo, Buffalo, NY) Jean Wactawski-Wende; (University of Florida, Gainesville/Jacksonville, FL) Marian Limacher; (University of Iowa, Iowa City/Davenport, IA) Jennifer Robinson; (University of Pittsburgh, Pittsburgh, PA) Lewis Kuller; (Wake Forest University School of Medicine, Winston-Salem, NC) Sally Shumaker; (University of Nevada, Reno, NV) Robert Brunner; (University of Minnesota, Minneapolis, MN) Karen L. Margolis. *Women's Health Initiative Memory Study:* (Wake Forest University School of Medicine, Winston-Salem, NC) Mark Espeland. *For a list of all the investigators who have contributed to WHI science, please visit* www.whi.org/researchers/Documents%20%20Write%20a%20Paper/WHI%20Investigator%20Long%20List.pdf.

References

[1] J. Y. Reginster, C. Cooper, R. Rizzoli et al., "Recommendations for the conduct of clinical trials for drugs to treat or prevent sarcopenia," *Aging Clinical and Experimental Research*, vol. 28, no. 1, pp. 47–58, 2016.

[2] D. Sumukadas, A. D. Struthers, and M. E. McMurdo, "Sarcopenia–a potential target for angiotensin-converting enzyme inhibition?," *Gerontology*, vol. 52, no. 4, pp. 237–242, 2006.

[3] A. V. Chobanian, G. L. Bakris, H. R. Black et al., "Seventh report of the Joint National Committee on prevention, detection, evaluation, and treatment of high blood pressure," *Hypertension*, vol. 426, no. 6, pp. 1206–1252, 2003.

[4] T. Yoshida, A. M. Tabony, S. Galvez et al., "Molecular mechanisms and signaling pathways of angiotensin II-induced muscle wasting: potential therapeutic targets for cardiac cachexia," *International Journal of Biochemistry and Cell Biology*, vol. 45, no. 10, pp. 2322–2332, 2013.

[5] C. S. Carter and L. Groban, "Role of the renin-angiotensin system in age-related sarcopenia and diastolic dysfunction," *Aging Health*, vol. 4, no. 1, pp. 37–46, 2008.

[6] M. Di Bari, L. V. van de Poll-Franse, G. Onder et al., "Antihypertensive medications and differences in muscle mass in older persons: the Health, Aging and Body Composition Study," *Journal of the American Geriatrics Society*, vol. 52, no. 6, pp. 961–966, 2004.

[7] S. L. Gray, A. Z. LaCroix, A. K. Aragaki et al., "Angiotensin-converting enzyme inhibitor use and incident frailty in women aged 65 and older: prospective findings from the Women's Health Initiative Observational Study," *Journal of the American Geriatrics Society*, vol. 57, no. 2, pp. 297–303, 2009.

[8] S. L. Gray, A. K. Aragaki, M. J. LaMonte et al., "Statins, angiotensin-converting enzyme inhibitors, and physical performance in older women," *Journal of the American Geriatrics Society*, vol. 60, no. 12, pp. 2206–2214, 2012.

[9] S. L. Gray, R. M. Boudreau, A. B. Newman et al., "Angiotensin-converting enzyme inhibitor and statin use and incident mobility limitation in community-dwelling older adults: the Health, Aging and Body Composition study," *Journal of the American Geriatrics Society*, vol. 59, no. 12, pp. 2226–2232, 2011.

[10] G. Onder, B. W. Penninx, R. Balkrishnan et al., "Relation between use of angiotensin-converting enzyme inhibitors and muscle strength and physical function in older women: an observational study," *The Lancet*, vol. 359, no. 9310, pp. 926–930, 2002.

[11] D. L. Blackwell and J. W. Lucas, *Tables of Summary Health Statistics for U.S. Adults: 2014 National Health Interview Survey*, 2015, Available from: http://www.cdc.gov/nchs/nhis/SHS/tables.htm.

[12] G. L. Anderson, J. Manson, R. Wallace et al., "Implementation of the Women's Health Initiative study design," *Annals of Epidemiology*, vol. 13, no. 9, pp. S5–S17, 2003.

[13] The Women's Health Initiative Study Group, "Design of the Women's Health Initiative clinical trial and observational study," *Controlled Clinical Trials*, vol. 19, no. 1, pp. 61–109, 1998.

[14] Z. Chen, T. J. Beck, J. A. Cauley et al., "Hormone therapy improves femur geometry among ethnically diverse postmenopausal participants in the Women's Health Initiative hormone intervention trials," *Journal of Bone and Mineral Research*, vol. 23, no. 12, pp. 1935–1945, 2008.

[15] J. Hays, J. R. Hunt, F. A. Hubbell et al., "The Women's Health Initiative recruitment methods and results," *Annals of Epidemiology*, vol. 13, no. 9, pp. S18–S77, 2003.

[16] Z. Chen, Z. Wang, T. Lohman et al., "Dual-energy X-ray absorptiometry is a valid tool for assessing skeletal muscle mass in older women," *Journal of Nutrition*, vol. 137, no. 12, pp. 2775–2780, 2007.

[17] Z. Chen, T. Bassford, S. B. Green et al., "Postmenopausal hormone therapy and body composition–a substudy of the estrogen plus progestin trial of the Women's Health Initiative," *American Journal of Clinical Nutrition*, vol. 82, no. 3, pp. 651–656, 2005.

[18] L. Qi, R. Nassir, R. Kosoy et al., "Relationship between diabetes risk and admixture in postmenopausal African-American and Hispanic-American women," *Diabetologia*, vol. 55, no. 5, pp. 1329–1337, 2012.

[19] R. E. Patterson, A. R. Kristal, L. F. Tinker, R. A. Carter, M. P. Bolton, and T. Agurs-Collins, "Measurement characteristics of the Women's Health Initiative food frequency questionnaire," *Annals of Epidemiology*, vol. 9, no. 3, pp. 178–187, 1999.

[20] P. M. Guenther, J. Reedy, S. M. Krebs-Smith, and B. B. Reeve, "Evaluation of the Healthy Eating Index-2005," *Journal of the American Dietetic Association*, vol. 108, no. 11, pp. 1854–1864, 2008.

[21] B. E. Ainsworth, W. L. Haskell, A. S. Leon et al., "Compendium of physical activities: classification of energy costs of human physical activities," *Medicine and Science in Sports and Exercise*, vol. 25, no. 1, pp. 71–80, 1993.

[22] J. E. Ware and C. D. Sherbourne, "The MOS 36-item short-form health survey (SF-36). I. Conceptual framework and item selection," *Medical Care*, vol. 30, no. 6, pp. 473–483, 1992.

[23] M. J. Azur, E. A. Stuart, C. Frangakis, and P. J. Leaf, "Multiple imputation by chained equations: what is it and how does it work?," *International Journal of Methods in Psychiatric Research*, vol. 20, no. 1, pp. 40–49, 2011.

[24] I. Janssen, S. B. Heymsfield, Z. M. Wang, and R. Ross, "Skeletal muscle mass and distribution in 468 men and women aged 18–88 yr," *Journal of Applied Physiology*, vol. 89, no. 1, pp. 81–88, 2000.

[25] M. D. Witham, H. E. Syddall, E. Dennison, C. Cooper, M. E. McMurdo, and A. A. Sayer, "ACE inhibitors, statins and thiazides: no association with change in grip strength among community dwelling older men and women from the Hertfordshire Cohort Study," *Age and Ageing*, vol. 43, no. 5, pp. 661–666, 2014.

[26] P. A. James, S. Oparil, B. L. Carter et al., "2014 evidence-based guideline for the management of high blood pressure in adults: report from the panel members appointed to the Eighth Joint National Committee (JNC 8)," *JAMA*, vol. 311, no. 5, pp. 507–520, 2014.

[27] S. Wassertheil-Smoller, G. Anderson, B. M. Psaty et al., "Hypertension and its treatment in postmenopausal women: baseline data from the Women's Health Initiative," *Hypertension*, vol. 36, no. 5, pp. 780–789, 2000.

[28] A. S. Go, M. A. Bauman, S. M. Coleman King et al., "An effective approach to high blood pressure control: a science advisory from the American Heart Association, the American College of Cardiology, and the Centers for Disease Control and Prevention," *Hypertension*, vol. 63, no. 4, pp. 878–885, 2014.

[29] C. W. Yancy, M. Jessup, B. Bozkurt et al., "2013 ACCF/AHA guideline for the management of heart failure: a report of the American College of Cardiology Foundation/American Heart

Association Task Force on Practice Guidelines," *Journal of the American College of Cardiology*, vol. 62, no. 16, pp. e147–e239, 2013.

[30] C. W. Yancy, M. Jessup, B. Bozkurt et al., "2016 ACC/AHA/HFSA focused update on new pharmacological therapy for heart failure: an update of the 2013 ACCF/AHA Guideline for the Management of Heart Failure: A Report of the American College of Cardiology/American Heart Association Task Force on Clinical Practice Guidelines and the Heart Failure Society of America," *Journal of the American College of Cardiology*, vol. 68, no. 13, pp. 1476–1488, 2016.

[31] M. Volpe, G. Tocci, A. Battistoni, and S. Rubattu, "Angiotensin II Receptor Blocker Neprilysin Inhibitor (ARNI): new avenues in cardiovascular therapy," *High Blood Pressure & Cardiovascular Prevention*, vol. 22, no. 3, pp. 241–246, 2015.

19

The Impact of Social and Cultural Engagement and Dieting on Well-Being and Resilience in a Group of Residents in the Metropolitan Area of Naples

Antonio Rapacciuolo,[1] Pasquale Perrone Filardi,[1] Rosario Cuomo,[2] Vincenzo Mauriello,[3] Maria Quarto,[4] Annamaria Kisslinger,[5,6] Gianluigi Savarese,[1] Maddalena Illario,[7,8] and Donatella Tramontano[6,9]

[1]*Department of Advanced Biomedical Science, University of Naples Federico II, 80131 Naples, Italy*
[2]*Department of Clinical Medicine and Surgery, University of Naples Federico II, 80131 Naples, Italy*
[3]*Arci Movie, 80147 Naples, Italy*
[4]*Department of Physics, University of Naples Federico II, 80131 Naples, Italy*
[5]*IEOS-CNR, Naples, Italy*
[6]*Fondazione GENS Onlus, 80121 Naples, Italy*
[7]*Department of Translational Medical Sciences, University of Naples Federico II, 80131 Naples, Italy*
[8]*R&D Unit, Federico II University Hospital, 80131 Naples, Italy*
[9]*Department of Molecular Medicine and Medical Biotechnology, University of Naples Federico II, 80131 Naples, Italy*

Correspondence should be addressed to Maddalena Illario; illario@unina.it and Donatella Tramontano; dtramont@unina.it

Academic Editor: F. R. Ferraro

Social isolation and exclusion are associated with poor health status and premature death. A number of related isolation factors, inadequate transportation system and restrictions in individuals' life space, have been associated with malnutrition in older adults. Since eating is a social event, isolation can have a negative effect on nutrition. Cultural involvement and participation in interactive activities are essential tools to fight social isolation, and they can counteract the detrimental effects of social isolation on health. To provide data supporting the hypothesis that encouraging participation might represent an innovative preventive and health promoting strategy for healthy living and aging, we developed an *ad hoc* questionnaire to investigate the relationship between cultural participation, well-being, and resilience in a sample of residents in the metropolitan area of Naples. The questionnaire includes a question on adherence to diet or to a special nutritional regimen; in addition, the participants are asked to mention their height and weight. We investigated the relationship between BMI, adherence to diet, and perceived well-being (PWB) and resilience in a sample of 571 subjects over 60 years of age. Here, we present evidence that engagement into social and cultural activities is associated with higher well-being and resilience, in particular in females over 60 years of age.

1. Introduction

Social isolation and exclusion are associated with poor health status and premature death, while social cohesion, the quality of social relationships and the existence of trust, mutual obligations, and respect in communities, helps to protect people and their health. Since social and family relationships are embedded within the definition of a "good quality of life" for all age groups, and particularly for older adults, it is social isolation inversely correlates with well-being [1–5]. A number of social isolation factors, inadequate transportation system and restrictions in individuals' life–space, have been associated with poor nutrition in older adults. Good nutrition is important for health and well-being at all stages of the life course; however, its determinants change with age. Older adults are particularly prone to slipping into a pattern of an inadequate diet because of decreased mobility associated with physical disabilities and/or fewer financial resources to spend on food [6, 7]. Moreover, past evidence support that socially isolated older adults are at a greater risk of dietary inadequacy because they lack social support, which promotes good diet. In recent years, several studies focused on the relationship between cultural access and physical and psychological health. Their results suggest that participation in social and cultural activities is beneficial for health, since it helps people to remain active and socially connected, avoiding social isolation and loneliness [8, 9]. In elderly people, participation in social and cultural activities correlates with decreased medication consumption and hospitalization. The association between cultural activities and health outcomes has been analyzed in the medical field, in the context of mental health, cognitive decline, onset of dementia, and related disorders [10–16].

Moreover, data are growing in support of the relationship between cultural and social engagement and well-being [17–23]. Well-being is shaped by not only the absence of disease and reduced physical functioning, but also by the presence of positive physical, mental, and psychosocial state. In this view, well-being is crucial to many aspects of our daily lives, since it includes global judgments such as emotions and resilience, quality of relationships, and overall life satisfaction [24–27]. In particular, cultural participation is the second predictor of psychological well-being after (presence/absence of) major diseases, and in this respect, it has a significantly stronger impact than variables such as income, place of residence, age, gender, or occupation. Finally, links have been documented between well-being and multiple aspects of physical health and mortality, cardiovascular disease, biological risk factors for infectious diseases, dementia, and disability in later life [28–31]. Considering the close relationship of high well-being with key health outcomes, tracking and improving well-being is becoming increasingly important for global organizations, governments, companies, and communities worldwide [31, 32].

Therefore, recently a number of studies explored losses in well-being caused by 2008 economic crisis. The findings reveal the negative impact of GDP fall, unemployment rising, and banking crashes on subjective and psychological well-being [33–38]. In addition, several reports provide evidence of an increased prevalence of suicides because of the recent great recession [39–41].

Finally, according to the United Nations Interregional Crime and Justice Research Institute, the global economic crisis has disproportionate effects on women [42].

The average Italian household has been severely affected by the crisis, with impacts that are particularly visible when looking at household income, jobs, life satisfaction, and civic engagement. From 2007 to 2011, Italy recorded a cumulative decline in real household disposable income of around 7%, one of the largest declines among the OECD countries. Market income inequality (before taxes and transfers) increased by 2% between 2007 and 2010, well above the OECD average of 1.2%. The largest impact of the crisis on people's well-being has come through lower employment and deteriorating labour market conditions. Between 2007 and 2012, the employment rate decreased by more than 1 percentage point in Italy, while the long-term unemployment rate increased by almost 3 percentage points. The poor employment situation had a major impact on life satisfaction. From 2007 to 2013, the percentage of Italian people declaring being very satisfied with their lives fell from 58% to 40% [42]. Moreover, according to data from the Italian Institute of Statistics (ISTAT), the crisis have worsened both the north–south and the gender gap in in terms of life satisfaction. The data indicate that in Italy the males are on average more satisfied of their life than females (M 36% > F 34%) and in addition that both males and females living in the north, that is, Lombardy region, are more satisfied of their life than those living in the south, that is, Campania region, (Lombardy: males 42%, females 41%; Campania: males 21,9%, females 19,4%). The 2008 crisis has deeply affected the city of Naples, the capital of the Campania region, and its metropolitan area worsening both the north > south gap and the chronic structural local problems. In that, the report of the Italian Institute of Statistics (ISTAT) shows that in 2014 Naples ranks 101 over the 107 Italian province in terms of quality of life. In addition, ISTAT reports that in 2014 the unemployment rate in Italy was 12,4% and in Naples 24,26% and that in the same year employment rate was slowly growing in Northern (+0,4%) and Central (+1,8%) Italy, while further declining in the South (−0,8%, −45.000 units) [43].

Long-lasting progressive and strong deindustrialization, high level of unemployment, and a large influx of illegal immigrants had explosive consequences on the breakdown of the social fabric that from the specific suburbs spreads like wildfire to the entire city of Naples. At present, local degradation and impoverishment, overlapping with welfare cut, consequent to nation-wide crisis, make day-by-day life difficult, in particular for the more fragile part of the population such as the elderly people living in the metropolitan area of Naples. On the other hand, Naples and its surrounding areas display an extraordinary richness of both tangible and intangible cultural heritage. The value of Naples monuments building, ancient ruins together with its location on the Mediterranean sea, gained the city to be listed by Unesco as a World Heritage Site in 1995 (http://whc.unesco.org/en/list/726/). Moreover, a number of artists, actors, directors, writers, and gallerists, some of them well-recognized world-wide, struggle every day to keep the city long history of creativity alive that represents the worldwide recognized Naples intangible heritage.

In this scenario, we considered the investigation of how citizens of the Metropolitan area of Naples react to adversities and how and if cultural tangible and intangible heritage would influence their subjective well-being valuable. The oldest-old are the fastest-growing sector in society, due to life expectancy increases and improved treatments for life-threatening diseases. Understanding the determinants of psychological well-being and their relationship with health outcomes at older ages is particularly important, since a high proportion of the budget for health and social care is devoted to the care of older people.

Due to the particularly high ageing index (A.I. = 120,3 in 2014) [43] and to the economic difficulties of the Metropolitan area of Naples, it is important to consider new affordable tools and strategies to promote a healthy ageing and to face the "burden" of this demographic change.

On these bases, we decided to take a snapshot of the metropolitan area of the city of Naples investigating the relationship between adherence to diet or nutritional regimen, BMI, and subjective well-being and the impact of social and cultural participation. In particular, we focused on the population over 60 years of age and on gender difference. To our knowledge, this is the first survey investigating subjective well-being in the metropolitan area of the city of Naples.

2. Methods

Within the framework of the A3 Action Group of the European Innovation Partnership on Active and Healthy Ageing and of the "Getting Optimize Aging Life Quality" (GOAL) project, Fondazione GENS Onlus developed an *ad hoc* anonymous questionnaire to assess perceived well-being, resilience, and perceived health and their relation with engagement into social and cultural experiences. The questionnaire comprises the following sections:

(a) Sociodemographic information, age, sex, place of birth, education, employment, and marital status.

(b) Psychological well-being: investigated by means of Psychological General Well-Being-Short (PGWB-S) questionnaire developed and validated in the Italian version by Grossi and coworkers in 2006 [44]. Grossi and coworkers reduced the number of items from the original 22-item PGWBI to 6 items to achieve a higher acceptability of the questionnaire in the population, to shorter time of administration and to obtain a better response rate together with lower rate of missing data. The authors reported that PGWB-S 6 showed that the PGWB-S maintained validity, reliability, and good acceptability for the use in various settings in Italy [44]. PGWB-S 6-item questionnaire analyzes the following domains: Anxiety, Vitality (positive), Depressed Mood, Self-Control, Positive Well-Being, and Vitality (negative) on a 0 to 5 scale referring to the four weeks before the date of the survey [44].

(c) Resilience according to Connor-Davidson resilience scale CD-RISC2 2 items: item 1 ("able to adapt to change") and item 8 ("tend to bounce back after illness or hardship") on a scale from 0 to 4 [45].

(d) Extent of social network.

(e) Participation in cultural and social activities.

(f) Life-style habits, PC use, smoke, diet, physical activity, transportation, number and type of diagnosed diseases, and self-reported perceived health status.

The anonymous questionnaire was submitted to volunteer participants covering wealthy, middle class, and poor neighborhoods of the metropolitan area of Naples. Trained GENS personnel explained the questionnaire and assisted volunteer participants while filling the questionnaire.

2.1. Statistical Analysis. Descriptive statistics were computed for all the indicators analyzed. Student's t-test and ANOVA with Bonferroni correction were performed to test continuous variables. Chi-square was used to test categorical variables. Linear regression analysis was performed to test the relationship between two variables. All statistical analysis were performed using Stata software (Stata Corp., College Station, TX, USA).

3. Results

3.1. Analysis of the Sample Population. Within 2014, we have collected 571 questionnaires of subjects over 60 years of age and this sample population is the object of the present work. Mean age of the 571 subjects over 60 years of age (from now on >60) is 70,05 ± 6,94 years. The >60 sample consists of 285 males and 286 females with a mean age of 70,35 ± 6,923 and 69,78 ± 6,980 years, respectively. The Subjective Well-Being (SWB) was assessed by measuring both psychological well-being and resilience. Self-reported psychological well-being referred to the past 4 weeks according to 6-item PGWB-S analyzing the following domains: Anxiety, Vitality (positive), Depressed Mood, Self-Control, Positivity, and Vitality (negative) on a 0 to 5 scale [45]. In physics, the term "resilience" indicates the power or the ability of a material to return to the original form, position, and so forth, after being bent, compressed, or stretched, and also elasticity. In the health field, resilience applies to the ability to adapt to changes and to readily recover from stressful situation like illness, depression, adversity, or the like. Thus, resilience is a key part of SWB. Resilience was assessed according to Connor-Davidson resilience scale, 2-item CD-RISC2, on a scale of 0 to 4 [45]. According to Chassany et al. and Grossi et al., PGWB scores have been grouped into the following divided categories: 0–60 Severe Distress, 61–71.0 Moderate Distress, 72–92 No Distress, and 93–110 Positive Well-Being [46, 47]. PWB score for all 571 >60 subjects was 68,22 ± 19,71, falling in the area of Moderate Distress. Males and females differently contribute to the PWB score of the whole >60 group, where the PWB score for >60 males is 71,61 ± 18,83 while that for >60 females is 64,92 ± 20,11 ($P < 0,0001$). Our results indicate that the PWB score of >60 males falls borderline between the area of No Distress and Moderate Distress, while that of the >60 female population falls within the area of Moderate Distress. It is interesting to note that PWB score of both >60 males and females, living in metropolitan area of the city of Naples, is largely below that reported for males and females living in Northern and Central Italy and in particularly in the city of Milan [47, 48]. To get a better insight in the PWB score gender difference, we analyzed the six PWB dimensions separately in males and females. The results reported in Table 1 show that females score is lower than that of males in all dimensions but Vitality (positive). On the other hand, resilience score of the whole >60 group was 5,867 ± 1,687, which resulted to be similar in >60 males and females, 5,91 ± 1,57 and 5,84 ± 1,8 respectively. However, when we analyzed resilience item 1 and item 2 separately, it came out that item (1) "able to adapt to change" and item (2) "tend to bounce back after illness or hardship" differently contribute to the cumulative resilience

Table 1: Comparison of the six dimensions of PWB, between females and males. Results are reported as mean ± SD. *P* value has been calculated by Student's *t*-test between each two groups.

PWB dimensions	Females	Males	*P* value
Anxiety	3,34 ± 1,311	3,63 ± 1,19	0,003
Vitality (positive)	3,16 ± 1,229	3,18 ± 1,191	0,835
Depressive mood	3,10 ± 1,237	3,44 ± 1,161	0,0004
Self-control	2,71 ± 1,293	3,14 ± 1,358	<0,0001
Positive WB	2,59 ± 1,139	2,84 ± 1,238	0,008
Vitality (negative)	3,03 ± 1,103	3,21 ± 1,16	0,0423

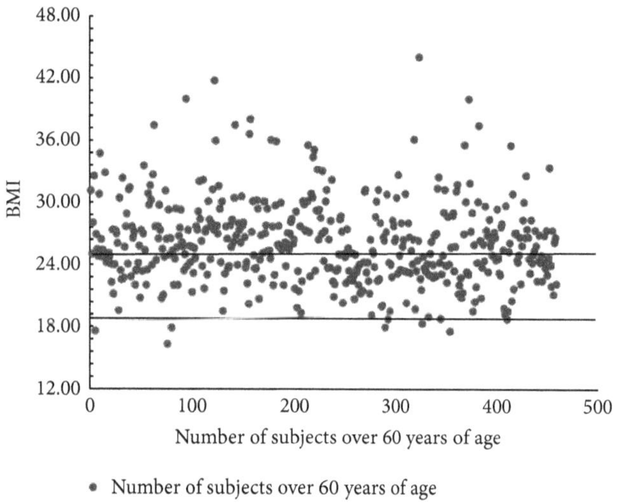

Figure 1: BMI values of all subjects over 60 years of age examined in the study.

score. In particular, both males and females >60 are less "able to adapt to change" (resilience item 1 score, females 2,71 ± 1,08 and males 2,728 ± 1,03) but "tend to bounce back after illness or hardship" more easily (resilience item 2 score, females 3,15 ± 0,9710 and males 3,20 ± 0,87). The difference between item 1 and item 2 score resulted to be statistically significant ($P < 0,0001$) both in >60 males and females. Finally, our data indicate a correlation between resilience and PWB (*R* 0,4708, *R* square 0,2217, *P* value < 0,0001). Same correlation was observed when >60 females and males were analyzed separately (F = *R* 0,418, *R* square 0,1810, *P* value < 0,0001; M = *R* 0,545, *R* square 0,2891, *P* value (two-tailed) < 0,0001).

3.2. Body Mass Index. Within the section related to perceived health status, participants indicated their weight and height. Body mass index (BMI), computed by dividing weight in kilograms by height in meters squared, was categorized according to WHO guidelines, underweight: BMI less than 18.5 kg/m^2; normal weight: BMI 18.5–24.9 kg/m^2 (reference category); overweight: BMI 25–29.9 kg/m^2; obesity: BMI 30–40+ kg/m^2 [49]. All subjects were requested to indicate weight and height. Mean BMI for all subjects resulted to be 25.58 ± 4.20 which falls in the range of overweight, according to the NIH indication [49]. BMI distribution of the all >60 subjects is depicted in Figure 1, and it indicates that 60%

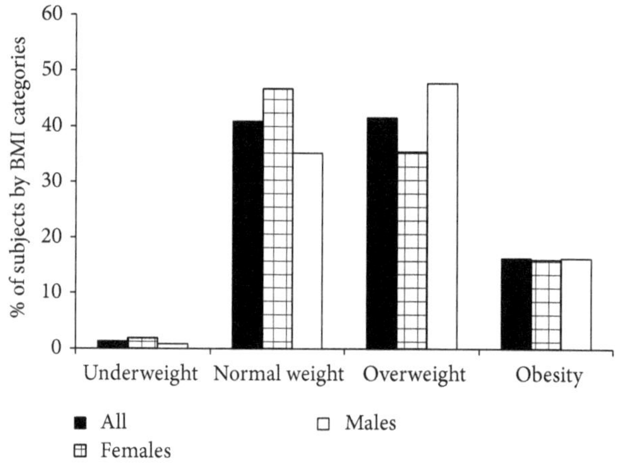

Figure 2: Distribution of >60 all, females, and males by BMI categories. Percentage per each group has been calculated over the total number of >60 years of age in all, females, and males groups separately.

of the >60 subjects fall within the overweight and obesity category, 40% are in the range of normal weight, and only 1% are underweight.

Then we examined all females and males distribution BMI classes and the results indicated that 51% of the >60 female subjects and 64% of the >60 male subjects fall in the range of overweight and obesity (Figure 2) while 47% of female and 35% of male subjects were in the range of normal weight. Since the relation between obesity and psychological and subjective well-being is becoming a hot issue, in both the health and the economic field, we compared the BMI, well-being, and resilience in the obese group versus the normal weight one. As it is shown in Table 2(a), in all the >60 subjects, there was no significant difference in PWB and resilience score according to BMI categories. On the other hand, when we analyzed women and men separately, we found that both PWB and resilience decrease in >60 obese females with respect to normal weight group, while BMI increases (Table 2(b)). Also, in >60 males, PWB and resilience score are almost superimposable in both the normal weight and the obesity group (Table 2(c)), while BMI increases. In addition, the opposite trend of PWB and resilience score between obese males and females amplifies the gender difference that remained significant ($P < 0,05$).

Moreover, correlation analysis between BMI and PWB and resilience indicates no correlation in all the population (BMI > PWB = *R* 0,049, *R* square 0,002, *P* value = 0,299; BMI > resilience = *R* 0,056, *R* square 0,003, *P* value 0,231) and in the male population (BMI > PWB *R* 0,085, *R* square 0,007, *P* value = 0,191; BMI > resilience = *R* 0,114, *R* square, 0,013, *P* value 0,081). On the contrary, in the female population a significant correlation was found both between BMI and PWB and between BMI and resilience (BMI > PWB = *R* 0,171, *R* square 0,029, *P* value 0,012; BMI > resilience = *R* 0,173, *R* square 0,029, *P* value 0,011).

Subjects indicate eventual diagnosed disease/s within the following list of diseases: diabetes, respiratory diseases, skin diseases, gastritis, anemia, depression, osteoporosis,

TABLE 2: *Panel a*: comparison of PWB and resilience scores between normal weight and obese all > 60 subjects. Results are reported as mean ± SD. *P* value has been calculated by Student's *t*-test between each two groups. *Panel b*: comparison of PWB and resilience scores between normal weight and obese > 60 Females results are reported as mean ± SD. *P* value has been calculated by Student's *t*-test between each two groups. *Panel c*: comparison of PWB and resilience scores between normal weight and obese > 60 males. Results are reported as mean ± SD. *P* value has been calculated by Student's *t*-test between each two groups.

	BMI categories	All > 60					
		BMI	*P* value	Resilience	*P* value	PWB	*P* value
a	Normal weight	22,57 ± 1,77	<0,0001	6,09 ± 1,52	NS	70,11 ± 18,48	NS
	Obesity	32,79 ± 3,06		5,85 ± 1,89		66,99 ± 23,44	
	BMI categories	Females > 60					
		BMI	*P* value	Resilience	*P* value	PWB	*P* value
b	Normal weight	22,33 ± 1,7	<0,0001	6,25 ± 1,45	<0,05	69,63 ± 16,95	0,0093
	Obesity	33,72 ± 3,4		5,36 ± 2,19		55,61 ± 22,18	
	BMI categories	Males > 60					
		BMI	*P* value	Resilience	*P* value	PWB	*P* value
c	Normal weight	23,22 ± 1,23	<0,0001	5,98 ± 1,54	NS	72,15 ± 18,89	NS
	Obesity	31,75 ± 1,76		6,17 ± 1,55		72,86 ± 21,78	

TABLE 3: The table depicts the number of >60 male and female subjects distributed according to self-reported diagnosed diseases.

BMI distribution	Females > 60					Males > 60				
	Diabetes	Hypertension	Obesity	CVD	Depression	Diabetes	Hypertension	Obesity	CVD	Depression
Normal weight	9	32	1	23	5	17	28	1	45	7
Overweight	12	31	2	16	9	21	38	2	56	7
Obesity	6	16	16	14	8	10	19	16	20	3

kidney diseases, migraine, anxiety, heart failure, arrhythmias, ischemic heart diseases, cancer, allergy, arthrosis, myocardial infarction, hypertension, obesity, liver disease, back pain, and colitis. The frequency of diabetes, hypertension, obesity, cardiovascular diseases (CVD), comprising heart failure, arrhythmias, ischemic heart disease, and myocardial infarction and depression, categorized according to BMI classes, is shown in Table 3. Hypertension resulted to be the most reported diagnosed disease within normal weight, overweight, and obesity classes in >60 females, while CVD was the most frequently reported by the >60 male group.

3.3. BMI, Resilience, and PWB in >60 Females and Males Participating and Nonparticipating in Cultural and Social Activities. Among the 571 >60 subjects, 78,45% are engaged into cultural and social activities, while 21,54% are not. Within the P population 52% are women and 48% are men, while in the NP population 57% are women and 43% are men. Interestingly, when we compared BMI of subjects participating (P) and nonparticipating (NP) to cultural and social activities, we observed that BMI was higher in females NP versus females P (<0,05) (Table 4(b)). On the other hand, no difference in BMI is observed between >60 males P and NP. More importantly, the >60 NP population displays PWB and resilience score significantly lower the >60 P. In particular, the >60 P male population frankly falls into the area of positive well-being, while that of NP goes in the area of moderate distress (Table 4). As for women, the PWB of the NP population dramatically crashes in the area of severe distress. These observations show an association between participation in cultural and social activities and subjective well-being, by means of PWB and resilience score. In addition, in the case of the female group, and in particular the NP females, we observed an inverse relation between BMI and PWB and resilience, since BMI increases while PWB and resilience decrease. The last observation suggests an intriguing and apparently new association between BMI, subjective well-being indicators, and participation in cultural and social activities.

3.4. Adherence to a Diet or a Nutritional Regimen. We then analyzed answers of >60 subjects to the question: Do you follow a diet or a nutritional regimen? The results indicate that 35% of males > 60 and 43% of females > 60 follow a diet or a nutritional regimen. Thereafter, we investigated the relation between perceived well-being and resilience and adherence to diet or nutritional regimen. Interestingly, women P adhering to diet display significantly higher PWB ($P = 0,013$) and resilience ($P = 0,043$) than the NP following diet (Table 5). In addition, a significant difference was observed in PWB and resilience between >60 female P and NP ($P < 0,0001$) nondieting. On the other hand, while PWB was higher in the >60 males of the P group with respect to the NP following a diet, resilience was similar in the two groups (Table 5). In addition, differently from females, NP males who do not follow a diet or nutritional regimen apparently are overall "happier" then NP following a diet. We then analyzed obese females and males dieting and nondieting. The results show

Table 4: *Panel a*: comparison of BMI, PWB, and resilience between >60 P and NP. Results are reported as mean ± SD. *P* value has been calculated by Student's t-test between each two groups. *Panel b*: comparison of BMI, PWB, and resilience between >60 P and NP Females. Results are reported as mean ± SD. *P* value has been calculated by Student's t-test between each two groups. *Panel c*: comparison of BMI, PWB, and resilience between >60 P and NP males. Results are reported as mean ± SD. *P* value has been calculated by Student's t-test between each two groups.

	>60 all	BMI	*P* value	Resilience	*P* value	PWB	*P* value
a	P	25,8 ± 3,932	0,004	6,07 ± 1,581	<0,0001	70,53 ± 17,98	<0,0001
	NP	27,1 ± 4,21		5,14 ± 1,83		58,95 ± 23,2	
	>60 males	BMI	*P* value	Resilience	*P* value	PWB	*P* value
b	P	26,18 ± 3,31	NS	6,02 ± 1,53	0,009	73,05 ± 16,93	0,015
	NP	26,6 ± 3,30		5,41 ± 1,64		65,38 ± 18,67	
	>60 females	BMI	*P* value	Resilience	*P* value	PWB	*P* value
c	P	25,25 ± 4,36	0,008	6,11 ± 1,53	<0,0001	68,16 ± 18,67	<0,0001
	NP	27,42 ± 5,25		4,75 ± 2,02		50,31 ± 20,48	

Table 5: *Panel a*: BMI, PWB, and resilience in >60 subjects following or nonfollowing a diet in relation to participation to cultural and social activities. Results are reported as mean ± SD. *P* value has been calculated by Student's t-test between each two groups. *Panel b*: BMI, PWB, and resilience in females >60 following or nonfollowing a diet in relation to participation in cultural and social activities. Results are reported as mean ± SD. *P* value has been calculated by Student's t-test between each two groups. *Panel c*: BMI, PWB, and resilience in males >60 following or nonfollowing a diet in relation to participation in cultural and social activities. Results are reported as mean ± SD. *P* value has been calculated by Student's t-test between each two groups.

		All > 60							
		Yes diet				No diet			
		PWB	*P* value	Resilience	*P* value	PWB	*P* value	Resilience	*P* value
a	P	70,79 ± 18,56	0,001	6,10 ± 1,58	0,02	70,08 ± 17,92	0,002	6,04 ± 1,58	<0,001
	NP	57,73 ± 22,47		5,43 ± 1,66		59,78 ± 23,69		5,05 ± 1,92	
		Males > 60							
		Yes diet				No diet			
		PWB	*P* value	Resilience	*P* value	PWB	*P* value	Resilience	*P* value
b	P	73,33 ± 18,59	0,028	6,15 ± 1,57	0,192	72,68 ± 16,34	NS	5,94 ± 1,54	NS
	NP	57,59 ± 26,01		5,59 ± 1,66		71,94 ± 19,83		5,65 ± 1,53	
		Females > 60							
		Yes diet				No diet			
		PWB	*P* value	Resilience	*P* value	PWB	*P* value	Resilience	*P* value
c	P	68,35 ± 18,22	0,013	6,05 ± 1,60	0,043	67,60 ± 19,05	<0,001	6,13 ± 1,63	<0,001
	NP	57,09 ± 20,14		5,24 ± 1,70		43,73 ± 19,27		4,22 ± 2,17	

that obese females dieting present both PWB and resilience scores higher than the nondieting obese females (PWB 61,69 ± 17,26 > 54,72 ± 16,69, $P < 0,009$; resilience 6 ± 1,57 > 5,429 ± 1,4, $P < 0,003$). Conversely, obese males dieting show both PWB and resilience scores lower than the nondieting obese males (PWB 67,35 ± 16,43 > 81,53 ± 17,18, $P < 0,05$; resilience 5,842 ± 1,46 > 6,706 ± 1,44, $P < 0,05$).

4. Discussion

To our knowledge, this is the first assessment of PWB and resilience conducted in the Metropolitan area of Naples. Our data show that a sample of 571 subjects over 60 years of age resident in the Metropolitan area of Naples display a PWB score of 68,22 ± 19,71 on a scale of 0 > 110, largely below PWB scores previously reported for the Italian population. In particular, Grossi et al. [47–50] reported a PWB score of 77.76 (17.73 SD) for the Italian population (1500 subjects) in 2011. The PWB score was geographically distributed as follows: north (696 subjects) 79.34 (17.71 SD), centre (293 subjects) 78.04 (17.12 SD), south (511 subjects) 75.47 (17.91 SD). Moreover, in 2013 the same authors reported that a sample of 1000 citizens of Milan displayed a PWB score of 82, 14 (15.63 SD) while that of the population over 60 years was 80,39.

The questionnaires analyzed here have been collected within 2014 when, as reported above [43], the Metropolitan area of Naples was still suffering for the economic crisis. Our results are in agreement with those reporting a relationship between unemployment and low level of PWB. Thus, we cannot exclude that the low PGWB score of this sample population of residents in the Metropolitan area of Naples reflects the detrimental effects of the economic and social crisis at local level. In particular, of note 50% of the 571 subjects over 60 years of age are retired, and retirement benefits represent for most families in the area, in a time of high unemployment, the only income to count on.

When PWB score was measured in >60 males and females separately, a gender difference was observed. It is generally reported that women have a score higher than men do in happiness, when happiness is measured as life satisfaction. It is also reported that the advantage of women in terms of happiness and life satisfaction is not uniform along the life cycle: women are less happy than men before the age of 18, happier than men until their fifties, and less happy again thereafter [51]. Moreover, the "paradox of declining female happiness" seems to indicate that the traditional gender gap in happiness (in favour of women) is progressively shrinking since the 1970s in spite of the type of technological progress, civil liberties, and gender-conscious policies that characterize modern Western societies [52].

On the other hand, it is well recognized that women score lower than men do, on measures that capture short-term positive and negative emotions and are more subject to depression symptoms [51].

The gender difference observed in PWB score in the sample of women >60 analyzed here is in line with results already reported by Grossi et al., using the same PGWB questionnaires we have used. Grossi and coworkers reported gender difference PWB scores in 2011 for the Italian population (PWB score females 74.82 and males 81) and in 2013 for citizens of Milan (PWB score females 78.32 and males 83) [47, 48]. We have reported that in a sample population of people nonparticipating in social and cultural activities, women PWB and resilience scores are lower than that of nonparticipating men [50] Moreover, in 2003, Ruini et al. reported a gender difference in favour of men by assessing well-being by means of different questionnaire [53]. Psychological well-being gender gap in favour of men was also reported by Pinquart and Sörensen in elderly [54] and by Hori and Kamo in their comparison of 33 countries [55] The latter authors as well as Ruini et al. suggest that different socialization and expectations by gender and different role of men and women in society explain gender gap in psychological well-being.

Biological factors such as hormones, neurotransmitter, and cytokines have been associated to well-being, differently in men and women [56–61]. Taking into account that, in the present work, we examined a female population with mean age 69,78 ± 6,980 living in the Metropolitan area of city of Naples, located in the South of Italy, we cannot exclude that the PWB gender gap mainly reflects women's "traditional" social role in this area.

According to Havighurst "activity theory," higher levels of participation in social and leisure activities, and role replacement when roles must be relinquished, promote well-being in older adults [62]. Thus, to achieve a healthy aging it is crucial to have equal opportunities for health, follow healthy diets, maintain social relations, participate in meaningful activities, and enjoy financial security. Participation in social and leisure activities means being willing to reach people, to stay connected, to keep learning, and to be curios, in one word to stay alive [17–23]. Social participation is closely linked to self-esteem, life satisfaction, and mental health status, which makes it a very important factor for quality of life. Engagement with community activities, friendships, and meaningful volunteer work are perceived as strategies for maintaining social participation, especially for people with a chronic disease [9]. Thus, encouraging participation in social and cultural activities could be a key tool to fight social isolation and its health detrimental outcomes.

Our results are in line with data in the literature showing positive association between engaging in leisure and well-being [17–23, 47–63]. In addition, some intervention studies seem to strengthen this observation. In particular, through interventions focused on the development of positive emotions, it is possible to improve well-being and reduce disability in the general population, and in most, if not all, mental disorders. These data indicate that well-being can be modified and that leisure and social activities may be affordable tools to improve well-being [64–72]. Moreover, data coming from research on "happiness genes," suggesting a genetic root of happiness/well-being, do not rule out gene-environment interaction on the expression "happiness genes." Availability and access to cultural and social activities are a key element of healthy environment and especially of urban environment [73–75].

Social isolation has been associated with malnutrition in older adults. Since eating is a social event, social isolation can have a negative effect on nutrition, and thus we speculated that social and cultural participation might influence adherence to diet [76–78]. Adequate nutrition is a key factor to healthy aging and to preventing disease onset; nevertheless eating appropriately and, even more, following a diet or a nutritional regimen are never an easy task. Motivations are important factors to eat healthy or to stay on a diet, and they change with age. In >60 subjects, dieting, by-and-large required by health problem, is perceived as a punishment. Social and cultural participation, fighting social isolation, may help >60 to follow healthier life styles, among which is healthy eating, or to accept more "easily" to face stressful situation, like being forced to diet. The results presented here suggest that >60 subjects, in particular females, participating in cultural and social activities, apparently "accept" diet or nutritional regimen better then NP subjects as it is shown by an overall higher score in both PWB and resilience. The higher PWB score observed in P females >60 following a diet deserves, in our view, a special consideration. Pampel in 2012 reported a more consistent association between cultural activities and low body weight in the Western country than elsewhere and that the relationship emerges more consistently for women than men [79].

Subjective well-being significantly correlates with high self-esteem, and self-esteem shares significant variance in both mental well-being and happiness. Self-esteem has been found to be the most dominant and powerful predictor of happiness. Quoting Mann, "Indeed, while low self-esteem leads to maladjustment, positive self-esteem, internal standards and aspirations actively seem to contribute to 'well-being'" [80]. Body image bears relationship to self-esteem and psychosocial adjustment (e.g., eating disturbances, depression, social anxiety, and sexual functioning) [81]. The association between body image and women's mental and physical health has been investigated with mainly focusing on young women's appearance concerns. However, in the "aging society" body concerns are becoming an issue also for older women, because of age-related changes in both appearance and functioning. In particular, aesthetic appearance is becoming relevant to older women and may lead some women to feel that their bodies are inadequate or lacking. Because of the association between beauty and youth, women lose their social value simply by growing old [82, 83]. The ideal of a thinner body image persists in older adult females, as also suggested by the observation that higher BMI predicts lower psychological well-being only among women. Moreover, body-image concerns are significant to self-esteem in older adulthood [84–86].

Conversely, improvements in body image are related to improvements in self-esteem and psychological well-being [87, 88]. On this basis, we cannot rule out that an "esthetic element" may play a role in the higher score in PWB and resilience reported by this sample of over 60 women participating in cultural and social activities and dieting, independently and far beyond health consciousness.

5. Conclusion

The aim of the study presented here was to assess subjective well-being in a sample of residents of the Metropolitan area of Naples, when the city is going through a very difficult time of its long history. To our knowledge, this is the first survey on this topic, and our data represent a suggestive baseline.

The present study has been designed to explore the possible association between cultural and social participation and well-being, which our results apparently support. Much larger and more in-depth studies than ours failed to find a causal link between cultural and social participation and well-being and health [29–89]. However, the association is well-documented and apparently is so appealing that several governments include engagement in cultural and social activities among their strategies to improve well-being and health [90–92]. Since welfare costs are one of the major sources of public finance deficits in the EU, investing in "cultural welfare," an affordable health preventive and promoting strategy for healthy living and aging, could result in a substantial saving of public resources [93].

Competing Interests

The authors declare that there are no competing interests.

Acknowledgments

The authors would like to thank Professors Giovanni Esposito, Vincenzo Canonico, and Patrizia Morrica, Drs. Aurelio Catalano and Maria Corbi, and Mrs. Fulvia Frallicciardi and Mrs. Rosa Anna Pironti for their invaluable help and support. This work was partially supported by Reference Sites Network for Prevention and Care of Frailty and Chronic Conditions in community dwelling persons of EU Countries, SUNFRAIL, Call for Proposal H2020-HP-PJ-2014, Project no. 664291.

References

[1] S. Cacioppo, A. J. Grippo, S. London, L. Goossens, and J. T. Cacioppo, "Loneliness: clinical Import and Interventions," *Perspectives on Psychological Science*, vol. 10, no. 2, pp. 238–249, 2015.

[2] J. T. Cacioppo and S. Cacioppo, "Social relationships and health: the toxic effects of perceived social isolation," *Social and Personality Psychology Compass*, vol. 8, no. 2, pp. 58–72, 2014.

[3] A. Steptoe, A. Shankar, P. Demakakos, and J. Wardle, "Social isolation, loneliness, and all-cause mortality in older men and women," *Proceedings of the National Academy of Sciences of the United States of America*, vol. 110, no. 15, pp. 5797–5801, 2013.

[4] J. Holt-Lunstad, T. B. Smith, M. Baker, T. Harris, and D. Stephenson, "Loneliness and social isolation as risk factors for mortality: a meta-analytic review," *Perspectives on Psychological Science*, vol. 10, no. 2, pp. 227–237, 2015.

[5] J. H. Fowler and N. A. Christakis, "Dynamic spread of happiness in a large social network: longitudinal analysis over 20 years in the Framingham Heart Study," *The British Medical Journal*, vol. 2008, article 337, 2008.

[6] S. Brownie, "Why are elderly individuals at risk of nutritional deficiency?" *International Journal of Nursing Practice*, vol. 12, no. 2, pp. 110–118, 2006.

[7] M. Dean, M. M. Raats, K. G. Grunert, and M. Lumbers, "Factors influencing eating a varied diet in old age," *Public Health Nutrition*, vol. 12, no. 12, pp. 2421–2427, 2009.

[8] T. J. VanderWeele, L. C. Hawkley, and J. T. Cacioppo, "On the reciprocal association between loneliness and subjective well-being," *American Journal of Epidemiology*, vol. 176, no. 9, pp. 777–784, 2012.

[9] V. Toepoel, "Ageing, leisure, and social connectedness: how could leisure help reduce social isolation of older people?" *Social Indicators Research*, vol. 113, no. 1, pp. 355–372, 2013.

[10] H. X. Wang, W. Xu, and J. J. Pei, "Leisure activities, cognition and dementia," *Biochimica et Biophysica Acta*, vol. 1822, no. 3, pp. 482–491, 2012.

[11] F. Takeda, H. Noguchi, T. Monma, N. Tamiya, and T. Ojima, "How possibly do leisure and social activities impact mental health of middle-aged adults in japan?: an evidence from a national longitudinal survey," *PLoS ONE*, vol. 10, no. 10, Article ID e0139777, 2015.

[12] C. Chiao, L.-J. Weng, and A. L. Botticello, "Social participation reduces depressive symptoms among older adults: an 18-year longitudinal analysis in Taiwan," *BMC Public Health*, vol. 11, article 292, 2011.

[13] Y. Iwasaki, C. P. Coyle, and J. W. Shank, "Leisure as a context for active living, recovery, health and life quality for persons with mental illness in a global context," *Health Promotion International*, vol. 25, no. 4, pp. 483–494, 2010.

[14] N. Agahi, "Leisure in late life: pattern of participation and relationship to health," in *Neurobiology, Care Sciences and Society*, Karolinska Institutet, Stockholm, Sweden, 2008.

[15] I. Nilsson, F. Nyqvist, Y. Gustafson, and M. Nygard, "Leisure engagement: medical conditions, mobility difficulties, and activity limitations—a later life perspective," *Journal of Aging Research*, vol. 2015, Article ID 610154, 8 pages, 2015.

[16] C. Opdebeeck, C. Quinn, S. M. Nelis, and L. Clare, "Is cognitive lifestyle associated with depressive thoughts and self-reported depressive symptoms in later life?" *European Journal of Ageing*, vol. 13, no. 1, pp. 63–73, 2016.

[17] E. Grossi, P. L. Sacco, G. T. Blessi, and R. Cerutti, "The impact of culture on the individual subjective well-being of the Italian population: an exploratory study," *Applied Research in Quality of Life*, vol. 6, no. 4, pp. 387–410, 2011.

[18] W. R. Holmes and J. Joseph, "Social participation and healthy ageing: a neglected, significant protective factor for chronic non communicable conditions," *Globalization and Health*, vol. 7, article 43, 2011.

[19] P.-J. Chang, L. Wray, and Y. Lin, "Social relationships, leisure activity, and health in older adults," *Health Psychology*, vol. 33, no. 6, pp. 516–523, 2014.

[20] C. F. Mendes de, T. A. Leon, and L. F. Berkman, "Social engagement as a longitudinal predictor of objective and subjective health," *European Journal of Ageing*, vol. 2, no. 1, pp. 48–55, 2005.

[21] K. M. Bennett, "Social engagement as a longitudinal predictor of objective and subjective health," *European Journal of Ageing*, vol. 2, no. 1, pp. 48–55, 2005.

[22] L. Kuykendall, L. Tay, and V. Ng, "Leisure engagement and subjective well-being: a meta-analysis," *Psychological Bulletin*, vol. 141, no. 2, pp. 364–403, 2015.

[23] V. Ateca-Amestoy, M. Gerstenblüth, I. Mussio, and M. Rossi, "How do cultural activities influence happiness? The relation between self-reported well-being and leisure," (working papers) 0614, Department of Economics—dECON, 2014, http://cienciassociales.edu.uy/departamentodeeconomia/wp-content/uploads/sites/2/2014/11/0614.pdf.

[24] G. V. Ostir, K. S. Markides, S. A. Black, and J. S. Goodwin, "Emotional well-being predicts subsequent functional independence and survival," *Journal of the American Geriatrics Society*, vol. 48, no. 5, pp. 473–478, 2000.

[25] G. V. Ostir, K. S. Markides, M. K. Peek, and J. S. Goodwin, "The association between emotional well-being and the incidence of stroke in older adults," *Psychosomatic Medicine*, vol. 63, no. 2, pp. 210–215, 2001.

[26] E. Diener, "Subjective well-being: the science of happiness and a proposal for a national index," *American Psychologist*, vol. 55, no. 1, pp. 34–43, 2000.

[27] D. Kahneman and J. Riis, "Living and thinking about it: two perspectives on life," in *The Science of Well-Being*, F. A. Huppert, N. Baylis, and B. Keverne, Eds., pp. 285–304, Oxford University Press, New York, NY, USA, 2006.

[28] C. D. Ryff, B. T. Radler, and E. M. Friedman, "Persistent psychological well-being predicts improved self-rated health over 9-10 years: longitudinal evidence from MIDUS," *Health Psychology Open*, vol. 2, no. 2, 2015.

[29] A. Steptoe, A. Deaton, and A. A. Stone, "Subjective wellbeing, health, and ageing," *The Lancet*, vol. 385, no. 9968, pp. 640–648, 2015.

[30] L. E. Sears, S. Agrawal, J. A. Sidney et al., "The well-being 5: development and validation of a diagnostic instrument to improve population well-being," *Population Health Management*, vol. 17, no. 6, pp. 357–365, 2014.

[31] F. A. Huppert and T. T. C. So, "Flourishing across Europe: application of a new conceptual framework for defining well-being," *Social Indicators Research*, vol. 110, no. 3, pp. 837–861, 2013.

[32] J. Burton, "WHO healthy workplace framework and model: background and supporting literature and practices," http://www.who.int/occupational_health/healthy_workplace_framework.pdf.

[33] A. Deaton, "The financial crisis and the well-being of Americans," *Oxford Economic Papers*, vol. 64, pp. 1–26, 2014.

[34] A. Montagnoli and M. Moro, *Everybody Hurts: Banking Crises and Individual Wellbeing*, Sheffield economic Research Paper Series no. 2014010, 2014.

[35] N. Drydakis, "The effect of unemployment on self-reported health and mental health in Greece from 2008 to 2013: a longitudinal study before and during the financial crisis," IZA Discussion Paper 8742, 2014, http://ftp.iza.org/dp8742.pdf.

[36] E. Flint, M. Bartley, N. Shelton, and A. Sacker, "Do labour market status transitions predict changes in psychological well-being?" *Journal of Epidemiology and Community Health*, vol. 67, no. 9, pp. 796–802, 2013.

[37] G. Van Hal, "The true cost of the economic crisis on psychological well-being: a review," *Psychology Research and Behavior Management*, vol. 8, pp. 17–25, 2015.

[38] WHO Regional Office for Europe report Impact of economic crisis on mental health, http://www.euro.who.int/__data/assets/pdf.../e94837.pdf.

[39] R. De Vogli, M. Marmot, and D. Stuckler, "Strong evidence that the economic crisis caused a rise in suicides in Europe: the need for social protection," *Journal of Epidemiology and Community Health*, vol. 67, no. 4, pp. 298–307, 2013.

[40] R. De Vogli, M. Marmot, and D. Stuckler, "Excess suicides and attempted suicides in Italy attributable to the great recession," *Journal of Epidemiology and Community Health*, vol. 67, no. 4, pp. 378–379, 2013.

[41] "The Impacts of the Crisis on Gender Equality and Women's Wellbeing in European Union (EU) Mediterranean Countries," 2014, http://www.unicri.it/news/files/VAW_draft_last_lowq.pdf.

[42] http://www.oecd.org/statistics/BLI%202014%20Italy%20country%20report.pdf.

[43] ISTAT, http://www.istat.it.

[44] E. Grossi, N. Groth, P. Mosconi et al., "Development and validation of the short version of the Psychological General Well-Being Index (PGWB-S)," *Health and Quality of Life Outcomes*, vol. 4, article 88, 2006.

[45] S. Vaishnavi, K. Connor, and J. R. T. Davidson, "An abbreviated version of the Connor-Davidson Resilience Scale (CD-RISC), the CD-RISC2: psychometric properties and applications in psychopharmacological trials," *Psychiatry Research*, vol. 152, no. 2-3, pp. 293–297, 2007.

[46] A. Chassany, E. Dimenäs, D. Dubois et al., *The Psychological General Well-Being Index (PGWBI) Manual User*, MAPI Research Institute, Lyon, France, 2004.

[47] E. Grossi, G. T. Blessi, P. L. Sacco, and M. Buscema, "The interaction between culture, health and psychological well-being: data mining from the Italian culture and well-being project," *Journal of Happiness Studies*, vol. 13, no. 1, pp. 129–148, 2012.

[48] E. Grossi, A. Compare, C. Lonardi, R. Cerutti, E. Callus, and M. Niero, "Gender-related effect of cultural participation in psychological well-being: Indications from the well-being project in the municipality of Milan," *Social Indicators Research*, vol. 114, no. 2, pp. 255–271, 2013.

[49] BMI WHO, "World Health Organization (WHO) expert committee on physical status. The use and interpretation of anthropometry," in *Report of a World Health Organization Expert Committee*, Series 854, WHO Technical Support, Geneva, Switzerland, 1995.

[50] M. Quarto, A. Kisslinger, and D. Tramontano, "The sick city sickens," in *Urbanistica Informazioni*, M. Sepe, Ed., Happiness and Public Space, pp. 111–115, 2015.

[51] C. Senik, "Gender Gaps in Subjective Wellbeing European Commission—Directorate-General for Justice," European Union, 2015, http://ec.europa.eu/justice/gender-equality/files/equal_economic_independence/160129_happiness_report_en.pdf.

[52] B. Stevenson and J. Wolfers, "The paradox of declining female happiness," IZA Discussion Paper 4200, 2009, http://ftp.iza.org/dp4200.pdf.

[53] C. Ruini, F. Ottolini, C. Rafanelli, E. Tossani, C. D. Ryff, and G. A. Fava, "The relationship of psychological well-being to distress and personality," *Psychotherapy and Psychosomatics*, vol. 72, no. 5, pp. 268–275, 2003.

[54] M. Pinquart and S. Sörensen, "Gender differences in self-concept and psychological well-being in old age: a meta-analysis," *Journals of Gerontology B: Psychological Sciences and Social Sciences*, vol. 56, no. 4, pp. P195–P213, 2001.

[55] M. Hori and Y. Kamo, "A multi-level analysis of psychological well-being related to work and family in 33 countries," in *Family and Health: Evolving Needs, Responsibilities, and Experiences*, vol. 8 of *Contemporary Perspectives in Family Research*, pp. 1–25, Emerald Group Publishing Limited, 2014.

[56] A. Steptoe, P. Demakakos, C. de Oliveira, and J. Wardle, "Distinctive biological correlates of positive psychological well-being in older men and women," *Psychosomatic Medicine*, vol. 74, no. 5, pp. 501–508, 2012.

[57] A. Steptoe, J. Wardle, and M. Marmot, "Positive affect and health-related neuroendocrine, cardiovascular, and inflammatory processes," *Proceedings of the National Academy of Sciences of the United States of America*, vol. 102, no. 18, pp. 6508-6512, 2005.

[58] A. Steptoe, K. O'Donnell, E. Badrick, M. Kumari, and M. Marmot, "Neuroendocrine and inflammatory factors associated with positive affect in healthy men and women: the Whitehall II study," *American Journal of Epidemiology*, vol. 167, no. 1, pp. 96–102, 2008.

[59] B. E. Kok, K. A. Coffey, M. A. Cohn et al., "How positive emotions build physical health: perceived positive social connections account for the upward spiral between positive emotions and vagal tone," *Psychological Science*, vol. 24, no. 7, pp. 1123–1132, 2013.

[60] E. M. Friedman, M. Hayney, G. D. Love, B. H. Singer, and C. D. Ryff, "Plasma interleukin-6 and soluble IL-6 receptors are associated with psychological well-being in aging women," *Health Psychology*, vol. 26, no. 3, pp. 305–313, 2007.

[61] C. D. Ryff, G. Dienberg Love, H. L. Urry et al., "Psychological well-being and ill-being: do they have distinct or mirrored biological correlates?" *Psychotherapy and Psychosomatics*, vol. 75, no. 2, pp. 85–95, 2006.

[62] R. Havighurst, "Successful aging," in *Processes of Aging*, R. Williams, C. Tibbits, and W. Donahue, Eds., vol. 1, Atherton Press, New York, NY, USA, 1963.

[63] G. Fernández-Mayoralas, F. Rojo-Pérez, P. Martínez-Martín et al., "Active ageing and quality of life: factors associated with participation in leisure activities among institutionalized older adults, with and without dementia," *Aging & Mental Health*, vol. 19, no. 11, pp. 1031–1041, 2015.

[64] M. J. Zawadzki, J. M. Smyth, and H. J. Costigan, "Real-time associations between engaging in leisure and daily health and well-being," *Annals of Behavioral Medicine*, vol. 49, no. 4, pp. 605–615, 2015.

[65] L. Becchetti, E. Giachin Ricca, and A. Pelloni, "The relationship bethween social leisure and life satisfaction: causality and policy implications," *Social Indicators Research*, vol. 108, no. 3, pp. 453–490, 2015.

[66] E. M. Friedman, C. Ruini, R. Foy, L. Jaros, H. Sampson, and C. D. Ryff, "Lighten UP! A community-based group intervention to promote psychological well-being in older adults," *Aging and Mental Health*, vol. 13, pp. 1–7, 2015.

[67] M. Levasseur, H. Lefebvre, M. Levert et al., "Personalized citizen assistance for social participation (APIC): a promising intervention for increasing mobility, accomplishment of social activities and frequency of leisure activities in older adults having disabilities," *Archives of Gerontology and Geriatrics*, vol. 64, pp. 96–102, 2016.

[68] C. R. Cloninger, "The science of wellbeing: an integrated approach to mental health and its disorders," *Psychiatria Danubina*, vol. 18, no. 3-4, pp. 218–224, 2006.

[69] L. Bolier, M. Haverman, G. J. Westerhof, H. Riper, F. Smit, and E. Bohlmeijer, "Positive psychology interventions: a meta-analysis of randomized controlled studies," *BMC Public Health*, vol. 13, article 119, 2013.

[70] S. Ballesteros, E. Kraft, S. Santana, and C. Tziraki, "Maintaining older brain functionality: a targeted review," *Neuroscience and Biobehavioral Reviews*, vol. 55, pp. 453–477, 2015.

[71] M. E. Paggi, D. Jopp, and C. Hertzog, "The importance of leisure activities in the relationship between physical health and well-being in a life span sample," *Gerontology*, 2016.

[72] L. Tay and L. Kuykendall, "Promoting happiness: the malleability of individual and societal subjective wellbeing," *International Journal of Psychology*, vol. 48, no. 3, pp. 159–176, 2013.

[73] J. E. De Neve, N. A. Christakis, J. H. Fowler, and B. S. Frey, "Genes, economics, and happiness," *Journal of Neuroscience, Psychology, and Economics*, vol. 5, no. 4, 2012.

[74] M. Bartels, "Genetics of wellbeing and its components satisfaction with life, happiness, and quality of life: a review and meta-analysis of heritability studies," *Calcified Tissue International*, vol. 96, no. 3, pp. 137–156, 2015.

[75] A. Okbay, B. M. Baselmans, J. E. De Neve et al., "Genetic variants associated with subjective well-being, depressive symptoms, and neuroticism identified through genome-wide analyses," *Nature Genetics*, 2016.

[76] V. H. Taylor, M. Forhan, S. N. Vigod, R. S. McIntyre, and K. M. Morrison, "The impact of obesity on quality of life," *Best Practice and Research: Clinical Endocrinology and Metabolism*, vol. 27, no. 2, pp. 139–146, 2013.

[77] M. L. Yan, K. Daviglus, K. Liu et al., "BMI and health-related quality of life in adults 65 years and older," *Obesity Research*, vol. 12, no. 1, pp. 69–76, 2004.

[78] H. A. Doll, S. E. K. Petersen, and S. L. Stewart-Brown, "Obesity and physical and emotional well-being: associations between body mass index, chronic illness, and the physical and mental components of the SF-36 questionnaire," *Obesity Research*, vol. 8, no. 2, pp. 160–170, 2000.

[79] F. C. Pampel, "Does reading keep you thin? Leisure activities, cultural tastes, and body weight in comparative perspective," *Sociology of Health and Illness*, vol. 34, no. 3, pp. 396–411, 2012.

[80] M. Mann, C. M. H. Hosman, H. P. Schaalma, and N. K. de Vries, "Self-esteem in a broad-spectrum approach for mental health promotion," *Health Education Research*, vol. 19, no. 4, pp. 357–372, 2004.

[81] J. K. Thompson, M. D. Coovert, and S. M. Stormer, "Body image, social comparison, and eating disturbance: a covariance structure modeling investigation," *International Journal of Eating Disorders*, vol. 26, no. 1, pp. 43–51, 1999.

[82] C. M. Peat, N. L. Peyerl, and J. J. Muehlenkamp, "Body image and eating disorders in older adults: a review," *Journal of General Psychology*, vol. 135, no. 4, pp. 343–358, 2008.

[83] J. D. Garner, "Feminism and feminist gerontology," *Journal of Women and Aging*, vol. 11, no. 2–23, pp. 3–12, 1999.

[84] F. R. Ferraro, J. J. Muehlenkamp, A. Paintner, K. Wasson, T. Hager, and F. Hoverson, "Aging, body image, and body shape," *Journal of General Psychology*, vol. 135, no. 4, pp. 379–392, 2008.

[85] L. Baker and E. Gringart, "Body image and self-esteem in older adulthood," *Ageing & Society*, vol. 29, no. 6, pp. 977–995, 2009.

[86] J. Bookwala and J. Boyar, "Gender, excessive body weight, and psychological well-being in adulthood," *Psychology of Women Quarterly*, vol. 32, no. 2, pp. 188–195, 2008.

[87] A. L. Palmeira, T. L. Branco, S. C. Martins et al., "Change in body image and psychologicalwell-being during behavioral obesity treatment: associations with weight loss and maintenance," *Body Image*, vol. 7, no. 3, pp. 187–193, 2010.

[88] P. N. Vieira, J. Mata, M. N. Silva et al., "Predictors of psychological well-being during behavioral obesity treatment in women," *Journal of Obesity*, vol. 2011, Article ID 936153, 8 pages, 2011.

[89] K. Cuypers, S. Krokstad, T. L. Holmen, M. S. Knudtsen, L. O. Bygren, and J. Holmen, "Patterns of receptive and creative cultural activities and their association with perceived health, anxiety, depression and satisfaction with life among adults: The HUNT study, Norway," *Journal of Epidemiology and Community Health*, vol. 66, no. 8, pp. 698–703, 2012.

[90] The European Commission: Quality of life in Europe: Subjective wellbeing Luxembourg: Publications Office of the European Union 2013, http://digitalcommons.ilr.cornell.edu/cgi/viewcontent.cgi?article=1318&context=intl.

[91] https://www.gov.uk/government/publications/quantifying-the-social-impacts-of-sport-and-culture.

[92] http://www.statcan.gc.ca/pub/82-003-x/2012004/article/11720/ref-eng.htm#n33.

[93] P. L. Sacco, "Culture 3.0: A new perspective for the EU 2014-2020 structural funds programming, on behalf of the European Expert Network on Culture (EENC)," Produced for the OMC Working Group on Cultural and Creative Industries, April 2011.

The Emerging Roles of the Calcineurin-Nuclear Factor of Activated T-Lymphocytes Pathway in Nervous System Functions and Diseases

Maulilio John Kipanyula,[1] Wahabu Hamisi Kimaro,[1] and Paul F. Seke Etet[2]

[1]*Department of Veterinary Anatomy, Faculty of Veterinary Medicine, Sokoine University of Agriculture, P.O. Box 3016, Chuo Kikuu, Morogoro, Tanzania*
[2]*Department of Basic Health Sciences, Qassim University, Buraydah, Al-Qassim 51452, Saudi Arabia*

Correspondence should be addressed to Maulilio John Kipanyula; kipanyula@suanet.ac.tz

Academic Editor: Elke Bromberg

The ongoing epidemics of metabolic diseases and increase in the older population have increased the incidences of neurodegenerative diseases. Evidence from murine and cell line models has implicated calcineurin-nuclear factor of activated T-lymphocytes (NFAT) signaling pathway, a Ca^{2+}/calmodulin-dependent major proinflammatory pathway, in the pathogenesis of these diseases. Neurotoxins such as amyloid-β, tau protein, and α-synuclein trigger abnormal calcineurin/NFAT signaling activities. Additionally increased activities of endogenous regulators of calcineurin like plasma membrane Ca^{2+}-ATPase (PMCA) and regulator of calcineurin 1 (RCAN1) also cause neuronal and glial loss and related functional alterations, in neurodegenerative diseases, psychotic disorders, epilepsy, and traumatic brain and spinal cord injuries. Treatment with calcineurin/NFAT inhibitors induces some degree of neuroprotection and decreased reactive gliosis in the central and peripheral nervous system. In this paper, we summarize and discuss the current understanding of the roles of calcineurin/NFAT signaling in physiology and pathologies of the adult and developing nervous system, with an emphasis on recent reports and cutting-edge findings. Calcineurin/NFAT signaling is known for its critical roles in the developing and adult nervous system. Its role in physiological and pathological processes is still controversial. However, available data suggest that its beneficial and detrimental effects are context-dependent. In view of recent reports calcineurin/NFAT signaling is likely to serve as a potential therapeutic target for neurodegenerative diseases and conditions. This review further highlights the need to characterize better all factors determining the outcome of calcineurin/NFAT signaling in diseases and the downstream targets mediating the beneficial and detrimental effects.

1. Introduction

Cellular responses to calcium (Ca^{2+}) mobilization are highly versatile due to the ability of intracellular Ca^{2+} signaling to activate an extensive repertoire of downstream signaling targets [1, 2]. Among such molecules, the calmodulin- (CaM-) dependent phosphatase calcineurin and its transcription factors termed nuclear factors of activated T cells (NFATs) are reported as pivotal in a wide range of physiological processes, including homeostasis, angiogenesis, myogenesis, adipogenesis, osteogenesis, chondrocyte differentiation, cardiovascular system development, pancreatic β-cell proliferation, hair follicle cell differentiation and remodeling, and activities of cells of the immune and nervous systems [3–12]. Overexpressed and decreased activities of calcineurin/NFAT pathway were also reported in pathologies affecting these functions [3, 6, 13–18].

A growing body of evidence suggests that calcineurin/NFAT pathway plays critical roles in normal and pathological nervous system. Over the last decade, this signaling pathway was reported as major player in corticogenesis, synaptogenesis, and neuritogenesis during mammalian nervous system development [19–23], as well as myelination, synaptic plasticity, neurotransmission, and central and peripheral nervous system cell proliferation, migration, and differentiation in the mature nervous system [24–26]. Altered calcineurin/NFAT activation is increasingly linked to pathological features of neurodegenerative diseases such as amyotrophic lateral sclerosis, Huntington's, Parkinson's, and Alzheimer's diseases, characterized by massive synaptic dysfunction, glial activation, and neuronal death in some regions of the brain [26–29]. Calcineurin/NFAT involvement has also been reported in psychiatric disorders, epilepsy, and traumatic brain and spinal cord injuries [30–35]. Moreover, recent data also suggest that NFAT isoforms are selectively activated in neurons and glial cells in nervous system diseases [36, 37] and animal models [38–41].

Herein, we discuss the current understanding of the role of calcineurin/NFAT signaling pathway in both physiology and pathologies of the adult and developing nervous system, with an emphasis on recent reports and cutting-edge findings.

2. Calcineurin/NFAT Pathway

2.1. Calcineurin. Calcineurin, also termed as protein phosphatase B (PP2B), is a Ca^{2+}/CaM-dependent serine/threonine phosphatase. It was described for the first time in the bovine brain about 40 years ago [42, 43]. Calcineurin is made up of a 61 kD CaM-binding catalytic subunit termed calcineurin A (CnA) and a 19 kD Ca^{2+}-binding regulatory subunit named calcineurin B (CnB) stably associated (noncovalently) [44, 45]. To date three isozymes of the catalytic subunit (CnAα, CnAβ, and CnAγ) have been reported. There are two isoforms of the regulatory subunit, namely, CnB1 and CnB2. In vertebrates, each subunit is encoded by a separate gene PPP3CA, PPP3CB, and PPP3CC for CnB1 and PPP3R1, PPP3R2 for CnB2 [46, 47]. The two calcineurin isoforms are widely distributed in mammalian tissues. Immunohistochemical studies showed that under normal conditions calcineurin isoforms are highly expressed in neuroinflammation-sensible neurons like corticohypothalamic pyramidal cells and cerebellar Purkinje cells, as well as in peripheral nervous system (PNS) glia like Schwann cells, but not in central nervous system (CNS) glia [37, 48, 49].

The subcellular distribution of calcineurin is an important control point in regulating its activity. Various studies addressed the subcellular localization of calcineurin in various mammalian cells [2, 50, 51]. In neurons, calcineurin was found in the cytoplasm, endoplasmic reticulum, Golgi apparatus, nucleus, synaptic vesicles, microsomes, mitochondrion outer membrane, and plasma membrane [2, 48, 49, 51, 52].

2.2. NFAT Transcription Factors. NFAT proteins are a family of transcription factors normally found in the cytoplasm in a hyperphosphorylated (inactive) state [53–55]. This family comprises five distinct gene products termed (i) NFATc, NFAT2, or NFATc1; (ii) NFATp, NFAT1, or NFATc2; (iii) NFATx, NFAT4, or NFATc3; (iii) NFAT3 or NFATc4; and (iv) osmotic response element-binding protein (OREBP), tonicity-responsive binding-protein (TonEBP), or NFAT5 [56, 57]. In the context of this review, nomenclature of NFATc1-c4 and NFAT5 will be used.

NFATc1–c4 occur as monomers with unique amino and carboxyl termini containing transcription activation domains (TADs) and two conserved domains: (i) a regulatory domain termed NFAT homology region (NHR), which shows a lesser degree of pair-wise sequence identity but has several strongly conserved sequence motifs characteristic of the NFAT family; and (ii) the Rel homology region (RHR) in the C-terminus, where the DNA binding domain (DBD) is located [14, 56]. The NHR encompasses calcineurin docking sites, a nuclear localization signal (NLS) responsible for calcineurin-mediated nuclear translocation, and an extended serine-rich region [44, 58–61]. On the other hand, the DBD binds DNA and interacts with partner proteins to transactivate gene transcription. Examples of partner transcription factors include AP-1 cell life and death regulators [dimeric transcription factors composed of activating transcription factor (ATF), Fos, or Jun subunits] and important oncogenic regulators like myocyte enhancer factor-2 (MEF2) and GATA binding protein 4 (GATA4) [60, 62]. Regions out of the regulatory and DNA binding domains like TADs demonstrate relatively little sequence conservation [57, 59]. NFAT5 is a homodimer with a distinct domain structure. This isoform retains only the RHR region of homology to the Ca^{2+}-regulated isoforms, whilst the remaining 600 amino acids are completely different. The DBD of NFATs is distantly related to the DBD of nuclear factor kappa B (NF-κB)/Rel family, allowing them to be classified sometimes as members of this extended family [63, 64].

NFATs regulate the transcriptional induction of genes encoding for immune modulators/activators such as granulocyte-macrophage colony-stimulating factor (GM-CSF), forkhead box P3 (FOXP3), immunoglobulin kappa (Igκ), gamma interferon (IFNγ), CD5, CD25, CD28, CD40, interleukin- (IL-) 2, IL-3, IL-4, IL-5, IL-13, IL-8, Th2-type cytokine IL-31, Fas ligand, macrophage inflammatory protein 1 alpha (MIP-1α), protein tyrosine kinase Syk, cyclooxygenase 2 (COX-2), and tumor necrosis factor alpha (TNF-α) and its family member BlyS. NFATs may also control genes encoding signaling molecules as variate as Ca^{2+} regulators [inositol 1,4,5-trisphosphate (IP_3) receptor (IP_3R), regulator of calcineurin 1 (RCAN1)], growth factors (VEGF, neurotrophins), myelination genes (P0 and Krox-20), glucose regulation genes (insulin, HNF1, PDX, and GLUT2), cell cycle and death regulator/activators [$p21^{Waf1}$, c-Myc, cyclin-dependent kinase 4 (CDK4), B-cell lymphoma 2 (Bcl-2), and cyclins A2, D1, and D2], oncogenes (Wnt, β-catenin), microRNAs (miR-21, miR-23, miR-24, miR-27, miR-125, miR-195, miR-199, and miR-224), and surfactants (sftpa, sftpb, sftpc, and abca3) [9, 65–74]. NFAT isoforms are ubiquitously expressed and are generally regulated by Ca^{2+} signaling, with exception of NFAT5 [59, 75, 76]. NFAT5 regulates hypertonic stress-induced gene transcription, whereas the other NFATs act as integrators of Ca^{2+} driven signaling pathways in gene expression and cell differentiation programs [57, 77, 78].

All Ca^{2+}-regulated NFATs (NFATc1–c4) are expressed in neurons [79]. The previously assumed functional redundancy of NFAT functions was proved wrong by their wide-ranging expression profile among cell types under both physiological and pathological conditions. For example, loss of specific NFAT subtypes resulted in cardiovascular, skeletal muscle, cartilage, neuronal, and/or immune system defects [54, 59, 80, 81]. In addition, Vihma and colleagues reported that NFAT subcellular localizations and transcriptional activities are isoform- and cell type-specific [37]. In that context, the strongest transcriptional activators were NFATc3 and NFATc4 in primary hippocampal neurons and NFATc1 and NFATc3 in human embryonic kidney-derived HEK293 cells.

2.3. Signaling Activation. The activation of calcineurin/NFAT signaling pathway involves three key steps: (i) NFAT protein dephosphorylation by calcineurin; (ii) nuclear translocation of NFATs; and (iii) increased affinity for DNA. Ligand-receptor interaction activates phospholipase C (PLC) resulting in the release of IP_3, which in turn leads to the release of Ca^{2+} from intracellular stores through IP_3Rs [59, 82]. Notably, Ca^{2+} release from the intracellular stores requires a stimulus capable of generation of second messengers that trigger Ca^{2+} release from intracellular stores in the endoplasmic/sarcoplasmic reticulum, via channels of IP_3R1–3 and ryanodine receptors (RyR1–3) [59, 83–87]. Like for other Ca^{2+}/CaM-dependent enzymes, calcineurin activation requires increase in cytosolic Ca^{2+} levels. Such activation may result from the binding of Ca^{2+} to calcineurin B subunit or from the binding of Ca^{2+}-activated CaM to calcineurin [50]. In turn, calcineurin activates NFATs by dephosphorylating multiple N-terminal phosphoserine residues in the regulatory domain. Such dephosphorylation increases NFAT affinity for DNA [59]. The dephosphorylation results in a conformational change in the NFAT molecule that exposes the nuclear localization signal, allowing NFAT nuclear translocation to take place, presumably through nuclear pores [88]. In the nucleus NFATs become transcriptionally active by forming complexes with other factors and coactivators, providing a direct link between intracellular Ca^{2+} signaling and gene expression. Calcineurin also promotes nuclear retention of NFAT by masking nuclear export signals (NES) and preventing NES-dependent nuclear export [88, 89]. Moreover, calcineurin mediated NFAT activation is mainly required at resting state (resting membrane potential), where the amount of Ca^{2+} released from intracellular stores is not sufficient for direct NFAT activation [75, 90].

2.4. Regulation and Pharmacology

2.4.1. Endogenous Regulation. Regulators of calcineurin (RCANs) or modulatory calcineurin-interacting proteins (MCIPs; MCIP1–3) belonging to the calcipressin family of proteins play a pivotal role in regulating calcineurin activity. The RCANs are evolutionarily conserved proteins that can directly bind and inhibit calcineurin. The RCAN1 genes are found on chromosome 21. The RCAN gene encodes different isoforms of protein, namely, RCAN1, RCAN2, RCAN3, and RCAN4 where RCAN1 and RCAN4 are the main isoforms. Furthermore, it appears that RCAN1 has two RCAN1 isoforms: 1S with 197 amino acids and RCAN.1L with 252 amino acids. Previous studies have shown that an aberration in RCANs activities decreases calcineurin-NFAT signaling activities. Recent studies have shown that RCANs can show both inhibitory and facilitatory roles in activation of the calcineurin-NFAT signaling pathway. A mechanistic explanation on how RCAN proteins precisely modulate calcineurin function is still debatable. Overall RCANs have been implicated to function primarily as chaperones for calcineurin biosynthesis or recycling, requiring binding, phosphorylation, ubiquitylation, and proteasomal degradation for their stimulatory effect [50, 91, 92]. Other regulators including scaffolding proteins, CAIN/CABIN-1, and A-kinase anchoring protein 79 (AKAP79) have also been identified to interact and inhibit calcineurin function in a phosphorylation-dependent manner in mammalian cells (details given below).

2.4.2. Endogenous Inhibition. The regulation of calcineurin/NFAT activity is achieved: (i) in the nucleus by activities of serine/threonine kinases promoting the export of nuclear NFAT; (ii) in the cytoplasm, through phosphorylation of NFAT serine (SP) repeats and N-terminal domain, which are critical for NFAT activation and nuclear import [88, 93, 94]. Various kinases were implicated in NFAT nuclear export. Examples include glycogen synthase kinase (GSK), protein kinase A (PKA), casein kinase, and also mitogen-activated protein kinases (MAPKs) like c-Jun NH_2- terminal kinases (JNKs) and cellular stress-associated p38 kinase [14, 54]. Although different kinases have been implicated in regulating NFAT activity, the distinction between drivers and passengers in the cytoplasm and in the nucleus is still puzzling. Notably, it is not clearly understood whether the kinases which mediate rephosphorylation of nuclear or activated NFATs are similar to those that phosphorylate NFATs under basal state conditions [14, 54]. Other early reports from targeted genetic and pharmacological manipulations suggest that members of the JNK family regulate both the import and export of NFATs while p38 MAPKs mediate NFAT rephosphorylation, thus NFAT nuclear export [13, 89, 95].

Calcineurin/NFAT signaling blocking agents mainly act at calcineurin and NFAT levels. They include cellular (protein inhibitors) and pharmacological inhibitors. Although numerous endogenous proteins may have potential to inhibit calcineurin or NFAT activities, only four are well-characterized: (i) A-kinase anchoring protein 79 (AKAP79), a scaffold protein that prevents calcineurin-substrate interactions [96, 97]; (ii) calcineurin inhibitor (CAIN) or calcineurin-binding (CABIN) proteins, which block calcineurin activity [98, 99]; (iii) calcineurin homologous protein (CHP); and (vi) modulatory calcineurin-interacting proteins (MCIP1–3), which prevent NFAT nuclear import by preventing its phosphorylation [94, 100–103].

2.4.3. Pharmacological Inhibition. Two pharmacological inhibitors of NFAT translocation, namely, cyclosporine A, FK506 (tacrolimus), and its ethyl analog ascomycin, are commonly used as immunosuppressants, particularly in organ transplantation [104–107]. These chemically distinct microbial products inhibit calcineurin activity by binding with subnanomolar affinity to cytosolic proteins called immunophilins. The resultant drug-protein composite binds tightly to calcineurin and blocks its phosphatase activity by preventing substrate access [14, 59]. Cyclosporine A binds to cyclophilin and FK506 binds to FK506-binding protein (FKBP) [88, 108]. These inhibitors indiscriminately block all downstream calcineurin signaling, including various signaling pathways collaborating with calcineurin/NFAT signaling pathway [39, 93]. Such complete blockade of calcineurin activities may explain at least partly the serious side effects of cyclosporine A and FK506 [104, 105], particularly in pediatric patients [106, 107].

Recent studies in rat brain slices and cultured astrocytes revealed that cyclosporine A increases reactive oxygen species (ROS) formation and alters glucose and energy metabolism partly by Krebs cycle inhibition and anaerobic glycolysis activation [109]. These detrimental effects probably participate in cyclosporine A neurotoxicity. Additionally, inhibition of NFAT activity suppressor GSK-3 mediated by wild-type mice chronic treatment with lithium or cyclosporine A resulted in increases in nuclear translocation of NFATc3 and Fas-dependent apoptosis in brain neurons, accompanied by pronounced motor deficits [110]. In the same study, neither neuronal loss nor motor deficits were observed in Fas deficient Tet/DN-GSK-3 mice, suggesting that GSK-3 contributes to the neurological toxicity induced by cyclosporine A. Therefore, GSK-3 inhibitors may improve calcineurin inhibitor neurotoxicity. Cyclosporine A may also mediate neuronal affection by decreasing biometal availability [111–113].

Moreover, experimental evidence has shown increases in spinal NMDA receptor activity as a result of calcineurin inhibitor induced pain syndrome (CIPS) [114–116]. A whole-cell patch-clamp study in spinal cord slices revealed that the effect may be mediated by the potentiation of pre- and postsynaptic NMDA receptor activity in the spinal cord [114]. In the same study, it was shown that FK506 treatment increased drastically the amplitude of excitatory postsynaptic currents mediated by NMDA receptor in dorsal horn neurons. Inhibitors of the serine/threonine protein kinase casein kinase II (CK2) involved in the upregulation of synaptic NMDAR activity in neurons abrogated pain hypersensitivity caused by FK506 [117, 118]. Nonetheless, cyclosporine A also mediated neuropathic pain independently of NMDA receptor [108, 118], suggesting that the processes mediating CIPS are complex and warrant further studies.

Interestingly, inhibitors that do not block calcineurin enzymatic activity *per se*, but rather interfere with enzyme targeting of one or more of its substrates, have recently been developed and used. For instance, the inhibitors of NFAT-calcineurin association (INCA) compounds may interfere selectively with calcineurin/NFAT interaction without preventing dephosphorylation of other calcineurin substrates [119, 120]. Substrate-selective enzyme inhibition represents an important progress over cyclosporine A or FK506-mediated complete blockade of calcineurin/NFAT signaling. This development is expected to lead to the development of safer classes of calcineurin/NFAT inhibitors. Certainly, the beneficial actions of cyclosporin A and FK506 are counterbalanced by serious toxicities attributed partly to their interference with calcineurin signaling in other cells and tissues. Although INCA have nonspecific cytotoxic effects, they are generally considered to be less toxic than treatment with cyclosporine A or FK506.

3. Nervous System Development

Calcineurin/NFAT signaling pathway is multifunctional. In the PNS, calcineurin/NFAT signaling was reported to have critical roles in the survival, proliferation, and differentiation of both neural and glial precursor cells [22], highlighting its potential role in tissue regeneration. Similar lines of evidence suggest that calcineurin/NFAT plays critical roles in the regulation of the CNS development, including corticogenesis and synaptogenesis.

3.1. Corticogenesis. Evidence supporting the involvement of the calcineurin/NFAT4 signaling pathway in corticogenesis includes a study in developing mouse cerebellar granule neurons that reported a pivotal role in controlling the temporal regulation of nuclear factor 1 occupancy. This serves as a key link between membrane potential and dendritic maturation, by a voltage-sensitive developmental switch [121]. In addition, the multifunctional HMG-box transcription factor Tox, a novel regulator of mammalian corticogenesis, is regulated by calcineurin/NFAT signaling [19]. Genetic and biochemical analyses in the developing embryo revealed that fibroblast growth factor- (FGF-) mediated calcineurin signaling may trigger neural induction by increasing Smad1/5 transcription via silencing of bone morphogenetic protein (BMP) signaling [122]. Furthermore, store-operated Ca^{2+} entry (SOCE) activation regulates gene transcription in the developing nervous system and mediates neural progenitor cell proliferation through calcineurin/NFAT signaling [123–125].

The role of the calcineurin/NFAT signaling in corticogenesis is probably mediated by NFATc3, the predominant NFAT isoform in neural progenitor cell cultures, which is also a potent inducer of neural progenitor cell differentiation into neurons and astrocytes [22, 126]. Interestingly, activity-dependent NFATc3 accumulation in the nucleus was reported in pericytes from cortical parenchymal microvessels [127], and differential expressions of NFATc3 and NFATc4 were reported in developing rat brain and traumatic brain injury models, where NFATc4 was primarily expressed by neurons and NFATc3 by astrocytes [125, 128]. These observations suggest that different NFATs are recruited at the same time in resident cells of damaged and growing nervous tissue, indicating that characterizing the effects of such NFAT changes in specific cell types may provide new therapeutic targets for neurodevelopmental disorders.

3.2. Synaptogenesis. The complex interactions between inhibitory gamma-aminobutyric acid (GABA) and excitatory NMDA receptor activities are required during synaptogenesis. Furthermore, this interaction plays an important role in the induction of immediate early genes necessary for effective changes in synaptic plasticity and long-term memory formation through calcineurin-dependent transcription of the key brain-derived neurotrophic factor (BDNF) [20, 23, 129, 130]. Of particular interest for neurodevelopmental treatments is a recently reported novel synthetic neurotrophic (BDNF and neurotrophin-like) compound that is able to induce neurite growth and confer neuroprotection [21]. In addition, the neurotrophin nerve growth factor (NGF) is known to upregulate the key regulator of plasminogen activation system and synaptogenic protein plasminogen activator inhibitor 1 (PAI-1) in primary mouse hippocampal neurons via calcineurin/NFAT signaling [131]. Protein kinase C (PKC)/calcineurin signaling-mediated dephosphorylation of axon growth regulatory molecule growth-associated protein 43 (GAP43) at developing GABAergic synapses resulted in pathological processing mimicking neonatal hypoxia, including misfolding of gephyrin, a protein critical for the organization of GABA receptors [132]. Calcineurin signaling also mediates the GABAergic synaptic modulation induced by transient receptor potential vanilloid type 1 (TrpV1), a ligand-gated channel abundantly expressed in developing primary sensory neurons [133, 134]. Certainly, these observations suggest that calcineurin signaling is involved in the development of GABAergic synaptic functions in the CNS.

Moreover, GABA promoted the shrinkage and elimination of synapses by suppressing local dendritic Ca^{2+} signaling in rat hippocampal CA1 pyramidal neurons via a mechanism depending on calcineurin and on actin-binding protein cofilin [135]. Similarly, more recent studies also suggested that calcineurin is a major signaling molecule in the selection of synapses, a critical mechanism in the reorganization of the developing and adult CNS mediated by the major inhibitory neurotransmitter GABA [132, 135, 136].

3.3. Endosome Trafficking. It is now widely accepted that calcineurin signaling is a major player in the control of the trafficking and signaling of endosomes performing the retrograde signaling, an event critical for the development, but also for the nervous system function [2, 137, 138]. Calabrese and colleagues reported calcineurin signaling modulation as a key event in the differential regulation of dynamins, major players of synaptic vesicle recycling in nerve terminals of developing neurons [137]. Notably, these authors observed that tetrodotoxin- (TTX-) mediated chronic suppression of neuronal activity results in the suppression of dynamin 1 clustering at nerve terminals and in an increase of clustering of dynamin 3, partly mediated by calcineurin signaling silencing. In addition, NGF-mediated calcineurin/NFAT signaling is critical for the control of endosome trafficking in neurons [77, 131, 138]. Such NGF/calcineurin/NFAT control of the trafficking of endosomes is under the control of the effector protein coronin-1 and regulatory events such as the phosphorylation of cAMP responsive element binding protein (CREB), which are also mediated by NGF receptor tropomyosin receptor kinase type 1 (TrkA) [138].

Notably, as other tyrosine kinase receptors, the receptors of neurotrophins may also activate NFATs via inhibition of the promoter of NFAT nuclear export GSK-3β, independent of Ca^{2+} and calcineurin signaling. For instance, a study assessing the physiological roles of estrogen-related receptor gamma (ERRγ), an orphan nuclear receptor highly expressed in the nervous system during embryogenesis and over lifespan, revealed its involvement in the regulation of dopaminergic neuronal phenotype. Such effect was mediated by GSK-3β-NFAT interactions, independently of Ca^{2+}/calcineurin signaling [139]. Similar, NGF facilitated NFAT-mediated gene expression induced by mild depolarization in dorsal root ganglion sensory neurons without changes in PLC activity-dependent events, including Ca^{2+}/calcineurin signaling. Instead, NGF effects were induced by phosphoinositide 3-kinase (PI3K)/Akt signaling triggered by TrkA receptor activation, which abrogated GSK-3β activity [77].

Furthermore, calcineurin is universally involved in vesicle endocytosis [12], and alterations in its endocytic activity may participate in the pathogenic processes of various psychiatric diseases. For instance, alterations in presynaptic functions of the γ isoform of the calcineurin catalytic subunit, such as synaptic vesicle cycling, have been suggested to contribute to schizophrenia, where variations in calcineurin Aγ gene *PPP3CC* are common in neurons [140]. Deregulation of intracellular Ca^{2+} also associates with the disruption of fast axonal transport (FAT) in the pathogenesis of Alzheimer's disease (AD) [141–144].

4. Nervous System Function

Calcineurin/NFAT has critical roles in neuronal and glial cell activity and survival, as well as resulting events, fundamental for nervous system function like neurotransmission and synaptic plasticity, and myelination as summarized in Figure 1.

4.1. Synaptic Plasticity and Neurotransmission

4.1.1. Synaptic Connectivity and Plasticity. Calcineurin/NFAT signaling and other pathways activated by T-type Ca^{2+} channel activation play critical roles in the shaping of synaptic connectivity of thalamocortical and nucleus reticularis thalami GABAergic neurons mediated by slow wave sleep [145], a process pivotal for the consolidation of recently acquired memories and for the restoration of synaptic homeostasis. This mechanism may be evolutionary conserved [54, 146, 147]. PLC/calcineurin signaling has been reported to regulate the trafficking of GABA A receptor in layer 3 pyramidal cells of murine barrel cortex [136]. Furthermore, the inhibition of group I metabotropic glutamate receptors (mGluRs), IP3Rs, or calcineurin in CA1 neurons resulted in the blockade of the heterosynaptic shrinkage [85, 87] that drives circuit remodeling during activity-dependent refinement of the developing nervous system and during experience-dependent plasticity in the hippocampus. This inhibition has been reported to negatively affect long-term potentiation (LTP) [87].

Experimental evidence also suggests that calcineurin is a regulator of synaptic plasticity. For instance, axon initial segment rapid shortening was partly mediated by calcineurin-dependent mechanisms, including phosphorylation of voltage-gated Na^{+} channels, in dentate granule cells [148]. Rapid modulation of the axon initial segment, the site of action potential initiation, is the major plasticity mechanisms used by neurons to control their excitability time from

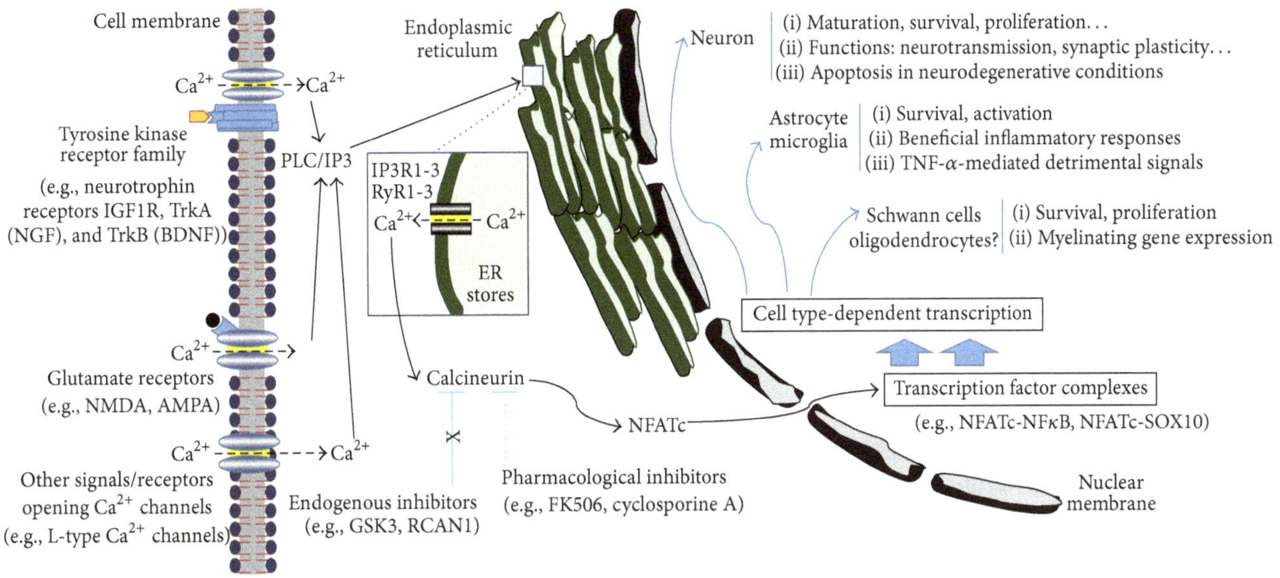

FIGURE 1: Calcineurin/NFAT signaling pathway. Calcineurin/nuclear factor of activated T-lymphocytes (NFAT) signaling activation in the nervous system is mainly induced by neurotrophins via their tyrosine kinase receptors, glutamate receptors, and nonligand-dependent receptors, such as voltage-gated Ca^{2+} channels in hippocampal neurons. The genes transcribed and the effects of these signaling pathways are cell-type dependent. Abbreviations: AMPA, α-amino-3-hydroxy-5-methyl-4-isoxazolepropionic acid; BDNF, brain-derived neurotrophic factor; GSK3, glycogen synthase kinase 3; IGF1R, insulin-like growth factor 1 receptor; IP_3R, inositol 1,4,5-trisphosphate receptor; NF-κB, nuclear factor kappa B; NFATc, Ca^{2+}-regulated NFATs; NGF, neurotrophin nerve growth factor; NMDA, N-methyl-D-aspartic acid; RCAN1, regulator of calcineurin 1; RyR; ryanodine receptor; TrkA, tropomyosin receptor kinase type 1; TrkB, tropomyosin receptor kinase type 2.

seconds to days. In another study, decreases in resting Ca^{2+} levels associated with prolonged blockade of synaptic activity resulted in the synthesis of retinoic acid, which triggered the related homeostatic synaptic plasticity, via a calcineurin-dependent mechanism in neurons [149]. Moreover, spinogenesis enhancement in hippocampal neurons by the steroid hormones dihydrotestosterone and testosterone was blocked by individual antagonism of PKC, PKA, calcineurin, LIM kinase (LIMK), or the MAPKs Erk and p38 [150]. Similar, estradiol-mediated rapid modulation of synaptic plasticity, an essential process for synaptic regulation, was abrogated by individual targeting of PI3K, PKC, PKA, calcineurin, CaM kinase II (CaMKII), LIMK, Erk, or p38, in hippocampal neurons [151].

4.1.2. Learning and Neurotransmission. Evidence of calcineurin/NFAT involvement in learning and memory processes was provided by experimental models of neurodegenerative disorders. A study in PS1-M146V knock-in FAD mice showed that decreased calcineurin activity is a common phenomenon in aging-related memory decline and may account for memory defects in AD, together with mutations in the gene encoding for GSK-3β substrate presenilin 1 (PS1) [152], which are critical for amyloid-β (Aβ) generation. In a study using a spinocerebellar ataxia type 3 (SCA3) transgenic mouse model, typical impairments of motor learning and cerebellar motor coordination resulted from altered long-term depression (LTD) of glutamatergic transmission in parallel fiber-Purkinje neurons [153]. Such alteration resulted mainly from transcriptional downregulation of PLC β4, IP3R1, and calcineurin B, suggesting that PLC/IP_3-Rs/calcineurin signaling is required for cerebellar LTD induction, thus motor learning and coordination.

Calcineurin/NFAT signaling is also involved in neuronal excitability and neurotransmission. Under physiological conditions, AKAP79/150-mediated calcineurin/NFAT signaling may prevent neuronal hyperexcitability in hippocampal neurons by increasing the transcriptional expression of key regulators of neuronal excitability like M-type K^+ channels [154]. PKC/calcineurin/NFAT signaling contributes to the maintenance of cyclic nucleotide-gated (HCN) channels in the hyperpolarized status critical for their mediation of neuronal excitability decrease in the distal dendrites of hippocampal CA1 pyramidal neurons [155], and membrane-derived bioactive phospholipid lysophosphatidic acid type 1 (LPA1) triggers RhoA/Rho kinase (ROCK)/calcineurin signaling to induce the internalization of the GABAAγ2 subunit at inhibitory synapses [156].

4.2. Calcineurin-PKA Interactions. The interplay between calcineurin and PKA signaling plays a critical role in the negative-feedback mechanism driving homeostatic synaptic plasticity [157], that is, accounting for the compensation of excessive inhibition or excitation of neuronal activity. Although calcineurin/NFAT signaling mainly regulates axon terminal remodeling, while PKA/CREB signaling controls synaptic vesicle accumulation [158], many lines of evidence suggest mutual inhibitory interactions between the activities of these signaling pathways. Examples include the activity of these signaling molecules when anchored to AKAP79/150. PKA kinase activity triggered by anchoring to AKAP79/150 resulted in the enhancement of Ca^{2+}-dependent inactivation of L-type Ca^{2+} channels, while the activation of the phosphatase activity of AKAP79/150-anchored calcineurin reversed such PKA action, reducing Ca^{2+}-dependent inactivation [96, 159]. The basal activity of AKAP79/150-anchored PKA maintained L-type Ca^{2+} channel-calcineurin/NFAT signaling functional coupling by preserving the phosphorylation of these channels, contrary to anchored calcineurin [159, 160]. Interestingly, such AKAP79/150 activity mediated the modulation of roundabout axonal guidance receptors Robo2/3 and ligands Slit2/3 in brain regions involved in reward, learning, and memory processes like islands of Calleja and the hippocampus [97].

Furthermore, PKA can induce NFAT nuclear export [14, 54]. PKA activation by forskolin-stimulated cAMP increased the stability and half-life of RCAN1 protein, enhancing its inhibitory effects on calcineurin [161]. In a recent study in pilocarpine-induced status epilepticus, a murine model of temporal lobe epilepsy (TLE), the nuclear translocation of CREB-regulated transcription coactivator 1 (CRTC1), which is a key regulator of CREB activity, was regulated by calcineurin activity in hippocampal neurons [24].

Opposite effects of calcineurin and PKA were also reported as key events in (i) the dynamic fission-fusion events that determine the shape and function of mitochondria [162, 163], thus cell survival; (ii) neuronal output stabilization induced by tonic dopamine via type 1 dopaminergic receptors [164]; and (iii) the phosphorylation/dephosphorylation of serine 897 in the NR1 subunit of the NMDA receptor (pNR1), whose increases in phosphorylation were reported in acute morphine withdrawal [30].

4.3. Myelination. Available data suggest that calcineurin/NFAT pathway participates in signaling cascades pivotal for Schwann cell myelination. Early studies reported that (i) murine Schwann cells express all Ca^{2+}-dependent NFAT isoforms; (ii) the promoter and upstream enhancer elements of the myelinating factor Krox-20 contain NFAT binding sites; and (iii) NFATs recruited by Ca^{2+}-dependent signaling can make transcriptionally active complexes with Krox-20 [9, 93, 165]. Reporter assays showed that Krox-20 is NFAT target gene and that calcineurin is upregulated in Schwann cells expressing Krox-20 [8, 166]. Moreover, we reported using rat Schwann cell cultures and an *in vitro* model of myelination that promyelinating actions of calcineurin/NFAT signaling, including increases in the expression of the myelinating genes *Krox-20, Periaxin,* and *P0*, require cAMP elevation [9]. Notably, in the absence of cAMP elevation, increase in cytosolic Ca^{2+} failed to induce Krox-20 expression. Furthermore, cyclosporine A and FK506 abrogated Krox-20 expression. Comparable observations were reported more recently by other authors [165, 167].

Experimental evidence also suggests that the activation of calcineurin/NFAT required for Schwann cell myelination occurs partly through neuregulin 1 (NRG1) stimulation [8, 168–170]. A study in mice lacking calcineurin B in cells of the neural crest lineage showed that calcineurin/NFAT signaling is required for NRG1-mediated Schwann cell myelination [170]. In this model NFAT activation failed, Krox-20 levels in Schwann cell were decreased, and radial sorting and myelination were markedly delayed [8, 170]. NRG1 addition to neuron-Schwann cell cocultures promoted the activation of NFAT isoforms and cooperative transcriptional activities of NFATc4 and SOX10 required for Krox-20 upregulation [168, 169]. In addition, NRG1/calcineurin/NFAT signaling upregulates myelinating genes in Schwann cells [8, 168, 171].

Unexpectedly, FK506 stimulated Schwann cell proliferation and promoted the survival of oligodendrocyte in murine models of traumatic spinal cord injury [172–174], suggesting that this signaling pathway is involved in the maintenance, thus activity, of myelinating cells in both peripheral and central nervous systems. Moreover, NFAT1 hyperactivation decreased experimental autoimmune encephalomyelitis induced by myelin oligodendrocyte glycoprotein (MOG), a key regulator of CNS myelination [175, 176].

5. Controversial Roles in Nervous System Diseases

5.1. Neurodegenerative Diseases

5.1.1. Pathogenic Roles. Increased calcineurin activity was reported in both aging and AD models [27, 177, 178]. For instance, calcineurin/NFAT signaling may mediate the aberrant activity of deregulated plasma membrane Ca^{2+} pumps (PMCAs), a suggested link between brain aging and the onset of neurodegenerative diseases [27, 179, 180]. The strongest AD genetic risk factor, the apoE4 allele, encodes for apolipoprotein E4 that has poor inhibitory abilities on calcineurin activity, unlike the neuroprotective apolipoproteins E2 and E3 [181–183]. Apolipoprotein E4 also drives CNS functional alterations associated with normal aging such as disturbed sleep [28, 29].

Overactivated calcineurin/NFAT signaling may contribute to synaptic plasticity affection in pathological conditions. Notably, in a postmortem study in human hippocampi, high nuclear levels of NFATs observed at the early stage of AD increased with cognitive decline severity [177]. Additionally, short exposure to $A\beta$ oligomers resulted in calcineurin activation with transient changes in postsynaptic proteins and morphological in spines, while longer exposure resulted in NFAT activation and marked spine loss in primary cortical neurons of wild-type mice [184]. $A\beta$-treatment of murine hippocampal neurons also resulted in Ca^{2+} signaling-dependent defects in BDNF transport first in dendrites and then in axons [40]. Studies in mouse and rat models of severe childhood epilepsy revealed that calcineurin/NFAT signaling mediates seizure-induced dendrite growth suppression in pyramidal neurons and thus the resulting learning and memory impairment associated with this intractable condition [185].

NFAT signaling alterations in neurodegenerative diseases are selective. A report by Abdul and colleagues strongly suggested that such selective alteration may play a key role in $A\beta$-induced neurodegeneration [186]. These authors observed increases in calcineurin A activity and more marked shifts of NFATc2 and NFATc4 to nuclear compartments in human hippocampus with increased dementia severity, while even in rapid-autopsy postmortem human brain tissue NFATc1 was unchanged. NFATc2 was more active in AD patients with mild cognitive impairment, contrary to NFATc4 whose expression was mostly associated with severe dementia. Still in the same study, changes in calcineurin/NFAT4 were directly correlated to soluble Aβ levels in postmortem hippocampus, while oligomeric Aβ strongly stimulated NFAT activation in primary rat astrocyte cultures. In another study, NFATc4 levels were significantly increased in brains of APP/PS1 transgenic mice (AD model) and NFATc4 overexpression increased Aβ production in human myeloid leukemia SAS-1 cells [36], suggesting a role for NFATc4 in amyloidogenesis. Mechanisms proposed for NFAT-mediated amyloidogenesis in human and murine astrocytes include increases in the expression of the gene encoding for TMP21, a p24 cargo protein involved in Aβ and Aβ precursor protein (APP) trafficking [187–190].

5.1.2. Beneficial Effects. The role of calcineurin in aberrant α-synuclein-mediated midbrain dopaminergic neuron toxicity, a hallmark of Parkinson's disease (PD), is controversial. In a study addressing the underlying intracellular mechanisms driving α-synuclein-mediated neurodegeneration, transgenic expression of PD α-synuclein A53T missense mutation promoted calcineurin/NFAT signaling, suggesting that this signaling pathway may contribute to the neurotoxic effects of aberrant α-synuclein [191]. Surprisingly, in a study using cells from various models (ranging from yeast to neurons), although aberrant α-synuclein also seemed to induce cellular toxicity via overactivation of Ca^{2+}-dependent signaling pathways, calcineurin inhibition with FK506 also resulted in toxicity [192], suggesting that calcineurin may mediate both beneficial and toxic effects under stimulation by aberrant α-synuclein. Characterizing the precise downstream targets mediating calcineurin beneficial or toxic effects may provide more insights of the novel therapeutic targets for synucleinopathies.

Calcineurin also mediates some beneficial and toxic effects of AMPA and NMDA receptors, which are postsynaptic site-located glutamate-gated ion channels critical for synaptic plasticity. Calcineurin translocation to synapses and increases in its activity mediated by NMDA receptor trafficking were reported as critical components of mechanisms driving rapid compression-induced dendritic spine plasticity in cortical pyramidal neurons, that is, the rapid trimming of dendritic spines occurring about 12 hours after mechanical compression [38]. A study using soluble Aβ treated in cultured rat hippocampal neurons and cultured hippocampal neurons from APPSwe AD-transgenic mice suggested that calcineurin signaling mediates AD-like synaptic dysfunction induced by tau protein partly via AMPA receptor downregulation [193]. In that study, soluble Aβ oligomer-induced deficits in AMPA receptor trafficking were mediated by tau phosphorylation and mislocalization to dendritic spines. FK506 abrogated all these alterations. Concomitant tau hyperphosphorylation and calcineurin overactivation were also reported in mouse models of Huntington's disease [41]. On the other hand, IL-6/Janus kinase (JAK) signaling induced neuroprotective anti-NMDA activities in cultured cerebellar granule neurons via calcineurin-dependent inhibition of activities of NMDA receptor subunits NR2B and NR2C and concomitant inhibitions of NMDA-induced L-type voltage-gated Ca^{2+} channel activity and intracellular Ca^{2+} store release [194].

Moreover, in AD pathogenesis, insulin-like growth factor 1 (IGF-1) that acts as a regulator of tau phosphorylation is silenced in activated astrocytes by Aβ/calcineurin-induced release of IGF-1-binding protein 3 (IGFBP-3); but intriguingly, Aβ directly induces increases in tau phosphorylation, and resulting neuronal death, via a mechanism involving the silencing of NFAT export kinase GSK-3β [195], suggesting opposite roles for calcineurin in AD pathogenesis. IGF-1 also protected motor neurons in SOD1 transgenic mice, a widely used model of amyotrophic lateral sclerosis, via a calcineurin-dependent mechanism [196]. Although it is now widely accepted that therapeutic benefits of IGF-1 treatment in neurodegenerative conditions may emerge partly from calcineurin-dependent inhibition of glial inflammatory reaction mediated by preventing TNF-α-induced nuclear translocation of NF-κB [197–199], it is also clear that the expression of TNF-α, resulting in detrimental neuroinflammation and functional alterations in neurons, is mediated by astrocytic and microglial calcineurin/NFAT signaling [200–202]. Studies in transgenic mice and *in vitro* models of neuroinflammatory diseases provided mechanistic insights into the context of these opposite roles. These studies showed that TNF-α activate calcineurin/NFAT/NF-κB canonical inflammatory pathway in quiescent astrocytes, while in activated astrocytes, IGF-1 released locally recruited calcineurin signaling to inhibit NF-κB-NFAT transcriptional activity through activation of the purinergic receptor P2Y6 [203, 204], suggesting that the activation status of the cell is an important determinant of calcineurin/NFAT activity, that is, downstream targets.

5.1.3. Pharmacological Inhibition and Endogenous Regulation. The pharmacological inhibition of calcineurin/NFAT signaling improved animal condition in a number of studies in neurodegenerative diseases and models. Examples include AD mouse models where pharmacological inhibition of this signaling pathway decreased Aβ plaques, reduced glial activation, alleviated both Aβ synaptotoxicity and neurotoxicity, and improved synaptic function [25, 205–207], suggesting a therapeutic potential for calcineurin inhibitors in AD. Reports by Kim and colleagues from studies performed in presenilin 1-mutant model of AD provided some mechanistic insights into the cognitive decline improvement resulting from reducing calcineurin activation in affected brains [25, 208]. These authors observed that the inhibition of abnormally increased calcineurin activity characteristic of the disease resulted in the stabilization of the phosphorylation of GluA1, a subunit of Ca^{2+}-permeable AMPA receptors, and promoted synaptic trafficking of Ca^{2+}-permeable AMPA receptors, as well as the resulting improvement in animal cognition [25]. Such improvement resulted at least partly from the restoration of Ca^{2+}-permeable AMPA receptor-mediated hippocampal LTP [208]. Decrease in calcineurin complexes with transmembrane AMPA receptor regulatory proteins (TARPs) like γ-8, which can stop the trafficking of both AMPA and to a lesser extent NMDA receptors [209–211], may also participate in this process. Furthermore, biometal mediated neurite elongation and neuritogenesis in neuron cultures via calcineurin silencing [111] and calcineurin/NFAT signaling induced a reduction in NGF expression and neurite outgrowth in rat neonatal ventricular cardiomyocytes and cultured sympathetic neurons [212, 213].

Not surprisingly considering the aforementioned observations in studies assessing the roles of calcineurin in neurodegenerative disorders (Section 5.1.2), endogenous regulators like plasma membrane calcium ATPase (PMCA) and RCAN1 mediate opposite effects in inflammatory processes. RCAN1 overexpression was reported to be pivotal in the prevention of sepsis and LPS-induced lethality [214] and in the protection against brain ischemia/reperfusion injury in murine models [215]. However, interactions of PMCA and vascular endothelial growth factor (VEGF), which dampened calcineurin/NFAT signaling, also induced the overexpression of both the counter-inflammatory factor RCAN1.4 and the proinflammatory factor COX-2 in activated murine endothelia [214, 216, 217]. Additionally, RCAN1 overexpression increased the susceptibility to oxidative stress in primary neurons [218] and exacerbated Ca^{2+} overloading-induced neuronal apoptosis [219], suggesting that the overexpression of calcineurin regulator RCAN1 may link Ca^{2+} overloading and oxidative stress in neurodegenerative disorders (Figure 1). Such detrimental effects of RCAN1 were mediated by RCAN1.4, and not by the other isoforms detected in human brain RCAN1.1 [91, 219], probably via PI3K/Akt/mTOR signaling [220, 221]. Such mechanistic insight was provided by a system study based on combinations of single-cell experimentation and *in silico* simulations where RCAN1 effect on inflammation mediated by calcineurin/NFAT appeared to change according to cellular levels, from inhibitory activity at low levels to facilitative activity at high levels [221]. Notably, in that study RCAN1 facilitative activity was switched on by nuclear export of GSK-3β, indicating that targeting the factors involved in this inhibitory mechanism of GSK-3β-mediated NFAT nuclear export may have a therapeutic potential in neurodegenerative diseases.

Considering that RCAN1 overexpression is a hallmark of Down syndrome [219, 222], it can be hypothesized that this event also contributes to the pathogenesis of AD-like neuropathology typically observed in Down syndrome patients after their middle age [223, 224]. In addition, the activity of pituitary adenylate cyclase-activating peptide (PACAP), a neurotrophic peptide involved in nervous system development, learning, and memory, was significantly disturbed by changes in RCAN1 expression [225]. RCAN1 overexpression impaired neurotrophic support of sympathetic neurons by inhibiting TrkA endocytosis, resulting in NGF signaling silencing and associated neurodevelopmental deficits [92]. Furthermore, overexpression of RCAN1 or dual-specificity tyrosine-(Y)-phosphorylation regulated kinase 1A (DYRK1A), another Down syndrome-associated protein, negatively regulated NFAT-dependent transcriptional activity and decreased NGF-mediated upregulation of PAI-1 levels [131], a key synaptogenic mechanism. Intriguingly, deficiency of RCAN1.1, but not RCAN1.4, affected radial migration of rat cortical neurons and caused periventricular heterotopia [226], suggesting that this RCAN1.1 isoform may mediate positive RCAN1 effects in developing cortex. Future studies using selective activations and inhibitions of RCAN1 isoforms may reveal the mechanisms accounting for isoform-specific effects in the developing cortex.

5.2. Neurodegenerative Conditions and Other Nervous System Diseases

5.2.1. Neurodegenerative Conditions. Alterations in the autophagy of mitochondria, the process that normally triggers damaged organelle elimination, are common in neurodegenerative diseases and conditions [227–230]. In a study using axotomized precerebellar neurons, a model of focal cerebellar lesion-induced remote degeneration, rapamycin-mediated autophagy, resulted in an aberrant mitochondrial fission partly caused by increased calcineurin activity [227]. The activity of a calcineurin docking motif present in the mitochondrial fission mechanoenzyme dynamin-related protein 1 (Drp1) contributed to mitochondrial fragmentation and ischemic neuronal injury in neuronal and nonneuronal cells [163]. Additionally, calcineurin inhibitors mitigated mitochondrial fragmentation in ferric ammonium citrate-exposed HT-22 hippocampal neurons, a model of iron overload and neurodegeneration [231].

Further evidence for calcineurin involvement in ischemic injury includes reports suggesting that abnormal increases in the activity of this phosphatase, mediated by disturbances in axonal Ca^{2+} homeostasis, may play a key role in secondary damage of neurons and capillary vessels observed during acute phase of diffuse axonal injury [173, 232]. Calcineurin signaling also mediated the activation of the cytoskeletal actin severing protein cofilin and the resulting neuronal death in oxygen-glucose deprivation/reperfusion and chemical induced oxidative stress, to *in vitro* models of ischemia [34]. Moreover, cyclosporine A prevented the apoptosis of astrocytes exposed to simulated ischemia *in vitro* via a calcineurin and Erk1/2-dependent mechanism [233] and through the inhibition of cytosolic phospholipase A2-(PLA2-) mediated release of arachidonic acid [234].

Selective calcineurin signaling in neurons and astrocytes is a key player in neurodegenerative conditions. An early study addressing neuronal apoptosis induced by the abused psychostimulant methamphetamine revealed pivotal roles for calcineurin activation and resulting Fas ligand upregulation mediated by nuclear translocations of NFATc3 and NFATc4 in rats [235]. The potent hepatotoxin microcystin-LR (MCLR) mediated an upregulation of calcineurin and NFATc3 levels in rat hippocampal neurons that resulted in marked increases in apoptotic and necrotic cell death [32]. MCLR effect was prevented by FK506 treatment. In addition, NFATc4 mediated light-induced retinal ganglion cell apoptosis by upregulating Fas ligand (FasL) expression on retinal neurons [236], and the overactivation of calcineurin/NFATc3 signaling induced the typical neuronal toxicity and functional alterations observed in murine developing hippocampal neurons following the inhalation of anesthetic isoflurane, including cognitive impairment [237]. A recent study in this model of postoperative cognitive dysfunction revealed that abnormal calcineurin/NFAT signaling associated with isoflurane exposure may mediate its detrimental effects by promoting the degradation of the survival molecule signal transducer and activator of transcription 3 (STAT3) [238]. Moreover, calcineurin/NFATc3 signaling in activated astrocytes played a key role in the induction of alterations in synaptic remodeling and homeostasis observed in the hippocampus in controlled cortical impact injury in rats [39, 128, 239]. As expected, calcineurin inhibition restored synaptic function and plasticity in the latter murine model of traumatic brain injury and in murine models of traumatic spinal cord injury [172–174] partly by abrogating astrocyte activation and reactive gliosis, which are pivotal events in neuroinflammation-mediated neuronal loss. Notably, calcineurin/NFAT signaling is critical for astrocyte activation [205, 240]. In another study in ischemic striatum and cortex and in cultured astrocytes where FK506 also induced neuroprotective effects, the calcineurin inhibitor prevented astrocyte apoptosis mediated by glutamate signaling [241].

Altogether, these observations suggest a role for calcineurin/NFAT signaling in astrocyte and neuronal losses observed in nervous system injury. Unexpectedly, sublethal ischemia increased neuronal resistance to excitotoxicity via calcineurin-dependent mechanisms including cyclin E1 protein increased expression and declustering of the delayed rectifying K^+ channel Kv2.1 at highly phosphorylated somatodendritic clusters [242]. In addition, preconditioning of neurons with biometal ions (Cu^{2+}, Zn^{2+}) protected these cells against NMDA receptor-induced excitotoxicity, through metal chaperone PBT2-induced calpain cleavage of calcineurin [111, 112]. Thus, calcineurin/NFAT pathway participates in the interplay between proinflammatory and counter-inflammatory signals in the nervous system, further suggesting that unraveling the downstream targets accounting for beneficial and neurotoxic effects of this signaling pathway may have a therapeutic potential in neurodegenerative conditions.

5.2.2. Psychotic Disorders. Early genetic studies showed that polymorphisms of the genes coding for either the catalytic or regulatory subunit of calcineurin isoenzymes are strongly associated with the risk for developing schizophrenia and other psychotic disorders whose pathological features include disturbances in Ca^{2+} signaling [46, 243–246]. A more recent genome-wide weighted coexpression network analysis on neural progenitors and neurons from individuals with Timothy syndrome, an autism spectrum disorder resulting from mutations in the gene encoding L-type CaV1.2 Ca^{2+} channels, suggested that the disease may be caused by disturbances in transcriptional activities of Ca^{2+}-dependent signaling molecules like FOX proteins, MEF2, CREB, and NFATs [247].

Furthermore, GABA A receptor activation promoted a decrease in anxiety indicators and hippocampal neurogenesis via the calcineurin/NFAT4 signaling in mice, suggesting that pharmacological targeting of this signaling pathway may improve emotional disorders [248]. Similar evidence from pharmacological and postmortem studies suggests that treatment with antipsychotics aimed at ameliorating some of the symptoms of the CNS disorders leads to alterations of the calcineurin expression pattern in the human brain [249–253]. Decreased calcineurin levels in the nucleus accumbens were reported in opioid withdrawal, a dysphoric state associated with complications in patient pain and increased risk of drug abuse and addiction [30], suggesting a role for calcineurin in long-lasting behaviors associated with reward. Furthermore, in a patch-clamp electrophysiology and fast-scan cyclic voltammetry study in mouse brain slices, the endogenous modulatory peptide neurotensin induced a long-term prevention of pathogenic increases in presynaptic dopamine release, characteristic of schizophrenia and other severe mesencephalic pathologies, by increasing inhibitory D2 dopamine autoreceptor function via a calcineurin-dependent mechanism [35].

5.2.3. Epilepsy. Many lines of evidence also support calcineurin involvement in nervous system diseases. Notably, various reports have suggested that calcineurin is likely to mediate physiological and pathological activities of GABA receptors. For instance, complex interactions between PKC and calcineurin may play a key role in GABA B autoreceptor-mediated functional regulation of nicotinic acetylcholine receptors (nAChRs), whose activation triggers the release of neurotransmitters from presynaptic nerve terminals, in mouse striatal GABAergic nerve terminals [254]. Somatic modulation of GABA A receptor-mediated fast inhibitory signaling in epileptiform activity was induced by calcineurin signaling in low-magnesium model of seizure in rat hippocampal neurons [31], suggesting a role of calcineurin in benzodiazepine resistance and the potential of its pharmacological targeting in status epilepticus.

Certainly, calcineurin/NFAT signaling involvement was also shown in pathogenic processes of other models of status epilepticus, including intracerebral injection of kainic acid [255], bicuculline [256], and pilocarpine [33]. Notably, calcineurin inhibitor ascomycin mediated anticonvulsant and neuroprotective effects, in different epilepsy models, including picrotoxin and latrunculin A models [257–259].

5.3. Emerging Challenge: Better Models? A growing number of studies are raising concerns about mechanistic reports of Ca^{2+}-dependent and other signaling pathways from currently used models of neurodegenerative diseases, in particular transgenic animals and cell lines. A study addressing the suitability of rat striatal primordia-derived ST14A cell line for the study of voltage-gated Ca^{2+} channel of striatal medium spiny neurons called for serious caution on the assumption of the presence of complete signaling cascades of G-protein coupled receptors in cell lines [260]. Notably, ST14A cells were reported to lack PLC-β1, a major effector of G-proteins for Ca^{2+} release from intracellular stores [59, 82], whose roles include (i) the regulation of forward locomotion in wild-type mice, among other dopamine receptor functions [261]; (ii) the mediation of Ca^{2+} flux required for mammalian sperm acrosome reaction [262]; and (iii) the mediation of the positive regulation of osteoblast differentiation [263]. In addition, most observations from studies in preclinical models of neurodegenerative diseases based on exogenous neurotoxins are not confirmed by clinical studies [264–266]. Similar observations emerge from studies in transgenic animals, where complex functional adaptations from gene knock-in or knock-out may limit the translational importance of findings [267–269]. In the case of neurodegenerative conditions, at least some of the controversy regarding changes in calcineurin/NFAT activity and/or expression appears to be due to the methodologies employed to measure activities and expression levels. Calcineurin, in particular, is highly sensitive to proteolysis during injury and neurodegeneration. However, most commercial antibodies to calcineurin only detect full-length calcineurin and miss the detection of high activity proteolytic fragments. Also, many studies have tended to measure calcineurin activity in whole brain tissue homogenates using commercially available phosphatase assays. While these kinds of assays are very good for kinetic analyses, they are very poor at assessing endogenous calcineurin activity toward endogenous substrates. Certainly, methodological challenges may have affected the quality of data generated by different groups. Although it appears that better models are needed, we also propose that better characterization of intracellular signaling in currently available and future experimental models may improve the translational importance of the findings.

6. Concluding Remarks

Calcineurin/NFAT pathway is pivotal during nervous system development and in various functions of mature central and peripheral nervous system. Notably, this signaling pathway is involved in myelination, corticogenesis, synaptogenesis, neuritogenesis, endosome trafficking, homeostatic synaptic plasticity, learning, and memory. Experimental evidence also shows that alterations in the activity of calcineurin/NFAT pathway and in activities of its endogenous regulators in the nervous system microvascular endothelial cells, astrocytes, microglia, Schwann cells, oligodendrocytes, and neurons participate in the pathogenesis of neurodegenerative diseases and conditions, but also psychotic disorders. Studies in transgenic animals and in cell lines also suggested that neurodegeneration-associated detrimental changes in calcineurin/NFAT signaling are NFAT isoform-selective as changes in NFATc3 and NFATc4, but not NFATc1 or NFATc2, are usually common. In addition pharmacological inhibition mitigated neuronal and astrocyte loss and improved cognitive functions in many models. However, other studies reported beneficial roles of calcineurin/NFAT in neurodegenerative diseases and conditions, in particular those reporting neurotoxic effects of pharmacological inhibition and increased endogenous regulation. These studies suggested that calcineurin can mediate both neuroprotective and neurodegenerative signals according to poorly understood determinant factors, which included the activation status of astrocytes in the central nervous system. Future studies should be devised to characterize better the factors determining the outcome of calcineurin/NFAT signaling in neurodegenerative diseases and conditions, as well as the downstream targets mediating the beneficial and detrimental effects of this signaling pathway, considering the implications for therapy.

Competing Interests

Authors have no conflict of interests.

References

[1] M. J. Berridge, M. D. Bootman, and H. L. Roderick, "Calcium signalling: dynamics, homeostasis and remodelling," *Nature Reviews Molecular Cell Biology*, vol. 4, no. 7, pp. 517–529, 2003.

[2] A. M. Cárdenas and F. D. Marengo, "How the stimulus defines the dynamics of vesicle pool recruitment, fusion mode, and vesicle recycling in neuroendocrine cells," *Journal of Neurochemistry*, vol. 137, no. 6, pp. 867–879, 2016.

[3] M. Buchholz and V. Ellenrieder, "An emerging role for Ca^{2+}/calcineurin/NFAT signaling in cancerogenesis," *Cell Cycle*, vol. 6, no. 1, pp. 16–19, 2007.

[4] A. Gafter-Gvili, B. Sredni, R. Gal, U. Gafter, and Y. Kalechman, "Cyclosporin A-induced hair growth in mice is associated with inhibition of calcineurin-dependent activation of NFAT in follicular keratinocytes," *American Journal of Physiology—Cell Physiology*, vol. 284, no. 6, pp. C1593–C1603, 2003.

[5] I. A. Graef, F. Chen, L. Chen, A. Kuo, and G. R. Crabtree, "Signals transduced by Ca^{2+}/calcineurin and NFATc3/c4 pattern the developing vasculature," *Cell*, vol. 105, no. 7, pp. 863–875, 2001.

[6] J. J. Heit, Å. A. Apelqvist, X. Gu et al., "Calcineurin/NFAT signalling regulates pancreatic β-cell growth and function," *Nature*, vol. 443, no. 7109, pp. 345–349, 2006.

[7] V. Horsley, A. O. Aliprantis, L. Polak, L. H. Glimcher, and E. Fuchs, "NFATc1 balances quiescence and proliferation of skin stem cells," *Cell*, vol. 132, no. 2, pp. 299–310, 2008.

[8] S.-C. Kao, H. Wu, J. Xie et al., "Calcineurin/NFAT signaling is required for neuregulin-regulated Schwann cell differentiation," *Science*, vol. 323, no. 5914, pp. 651–654, 2009.

[9] M. J. Kipanyula, A. Woodhoo, M. Rahman, D. Payne, K. R. Jessen, and R. Mirsky, "Calcineurin-nuclear factor of activated t cells regulation of Krox-20 expression in Schwann cells requires elevation of intracellular cyclic AMP," *Journal of Neuroscience Research*, vol. 91, no. 1, pp. 105–115, 2013.

[10] M. C. Lawrence, N. Borenstein-Auerbach, K. McGlynn et al., "NFAT targets signaling molecules to gene promoters in pancreatic β-cells," *Molecular Endocrinology*, vol. 29, no. 2, pp. 274–288, 2015.

[11] C. Mammucari, A. T. D. Vignano, A. A. Sharov et al., "Integration of Notch 1 and calcineurin/NFAT signaling pathways in keratinocyte growth and differentiation control," *Developmental Cell*, vol. 8, no. 5, pp. 665–676, 2005.

[12] X.-S. Wu, Z. Zhang, W.-D. Zhao, D. Wang, F. Luo, and L.-G. Wu, "Calcineurin is universally involved in vesicle endocytosis at neuronal and nonneuronal secretory cells," *Cell Reports*, vol. 7, no. 4, pp. 982–988, 2014.

[13] J. C. Braz, O. F. Bueno, Q. Liang et al., "Targeted inhibition of p38 MAPK promotes hypertrophic cardiomyopathy through upregulation of calcineurin-NFAT signaling," *The Journal of Clinical Investigation*, vol. 111, no. 10, pp. 1475–1486, 2003.

[14] G. R. Crabtree and E. N. Olson, "NFAT signaling: choreographing the social lives of cells," *Cell*, vol. 109, no. 2, supplement 1, pp. S67–S79, 2002.

[15] T. Minami, S. Jiang, K. Schadler et al., "The calcineurin-NFAT-angiopoietin-2 signaling axis in lung endothelium is critical for the establishment of lung metastases," *Cell Reports*, vol. 4, no. 4, pp. 709–723, 2013.

[16] E. N. Olson and R. S. Williams, "Calcineurin signaling and muscle remodeling," *Cell*, vol. 101, no. 7, pp. 689–692, 2000.

[17] B. Pyrzynska, A. Lis, G. Mosieniak, and B. Kaminska, "Cyclosporin A-sensitive signaling pathway involving calcineurin regulates survival of reactive astrocytes," *Neurochemistry International*, vol. 38, no. 5, pp. 409–415, 2001.

[18] R. P. Sah, R. K. Dawra, and A. K. Saluja, "New insights into the pathogenesis of pancreatitis," *Current Opinion in Gastroenterology*, vol. 29, no. 5, pp. 523–530, 2013.

[19] B. Artegiani, A. M. de Jesus Domingues, S. Bragado Alonso et al., "Tox: a multifunctional transcription factor and novel regulator of mammalian corticogenesis," *The EMBO Journal*, vol. 34, no. 7, pp. 896–910, 2015.

[20] M. Fukuchi, A. Tabuchi, Y. Kuwana et al., "Neuromodulatory effect of Gαs- or Gαq-coupled G-protein-coupled receptor on NMDA receptor selectively activates the NMDA receptor/Ca^{2+}/calcineurin/cAMP response element-binding protein-regulated transcriptional coactivator 1 pathway to effectively induce brain-derived neurotrophic factor expression in neurons," *The Journal of Neuroscience*, vol. 35, no. 14, pp. 5606–5624, 2015.

[21] S. Sawamura, M. Hatano, Y. Takada et al., "Screening of transient receptor potential canonical channel activators identifies novel neurotrophic piperazine compounds," *Molecular Pharmacology*, vol. 89, no. 3, pp. 348–363, 2016.

[22] M. C. Serrano-Pérez, M. Fernández, F. Neria et al., "NFAT transcription factors regulate survival, proliferation, migration, and differentiation of neural precursor cells," *Glia*, vol. 63, no. 6, pp. 987–1004, 2015.

[23] M. Tsuda, "Gene regulation involved in the formation of long-term memory," *Yakugaku Zasshi*, vol. 135, no. 4, pp. 597–617, 2015.

[24] D. Dubey and B. E. Porter, "CRTC1 nuclear localization in the hippocampus of the pilocarpine-induced status epilepticus model of temporal lobe epilepsy," *Neuroscience*, vol. 320, pp. 43–56, 2016.

[25] S. Kim, C. J. Violette, and E. B. Ziff, "Reduction of increased calcineurin activity rescues impaired homeostatic synaptic plasticity in presenilin 1 M146V mutant," *Neurobiology of Aging*, vol. 36, no. 12, pp. 3239–3246, 2015.

[26] B. Mojsa, S. Mora, J. P. Bossowski, I. Lassot, and S. Desagher, "Control of neuronal apoptosis by reciprocal regulation of NFATc3 and Trim17," *Cell Death and Differentiation*, vol. 22, no. 2, pp. 274–286, 2015.

[27] T. Boczek, B. Ferenc, M. Lisek, and L. Zylinska, "Regulation of GAP43/calmodulin complex formation via calcineurin-dependent mechanism in differentiated PC12 cells with altered PMCA isoforms composition," *Molecular and Cellular Biochemistry*, vol. 407, no. 1-2, pp. 251–262, 2015.

[28] R. S. Osorio, E. L. Ducca, M. E. Wohlleber et al., "Orexin-A is associated with increases in cerebrospinal fluid phosphorylated-tau in cognitively normal elderly subjects," *Sleep*, vol. 39, no. 6, pp. 1253–1260, 2016.

[29] A. P. Spira, C. E. Gonzalez, V. K. Venkatraman et al., "Sleep duration and subsequent cortical thinning in cognitively normal older adults," *Sleep*, vol. 39, no. 5, pp. 1121–1128, 2016.

[30] E. M. Anderson, T. Reeves, K. Kapernaros, J. K. Neubert, and R. M. Caudle, "Phosphorylation of the *N*-methyl-D-aspartate receptor is increased in the nucleus accumbens during both acute and extended morphine withdrawal," *Journal of Pharmacology and Experimental Therapeutics*, vol. 355, no. 3, pp. 496–505, 2015.

[31] R. Eckel, B. Szulc, M. C. Walker, and J. T. Kittler, "Activation of calcineurin underlies altered trafficking of $\alpha 2$ subunit containing GABAA receptors during prolonged epileptiform activity," *Neuropharmacology*, vol. 88, pp. 82–90, 2015.

[32] G. Li, W. Yan, Y. Dang, J. Li, C. Liu, and J. Wang, "The role of calcineurin signaling in microcystin-LR triggered neuronal toxicity," *Scientific Reports*, vol. 5, Article ID 11271, 2015.

[33] J. Liu, X. Li, L. Chen, P. Xue, Q. Yang, and A. Wang, "Increased calcineurin expression after pilocarpine-induced status epilepticus is associated with brain focal edema and astrogliosis," *International Journal of Neuroscience*, vol. 126, no. 6, pp. 560–567, 2016.

[34] A. Madineni, Q. Alhadidi, and Z. A. Shah, "Cofilin inhibition restores neuronal cell death in oxygen-glucose deprivation model of ischemia," *Molecular Neurobiology*, vol. 53, no. 2, pp. 867–878, 2016.

[35] E. Piccart, N. A. Courtney, S. Y. Branch, C. P. Ford, and M. J. Beckstead, "Neurotensin induces presynaptic depression of D_2 dopamine autoreceptor-mediated neurotransmission in midbrain dopaminergic neurons," *Journal of Neuroscience*, vol. 35, no. 31, pp. 11144–11152, 2015.

[36] Z. Mei, P. Yan, X. Tan, S. Zheng, and B. Situ, "Transcriptional regulation of BACE1 by NFAT3 leads to enhanced amyloidogenic processing," *Neurochemical Research*, vol. 40, no. 4, pp. 829–836, 2015.

[37] H. Vihma, M. Luhakooder, P. Pruunsild, and T. Timmusk, "Regulation of different human NFAT isoforms by neuronal activity," *Journal of Neurochemistry*, vol. 137, no. 3, pp. 394–408, 2016.

[38] L.-J. Chen, Y.-J. Wang, J.-R. Chen, and G.-F. Tseng, "NMDA receptor triggered molecular cascade underlies compression-induced rapid dendritic spine plasticity in cortical neurons," *Experimental Neurology*, vol. 266, pp. 86–98, 2015.

[39] J. L. Furman, P. Sompol, S. D. Kraner et al., "Blockade of astrocytic calcineurin/NFAT signaling helps to normalize hippocampal synaptic function and plasticity in a rat model of traumatic brain injury," *The Journal of Neuroscience*, vol. 36, no. 5, pp. 1502–1515, 2016.

[40] K. J. Gan and M. A. Silverman, "Dendritic and axonal mechanisms of Ca^{2+} elevation impair BDNF transport in $A\beta$ oligomer-treated hippocampal neurons," *Molecular Biology of the Cell*, vol. 26, no. 6, pp. 1058–1071, 2015.

[41] M. Gratuze, A. Noël, C. Julien et al., "Tau hyperphosphorylation and deregulation of calcineurin inmousemodels of Huntington's disease," *Human Molecular Genetics*, vol. 24, no. 1, pp. 86–99, 2015.

[42] H. C. Ho, T. S. Teo, R. Desai, and J. H. Wang, "Catalytic and regulatory properties of two forms of bovine heart cyclic nucleotide phosphodiesterase," *Biochimica et Biophysica Acta (BBA)—Enzymology*, vol. 429, no. 2, pp. 461–473, 1976.

[43] J. H. Wang and R. Desai, "A brain protein and its effect on the CA2+-and protein modulator-activated cyclic nucleotide phosphodiesterase," *Biochemical and Biophysical Research Communications*, vol. 72, no. 3, pp. 926–932, 1976.

[44] H. Li, A. Rao, and P. G. Hogan, "Interaction of calcineurin with substrates and targeting proteins," *Trends in Cell Biology*, vol. 21, no. 2, pp. 91–103, 2011.

[45] F. Rusnak and P. Mertz, "Calcineurin: form and function," *Physiological Reviews*, vol. 80, no. 4, pp. 1483–1521, 2000.

[46] F. Mathieu, S. Miot, B. Etain et al., "Association between the PPP3CC gene, coding for the calcineurin gamma catalytic subunit, and bipolar disorder," *Behavioral and Brain Functions*, vol. 4, article 2, 2008.

[47] C. R. Williams and J. L. Gooch, "Calcineurin inhibitors and immunosuppression—a tale of two isoforms," *Expert Reviews in Molecular Medicine*, vol. 14, article e14, 2012.

[48] R. J. Bram, D. T. Hung, P. K. Martin, S. L. Schreiber, and G. R. Crabtree, "Identification of the immunophilins capable of mediating inhibition of signal transduction by cyclosporin A and FK506: roles of calcineurin binding and cellular location," *Molecular and Cellular Biology*, vol. 13, no. 8, pp. 4760–4769, 1993.

[49] N. Usuda, H. Arai, H. Sasaki et al., "Differential subcellular localization of neural isoforms of the catalytic subunit of calmodulin-dependent protein phosphatase (calcineurin) in central nervous system neurons: immunohistochemistry on formalin-fixed paraffin sections employing antigen retrieval by microwave irradiation," *Journal of Histochemistry and Cytochemistry*, vol. 44, no. 1, pp. 13–18, 1996.

[50] S. Mehta, N.-N. Aye-Han, A. Ganesan, L. Oldach, K. Gorshkov, and J. Zhang, "Calmodulin-controlled spatial decoding of oscillatory Ca^{2+} signals by calcineurin," *eLife*, vol. 3, article e03765, 2014.

[51] S. Mehta and J. Zhang, "Using a genetically encoded FRET-based reporter to visualize calcineurin phosphatase activity in living cells," *Methods in Molecular Biology*, vol. 1071, pp. 139–149, 2014.

[52] F. A. Anthony, M. A. Winkler, H. H. Edwards, and W. Y. Cheung, "Quantitative subcellular localization of calmodulin-dependent phosphatase in chick forebrain," *The Journal of Neuroscience*, vol. 8, no. 4, pp. 1245–1253, 1988.

[53] M. Boothby, "Cracking the code without rosetta: molecular regulation of calcium-stimulated gene transcription after T cell activation," *The Journal of Immunology*, vol. 185, no. 9, pp. 4969–4971, 2010.

[54] R. A. Schulz and K. E. Yutzey, "Calcineurin signaling and NFAT activation in cardiovascular and skeletal muscle development," *Developmental Biology*, vol. 266, no. 1, pp. 1–16, 2004.

[55] J.-P. Shaw, P. J. Utz, D. B. Durand, J. J. Toole, E. A. Emmel, and G. R. Crabtree, "Identification of a putative regulator of early T cell activation genes," *Journal of Immunology*, vol. 185, no. 9, pp. 4972–4975, 2010.

[56] H. Vihma, P. Pruunsild, and T. Timmusk, "Alternative splicing and expression of human and mouse NFAT genes," *Genomics*, vol. 92, no. 5, pp. 279–291, 2008.

[57] L. Jin, P. Sliz, L. Chen et al., "An asymmetric NFAT1 dimer on a pseudo-palindromic κB-like DNA site," *Nature Structural Biology*, vol. 10, no. 10, pp. 807–811, 2003.

[58] J. Aramburu, F. García-Cózar, A. Raghavan, H. Okamura, A. Rao, and P. G. Hogan, "Selective inhibition of NFAT activation by a peptide spanning the calcineurin targeting site of NFAT," *Molecular Cell*, vol. 1, no. 5, pp. 627–637, 1998.

[59] M. R. Müller, Y. Sasaki, I. Stevanovic et al., "Requirement for balanced Ca/NFAT signaling in hematopoietic and embryonic development," *Proceedings of the National Academy of Sciences of the United States of America*, vol. 106, no. 17, pp. 7034–7039, 2009.

[60] Z. Qian, P. G. Dougherty, T. Liu et al., "Structure-based optimization of a peptidyl inhibitor against calcineurin-nuclear factor of activated T cell (NFAT) interaction," *Journal of Medicinal Chemistry*, vol. 57, no. 18, pp. 7792–7797, 2014.

[61] Q. Wang, Y. Zhou, P. Rychahou, C. Liu, H. L. Weiss, and B. M. Evers, "NFAT5 represses canonical Wnt signaling via inhibition of β-catenin acetylation and participates in regulating intestinal cell differentiation," *Cell Death and Disease*, vol. 4, article e671, 2013.

[62] D. V. Faget, P. I. Lucena, B. K. Robbs, and J. P. B. Viola, "NFAT1 C-terminal domains are necessary but not sufficient for inducing cell death," *PLoS ONE*, vol. 7, no. 10, article e47868, 2012.

[63] M. De Lumley, D. J. Hart, M. A. Cooper, S. Symeonides, and J. M. Blackburn, "A biophysical characterisation of factors controlling dimerisation and selectivity in the NF-κB and NFAT families," *Journal of Molecular Biology*, vol. 339, no. 5, pp. 1059–1075, 2004.

[64] S. A. Wolfe, P. Zhou, V. Dötsch et al., "Unusual rel-like architecture in the DNA-binding domain of the transcription factor NFATc," *Nature*, vol. 385, no. 6612, pp. 172–176, 1997.

[65] D. L. Bates, K. K. B. Barthel, Y. Wu et al., "Crystal structure of NFAT bound to the HIV-1 LTR tandem κB enhancer element," *Structure*, vol. 16, no. 5, pp. 684–694, 2008.

[66] C.-H. Chen, V. A. Martin, N. M. Gorenstein, R. L. Geahlen, and C. B. Post, "Two closely spaced tyrosines regulate NFAT signaling in B cells via Syk association with Vav," *Molecular and Cellular Biology*, vol. 31, no. 14, pp. 2984–2996, 2011.

[67] E. Dirkx, M. M. Gladka, L. E. Philippen et al., "Nfat and miR-25 cooperate to reactivate the transcription factor Hand2 in heart failure," *Nature Cell Biology*, vol. 15, no. 11, pp. 1282–1293, 2013.

[68] H. Hu, I. Djuretic, M. S. Sundrud, and A. Rao, "Transcriptional partners in regulatory T cells: Foxp3, Runx and NFAT," *Trends in Immunology*, vol. 28, no. 8, pp. 329–332, 2007.

[69] S.-H. Im and A. Rao, "Activation and deactivation of gene expression by Ca^{2+}/calcineurin-NFAT-mediated signaling," *Molecules and Cells*, vol. 18, no. 1, pp. 1–9, 2004.

[70] F. Macián, C. López-Rodríguez, and A. Rao, "Partners in transcription: NFAT and AP-1," *Oncogene*, vol. 20, no. 19, pp. 2476–2489, 2001.

[71] K. Park, J.-H. Park, W.-J. Yang, J.-J. Lee, M.-J. Song, and H.-P. Kim, "Transcriptional activation of the IL31 gene by NFAT and STAT6," *Journal of Leukocyte Biology*, vol. 91, no. 2, pp. 245–257, 2012.

[72] Y. J. Shyu, C. D. Suarez, and C.-D. Hu, "Visualization of AP-1-NF-κB ternary complexes in living cells by using a BiFC-based FRET," *Proceedings of the National Academy of Sciences of the United States of America*, vol. 105, no. 1, pp. 151–156, 2008.

[73] W. Wang, J. Lou, R. Zhong et al., "The roles of Ca^{2+}/NFAT signaling genes in kawasaki disease: single-and multiple-risk genetic variants," *Scientific Reports*, vol. 4, article 5208, 2014.

[74] J. Zuo, F. Wu, Y. Liu et al., "MicroRNA transcriptome profile analysis in porcine muscle and the effect of miR-143 on the MYH7 gene and protein," *PLoS ONE*, vol. 10, no. 4, Article ID e0124873, 2015.

[75] I. A. Graef, F. Wang, F. Charron et al., "Neurotrophins and netrins require calcineurin/NFAT signaling to stimulate outgrowth of embryonic axons," *Cell*, vol. 113, no. 5, pp. 657–670, 2003.

[76] G. L. Hernández, O. V. Volpert, M. A. Íñiguez et al., "Selective inhibition of vascular endothelial growth factor-mediated angiogenesis by cyclosporin A: roles of the nuclear factor of activated T cells and cyclooxygenase 2," *Journal of Experimental Medicine*, vol. 193, no. 5, pp. 607–620, 2001.

[77] M.-S. Kim, L. P. Shutov, A. Gnanasekaran et al., "Nerve growth factor (NGF) regulates activity of nuclear factor of activated T-cells (NFAT) in neurons via the phosphatidylinositol 3-kinase (PI3K)-Akt-glycogen synthase kinase 3β (GSK3β) pathway," *The Journal of Biological Chemistry*, vol. 289, no. 45, pp. 31349–31360, 2014.

[78] E. H. Y. Tong, J.-J. Guo, S.-X. Xu et al., "Inducible nucleosome depletion at OREBP-binding-sites by hypertonic stress," *PLoS ONE*, vol. 4, no. 12, article e8435, 2009.

[79] A. Canellada, B. G. Ramirez, T. Minami, J. M. Redondo, and E. Cano, "Calcium/calcineurin signaling in primary cortical astrocyte cultures: Rcan1-4 and cyclooxygenase-2 as NFAT target genes," *Glia*, vol. 56, no. 7, pp. 709–722, 2008.

[80] V. Horsley and G. K. Pavlath, "NFAT: ubiquitous regulator of cell differentiation and adaptation," *Journal of Cell Biology*, vol. 156, no. 5, pp. 771–774, 2002.

[81] S. Reppert, E. Zinser, C. Holzinger, L. Sandrock, S. Koch, and S. Finotto, "NFATc1 deficiency in T cells protects mice from experimental autoimmune encephalomyelitis," *European Journal of Immunology*, vol. 45, no. 5, pp. 1426–1440, 2015.

[82] D. Park, D.-Y. Jhon, C.-W. Lee, K.-H. Lee, and S. G. Rhee, "Activation of phospholipase C isozymes by G protein $\beta\gamma$ subunits," *The Journal of Biological Chemistry*, vol. 268, no. 7, pp. 4573–4576, 1993.

[83] D. Mandikian, E. Bocksteins, L. K. Parajuli et al., "Cell type-specific spatial and functional coupling between mammalian brain Kv2.1 K^+ channels and ryanodine receptors," *Journal of Comparative Neurology*, vol. 522, no. 15, pp. 3555–3574, 2014.

[84] F. J. Muñoz, J. A. Godoy, W. Cerpa, I. M. Poblete, J. P. Huidobro-Toro, and N. C. Inestrosa, "Wnt-5a increases NO and modulates NMDA receptor in rat hippocampal neurons," *Biochemical and Biophysical Research Communications*, vol. 444, no. 2, pp. 189–194, 2014.

[85] W. C. Oh, L. K. Parajuli, and K. Zito, "Heterosynaptic structural plasticity on local dendritic segments of hippocampal CA1 neurons," *Cell Reports*, vol. 10, no. 2, pp. 162–169, 2015.

[86] T. Vervliet, J. B. Parys, and G. Bultynck, "Bcl-2 and FKBP12 bind to IP_3 and ryanodine receptors at overlapping sites: the complexity of protein-protein interactions for channel regulation," *Biochemical Society Transactions*, vol. 43, pp. 396–404, 2015.

[87] Y. Yamazaki, S. Fujii, J.-I. Goto, H. Fujiwara, and K. Mikoshiba, "Activation of inositol 1,4,5-trisphosphate receptors during preconditioning low-frequency stimulation suppresses subsequent induction of long-term potentiation in hippocampal CA1 neurons," *Neuroscience*, vol. 311, pp. 195–206, 2015.

[88] H. Okamura, J. Aramburu, C. García-Rodríguez et al., "Concerted dephosphorylation of the transcription factor NFAT1 induces a conformational switch that regulates transcriptional activity," *Molecular Cell*, vol. 6, no. 3, pp. 539–550, 2000.

[89] Z.-H. Deng, T. S. Gomez, D. G. Osborne, C. A. Phillips-Krawczak, J.-S. Zhang, and D. D. Billadeau, "Nuclear FAM21 participates in NF-κB-dependent gene regulation in pancreatic cancer cells," *Journal of Cell Science*, vol. 128, no. 2, pp. 373–384, 2015.

[90] R. S. Lewis, "Calcium oscillations in T-cells: mechanisms and consequences for gene expression," *Biochemical Society Transactions*, vol. 31, no. 5, pp. 925–929, 2003.

[91] A. N. Mitchell, L. Jayakumar, I. Koleilat et al., "Brain expression of the calcineurin inhibitor RCAN1 (Adapt78)," *Archives of Biochemistry and Biophysics*, vol. 467, no. 2, pp. 185–192, 2007.

[92] A. Patel, N. Yamashita, M. Ascaño et al., "RCAN1 links impaired neurotrophin trafficking to aberrant development of the sympathetic nervous system in Down syndrome," *Nature Communications*, vol. 6, Article ID 10119, 2015.

[93] P. G. Hogan, L. Chen, J. Nardone, and A. Rao, "Transcriptional regulation by calcium, calcineurin, and NFAT," *Genes and Development*, vol. 17, no. 18, pp. 2205–2232, 2003.

[94] E. Kilanczyk, A. Filipek, and M. Hetman, "Calcyclin-binding protein/Siah-1-interacting protein as a regulator of transcriptional responses in brain cells," *Journal of Neuroscience Research*, vol. 93, no. 1, pp. 75–81, 2015.

[95] P. G. Del Arco, S. Martínez-Martínez, J. L. Maldonado, I. Ortega-Pérez, and J. M. Redondo, "A role for the p38 MAP kinase pathway in the nuclear shuttling of NFATp," *Journal of Biological Chemistry*, vol. 275, no. 18, pp. 13872–13878, 2000.

[96] P. J. Dittmer, M. L. Dell'Acqua, and W. A. Sather, "Ca^{2+}/calcineurin-dependent inactivation of neuronal L-type Ca^{2+} channels requires priming by AKAP-anchored protein kinase A," *Cell Reports*, vol. 7, no. 5, pp. 1410–1416, 2014.

[97] B. K. Samelson, B. B. Gore, J. L. Whiting et al., "A-kinase anchoring protein 79/150 recruits protein kinase C to phosphorylate roundabout receptors," *The Journal of Biological Chemistry*, vol. 290, no. 22, pp. 14107–14119, 2015.

[98] Y. Wen, P. Zhou, L. Liu, Z. Wang, Y. Zhang, and J. Liang, "Effect of the knockdown of Cabin1 on p53 in glomerular podocyte," *Journal of Receptors and Signal Transduction*, vol. 36, no. 2, pp. 173–180, 2016.

[99] J.-K. Yi, H.-J. Kim, D.-H. Yu et al., "Regulation of inflammatory responses and fibroblast-like synoviocyte apoptosis by calcineurin-binding protein 1 in mice with collagen-induced arthritis," *Arthritis and Rheumatism*, vol. 64, no. 7, pp. 2191–2200, 2012.

[100] F. Di Sole, K. Vadnagara, O. W. Moe, and V. Babich, "Calcineurin homologous protein: a multifunctional Ca^{2+}-binding protein family," *American Journal of Physiology—Renal Physiology*, vol. 303, no. 2, pp. F165–F179, 2012.

[101] Y. Kobayashi, R. da Silva, H. Kumanogoh et al., "Ganglioside contained in the neuronal tissue-enriched acidic protein of 22 kDa (NAP-22) fraction prepared from the detergent-resistant membrane microdomain of rat brain inhibits the phosphatase activity of calcineurin," *Journal of Neuroscience Research*, vol. 93, no. 9, pp. 1462–1470, 2015.

[102] X. Lin, R. A. Sikkink, F. Rusnak, and D. L. Barber, "Inhibition of calcineurin phosphatase activity by a calcineurin B homologous protein," *The Journal of Biological Chemistry*, vol. 274, no. 51, pp. 36125–36131, 1999.

[103] R. B. Vega, J. Yang, B. A. Rothermel, R. Bassel-Duby, and R. S. Williams, "Multiple domains of MCIP1 contribute to inhibition of calcineurin activity," *Journal of Biological Chemistry*, vol. 277, no. 33, pp. 30401–30407, 2002.

[104] C. Brandt, V. Pavlovic, A. Radbruch, M. Worm, and R. Baumgrass, "Low-dose cyclosporine A therapy increases the regulatory T cell population in patients with atopic dermatitis," *Allergy*, vol. 64, no. 11, pp. 1588–1596, 2009.

[105] J. Cury Martins, C. Martins, V. Aoki, A. F. T. Gois, H. A. Ishii, and E. M. K. da Silva, "Topical tacrolimus for atopic dermatitis," *The Cochrane Database of Systematic Reviews*, no. 7, Article ID CD009864, 2015.

[106] B. Höcker and B. Tönshoff, "Calcineurin inhibitor-free immunosuppression in pediatric renal transplantation: a viable option?" *Pediatric Drugs*, vol. 13, no. 1, pp. 49–69, 2011.

[107] J. M. Tredger, N. W. Brown, and A. Dhawan, "Calcineurin inhibitor sparing in paediatric solid organ transplantation: managing the efficacy/toxicity conundrum," *Drugs*, vol. 68, no. 10, pp. 1385–1414, 2008.

[108] B. Kaminska, I. Figiel, B. Pyrzynska, R. Czajkowski, and G. Mosieniak, "Treatment of hippocampal neurons with cyclosporin A results in calcium overload and apoptosis which are independent on NMDA receptor activation," *British Journal of Pharmacology*, vol. 133, no. 7, pp. 997–1004, 2001.

[109] J. Klawitter, S. Gottschalk, C. Hainz, D. Leibfritz, U. Christians, and N. J. Serkova, "Immunosuppressant neurotoxicity in rat brain models: oxidative stress and cellular metabolism," *Chemical Research in Toxicology*, vol. 23, no. 3, pp. 608–619, 2010.

[110] R. Gómez-Sintes and J. J. Lucas, "NFAT/Fas signaling mediates the neuronal apoptosis and motor side effects of GSK-3 inhibition in a mouse model of lithium therapy," *The Journal of Clinical Investigation*, vol. 120, no. 7, pp. 2432–2445, 2010.

[111] L. Bica, J. R. Liddell, P. S. Donnelly et al., "Neuroprotective copper bis(thiosemicarbazonato) complexes promote neurite elongation," *PLoS ONE*, vol. 9, no. 2, Article ID e90070, 2014.

[112] T. Johanssen, N. Suphantarida, P. S. Donnelly et al., "PBT2 inhibits glutamate-induced excitotoxicity in neurons through metal-mediated preconditioning," *Neurobiology of Disease*, vol. 81, pp. 176–185, 2015.

[113] F. Rapisarda, G. Portale, S. Ferrario et al., "Magnesium, calcium and potassium: 'no one was born alone,'" *Giornale Italiano di Nefrologia*, vol. 33, 2016.

[114] S.-R. Chen, Y.-M. Hu, H. Chen, and H.-L. Pan, "Calcineurin inhibitor induces pain hypersensitivity by potentiating pre- and postsynaptic NMDA receptor activity in spinal cords," *Journal of Physiology*, vol. 592, no. 1, pp. 215–227, 2014.

[115] S.-R. Chen, H.-Y. Zhou, H. S. Byun, H. Chen, and H.-L. Pan, "Casein kinase II regulates *N*-methyl-D-aspartate receptor activity in spinal cords and pain hypersensitivity induced by nerve injury," *The Journal of Pharmacology and Experimental Therapeutics*, vol. 350, no. 2, pp. 301–312, 2014.

[116] G. Miletic, J. L. Hermes, G. L. Bosscher, B. M. Meier, and V. Miletic, "Protein kinase C gamma-mediated phosphorylation of GluA1 in the postsynaptic density of spinal dorsal horn neurons accompanies neuropathic pain, and dephosphorylation by calcineurin is associated with prolonged analgesia," *PAIN*, vol. 156, no. 12, pp. 2514–2520, 2015.

[117] Y.-M. Hu, S.-R. Chen, H. Chen, and H.-L. Pan, "Casein kinase II inhibition reverses pain hypersensitivity and potentiated spinal N-methyl-D-aspartate receptor activity caused by calcineurin inhibitor," *Journal of Pharmacology and Experimental Therapeutics*, vol. 349, no. 2, pp. 239–247, 2014.

[118] H. J. Solinski, F. Petermann, K. Rothe, I. Boekhoff, T. Gudermann, and A. Breit, "Human Mas-related G protein-coupled receptors-X1 induce chemokine receptor 2 expression in rat dorsal root ganglia neurons and release of chemokine ligand 2 from the human LAD-2 mast cell line," *PLoS ONE*, vol. 8, no. 3, Article ID e58756, 2013.

[119] M. H. A. Roehrl, J. Y. Wang, and G. Wagner, "Discovery of small-molecule inhibitors of the NFAT-calcineurin interaction by competitive high-throughput fluorescence polarization screening," *Biochemistry*, vol. 43, no. 51, pp. 16067–16075, 2004.

[120] K. Takeuchi, M. H. A. Roehrl, Z.-Y. J. Sun, and G. Wagner, "Structure of the calcineurin-NFAT complex: defining a T cell activation switch using solution NMR and crystal coordinates," *Structure*, vol. 15, no. 5, pp. 587–597, 2007.

[121] B. Ding, W. Wang, T. Selvakumar et al., "Temporal regulation of nuclear factor one occupancy by calcineurin/NFAT governs a voltage-sensitive developmental switch in late maturing neurons," *The Journal of Neuroscience*, vol. 33, no. 7, pp. 2860–2872, 2013.

[122] A. Cho, Y. Tang, J. Davila et al., "Calcineurin signaling regulates neural induction through antagonizing the BMP pathway," *Neuron*, vol. 82, no. 1, pp. 109–124, 2014.

[123] M. D. Cahalan, "STIMulating store-operated Ca^{2+} entry," *Nature Cell Biology*, vol. 11, no. 6, pp. 669–677, 2009.

[124] R. Palty, A. Raveh, I. Kaminsky, R. Meller, and E. Reuveny, "SARAF inactivates the store operated calcium entry machinery to prevent excess calcium refilling," *Cell*, vol. 149, no. 2, pp. 425–438, 2012.

[125] A. Somasundaram, A. K. Shum, H. J. McBride et al., "Store-operated CRAC channels regulate gene expression and proliferation in neural progenitor cells," *The Journal of Neuroscience*, vol. 34, no. 27, pp. 9107–9123, 2014.

[126] J. D. Ulrich, M.-S. Kim, P. R. Houlihan et al., "Distinct activation properties of the nuclear factor of activated T-cells (NFAT) isoforms NFATc3 and NFATc4 in neurons," *Journal of Biological Chemistry*, vol. 287, no. 45, pp. 37594–37609, 2012.

[127] J. A. Filosa, M. T. Nelson, and L. V. Gonzalez Bosc, "Activity-dependent NFATc3 nuclear accumulation in pericytes from cortical parenchymal microvessels," *American Journal of Physiology—Cell Physiology*, vol. 293, no. 6, pp. C1797–C1805, 2007.

[128] H. Q. Yan, S. S. Shin, X. Ma, Y. Li, and C. E. Dixon, "Differential effect of traumatic brain injury on the nuclear factor of activated T Cells C3 and C4 isoforms in the rat hippocampus," *Brain Research*, vol. 1548, pp. 63–72, 2014.

[129] M. Fukuchi, Y. Kirikoshi, A. Mori et al., "Excitatory GABA induces BDNF transcription via CRTC1 and phosphorylated CREB-related pathways in immature cortical cells," *Journal of Neurochemistry*, vol. 131, no. 2, pp. 134–146, 2014.

[130] F. Niwa, H. Bannai, M. Arizono, K. Fukatsu, A. Triller, and K. Mikoshiba, "Gephyrin-independent $GABA_AR$ mobility and clustering during plasticity," *PLoS ONE*, vol. 7, no. 4, Article ID e36148, 2012.

[131] G. C. Stefos, U. Soppa, M. Dierssen, and W. Becker, "NGF upregulates the plasminogen activation inhibitor-1 in neurons via the calcineurin/NFAT pathway and the Down syndrome-related proteins DYRK1A and RCAN1 attenuate this effect," *PLoS ONE*, vol. 8, no. 6, Article ID e67470, 2013.

[132] C.-Y. Wang, H.-C. Lin, Y.-P. Song et al., "Protein kinase C-dependent growth-associated protein 43 phosphorylation regulates gephyrin aggregation at developing GABAergic synapses," *Molecular and Cellular Biology*, vol. 35, no. 10, pp. 1712–1726, 2015.

[133] F. J. Caballero, R. Soler-Torronteras, M. Lara-Chica et al., "AM404 inhibits NFAT and NF-κB signaling pathways and impairs migration and invasiveness of neuroblastoma cells," *European Journal of Pharmacology*, vol. 746, pp. 221–232, 2015.

[134] A. E. Chávez, V. M. Hernández, A. Rodenas-Ruano, C. Savio Chan, and P. E. Castillo, "Compartment-specific modulation of GABAergic synaptic transmission by TRPV1 channels in the dentate gyrus," *The Journal of Neuroscience*, vol. 34, no. 50, pp. 16621–16629, 2014.

[135] T. Hayama, J. Noguchi, S. Watanabe et al., "GABA promotes the competitive selection of dendritic spines by controlling local Ca^{2+} signaling," *Nature Neuroscience*, vol. 16, no. 10, pp. 1409–1416, 2013.

[136] H. Toyoda, M. Saito, H. Sato et al., "Enhanced desensitization followed by unusual resensitization in $GABA_A$ receptors in phospholipase C-related catalytically inactive protein-1/2 double-knockout mice," *Pflügers Archiv*, vol. 467, no. 2, pp. 267–284, 2014.

[137] B. Calabrese and S. Halpain, "Differential targeting of dynamin-1 and dynamin-3 to nerve terminals during chronic suppression of neuronal activity," *Molecular and Cellular Neuroscience*, vol. 68, pp. 36–45, 2015.

[138] D. Suo, J. Park, A. W. Harrington, L. S. Zweifel, S. Mihalas, and C. D. Deppmann, "Coronin-1 is a neurotrophin endosomal effector that is required for developmental competition for survival," *Nature Neuroscience*, vol. 17, no. 1, pp. 36–45, 2014.

[139] J. Lim, H.-S. Choi, and H. J. Choi, "Estrogen-related receptor gamma regulates dopaminergic neuronal phenotype by activating GSK3β/NFAT signaling in SH-SY5Y cells," *Journal of Neurochemistry*, vol. 133, no. 4, pp. 544–557, 2015.

[140] J. R. Cottrell, B. Li, J. W. Kyung et al., "Calcineurin Aγ is a functional phosphatase that modulates synaptic vesicle endocytosis," *The Journal of Biological Chemistry*, vol. 291, no. 4, pp. 1948–1956, 2016.

[141] D. C. Hondius, P. van Nierop, K. W. Li et al., "Profiling the human hippocampal proteome at all pathologic stages of Alzheimer's disease," *Alzheimer's & Dementia*, vol. 12, no. 6, pp. 654–668, 2016.

[142] G. Pigino, G. Morfini, Y. Atagi et al., "Disruption of fast axonal transport is a pathogenic mechanism for intraneuronal amyloid beta," *Proceedings of the National Academy of Sciences of the United States of America*, vol. 106, no. 14, pp. 5907–5912, 2009.

[143] E. M. Ramser, K. J. Gan, H. Decker et al., "Amyloid-β oligomers induce tau-independent disruption of BDNF axonal transport via calcineurin activation in cultured hippocampal neurons," *Molecular Biology of the Cell*, vol. 24, no. 16, pp. 2494–2505, 2013.

[144] P. Toglia, K. H. Cheung, D. D. Mak, and G. Ullah, "Impaired mitochondrial function due to familial Alzheimer's disease-causing presenilins mutants via Ca^{2+} disruptions," *Cell Calcium*, vol. 59, no. 5, pp. 240–250, 2016.

[145] R. Pigeat, P. Chausson, F. M. Dreyfus, N. Leresche, and R. C. Lambert, "Sleep slow wave-related homo and heterosynaptic LTD of intrathalamic $GABA_A$ergic synapses: involvement of T-type Ca^{2+} channels and metabotropic glutamate receptors," *The Journal of Neuroscience*, vol. 35, no. 1, pp. 64–73, 2015.

[146] D. M. Raizen, J. E. Zimmerman, M. H. Maycock et al., "Lethargus is a *Caenorhabditis elegans* sleep-like state," *Nature*, vol. 451, pp. 569–572, 2008.

[147] C.-O. Wong, K. Chen, Y. Lin et al., "A TRPV channel in drosophila motor neurons regulates presynaptic resting Ca^{2+} levels, synapse growth, and synaptic transmission," *Neuron*, vol. 84, no. 4, pp. 764–777, 2014.

[148] M. D. Evans, A. S. Dumitrescu, D. L. H. Kruijssen, S. E. Taylor, and M. S. Grubb, "Rapid modulation of axon initial segment length influences repetitive spike firing," *Cell Reports*, vol. 13, no. 6, pp. 1233–1245, 2015.

[149] K. L. Arendt, Z. Zhang, S. Ganesan et al., "Calcineurin mediates homeostatic synaptic plasticity by regulating retinoic acid synthesis," *Proceedings of the National Academy of Sciences of the United States of America*, vol. 112, no. 42, pp. E5744–E5752, 2015.

[150] Y. Hatanaka, Y. Hojo, H. Mukai et al., "Rapid increase of spines by dihydrotestosterone and testosterone in hippocampal neurons: dependence on synaptic androgen receptor and kinase networks," *Brain Research*, vol. 1621, pp. 121–132, 2015.

[151] Y. Hasegawa, Y. Hojo, H. Kojima et al., "Estradiol rapidly modulates synaptic plasticity of hippocampal neurons: involvement of kinase networks," *Brain Research*, vol. 1621, pp. 147–161, 2015.

[152] H. Zhang, J. Liu, S. Sun, E. Pchitskaya, E. Popugaeva, and I. Bezprozvanny, "Calcium signaling, excitability, and synaptic plasticity defects in a mouse model of Alzheimer's disease," *Journal of Alzheimer's Disease*, vol. 45, no. 2, pp. 561–580, 2015.

[153] A.-H. Chou, Y.-L. Chen, S.-H. Hu, Y.-M. Chang, and H.-L. Wang, "Polyglutamine-expanded ataxin-3impairslong-term depression in Purkinje neurons of SCA3 transgenic mouse byinhibiting HAT andimpairing histone acetylation," *Brain Research*, vol. 1583, no. 1, pp. 220–229, 2014.

[154] J. Zhang and M. S. Shapiro, "Activity-dependent transcriptional regulation of M-Type (Kv7) K^+ channels by AKAP79/150-mediated NFAT actions," *Neuron*, vol. 76, no. 6, pp. 1133–1146, 2012.

[155] A. D. Williams, S. Jung, and N. P. Poolos, "Protein kinase C bidirectionally modulates I_h and hyperpolarization-activated cyclic nucleotide-gated (HCN) channel surface expression in hippocampal pyramidal neurons," *Journal of Physiology*, vol. 593, no. 13, pp. 2779–2792, 2015.

[156] V. García-Morales, F. Montero, D. González-Forero et al., "Membrane-derived phospholipids control synaptic neurotransmission and plasticity," *PLoS Biology*, vol. 13, no. 5, Article ID e1002153, 2015.

[157] S. Kim and E. B. Ziff, "Calcineurin mediates synaptic scaling via synaptic trafficking of Ca^{2+}-permeable AMPA receptors," *PLoS Biology*, vol. 12, no. 7, Article ID e1001900, 2014.

[158] T. Yoshida and M. Mishina, "Distinct roles of calcineurin-nuclear factor of activated T cells and protein kinase A-cAMP response element-binding protein signaling in presynaptic differentiation," *Journal of Neuroscience*, vol. 25, no. 12, pp. 3067–3079, 2005.

[159] J. G. Murphy, J. L. Sanderson, J. A. Gorski et al., "AKAP-anchored PKA maintains neuronal L-type calcium channel activity and NFAT transcriptional signaling," *Cell Reports*, vol. 7, no. 5, pp. 1577–1588, 2014.

[160] H. Li, M. D. Pink, J. G. Murphy, A. Stein, M. L. Dell'Acqua, and P. G. Hogan, "Balanced interactions of calcineurin with AKAP79 regulate Ca^{2+}-calcineurin-NFAT signaling," *Nature Structural and Molecular Biology*, vol. 19, no. 3, pp. 337–345, 2012.

[161] S. R. Seo, S. S. Kim, and K. C. Chung, "Activation of adenylate cyclase by forskolin increases the protein stability of RCAN1 (DSCR1 or Adapt78)," *FEBS Letters*, vol. 583, no. 19, pp. 3140–3144, 2009.

[162] S. Deheshi, B. Dabiri, S. Fan, M. Tsang, and G. L. Rintoul, "Changes in mitochondrial morphology induced by calcium or rotenone in primary astrocytes occur predominantly through ros-mediated remodeling," *Journal of Neurochemistry*, vol. 133, no. 5, pp. 684–699, 2015.

[163] A. M. Slupe, R. A. Merrill, K. H. Flippo, M. A. Lobas, J. C. D. Houtman, and S. Strack, "A calcineurin docking motif (LXVP) in dynamin-related protein 1 contributes to mitochondrial

fragmentation and ischemic neuronal injury," *The Journal of Biological Chemistry*, vol. 288, no. 17, pp. 12353–12365, 2013.

[164] W.-D. C. Krenz, E. W. Rodgers, and D. J. Baro, "Tonic 5nM DA stabilizes neuronal output by enabling bidirectional activity-dependent regulation of the hyperpolarization activated current via PKA and calcineurin," *PLoS ONE*, vol. 10, no. 2, Article ID e0117965, 2015.

[165] K. Bacallao and P. V. Monje, "Requirement of cAMP signaling for Schwann cell differentiation restricts the onset of myelination," *PLoS ONE*, vol. 10, no. 2, Article ID e0116948, 2015.

[166] R. Nagarajan, J. Svaren, N. Le, T. Araki, M. Watson, and J. Milbrandt, "EGR2 mutations in inherited neuropathies dominant-negatively inhibit myelin gene expression," *Neuron*, vol. 30, no. 2, pp. 355–368, 2001.

[167] K. Bacallao and P. V. Monje, "Opposing roles of PKA and EPAC in the cAMP-dependent regulation of schwann cell proliferation and differentiation," *PLoS ONE*, vol. 8, no. 12, Article ID e82354, 2013.

[168] M. Finzsch, S. Schreiner, T. Kichko et al., "Sox10 is required for Schwann cell identity and progression beyond the immature Schwann cell stage," *Journal of Cell Biology*, vol. 189, no. 4, pp. 701–712, 2010.

[169] R. I. Peirano, D. E. Goerich, D. Riethmacher, and M. Wegner, "Protein zero gene expression is regulated by the glial transcription factor Sox10," *Molecular and Cellular Biology*, vol. 20, no. 9, pp. 3198–3209, 2000.

[170] A. Rao, "Signaling to gene expression: calcium, calcineurin and NFAT," *Nature Immunology*, vol. 10, no. 1, pp. 3–5, 2009.

[171] S.-W. Jang and J. Svaren, "Induction of myelin protein zero by early growth response 2 through upstream and intragenic elements," *The Journal of Biological Chemistry*, vol. 284, no. 30, pp. 20111–20120, 2009.

[172] H. Fansa, G. Keilhoff, T. Horn, S. Altmann, G. Wolf, and W. Schneider, "Stimulation of Schwann cell proliferation and axonal regeneration by FK 506," *Restorative Neurology and Neuroscience*, vol. 16, no. 2, pp. 77–86, 2000.

[173] M.-S. Guzmán-Lenis, C. Vallejo, X. Navarro, and C. Casas, "Analysis of FK506-mediated protection in an organotypic model of spinal cord damage: heat shock protein 70 levels are modulated in microglial cells," *Neuroscience*, vol. 155, no. 1, pp. 104–113, 2008.

[174] S. Nottingham, P. Knapp, and J. Springer, "Fk506 treatment inhibits caspase-3 activation and promotes oligodendroglial survival following traumatic spinal cord injury," *Experimental Neurology*, vol. 177, no. 1, pp. 242–251, 2002.

[175] L. Dietz, F. Frommer, A.-L. Vogel et al., "NFAT1 deficit and NFAT2 deficit attenuate EAE via different mechanisms," *European Journal of Immunology*, vol. 45, no. 5, pp. 1377–1389, 2015.

[176] S. Ghosh, S. B. Koralov, I. Stevanovic et al., "Hyperactivation of nuclear factor of activated T cells 1 (NFAT1) in T cells attenuates severity of murine autoimmune encephalomyelitis," *Proceedings of the National Academy of Sciences of the United States of America*, vol. 107, no. 34, pp. 15169–15174, 2010.

[177] H. M. Abdul, J. L. Furman, M. A. Sama, D. M. Mathis, and C. M. Norris, "NFATs and Alzheimer's disease," *Molecular and Cellular Pharmacology*, vol. 2, no. 1, pp. 7–14, 2010.

[178] C. M. Norris, I. Kadish, E. M. Blalock et al., "Calcineurin triggers reactive/inflammatory processes in astrocytes and is upregulated in aging and Alzheimer's models," *Journal of Neuroscience*, vol. 25, no. 18, pp. 4649–4658, 2005.

[179] M. Berrocal, I. Corbacho, M. Vázquez-Hernández, J. Ávila, M. R. Sepúlveda, and A. M. Mata, "Inhibition of PMCA activity by tau as a function of aging and Alzheimer's neuropathology," *Biochimica et Biophysica Acta—Molecular Basis of Disease*, vol. 1852, no. 7, pp. 1465–1476, 2015.

[180] M. Berrocal, D. Marcos, M. R. Sepúlveda, M. Pérez, J. Ávila, and A. M. Mata, "Altered Ca^{2+} dependence of synaptosomal plasma membrane Ca^{2+}-ATPase in human brain affected by Alzheimer's disease," *The FASEB Journal*, vol. 23, no. 6, pp. 1826–1834, 2009.

[181] C. Conejero-Goldberg, J. J. Gomar, T. Bobes-Bascaran et al., "APOE2 enhances neuroprotection against Alzheimer's disease through multiple molecular mechanisms," *Molecular Psychiatry*, vol. 19, no. 11, pp. 1243–1250, 2014.

[182] H. Hayashi, R. B. Campenot, D. E. Vance, and J. E. Vance, "Protection of neurons from apoptosis by apolipoprotein E-containing lipoproteins does not require lipoprotein uptake and involves activation of phospholipase Cγ1 and inhibition of calcineurin," *The Journal of Biological Chemistry*, vol. 284, no. 43, pp. 29605–29613, 2009.

[183] M. Shinohara, T. Kanekiyo, L. Yang et al., "*APOE2* eases cognitive decline during aging: clinical and preclinical evaluations," *Annals of Neurology*, vol. 79, no. 5, pp. 758–774, 2016.

[184] H.-Y. Wu, E. Hudry, T. Hashimoto et al., "Distinct dendritic spine and nuclear phases of calcineurin activation after exposure to amyloid-β revealed by a novel fluorescence resonance energy transfer assay," *Journal of Neuroscience*, vol. 32, no. 15, pp. 5298–5309, 2012.

[185] J. R. Casanova, M. Nishimura, and J. W. Swann, "The effects of early-life seizures on hippocampal dendrite development and later-life learning and memory," *Brain Research Bulletin*, vol. 103, pp. 39–48, 2014.

[186] H. M. Abdul, M. A. Sama, J. L. Furman et al., "Cognitive decline in Alzheimer's disease is associated with selective changes in calcineurin/NFAT signaling," *The Journal of Neuroscience*, vol. 29, no. 41, pp. 12957–12969, 2009.

[187] K. Bromley-Brits and W. Song, "The role of TMP21 in trafficking and amyloid-β precursor protein (APP) processing in Alzheimer's disease," *Current Alzheimer Research*, vol. 9, no. 4, pp. 411–424, 2012.

[188] A. A. Grolla, G. Fakhfouri, G. Balzaretti et al., "Aβ leads to Ca^{2+} signaling alterations and transcriptional changes in glial cells," *Neurobiology of Aging*, vol. 34, no. 2, pp. 511–522, 2013.

[189] D. Lim, A. Iyer, V. Ronco et al., "Amyloid beta deregulates astroglial mGluR5-mediated calcium signaling via calcineurin and Nf-kB," *Glia*, vol. 61, no. 7, pp. 1134–1145, 2013.

[190] S. Liu, S. Zhang, K. Bromley-Brits et al., "Transcriptional regulation of TMP21 by NFAT," *Molecular Neurodegeneration*, vol. 6, article 21, 2011.

[191] J. Luo, L. Sun, X. Lin et al., "A calcineurin- and NFAT-dependent pathway is involved in α-synuclein-induced degeneration of midbrain dopaminergic neurons," *Human Molecular Genetics*, vol. 23, no. 24, pp. 6567–6574, 2014.

[192] G. Caraveo, P. K. Auluck, L. Whitesell et al., "Calcineurin determines toxic versus beneficial responses to α-synuclein," *Proceedings of the National Academy of Sciences of the United States of America*, vol. 111, no. 34, pp. E3544–E3552, 2014.

[193] E. C. Miller, P. J. Teravskis, B. W. Dummer, X. Zhao, R. L. Huganir, and D. Liao, "Tau phosphorylation and tau mislocalization mediate soluble Aβ oligomer-induced AMPA glutamate receptor signaling deficits," *European Journal of Neuroscience*, vol. 39, no. 7, pp. 1214–1224, 2014.

[194] S.-H. Ma, Q.-X. Zhuang, W.-X. Shen, Y.-P. Peng, and Y.-H. Qiu, "Interleukin-6 reduces NMDAR-mediated cytosolic Ca^{2+} overload and neuronal death via JAK/CaN signaling," *Cell Calcium*, vol. 58, no. 3, pp. 286–295, 2015.

[195] K. Watanabe, K. Uemura, M. Asada et al., "The participation of insulin-like growth factor-binding protein 3 released by astrocytes in the pathology of Alzheimer's disease," *Molecular Brain*, vol. 8, article 82, 2015.

[196] G. Dobrowolny, C. Giacinti, L. Pelosi et al., "Muscle expression of a local Igf-1 isoform protects motor neurons in an ALS mouse model," *Journal of Cell Biology*, vol. 168, no. 2, pp. 193–199, 2005.

[197] A. M. Fernandez, S. Jimenez, M. Mecha et al., "Regulation of the phosphatase calcineurin by insulin-like growth factor I unveils a key role of astrocytes in Alzheimer's pathology," *Molecular Psychiatry*, vol. 17, no. 7, pp. 705–718, 2012.

[198] S. Pons and I. Torres-Aleman, "Insulin-like growth factor-I stimulates dephosphorylation of IκB through the serine phosphatase calcineurin (protein phosphatase 2B)," *Journal of Biological Chemistry*, vol. 275, no. 49, pp. 38620–38625, 2000.

[199] T. Takadera and T. Ohyashiki, "Caspase-dependent apoptosis induced by calcineurin inhibitors was prevented by glycogen synthase kinase-3 inhibitors in cultured rat cortical cells," *Brain Research*, vol. 1133, no. 1, pp. 20–26, 2007.

[200] S. Á. Álvarez, A. Blanco, M. Fresno, and M. Á. Muñoz-Fernández, "TNF-α contributes to caspase-3 independent apoptosis in neuroblastoma cells: role of NFAT," *PLoS ONE*, vol. 6, no. 1, Article ID e16100, 2011.

[201] A. Canellada, E. Cano, L. Sánchez-Ruiloba, F. Zafra, and J. M. Redondo, "Calcium-dependent expression of TNF-α in neural cells is mediated by the calcineurin/NFAT pathway," *Molecular and Cellular Neuroscience*, vol. 31, no. 4, pp. 692–701, 2006.

[202] B. Ma, J. Yu, C. Xie et al., "Toll-like receptors promote mitochondrial translocation of nuclear transcription factor nuclear factor of activated T-cells in prolonged microglial activation," *The Journal of Neuroscience*, vol. 35, no. 30, pp. 10799–10814, 2015.

[203] A. M. Fernandez, S. Fernandez, P. Carrero, M. Garcia-Garcia, and I. Torres-Aleman, "Calcineurin in reactive astrocytes plays a key role in the interplay between proinflammatory and anti-inflammatory signals," *The Journal of Neuroscience*, vol. 27, no. 33, pp. 8745–8756, 2007.

[204] B. Kim, H.-K. Jeong, J.-H. Kim, S. Y. Lee, I. Jou, and E.-H. Joe, "Uridine 5′-diphosphate induces chemokine expression in microglia and astrocytes through activation of the P2Y6 receptor," *Journal of Immunology*, vol. 186, no. 6, pp. 3701–3709, 2011.

[205] J. L. Furman, D. M. Sama, J. C. Gant et al., "Targeting astrocytes Ameliorates neurologic changes in a mouse model of Alzheimer's disease," *Journal of Neuroscience*, vol. 32, no. 46, pp. 16129–16140, 2012.

[206] H.-S. Hong, J.-Y. Hwang, S.-M. Son, Y.-H. Kim, M. Moon, and M.-J. Inhee, "FK506 reduces amyloid plaque burden and induces MMP-9 in AβPP/PS1 double transgenic mice," *Journal of Alzheimer's Disease*, vol. 22, no. 1, pp. 97–105, 2010.

[207] E. Hudry, H.-Y. Wu, M. Arbel-Ornath et al., "Inhibition of the NFAT pathway alleviates amyloid beta neurotoxicity in a mouse model of Alzheimer's disease," *Journal of Neuroscience*, vol. 32, no. 9, pp. 3176–3192, 2012.

[208] S. Kim, R. F. Titcombe, H. Zhang et al., "Network compensation of cyclic GMP-dependent protein kinase II knockout in the hippocampus by Ca^{2+}-permeable AMPA receptors," *Proceedings of the National Academy of Sciences of the United States of America*, vol. 112, no. 10, pp. 3122–3127, 2015.

[209] M. I. K. Hamad, A. Jack, O. Klatt et al., "Type I TARPs promote dendritic growth of early postnatal neocortical pyramidal cells in organotypic cultures," *Development*, vol. 141, no. 8, pp. 1737–1748, 2014.

[210] M. Itakura, I. Watanabe, T. Sugaya, and M. Takahashi, "Direct association of the unique C-terminal tail of transmembrane AMPA receptor regulatory protein γ-8 with calcineurin," *FEBS Journal*, vol. 281, no. 5, pp. 1366–1378, 2014.

[211] D. M. MacLean, S. S. Ramaswamy, M. Du, J. R. Howe, and V. Jayaraman, "Stargazin promotes closure of the AMPA receptor ligand-binding domain," *The Journal of General Physiology*, vol. 144, no. 6, pp. 503–512, 2014.

[212] O. R. Rana, E. Saygili, C. Meyer et al., "Regulation of nerve growth factor in the heart: the role of the calcineurin-NFAT pathway," *Journal of Molecular and Cellular Cardiology*, vol. 46, no. 4, pp. 568–578, 2009.

[213] E. Saygili, O. R. Rana, C. Günzel et al., "Rate and irregularity of electrical activation during atrial fibrillation affect myocardial NGF expression via different signalling routes," *Cellular Signalling*, vol. 24, no. 1, pp. 99–105, 2012.

[214] T. Minami, K. Yano, M. Miura et al., "The down syndrome critical region gene 1 short variant promoters direct vascular bed-specific gene expression during inflammation in mice," *Journal of Clinical Investigation*, vol. 119, no. 8, pp. 2257–2270, 2009.

[215] M. Sobrado, B. G. Ramirez, F. Neria et al., "Regulator of calcineurin 1 (Rcan1) has a protective role in brain ischemia/reperfusion injury," *Journal of Neuroinflammation*, vol. 9, article 48, 2012.

[216] R. R. Baggott, A. Alfranca, D. López-Maderuelo et al., "Plasma membrane calcium ATPase isoform 4 inhibits vascular endothelial growth factor-mediated angiogenesis through interaction with calcineurin," *Arteriosclerosis, Thrombosis, and Vascular Biology*, vol. 34, no. 10, pp. 2310–2320, 2014.

[217] C.-J. Liu, Y.-C. Cheng, K.-W. Lee et al., "Lipopolysaccharide induces cellular hypertrophy through calcineurin/NFAT-3 signaling pathway in H9c2 myocardiac cells," *Molecular and Cellular Biochemistry*, vol. 313, no. 1-2, pp. 167–178, 2008.

[218] S. Porta, S. A. Serra, M. Huch et al., "RCAN1 (DSCR1) increases neuronal susceptibility to oxidative stress: a potential pathogenic process in neurodegeneration," *Human Molecular Genetics*, vol. 16, no. 9, pp. 1039–1050, 2007.

[219] X. Sun, Y. Wu, B. Herculano, and W. Song, "RCAN1 overexpression exacerbates calcium overloading-induced neuronal apoptosis," *PLoS ONE*, vol. 9, no. 4, Article ID e95471, 2014.

[220] M. Perluigi, G. Pupo, A. Tramutola et al., "Neuropathological role of PI3K/Akt/mTOR axis in Down syndrome brain," *Biochimica et Biophysica Acta—Molecular Basis of Disease*, vol. 1842, no. 7, pp. 1144–1153, 2014.

[221] S.-Y. Shin, H. W. Yang, J.-R. Kim, W. D. Heo, and K.-H. Cho, "A hidden incoherent switch regulates RCAN1 in the calcineurin-NFAT signaling network," *Journal of Cell Science*, vol. 124, no. 1, pp. 82–90, 2011.

[222] Y. Wu, P. T. T. Ly, and W. Song, "Aberrant expression of RCAN1 in Alzheimer's pathogenesis: a new molecular mechanism and a novel drug target," *Molecular Neurobiology*, vol. 50, no. 3, pp. 1085–1097, 2014.

[223] X. Liogier d'Ardhuy, J. O. Edgin, C. Bouis et al., "Assessment of cognitive scales to examine memory, executive function and

language in individuals with down syndrome: implications of a 6-month observational study," *Frontiers in Behavioral Neuroscience*, vol. 9, article 300, 2015.

[224] F. Stagni, A. Giacomini, S. Guidi, E. Ciani, and R. Bartesaghi, "Timing of therapies for downsyndrome: the sooner, the better," *Frontiers in Behavioral Neuroscience*, vol. 9, article 265, 2015.

[225] E. H. Lee, S. S. Kim, S. Lee, K.-H. Baek, and S. R. Seo, "Pituitary Adenylate Cyclase-Activating Polypeptide (PACAP) targets down syndrome candidate region 1 (DSCR1/RCAN1) to control neuronal differentiation," *The Journal of Biological Chemistry*, vol. 290, no. 34, pp. 21019–21031, 2015.

[226] Y. Li, J. Wang, Y. Zhou, D. Li, and Z.-Q. Xiong, "Rcan1 deficiency impairs neuronal migration and causes periventricular heterotopia," *The Journal of Neuroscience*, vol. 35, no. 2, pp. 610–620, 2015.

[227] V. Cavallucci, E. Bisicchia, M. T. Cencioni et al., "Acute focal brain damage alters mitochondrial dynamics and autophagy in axotomized neurons," *Cell Death and Disease*, vol. 5, article e1545, 2014.

[228] B. M. Edens, N. Miller, and Y. Ma, "Impaired autophagy and defective mitochondrial function: converging paths on the road to motor neuron degeneration," *Frontiers in Cellular Neuroscience*, vol. 10, article 44, 2016.

[229] S. Ghavami, S. Shojaei, B. Yeganeh et al., "Autophagy and apoptosis dysfunction in neurodegenerative disorders," *Progress in Neurobiology*, vol. 112, pp. 24–49, 2014.

[230] V. G. Yerra and A. Kumar, "Adenosine monophosphate-activated protein kinase abates hyperglycaemia-induced neuronal injury in experimental models of diabetic neuropathy: effects on mitochondrial biogenesis, autophagy and neuroinflammation," *Molecular Neurobiology*, 2016.

[231] J. Park, D. G. Lee, B. Kim et al., "Iron overload triggers mitochondrial fragmentation via calcineurin-sensitive signals in HT-22 hippocampal neuron cells," *Toxicology*, vol. 337, pp. 39–46, 2015.

[232] J. Mu, Y. Song, J. Zhang, W. Lin, and H. Dong, "Calcium signaling is implicated in the diffuse axonal injury of brain stem," *International Journal of Clinical and Experimental Pathology*, vol. 8, no. 5, pp. 4388–4397, 2015.

[233] B. Gabryel, A. Pudelko, J. Adamczyk, I. Fischer, and A. Malecki, "Calcineurin and Erk1/2-signaling pathways are involved in the antiapoptotic effect of cyclosporin A on astrocytes exposed to simulated ischemia in vitro," *Naunyn-Schmiedeberg's Archives of Pharmacology*, vol. 374, no. 2, pp. 127–139, 2006.

[234] B. Gabryel, M. Chalimoniuk, A. Stolecka, K. Waniek, J. Langfort, and A. Malecki, "Inhibition of arachidonic acid release by cytosolic phospholipase A_2 is involved in the antiapoptotic effect of FK506 and cyclosporin A on astrocytes exposed to simulated ischemia in vitro," *Journal of Pharmacological Sciences*, vol. 102, no. 1, pp. 77–87, 2006.

[235] S. Jayanthi, X. Deng, B. Ladenheim et al., "Calcineurin/NFAT-induced up-regulation of the Fas ligand/Fas death pathway is involved in methamphetamine-induced neuronal apoptosis," *Proceedings of the National Academy of Sciences of the United States of America*, vol. 102, no. 3, pp. 868–873, 2005.

[236] Y. Xu, L. Yang, S. Yu et al., "Spatiotemporal changes in NFATc4 expression of retinal ganglion cells after light-induced damage," *Journal of Molecular Neuroscience*, vol. 53, no. 1, pp. 69–77, 2014.

[237] C. Ni, Z. Li, M. Qian, Y. Zhou, J. Wang, and X. Guo, "Isoflurane induced cognitive impairment in aged rats through hippocampal calcineurin/NFAT signaling," *Biochemical and Biophysical Research Communications*, vol. 460, no. 4, pp. 889–895, 2015.

[238] Y. Yang, S. Song, H. Min, X. Chen, and Q. Gao, "STAT3 degradation mediated by calcineurin involved in the neurotoxicity of isoflurane," *NeuroReport*, vol. 27, no. 2, pp. 124–130, 2016.

[239] F. Neria, M. del Carmen Serrano-Perez, P. Velasco, K. Urso, P. Tranque, and E. Cano, "NFATc3 promotes Ca^{2+}-dependent MMP3 expression in astroglial cells," *Glia*, vol. 61, no. 7, pp. 1052–1066, 2013.

[240] M. A. Sama, D. M. Mathis, J. L. Furman et al., "Interleukin-1β-dependent signaling between astrocytes and neurons depends critically on astrocytic calcineurin/NFAT activity," *Journal of Biological Chemistry*, vol. 283, no. 32, pp. 21953–21964, 2008.

[241] K. Szydlowska, M. Zawadzka, and B. Kaminska, "Neuroprotectant FK506 inhibits glutamate-induced apoptosis of astrocytes in vitro and in vivo," *Journal of Neurochemistry*, vol. 99, no. 3, pp. 965–975, 2006.

[242] N. H. Shah, A. J. Schulien, K. Clemens et al., "Cyclin E1 regulates Kv2.1 channel phosphorylation and localization in neuronal ischemia," *Journal of Neuroscience*, vol. 34, no. 12, pp. 4326–4331, 2014.

[243] D. J. Gerber, D. Hall, T. Miyakawa et al., "Evidence for association of schizophrenia with genetic variation in the 8p21.3 gene, PPP3CC, encoding the calcineurin gamma subunit," *Proceedings of the National Academy of Sciences of the United States of America*, vol. 100, no. 15, pp. 8993–8998, 2003.

[244] T. Miyakawa, L. M. Leiter, D. J. Gerber et al., "Conditional calcineurin knockout mice exhibit multiple abnormal behaviors related to schizophrenia," *Proceedings of the National Academy of Sciences of the United States of America*, vol. 100, no. 15, pp. 8987–8992, 2003.

[245] C. A. Ogden, M. E. Rich, N. J. Schork et al., "Candidate genes, pathways and mechanisms for bipolar (manic-depressive) and related disorders: an expanded convergent functional genomics approach," *Molecular Psychiatry*, vol. 9, no. 11, pp. 1007–1029, 2004.

[246] N. Park, S. H. Juo, R. Cheng et al., "Linkage analysis of psychosis in bipolar pedigrees suggests novel putative loci for bipolar disorder and shared susceptibility with schipzoprenia," *Molecular Psychiatry*, vol. 9, no. 12, pp. 1091–1099, 2004.

[247] Y. Tian, I. Voineagu, S. P. Paşca et al., "Alteration in basal and depolarization induced transcriptional network in iPSC derived neurons from Timothy syndrome," *Genome Medicine*, vol. 6, no. 10, article 75, 2014.

[248] G. Quadrato, M. Y. Elnaggar, C. Duman, A. Sabino, K. Forsberg, and S. Di Giovanni, "Modulation of GABAA receptor signaling increases neurogenesis and suppresses anxiety through NFATc4," *The Journal of Neuroscience*, vol. 34, no. 25, pp. 8630–8645, 2014.

[249] C. Crozatier, S. Farley, I. M. Mansuy, S. Dumas, B. Giros, and E. T. Tzavara, "Calcineurin (protein phosphatase 2B) is involved in the mechanisms of action of antidepressants," *Neuroscience*, vol. 144, no. 4, pp. 1470–1476, 2007.

[250] S. L. Eastwood, P. W. J. Burnet, and P. J. Harrison, "Decreased hippocampal expression of the susceptibility gene PPP3CC and other calcineurin subunits in schizophrenia," *Biological Psychiatry*, vol. 57, no. 7, pp. 702–710, 2005.

[251] N. Kozlovsky, E. Scarr, B. Dean, and G. Agam, "Postmortem brain calcineurin protein levels in schizophrenia patients are not different from controls," *Schizophrenia Research*, vol. 83, no. 2-3, pp. 173–177, 2006.

[252] H. K. Manji, I. I. Gottesman, and T. D. Gould, "Signal transduction and genes-to-behaviors pathways in psychiatric diseases," *Science's STKE*, vol. 2003, no. 207, article pe49, 2003.

[253] W. J. Rushlow, Y. H. Seah, D. J. Belliveau, and N. Rajakumar, "Changes in calcineurin expression induced in the rat brain by the administration of antipsychotics," *Journal of Neurochemistry*, vol. 94, no. 3, pp. 587–596, 2005.

[254] T. D. McClure-Begley, S. R. Grady, M. J. Marks, A. C. Collins, and J. A. Stitzel, "Presynaptic GABAB autoreceptor regulation of nicotinic acetylcholine receptor mediated [^{3}H]-GABA release from mouse synaptosomes," *Biochemical Pharmacology*, vol. 91, no. 1, pp. 87–96, 2014.

[255] T.-T. Tzeng, H.-J. Tsay, L. Chang et al., "Caspase 3 involves in neuroplasticity, microglial activation and neurogenesis in the mice hippocampus after intracerebral injection of kainic acid," *Journal of Biomedical Science*, vol. 20, no. 1, article 90, 2013.

[256] H. Tokuoka, T. Hatanaka, D. Metzger, and H. Ichinose, "Nurr1 expression is regulated by voltage-dependent calcium channels and calcineurin in cultured hippocampal neurons," *Neuroscience Letters*, vol. 559, pp. 50–55, 2014.

[257] C. Freire-Cobo, G. Sierra-Paredes, M. Freire, and G. Sierra-Marcuño, "The calcineurin inhibitor Ascomicin interferes with the early stage of the epileptogenic process induced by Latrunculin A microperfusion in rat hippocampus," *Journal of Neuroimmune Pharmacology*, vol. 9, no. 5, pp. 654–667, 2014.

[258] G. Sierra-Paredes and G. Sierra-Marcuño, "Ascomycin and FK506: pharmacology and therapeutic potential as anticonvulsants and neuroprotectants," *CNS Neuroscience and Therapeutics*, vol. 14, no. 1, pp. 36–46, 2008.

[259] A. Vázquez-López, G. Sierra-Paredes, and G. Sierra-Marcuño, "Seizures induced by microperfusion of glutamate and glycine in the hippocampus of rats pretreated with latrunculin A," *Neuroscience Letters*, vol. 388, no. 2, pp. 81–85, 2005.

[260] M. L. Roberts-Crowley and A. R. Rittenhouse, "Characterization of ST14A cells for studying modulation of voltage-gated calcium channels," *PLoS ONE*, vol. 10, no. 7, Article ID e0132469, 2015.

[261] I. O. Medvedev, A. J. Ramsey, S. T. Masoud et al., "D1 dopamine receptor coupling to PLCβ regulates forward locomotion in mice," *The Journal of Neuroscience*, vol. 33, no. 46, pp. 18125–18133, 2013.

[262] L. D. Walensky and S. H. Snyder, "Inositol 1,4,5-trisphosphate receptors selectively localized to the acrosomes of mammalian sperm," *Journal of Cell Biology*, vol. 130, no. 4, pp. 857–869, 1995.

[263] G. Ramazzotti, A. Bavelloni, W. Blalock, M. Piazzi, L. Cocco, and I. Faenza, "BMP-2 induced expression of PLCβ1 that is a positive regulator of osteoblast differentiation," *Journal of Cellular Physiology*, vol. 231, no. 3, pp. 623–629, 2016.

[264] J. Brotchie and P. Jenner, "New approaches to therapy," *International Review of Neurobiology*, vol. 98, pp. 123–150, 2011.

[265] S. N. A. Bukhari and I. Jantan, "Synthetic curcumin analogs as inhibitors of β-amyloid peptide aggregation: potential therapeutic and diagnostic agents for Alzheimer's disease," *Mini-Reviews in Medicinal Chemistry*, vol. 15, no. 13, pp. 1110–1121, 2015.

[266] J. Segura-Aguilar, P. Muñoz, and I. Paris, "Aminochrome as new preclinical model to find new pharmacological treatment that stop the development of Parkinsons disease," *Current Medicinal Chemistry*, vol. 23, no. 4, pp. 346–359, 2016.

[267] L. Brandenstein, M. Schweizer, J. Sedlacik, J. Fiehler, and S. Storch, "Lysosomal dysfunction and impaired autophagy in a novel mouse model deficient for the lysosomal membrane protein Cln7," *Human Molecular Genetics*, vol. 25, no. 4, pp. 777–791, 2016.

[268] G. Natale, P. Lenzi, G. Lazzeri et al., "Compartment-dependent mitochondrial alterations in experimental ALS, the effects of mitophagy and mitochondriogenesis," *Frontiers in Cellular Neuroscience*, vol. 9, article 434, 2015.

[269] D. M. Samy, C. A. Ismail, R. A. Nassra, T. M. Zeitoun, and A. M. Nomair, "Downstream modulation of extrinsic apoptotic pathway in streptozotocin-induced Alzheimer's dementia in rats: erythropoietin versus curcumin," *European Journal of Pharmacology*, vol. 770, pp. 52–60, 2016.

21

Age-Dependent Loss of Mitochondrial Function in Epithelial Tissue Can Be Reversed by Coenzyme Q_{10}

Daniel Schniertshauer, Daniel Gebhard, and Jörg Bergemann

Department of Life Sciences, Albstadt-Sigmaringen University of Applied Sciences, 72488 Sigmaringen, Germany

Correspondence should be addressed to Daniel Schniertshauer; schniertshauer@hs-albsig.de

Academic Editor: Carmela R. Balistreri

The process of aging is characterized by the increase of age-associated disorders as well as severe diseases. Due to their role in the oxidative phosphorylation and thus the production of ATP which is crucial for many cellular processes, one reason for this could be found in the mitochondria. The accumulation of reactive oxygen species damaged mitochondrial DNA and proteins can induce mitochondrial dysfunction within the electron transport chain. According to the "mitochondrial theory of aging," understanding the impact of harmful external influences on mitochondrial function is therefore essential for a better view on aging in general, but the measurement of mitochondrial respiration in skin cells from cell cultures cannot completely reflect the real situation in skin. Here, we describe a new method to measure the mitochondrial respiratory parameters in epithelial tissue derived from human skin biopsies using a XF24 extracellular flux analyzer to evaluate the effect of coenzyme Q10. We observed a decrease in mitochondrial respiration and ATP production with donor age corresponding to the "mitochondrial theory of aging." For the first time *ex vivo* in human epidermis, we could show also a regeneration of mitochondrial respiratory parameters if the reduced form of coenzyme Q10, ubiquinol, was administered. In conclusion, an age-related decrease in mitochondrial respiration and ATP production was confirmed. Likewise, an increase in the respiratory parameters by the addition of coenzyme Q10 could also be shown. The fact that there is a significant effect of administered coenzyme Q10 on the respiratory parameters leads to the assumption that this is mainly caused by an increase in the electron transport chain. This method offers the possibility of testing age-dependent effects of various substances and their influence on the mitochondrial respiration parameters in human epithelial tissue.

1. Introduction

Oxidative phosphorylation is the main metabolic pathway for the production of cellular energy. It is located at the inner mitochondrial membrane where a series of redox reactions convert dietary energy from organic acids and fats into utilizable energy in the form of ATP. This close proximity to reactive oxygen species (ROS) generation sites makes mitochondrial DNA (mtDNA) vulnerable to oxidative damages. Lack of protective histones and limited repair processes in mitochondria may thus promote a high mutation rate of mtDNA [1, 2]. Those mutations have been identified as an important factor in aging processes as well as pathogenesis of inherited and age-related diseases [3]. Being the main site of ROS generation, mitochondria are thought to be part of a process in which continuous accumulation of ROS damaged mtDNA and proteins induces electron transport chain (ETC) dysfunction, which in turn leads to an enhanced ROS production. According to the "mitochondrial theory of aging," this vicious cycle is a major cause for cellular aging, tissue dysfunction, and degeneration [4]. Indeed, ROS present a mutagenic exposure for (mt)DNA throughout the whole life span of an organism which have the potency to damage all sorts of cellular structures such as proteins, lipid membranes, or DNA [5, 6]. Damaged proteins have been shown to bind to mitochondria and disturb their function [7]. Oxidation of nucleic acids in DNA is the most problematic consequence of oxidative stress. ROS can cause single- and double-strand breaks, oxidation of DNA bases (e.g. 8-oxo-7,8-dihydroguanine (8-oxoG)), and DNA-protein interactions, among others [7, 8]. In addition to the harmful properties, ROS are essential for important physiological functions such as signal transduction or the defense against viruses and bacteria. Because of their crucial function and their role in ROS metabolism, mitochondria play a central role in most aging hypotheses. The "maximum metabolic slope theory" by Prinzinger suggests a correlation between life span and energy production [9]. It postulates that aging is a consequence of a limited capacity of mitochondria to produce energy. The "defective powerhouse model of premature skin aging" by Krutmann and Schroeder combines UV-induced mtDNA mutations and infrared-induced ETC dysfunction as corporate elicitors of mitochondrial dysfunction [6]. Aging is a continuous, multifaceted process. It is a complex combination of (mt)DNA mutation, oxidative stress, improper degradation of dysfunctional proteins and organelles and their subsequent accumulation in the cell, impairment of cellular metabolism, mitochondrial dysfunction, and compromised energy production. Even though aging has been studied extensively, it is still a matter of controversy whether observed cellular changes accompanied by aging are the cause for aging or its consequence. To break the process of ROS, DNA damage, and aging, the body tries to counteract with natural substances such as (coenzyme Q10) CoQ10, among others. CoQ10 is well characterized as intrinsic part of the ETC for its role in electron transport in mitochondrial respiratory chain between complexes I/II and III and the connected proton translocation from mitochondrial matrix to intermembrane space. However, CoQ10 is not only present in mitochondrial but all membranes throughout the cell [1]. Thereby, CoQ10 plays a pivotal role in various cellular processes such as cellular transport, regulation of cytosolic NAD+/NADH ratio, cell growth and differentiation, as well as degradation of cellular compounds. CoQ10 is a potent antioxidant and the only membrane-located antioxidant synthesized endogenously [1]. It prevents lipid peroxidation and efficiently protects DNA bases and proteins during oxidative stress, which is particularly important in the case of mtDNA [10, 11]. CoQ10 treatment was shown to induce increased activity of antioxidative enzymes such as superoxide dismutase and glutathione peroxidase [12]. CoQ10 is also involved in the prevention of mitochondrial ROS formation as an obligatory cofactor for mitochondrial uncoupling proteins [13, 14]. Activation of those proteins leads to uncoupling of oxidative phosphorylation and thereby reduces mitochondrial ROS generation. Regarding the versatile effects of CoQ10 on cell metabolism, it is no surprise that CoQ10 has been shown to be a beneficial therapeutic in various age-related and degenerative conditions such as neurodegeneration, mitochondrial myopathies, age-related macular degeneration, and cardiovascular diseases [15–18]. In all those disease patterns, low levels of endogenous CoQ10 in comparison with healthy subjects have been reported. Also aging has been shown to be accompanied by reduced CoQ10 levels in the body [10]. In this study, we examined the influence of CoQ10 on mitochondrial respiratory parameters *ex vivo* in epithelial tissue derived from human skin biopsies. To do so, we analyzed the mitochondrial respiration profile after treatment with or without CoQ10. We therefore established a Seahorse XF analyzer method to measure the mitochondrial respiration *ex vivo* directly in epidermis. We observed a decrease in mitochondrial respiration and ATP production with donor age corresponding to the "mitochondrial theory of aging" that says that the impairment of DNA repair and mitochondrial function might build a vicious cycle, contributing to the generally observed decrease in DNA repair capacity and mitochondrial function with age, and thereby accelerating (skin) aging and (skin) cancer development. We observed also a regeneration of mitochondrial respiratory parameters if the reduced form of CoQ10, ubiquinol, was administered.

2. Materials and Methods

2.1. Cell Culture. All experiments were conducted in accordance with the Declaration of Helsinki and approved by the Ethics Commission of the State Medical Association of Baden-Württemberg, Germany (187-03). Patients were informed in advance and gave their written consent to the use of their samples. Experiments were carried out with skin biopsies from donors of different ages, which were received from the Kreiskrankenhaus Sigmaringen, general surgery unit, or from Aesthetic Perfection Lake Constance, plastic surgery unit, Germany. The profiles of the donors are summarized in Table 1. Depending on the size of the biopsies, they have been used either for experiments with CoQ10 and placebo treatment or for untreated measured. After surgery, biopsies were kept in PBS at 4°C for a maximum of 24 h. The next day initially, the biopsies were washed with 70% isopropanol and then with PBS. After removal of fat and connective tissue adherent to the dermis, the biopsies were cut and incubated with Dispase II (Roche Diagnostics, Indianapolis, IN, United States) at 4°C for 16 h in keratinocyte growth medium (Lonza, Walkersville, MD, United States). Afterwards, epidermis and dermis were separated.

2.2. CoQ10 Supplementation. In order to investigate the effect of CoQ10 on the mitochondrial respiration parameters in epidermis, we applied an ubiquinol formulation (QuinoMit Q10 fluid; MSE Pharmazeutika GmbH, Bad Homburg, Germany). CoQ10 was always freshly weighted, diluted with ultrapure water (Millipore), and supplemented to the overnight-separation media with Dispase II. CoQ10 placebo formulation lacking CoQ10 (carrier control) was administrated exactly as described for QuinoMit. Preliminary studies with different CoQ10 concentrations showed high potency at a concentration of 100 μM CoQ10. Therefore, all experiments were performed using 100 μM CoQ10.

2.3. Mitochondrial Respiration Measurements. To get a mitochondrial respiration profile, epidermis was measured with a Seahorse Bioscience XF24 Extracellular Flux Analyzer (Agilent Technologies, Santa Clara, CA, United States). XF Flux-Plates (sensor cartridge) were incubated overnight at 37°C in calibrant solution. For each treatment, a minimum of three wells were analyzed in parallel. 16 hours prior to

Table 1: Summary of all donors.

Donor	Age (y)	Sex	Smoking/nonsmoking	Body site
1	29	F	s	Femoral
2	35	F	ns	Upper eyelids
3	45	M	ns	Foreskin
4	46	M	ns	Abdomen
5	46	F	ns	Upper eyelids
6	54	F	ns	Upper eyelids
7	55	F	ns	Upper eyelids
8	57	F	ns	Abdomen
9	57	M	ns	Upper eyelids
10	60	M	ns	Abdomen
11	62	F	ns	Abdomen
12	63	M	ns	Abdomen
13	64	M	s	Abdomen
14	64	M	s	Abdomen
15	68	F	ns	Abdomen
16	68	M	ns	Abdomen
17	71	M	ns	Abdomen
18	73	F	ns	Abdomen
19	74	F	s	Abdomen
20	75	F	s	Abdomen
21	76	M	ns	Abdomen
22	77	M	s	Abdomen
23	77	M	ns	Upper eyelids
24	77	M	s	Abdomen
25	78	M	ns	Abdomen
26	80	F	ns	Abdomen
27	83	M	ns	Abdomen
28	83	F	ns	Abdomen
29	84	M	ns	Abdomen

F: female; M: male; ns: nonsmoking; s: smoking.

measurement, biopsies were treated with or without 100 μM CoQ10 or CoQ10 carrier control and incubated at 4°C. To measure the change of oxygen consumption rate (OCR (pmol/min)) and pH in medium surrounding the epidermis, XF24 islet capture microplates (Agilent Technologies, Santa Clara, CA, United States) were used. In these plates, small nets can be fixed to the plate bottom. To measure the oxygen consumption of the vital layer of the epidermis (stratum basale), epidermis and dermis were enzymatically separated and the epidermis placed with the vital—basal—side on the net. This orientation was essential for the measurement because the facing side of the net gets detected by the sensor. The small nets were then fixed in the microplates. It was especially critical to ensure after detachment of the epidermis from the dermis that the basal side shows to the net. In addition, within the ring in the center of the net (Figure 1(a)), there should be no holes (Figure 1(b)) or air bubbles (Figure 1(c)). Samples are then incubated for 30 min in 450 μL unbuffered assay medium (D7777, pH 7.4; Sigma-Aldrich, St. Louis, MO) at 37°C without CO_2 for 1 h. During this 1 h preincubation phase, the Flux-Plate was loaded with the stress reagents (XF Cell Mito Stress Test Kit, Agilent Technologies) and instrument calibration started. Oligomycin, carbonyl cyanide-ptrifluoromethoxyphenylhydrazone (FCCP), and rotenone combined with antimycin A were all prepared to result in a 4 μM final concentration after injection. After the insertion of the microplate, a 15 min equilibration phase was implemented before measurements. First, the initial respiration (basal response) was measured. Then, the active ingredients in the three ports were injected consecutively to determine the effect of each compound. This makes it possible to determine the efficiency of the individual complexes within the respiratory chain. Oligomycin blocks the F_0 subunit of the ATP synthase. The decrease in respiration can thus be regarded as a measure of the ATP production of the mitochondria. The decoupling of the respiratory chain by the protonophore FCCP allows the maximal respiration to be determined independently of the proton gradient. Finally, complexes I and II are blocked by the addition of rotenone and antimycin and thus the mitochondrial respiration. The remaining oxygen consumption is thus attributable to the nonmitochondrial respiration. The measurement of the initial phase and after addition of FCCP was done in three all other phases in six cycles. Each cycle involved 4 min mixing, 2 min waiting, and 3 min oxygen consumption rate (OCR) measurement. OCR was reported in the unit of pM·min^{-1}. Normalization of the obtained data takes place over the surface within the inner ring of the net (Figure 1(d)). The difference between basal response (oxygen consumption of the third cycle) and the lowest oxygen consumption after the injection of rotenone and antimycin A gave information about the mitochondrial respiration. ATP-linked respiration was calculated from the rate of respiration inhibition by oligomycin. The maximal response was represented by the maximum respiration after FCCP injection. Proton leak was calculated by the subtraction of the lowest OCR signal after the injection of rotenone and antimycin A from the OCR signal after the addition of oligomycin.

2.4. Statistical Analysis. Statistical evaluation was performed using Prism 5.03 (GraphPad Software, Inc.). Values are presented as mean ± SEM or individual values. Comparison between multiple groups was performed by one-way ANOVA with Dunnett's multiple comparison test. Comparison between two columns was done by *t*-test. For correlation with age, linear regression was used. Statistical significance was defined as $p < 0.05$.

3. Results

3.1. Mitochondrial Respiration in Epithelial Tissue Depends on Donor Age. In this study, we investigated the effect of CoQ10 on respiratory parameters in epidermal biopsies of donors of various ages. First, we analyzed the mitochondrial respiration and ATP production as a function of age (Figure 2). To do so, we measured the respiration profile with a Seahorse XF analyzer. As shown, both the mitochondrial respiration and ATP production in the measured donor collective (Table 1) decrease drastically with increasing age. This results in a reduction of mitochondrial respiration by an average of approximately 10 percent per decade.

3.2. Effect of CoQ10 on Respiratory Parameters in Epithelial Tissue. In the next experiment, the impact of CoQ10 and

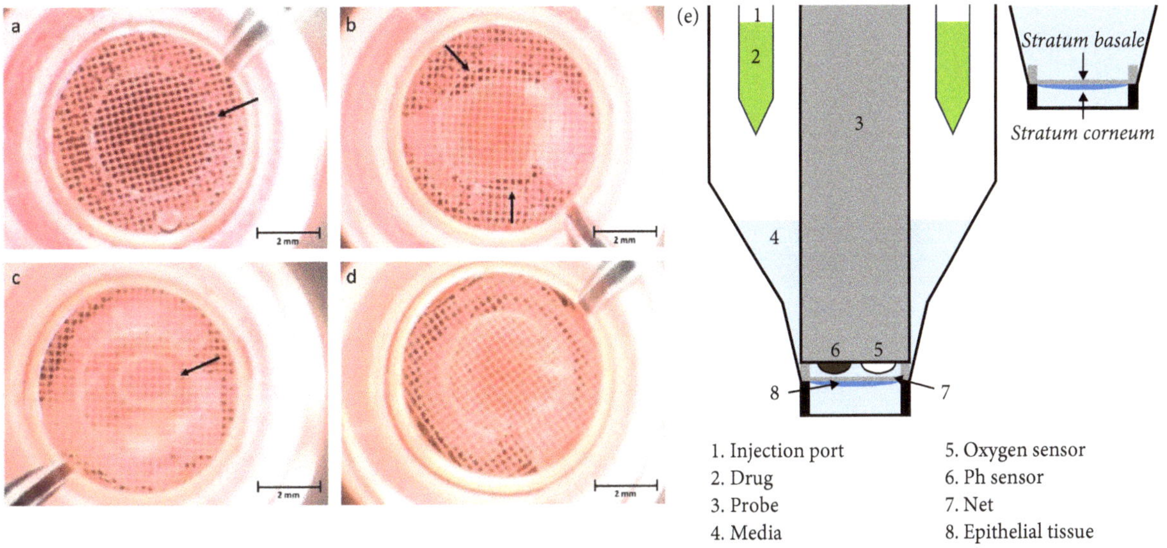

FIGURE 1: Microscopic image of an epidermis in an XF24 islet capture microplate. The epidermis was applied as flat as possible with the basal side on the net and then placed in the multiwell plate. The measurement of oxygen consumption takes place within the ring marked with the arrow (a). It was especially critical to ensure after detachment of the epidermis from the dermis that the basal side shows to the net. In addition, within the ring in the center of the net, there should be no holes (b) or air bubbles (c). Normalization of the obtained data takes place over the surface within the inner ring of the net (d). Schematic setup of the XF24 measuring system with an islet capture microplate (e).

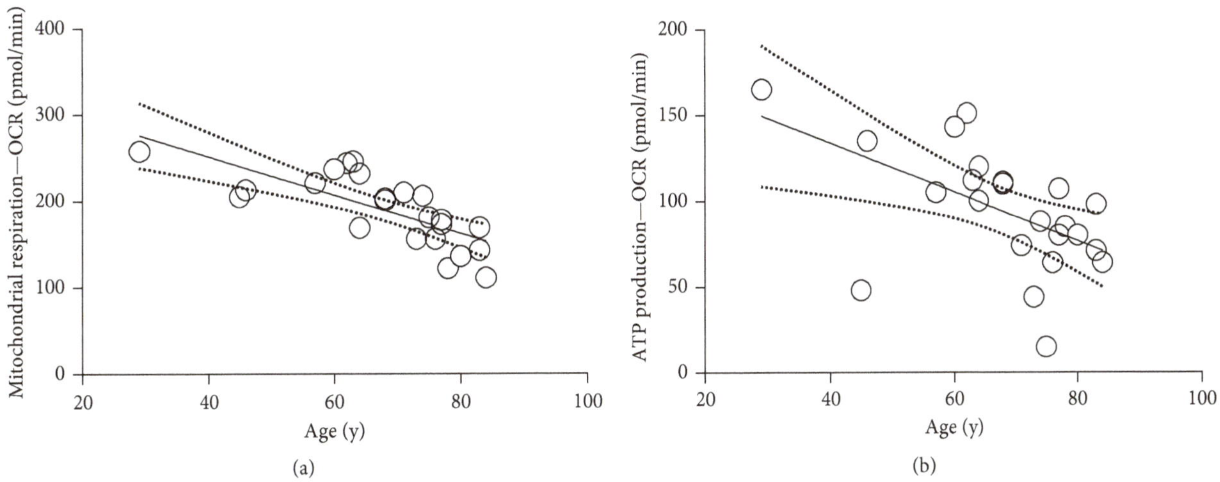

FIGURE 2: Mitochondrial respiration (a) and ATP production (b) in epithelial tissue depend on donor age. 16 hours prior to measurement, purified biopsies were stored overnight at 4°C in Dispase II. On the next day, the mitochondrial respiration of the separated epidermis was analyzed with an XF analyzer ($n = 23$, linear regression with 95% confidence interval, R^2 mitochondrial respiration $= 0.5487/p \leq 0.0001$, ATP production $= 0.2945/p \leq 0.01$, deviation from zero = significant).

CoQ10 carrier control treatment on respiratory parameters was examined. Therefore, 16 hours prior to measurement, biopsies were treated with or without 100 μM CoQ10 or CoQ10 carrier control and incubated at 4°C. Due to the small size of many biopsies, treatment with CoQ10 and carrier control could not be performed on all samples obtained. Preliminary studies with different CoQ10 concentrations showed high potency at a concentration of 100 μM CoQ10. Therefore, all experiments were performed using 100 μM CoQ10. To measure the change of OCR and pH in medium surrounding the epidermis, XF24 islet capture microplates (Agilent Technologies, Santa Clara, CA, United States) were used. CoQ10 supplementation induced an increase in mitochondrial respiration (Figure 3(a)) and also increased almost all key respiratory parameters, while there was no effect of CoQ10 carrier control (Figure 3(b)). A significant increase in basal response, maximal response, mitochondrial respiration, and proton leak with 100 μM CoQ10 was observed. ATP-linked respiration was also increased but not significantly. Carrier control-treated epidermis cells showed no significantly higher respiration parameters. Therefore, CoQ10 treatment had a positive effect on respiratory parameters in epithelial tissue.

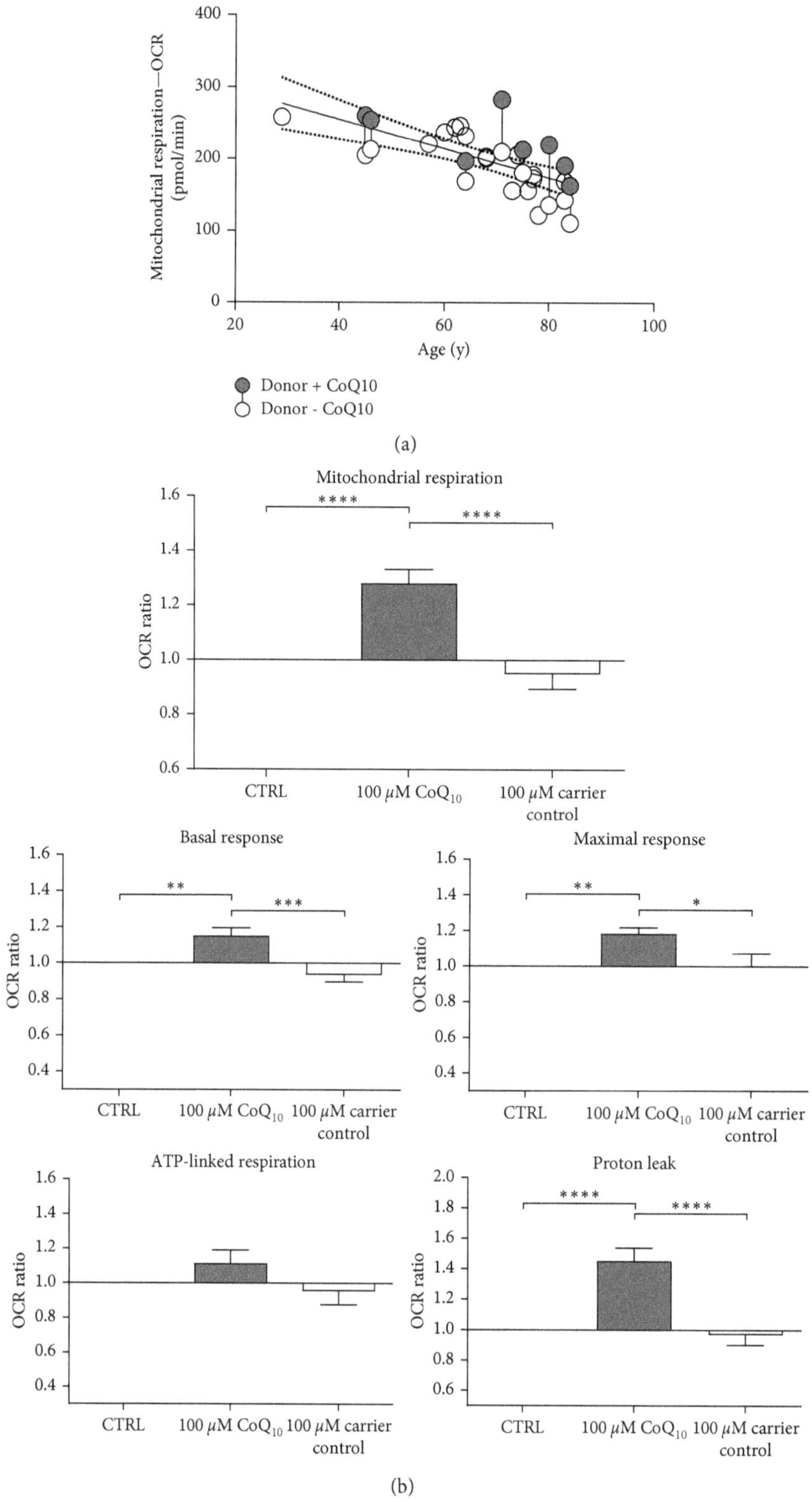

Figure 3: Effect of CoQ10 on respiratory parameters in epithelial tissue. 16 hours prior to measurement, purified biopsies were stored overnight at 4°C in Dispase II. During incubation with Dispase II, the samples were treated with or without 100 μM CoQ10 or CoQ10 carrier control. On the next day, the respiration profile of the separated dermis was analyzed with an XF analyzer. White circles represent untreated samples. CoQ10-treated samples are shown in dark gray circles. Connected circles represent the same donor. ((a) $n = 23$, linear regression with 95% confidence interval, $R^2 = 0.4354/p \leq 0.0001$, deviation from zero = significant; (b) $n = 8$, mean ± SEM, one-way ANOVA with Dunnett's multiple comparison test versus control and CoQ10 carrier control, $****p < 0.0001$). Control cells correspond to 1.0. OCR = oxygen consumption rate.

3.3. Influence of Sampling Location of Biopsies on Mitochondrial Respiration. In order to exclude a photoaging effect on the values obtained, the mitochondrial respiration of biopsies from body regions with a high UV exposure (HE) (e.g., eyelids) and biopsies from low UV-exposed body regions (LE) (e.g., abdomen) were randomly compared (Figure 4). For this, we measured the mitochondrial respiration profile with a Seahorse XF analyzer. Samples with a high UV exposure showed a significantly lower mitochondrial respiration on average than samples with a low UV exposure. These samples (HE) were not included in the evaluation of age dependence.

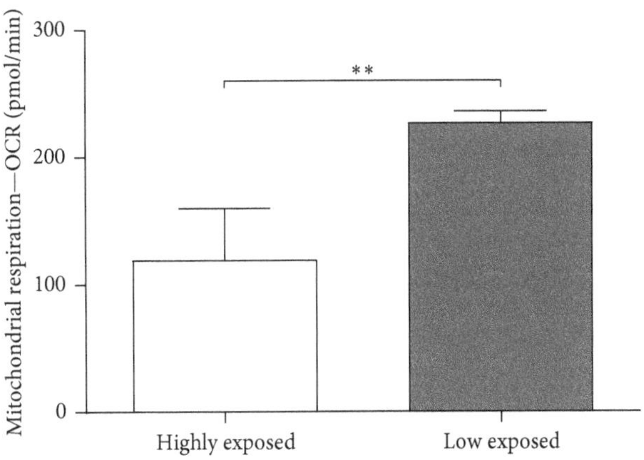

FIGURE 4: Influence of sampling location of biopsies on mitochondrial respiration. 16 hours prior to measurement, purified biopsies were stored overnight at 4°C in Dispase II. On the next day, the respiration profile of the separated dermis was analyzed with an XF analyzer. The range of age in both groups (HE and LE) was between 29 and 77 years ($n = 6$ highly exposed, $n = 6$ low exposed, linear regression, mean ± SEM, *t*-test, $**p < 0.05$).

4. Discussion

The term aging is often defined as the accumulation of damage and harmful changes within the cell over time, which can lead to an increased incidence of disease but in any case leads to death. The exact relationship between the accumulation of this damage and aging itself is not fully understood. It is assumed that a reduction of CoQ10 biosynthesis during aging as well as in age-related diseases plays a significant role in here [19, 20]. In addition, mitochondria and their role in energy production are increasingly becoming the main players in the process of aging [21, 22]. Therefore, CoQ10 has become a popular study object in recent years and the increasing evidence for its diverse positive properties has led to an increasing use of CoQ10 in mitochondrial medicine in the therapy of various (degenerative) diseases.

This study investigated the effect of CoQ10 on the mitochondrial respiratory parameters with increasing age directly in epithelial tissue, isolated from human skin biopsies. We observed a decrease in mitochondrial respiration as well as in ATP production with donor age and a regeneration of mitochondrial respiratory parameters by the addition of CoQ10. The observed decrease in mitochondrial respiration and ATP production with donor age in the first experiment, approximately ten percent per decade, corresponds to the "mitochondrial theory of aging" that says that the impairment of DNA repair and mitochondrial function might build a vicious cycle, contributing to the generally observed decrease in DNA repair capacity and mitochondrial function with age [18, 23–26]. With increasing age, the number of DNA damage in mitochondria increases. If these damages are not repaired, mutations occur. These mutations can lead to age-associated diseases, but at least to a loss of capacity in the ETC [9]. The results of this study correlate with the "maximum metabolic slope theory" by Prinzinger [9] that suggests a correlation between life span and energy production. According to this, aging is a consequence of the fact that the mitochondria can no longer provide sufficient energy. A decrease in mitochondrial respiration and ATP production with increasing age is a clear proof of this. In a further experiment, we could show that treatment with CoQ10 leads to a significant increase in most mitochondrial respiratory parameters in human epithelial tissue. Preliminary experiments tested cell viability and proliferation of fibroblasts using different CoQ10 concentrations in a range of 0–1000 μM. The experiments showed no toxic or antiproliferative effect of CoQ10 within this range. Furthermore, the safety of CoQ10 is well documented in rats and humans [27, 28]. The dosages chosen complied with dosages used in other in vitro studies [29–32]. 100 μM showed a significant change in most respiratory parameters and was therefore chosen for this study. CoQ10 carrier control in the same concentration as CoQ10 revealed no significant impact of the additives contained in QuinoMit Q10 fluid. Therefore, all results were related to CoQ10 administration. The age-related decrease in mitochondrial respiration was diminished by CoQ10 treatment. It could be shown that almost all key respiratory parameters were increased. An increase can be attributed to an enhanced ETC. Estornell et al. reported a correlation between CoQ10 concentration and respiratory rate which led to the assumption that physiological CoQ10 concentrations do not saturate the respiratory chain [33, 34]. Thus, CoQ10 administration was expected to induce an increase of mitochondrial respiration. These assumptions could be confirmed. It is assumed that the addition of CoQ10 results in improved electron transport and thus an increase in respiratory parameters. The "free radical theory of aging" by Harman says that the accumulation of mitochondrial damage leads to physiological dysfunctions and finally to pathological diseases [4]. It has been suggested that the mitochondrial respiratory chain become "leaky," releasing more ROS [35]. For the role of mitochondrial dysfunction and ROS release in age-related diseases, there is abundant evidence [36–38]. Also the accumulation of oxidative damage with age is proven [39].

We suppose that exogenously added CoQ10 acts as an "electron clamp" and thus enhances the electron transport between complexes I/II and III in the mitochondrial respiratory chain which has become "leaky" over the years. This could explain the increased mitochondrial respiration after CoQ10 treatment. On the other hand, the production of ROS could thereby be reduced and thus cellular damage, aging, and disease be attenuated.

5. Conclusions

In conclusion, an age-related decrease in mitochondrial respiration and ATP production in accordance with the mitochondrial theory of aging was confirmed. Likewise, an increase in the respiratory parameters by the addition of CoQ10 could also be shown. The fact that there is a significant effect of administered CoQ10 on the respiratory parameters leads to the assumption that this is mainly caused by an increase in the ETC. Low levels of endogenous CoQ10 have been implicated in various age-related and chronic diseases. Often, mitochondrial dysfunction and/or low antioxidant activity play an important role. The ability of CoQ10 to improve the electron transport chain and its antioxidant potential makes it an important therapeutic agent for influencing the development of some age-associated diseases and the aging process itself. Despite these facts, further studies performed on humans and in advance on human tissue are needed to better understand the promising effects of CoQ10 and before CoQ10 can be considered as an effective antiaging therapy. The mitochondrial respiration assay we established for this study offers the possibility of testing age-dependent effects of various substances and their influence on the mitochondrial respiration parameters in human epithelial tissue.

Conflicts of Interest

Jörg Bergemann has consulting contracts with MSE Pharmazeutika GmbH, Bad Homburg, Germany, and Beiersdorf AG, Hamburg, Germany.

Acknowledgments

The authors thank Dr. Hug, Dr. Huth, Dr. Astfalk, and Dr. Then-Schlagau for the kind supply of samples. They also thank Dr. Franz Enzmann and Dr. Alexander Bürkle for scientific advice. This study was supported by the BMBF-FHprofUnt2012 "MitoFunk" (03FH022PX2) and by the Baden-Württemberg Ministry of Science, Research and Art.

References

[1] M. Turunen, J. Olsson, and G. Dallner, "Metabolism and function of coenzyme Q," *Biochimica et Biophysica Acta (BBA)-Biomembranes*, vol. 1660, no. 1-2, pp. 171–199, 2004.

[2] D. C. Wallace, "A mitochondrial paradigm of metabolic and degenerative diseases, aging, and cancer: a dawn for evolutionary medicine," *Annual Review of Genetics*, vol. 39, no. 1, pp. 359–407, 2005.

[3] C. Desler, M. L. Marcker, K. K. Singh, and L. J. Rasmussen, "The importance of mitochondrial DNA in aging and cancer," *Journal of Aging Research*, vol. 2011, Article ID 407536, p. 9, 2011.

[4] D. Harman, "The biologic clock: the mitochondria?," *Journal of the American Geriatrics Society*, vol. 20, no. 4, pp. 145–147, 1972.

[5] D. A Clayton, J. N. Doda, and E. C. Friedberg, "The absence of a pyrimidine dimer repair mechanism in mammalian mitochondria," *Proceedings of the National Academy of Sciences*, vol. 71, no. 7, pp. 2777–2781, 1974.

[6] J. Krutmann and P. Schroeder, "Role of mitochondria in photoaging of human skin: the defective powerhouse model," *Journal of Investigative Dermatology Symposium Proceedings*, vol. 14, no. 1, pp. 44–49, 2009.

[7] U. T. Brunk and A. Terman, "The mitochondrial-lysosomal axis theory of aging: accumulation of damaged mitochondria as a result of imperfect autophagocytosis," *European Journal of Biochemistry*, vol. 269, no. 8, pp. 1996–2002, 2002.

[8] B. Demple and L. Harrison, "Repair of oxidative damage to DNA: enzymology and biology," *Annual Review of Biochemistry*, vol. 63, no. 1, pp. 915–948, 1994.

[9] R. Prinzinger, "Programmed ageing: the theory of maximal metabolic scope. How does the biological clock tick?," *EMBO Reports*, vol. 6, pp. S14–S19, 2005.

[10] M. Bentinger, M. Tekle, and G. Dallner, "Coenzyme Q-biosynthesis and functions," *Biochemical and Biophysical Research Communications*, vol. 396, no. 1, pp. 74–79, 2010.

[11] P. Forsmark-Andrée, G. Dallner, and L. Ernster, "Endogenous ubiquinol prevents protein modification accompanying lipid peroxidation in beef heart submitochondrial particles," *Free Radical Biology and Medicine*, vol. 19, no. 6, pp. 749–757, 1995.

[12] T. Blatt and G. P. Littarru, "Biochemical rationale and experimental data on the antiaging properties of CoQ(10) at skin level," *Biofactors*, vol. 37, no. 5, pp. 381–385, 2011.

[13] K. S. Echtay, E. Winkler, and M. Klingenberg, "Coenzyme Q is an obligatory cofactor for uncoupling protein function," *Nature*, vol. 408, no. 6812, pp. 609–613, 2000.

[14] K. S. Echtay, E. Winkler, K. Frischmuth, and M. Klingenberg, "Uncoupling proteins 2 and 3 are highly active H(+) transporters and highly nucleotide sensitive when activated by coenzyme Q (ubiquinone)," *Proceedings of the National Academy of Sciences*, vol. 98, no. 4, pp. 1416–1421, 2001.

[15] M. F. Beal, "Mitochondrial dysfunction and oxidative damage in Alzheimer's and Parkinson's diseases and coenzyme Q10 as a potential treatment," *Journal of Bioenergetics and Biomembranes*, vol. 36, no. 4, pp. 381–386, 2004.

[16] R. S. Chen, C. C. Huang, and N. S. Chu, "Coenzyme Q10 treatment in mitochondrial encephalomyopathies. Short-term double-blind, crossover study," *European Neurology*, vol. 37, no. 4, pp. 212–218, 1997.

[17] M. A. Blasi, C. Bovina, G. Carella et al., "Does coenzyme Q10 play a role in opposing oxidative stress in patients with age-related macular degeneration?," *Ophthalmologica*, vol. 215, no. 1, pp. 51–54, 2001.

[18] M. S. Damian, D. Ellenberg, R. Gildemeister et al., "Coenzyme Q10 combined with mild hypothermia after cardiac arrest: a preliminary study," *Circulation*, vol. 110, no. 19, pp. 3011–3016, 2004.

[19] M. Battino, A. Gorini, R. F. Villa et al., "Coenzyme Q content in synaptic and non-synaptic mitochondria from different brain regions in the ageing rat," *Mechanisms of Ageing and Development*, vol. 78, no. 3, pp. 173–187, 1995.

[20] M. Turunen, E. L. Appelkvist, P. Sindelar, and G. Dallner, "Blood concentration of coenzyme Q(10) increases in rats

when esterified forms are administered," *Journal of Nutrition*, vol. 129, no. 12, pp. 2113–2118, 1999.

[21] D. C. Wallace, "Mitochondrial diseases in man and mouse," *Science*, vol. 283, no. 5407, pp. 1482–1488, 1999.

[22] D. C. Wallace, W. Fan, and V. Procaccio, "Mitochondrial energetics and therapeutics," *Annual Review of Pathology: Mechanisms of Disease*, vol. 5, no. 1, pp. 297–348, 2010.

[23] F. Hazane, S. Sauvaigo, T. Douki, A. Favier, and J. C. Beani, "Age-dependent DNA repair and cell cycle distribution of human skin fibroblasts in response to UVA irradiation," *Journal of Photochemistry and Photobiology B: Biology*, vol. 82, no. 3, pp. 214–223, 2006.

[24] S. Sauvaigo, M. Bonnet-Duquennoy, F. Odin et al., "DNA repair capacities of cutaneous fibroblasts: effect of sun exposure, age and smoking on response to an acute oxidative stress," *British Journal of Dermatology*, vol. 157, no. 1, pp. 26–32, 2007.

[25] Y. H. Wei, S. B. Wu, Y. S. Ma, and H. C. Lee, "Respiratory function decline and DNA mutation in mitochondria, oxidative stress and altered gene expression during aging," *Chang Gung Medical Journal*, vol. 32, no. 2, pp. 113–132, 2009.

[26] S. Prahl, T. Kueper, T. Biernoth et al., "Aging skin is functionally anaerobic: importance of coenzyme Q10 for anti aging skin care," *Biofactors*, vol. 32, no. 1–4, pp. 245–255, 2008.

[27] K. D. Williams, J. D. Maneke, M. AbdelHameed et al., "52-week oral gavage chronic toxicity study with ubiquinone in rats with a 4-week recovery," *Journal of Agricultural and Food Chemistry*, vol. 47, no. 9, pp. 3756–3763, 1999.

[28] H. Ikematsu, K. Nakamura, S. Harashima, K. Fujii, and N. Fukutomi, "Safety assessment of coenzyme Q10 (Kaneka Q10) in healthy subjects: a double-blind, randomized, placebo-controlled trial," *Regulatory Toxicology and Pharmacology*, vol. 44, no. 3, pp. 212–218, 2006.

[29] U. Hoppe, J. Bergemann, W. Diembeck et al., "Coenzyme Q10, a cutaneous antioxidant and energizer," *Biofactors*, vol. 9, no. 2–4, pp. 371–378, 1999.

[30] D. A. Groneberg, B. Kindermann, M. Althammer et al., "Coenzyme Q10 affects expression of genes involved in cell signalling, metabolism and transport in human CaCo-2 cells," *International Journal of Biochemistry & Cell Biology*, vol. 37, no. 6, pp. 1208–1218, 2005.

[31] C. Schmelzer, I. Lindner, C. Vock, K. Fujii, and F. Döring, "Functional connections and pathways of coenzyme Q10-inducible genes: an in-silico study," *IUBMB Life*, vol. 59, no. 10, pp. 628–633, 2007.

[32] C. Schmelzer, G. Lorenz, G. Rimbach, and F. Döring, "In vitro effects of the reduced form of coenzyme Q(10) on secretion levels of TNF-alpha and chemokines in response to LPS in the human monocytic cell line THP-1," *Journal of Clinical Biochemistry and Nutrition*, vol. 44, no. 1, pp. 62–66, 2009.

[33] E. Estornell, R. Fato, C. Castelluccio, M. Cavazzoni, G. Parenti Castelli, and G. Lenaz, "Saturation kinetics of coenzyme Q in NADH and succinate oxidation in beef heart mitochondria," *FEBS Letters*, vol. 311, no. 2, pp. 107–109, 1992.

[34] G. P. Littarru and L. Tiano, "Bioenergetic and antioxidant properties of coenzyme Q10: recent developments," *Molecular Biotechnology*, vol. 37, no. 1, pp. 31–37, 2007.

[35] E. Samper, D. G. Nicholls, and S. Melov, "Mitochondrial oxidative stress causes chromosomal instability of mouse embryonic fibroblasts," *Aging Cell*, vol. 2, no. 5, pp. 277–285, 2003.

[36] M. Lagouge and N. G. Larsson, "The role of mitochondrial DNA mutations and free radicals in disease and ageing," *Journal of Internal Medicine*, vol. 273, no. 6, pp. 529–543, 2013.

[37] E. Marzetti, A. Csiszar, D. Dutta, G. Balagopal, R. Calvani, and C. Leeuwenburgh, "Role of mitochondrial dysfunction and altered autophagy in cardiovascular aging and disease: from mechanisms to therapeutics," *American Journal of Physiology-Heart and Circulatory Physiology*, vol. 305, no. 4, pp. H459–H476, 2013.

[38] S. Maynard, G. Keijzers, M. Gram et al., "Relationships between human vitality and mitochondrial respiratory parameters, reactive oxygen species production and dNTP levels in peripheral blood mononuclear cells," *Aging*, vol. 5, no. 11, pp. 850–864, 2013.

[39] E. K. Hudson, B. A. Hogue, N. C Souza-Pinto et al., "Age-associated change in mitochondrial DNA damage," *Free Radical Research*, vol. 29, no. 6, pp. 573–579, 1998.

22

Estimating Long-Term Care Costs among Thai Elderly: A Phichit Province Case Study

Pattaraporn Khongboon [1,2] **and Sathirakorn Pongpanich** [1]

[1] *College of Public Health Sciences, Chulalongkorn University, Pathumwan, Bangkok 10330, Thailand*
[2] *Prince Mahidol Award Foundation under the Royal Patronage, Faculty of Medicine, Siriraj Hospital, Bangkoknoi, Bangkok 10700, Thailand*

Correspondence should be addressed to Sathirakorn Pongpanich; sathirakorn.p@chula.ac.th

Academic Editor: Rainer Beurskens

Background. Rural-urban inequality in long-term care (LTC) services has been increasing alongside rapid socioeconomic development. This study estimates the average spending on LTC services and identifies the factors that influence the use and cost of LTC for the elderly living in urban and rural areas of Thailand. *Methods.* The sample comprised 837 elderly aged 60 years drawn from rural and urban areas in Phichit Province. Costs were assessed over a 1-month period. Direct costs of caregiving and indirect costs (opportunity cost method) were analyzed. Binary logistic regression was performed to determine which factors affected LTC costs. *Results.* The total annual LTC spending for rural and urban residents was on average USD 7,285 and USD 7,280.6, respectively. Formal care and informal care comprise the largest share of payments. There was a significant association between rural residents and costs for informal care, day/night care, and home renovation. *Conclusions.* Even though total LTC expenditures do not seem to vary significantly across rural and urban areas, the fundamental differences between areas need to be recognized. Reorganizing country delivery systems and finding a balance between formal and informal care are alternative solutions.

1. Introduction

Compared to other Asian developing countries, Thailand is in serious need of long-term care (LTC) due to its rapid aging population [1]. Since an average Thai survives beyond 80 years, LTC should be increased to nearly tenfold from 2000 to 2050. Unlike earlier cohorts, the population of Thailand and other developing countries, who would reach 70–80 years in the next few decades, are expected to be prone to noncommunicable diseases [2, 3]. According to the World Health Organization (WHO), LTC includes activities carried out by formal caretakers such as professionals; auxiliaries like social, health, or other workers; or informal caregivers like neighbors, friends, and family [4]. LTC policies are different in different nations and are influenced by culture, history, structure, and economic performance [5, 6].

The government of Thailand completely understands the challenge that LTC poses regarding the declining availability of family aid [7, 8]. In 2011, a new community care policy was developed as a part of a project in the district of Lam Sonthi, in Lopburi Province [9]. Additionally, a funding of USD 17.4 million was created by the National Health Security Office (NHSO) for LTC facilities for the elderly [10]. In the fiscal year 2016, a trial program announced by the government spread across 1,000 subdistricts, including 100,000 severely disabled individuals [11].

Previous studies in Thailand show that the average operating cost of NGOs' nursing homes in 2007 was USD 271 per resident, while the average monthly operating costs of government institutions were USD 313–361 per resident. The average monthly expenses were USD 748 per resident, which were paid by private nursing homes [1]. In Bangkok, the average monthly expenditure of private institutions' LTC was USD 464.45 per person–USD 406 in the northern areas and USD 638 in the southern areas [12]. According to Wongsin et al. [13], the total cost per day of LTC-dependent elderly citizens in hospitals in 2012 was USD 130,624 annually and that of formal care assistants was USD 12,191 annually. The average expenditure of institutional LTC for the elderly moderate ADL dependence was USD 13–13.35 per person daily.

Considering physical and social health, rural and urban residents receive different access to health care services [14, 15]. Due to dualistic urban-rural economic structure, there are vast inequalities among both rural and urban areas in spite of the rapid economic growth [16, 17]. The progress of health care expenditures is of particular concern to a rural population whose incomes are lower than their urban counterparts [17, 18].

Studies conducted in other countries show that health care and LTC costs were related to factors like age, gender, comorbidity, admission, dependence in personal activities of daily living (ADL), living arrangement, and health status among others [19–21]. To be specific, the aforementioned demographic factors may exert a significant influence on the scope of an individual's access to care, exclusively related to residential care placement. For example, an individual's income and health insurance might help them gain easier access to health care. Similarly, there are other sources of help such as social support networks and publicly financed LTC. Individuals who do not have the adequate economic backup or health insurance support can seek help from the aforementioned formal service providers within the health care service sector [22].

One can easily decipher that functional impairment is generally regarded as the factor behind the failure to indulge in ADLs. Against this backdrop, those who are in need of health or personal care services confront the problem of ADL impairment; for instance, those who deal with household works tend to depend on the aforementioned services. On the other hand, one can expect extreme ADL impairment and related assistance from formal and informal bases within the parlance of long-term health care [23]. Besides, senior citizens with ADL impairment, but living with their relatives, are less likely to be placed in any health care facility, including nursing homes. On the other side, loner unmarried senior citizens with ADL impairment are usually taken care of by their relatives or friends [24].

Regional differences can be seen in the context of utilizing health care facilities, especially within the supply of LTC choices like patient care facilities at nursing homes [25]. Research works conducted on elderly citizens who tend to live in their own homes prove that men usually seek help from informal sources, whereas women tend to seek help from formal sources [21]. Similarly, one's marital status can determine the range of assistance within ADL impairment treatment. In this scenario, research premised upon community involvement proves that family support is an essential factor which determines the level of assistance sought by married individuals, divorcees, and widowers. Besides, married individuals tend to seek formal assistance as compared to their unmarried counterparts in general [24].

The policy care for Thailand has been formed using a costing model that takes into account projected expenditure and actuarial estimates to bring about various LTC options [13, 26]. However, no research has been undertaken on the difference in LTC expenditures between rural and urban areas. In addition, when the LTC provisions for Thailand are planned, influencing factors should be understood together with LTC service costs. With this information, policy-makers can understand the health care needs of elderly citizens and their families and will be able to establish an appropriate LTC system.

This study is not focused on the LTC policy under the National Health Security funding. Assuming that the elderly are the primary payers and that the rural elderly have higher LTC spending than those in urban areas, the average spending on LTC services is estimated and the factors influencing the use of LTC in urban and rural areas are extracted.

2. Materials and Methods

2.1. Study Area. A transversal survey was conducted with the help of in-person interviews in Phichit Province during February to June 2016. Phichit is situated in the north of Thailand. Of its population, 21.1% are aged 60 years and over, which is higher than the national average (14.9%). Based on the 2015 National Civil Registration Systems [27], the area in Phichit with the highest percentage of people aged 60 and above was Bang Mun Nak subdistrict (19.44%) followed by Muang subdistrict (18.29%). So, in this study, Bangkmulnark subdistrict represents rural areas and Muang subdistrict represents urban areas.

2.2. The Number of Subjects or Sample Size. The sample size of the elderly was determined by adopting the Taro Yamane formula for minimum sample size [28]. The minimum sample size was 364 in the rural area and 333 in the urban area. The nonresponse rate was 20%, and thus, the sample size in the rural and urban area increased to 437 and 400 people, respectively.

2.3. Recruitment of Subjects. A simple random sampling was employed by computerized random selection of the elderly names from the National Civil Registration list. The subjects were recruited from the community in subdistrict (Tambon) areas, Phichit Province. The interviewing team made contact with the community headman prior to visiting each selected subject at their home. The subjects comprised elderly people and their main caregivers, all of whom were willing to participate and gave their consent. The inclusion criteria were (1) being 60 years old or above, having the ability to talk with clarity, and being in possession of one's senses and (2) living alone or with someone who was assumed to be a caregiver and had served in that role for at least 1 month.

2.4. Survey Tools and Data Collection. Suwanrada et al. [12] designed the structured interview-administered survey used in this study. The survey, which had open-ended as well as closed-ended queries, included queries regarding the sociodemographic characteristics of elderly people (age, place of stay, education, salary, gender, single or married, lifestyle, and health details). In addition, the survey asked whether elderly respondents had any sort of disability, which it described as problems carrying out any of 10 normal tasks (taking a bath, eating food, maintaining personal hygiene, going to the toilet, climbing stairs, getting dressed, walking 200 meters, moving in bed, urinary incontinence, and fecal incontinence). Moreover, the survey inquired about the caretakers' characteristics (education, age, salary, number of hours devoted to caregiving, and gender).

Furthermore, the survey asked subjects for the details of items bought in the previous month, including the price of medical equipment (e.g., hearing aid, glucometer, bedpan, bubble mattress, back brace, and bathing chair), the price of everyday goods (e.g., adult diapers), the cost of medical procedures (out of pocket), lifestyle, travel, and home renovation for elderly during the year.

2.5. Data Quality. Skilled research associates conducted the data collection. Data management tasks were carried out to monitor the quality of the information. At the end of every interview, the examiner checked whether the data collected were complete. The data were entered twice into SPSS 18 data. To enhance their quality, data-cleaning techniques were used. Moreover, where data were not included, SPSS 18 displayed the term "system-missing."

2.6. Cost Component. In this study, the cost component consisted of both direct and indirect costs:

(i) Direct costs are expenses that can be directly traced to a product. The direct costs that the elderly people incurred were out-of-pocket medical expenses for the previous month, which covered doctors' appointments and medications, medical devices, everyday necessities, and proper care.

(ii) The indirect costs associated with LTC are mainly related to the loss of human capital of carers. The indirect costs of the elderly were translated into the economic value of the informal care that relatives provided; even if no money was charged, the resource was not considered free.

(iii) Formal care was provided by experts in institutions, whether government-operated or handled by private organizations. The present research regarded formal caregivers as hired caretakers.

(iv) Informal care refers to unpaid caregivers providing constant care and support. It includes care provided by family members, neighbors, and volunteers in the community. The costs of informal care in this study are measured in terms of opportunity costs.

2.7. Cost Calculation. The total costs were evaluated by summing the direct and indirect costs that the caretakers paid for one month. The total cost excludes the elderly's earning loss due to their inability to work. It is assumed that the earning loss due to age-related bodily changes has a minimal effect. Cost variable descriptions are given in Table 1.

The direct costs including out-of-pocket expenses for daily supplies, those paid for hired caretakers, and those paid for day/night care in the last month were transformed into yearly expenditure through multiplication by 12.

Regarding medical devices (e.g., bathing chairs, wheelchairs, and canes), when an elderly person purchased them, we applied a 5-year useful life to the straight-line depreciation technique to evaluate the annual costs of the medical devices [29, 30].

The cost of home renovation for elderly in the previous year was divided by the number of people living in the home to calculate each person's expenditure. The price of home renovation for each person was then divided by 20 years of practical life [29, 30].

With respect to opportunity costs, Suwanrada et al. [12] calculated the salaries on a weekly basis in an effort to determine the value of the time of the respondents who were not working by assigning salaries to them. In this scenario, salary differences could have resulted from age-related and educational level-related differentiation in both genders; consequently, both constraints were used as predictors. Furthermore, Suwanrada et al. [12] considered the coefficients of all the constraints. Moreover, the antilog was multiplied by 52 to calculate the annual income of every subject.

The complete relationship between wage, age, gender, and education level is written as follows:

$$\text{Logit}(\text{WAGE}) = \beta_0 + \beta_1 \cdot (\text{AGE}) - \beta_2 \cdot \left(\text{AGE}^2\right) + \beta_3 \cdot (\text{GENDER}) + \beta_4 \cdot (\text{EDULEVEL}). \quad (1)$$

In addition, all estimated costs were further converted into 2017 USD using an exchange rate of USD 1 = THB 34.45 (the exchange rate as of March 31, 2017) [31].

2.8. Statistical Analysis. To summarize the features of people who took part in the research, descriptive statistics and sample probability weights were applied.

The entire direct and indirect costs that the aged individual, relative, and caretaker incurred were said to be equal to the price of care of a single individual for 1 month. According to the following theoretical viewpoint and general method, the LTC expenses of a person were considered to entail operational parameters (e.g., gender, education, single or married, lifestyle, disabled or not, income, and any persistent sickness).

Dependent variables were found to be dichotomous as, during the study, the investigators observed a large mass of zero-costs. It presented a skewed distribution, skewed to the right by rare but extremely high-cost events. In addition, applying linear model can result in biased parameters. Subsequently, in this study, the investigators employed a logistic regression instead of the linear model towards the determination of the probability of LTC services [32–34].

Table 1: Description of cost variables.

Cost type	Cost categories	Description
Direct costs	Daily supplies	Costs associated with medication, special testing, material supplies (feeding tubes, nasal oxygen, urinary catheters, etc.), dressing set, bed pads, adult diapers, tissue paper care, transportation, medical procedure, and physical therapy
	Day/night care	Costs associated with paying for adult day health/day care or overnight care
	Formal care	Costs associated with paying for a licensed practical nurse, a certified nursing assistant, trained caregivers, untrained caregivers, or any kind of paid providers
	Home renovation	Costs associated with various modifications that can make it easier for aging residents to navigate through and live in their homes, including brighter lighting, handrails, stair lifts, and accessible workspaces. These home modifications can range in cost from a few baht for a brighter light bulb to thousands of baht for significant remodeling (stair lifts, etc.)
	Medical devices	Costs associated with back brace, bedpan, blood sugar testing, bubble mattress, chair for bathing, hearing aid, manual home care bed, nebulizers, overbed table, oxygen saturation monitor, oxygen tanks, single cane, suction, tripod cane, walker, and wheelchair
Indirect cost	Informal care (opportunity cost)	The cost of informal care that family members offered without payment. It constituted productivity losses due to lost work time and was estimated using the human capital approach, which measured output losses in lost earnings

Correspondingly, during the study, a binary logistic regression and maximum likelihood function were used for calculation of the log odds ratio: $y = 0$ if no costs were incurred and $y = 1$ if costs were incurred. It was presumed for the analysis that a parametric binary probability model directed the probability of positive expenses Pr $(Y > 0\ X)$.

We selected independent variables potentially associated with LTC costs based on literature reviews. It was presumed that the following factors determine a person's probability of incurring care expenses: age, gender, education, living arrangement, marital status, region, extent of disability, income, and persistent sickness [21, 24, 35–40]. The independent variables were found to be dichotomous. Table 2 displays the values and corresponding labels.

2.9. Ethical Considerations. This research was approved by the Ethics Review Committee for Research Involving Human Research Subjects, Health Sciences Group, Chulalongkorn University, Certificate of Approval number 170/2558. The authors obtained written consent from all participants prior to their involvement in this study.

3. Results

3.1. Sample Characteristics. Of the rural participants, the mean age was 71.44 years; 47.6% were aged 60–69 years. Of them, 69.1% were accounted for by women; 46% were married but without spouses, while 17.8% were living alone. Around 83.5% alongside half of caregivers had primary education, with 67.3% of them being workless. Nearly 77.8% along with 62.9% of caregivers had an annual income of less than USD 4,354, whereas 90.2% used old age allowance (OAA) for support; 24.9% suffered from a disability, while 81.5% had a chronic disease. About 74.8% had caregivers, with the mean age being 52.82 years; 44.6% were aged 41–60 years. Of the 80% women, 24.5% were unmarried, 85.6% lived with recipients, and 43.9% spent 5–8 hours daily.

Of the urban participants, the mean age was 68.58 years; 59.3% were aged 60–69 years; 65.5% of them were women. Close to 51% were married and had spouses, while 18.8% were single. Also, 63.3% alongside 32.6% of their caregivers had primary education, while 62.3% were workless. Meanwhile, 55.6% had an annual income of less than USD 4,354, while 71.5% depended on OAA; 9.8% had a disability, whilst 75.8% had a chronic disease. In addition, 33.8% of them had caregivers with the mean age of 52.50 years; 48.1% were aged 41–60 years. Nearly 65.2% were women; 57% were married and had spouses, 83% lived with recipients, and 42.2% were workless and without income, whereas 60% spent 5–8 hours daily.

The elderly in the rural area were more likely to have primary education ($\chi^2 = 44.93$, $p < 0.001$) and less likely to be aged 60–69 ($\chi^2 = 50.32$, $p < 0.001$). They were more likely to have an annual income of less than USD 4,345 than those elderly in urban areas (x^2 = 52.84, p < 0.001). Moreover, the elderly in the rural areas were more likely to have caregivers

Table 2: Study variables for logistic regression.

	Value label
Dependent variables	
Daily supplies	0 = did not pay, 1 = did pay
Day/night care cost	0 = did not pay, 1 = did pay
Formal care	0 = did not pay, 1 = did pay
Home renovation	0 = did not pay, 1 = did pay
Informal care (opportunity cost)	0 = did not pay, 1 = did pay
Medical devices	0 = did not pay, 1 = did pay
Independent variables	
Age	Continuous
Area	0 = rural, 1 = urban
Annual income ≥ USD 4,354	0 = no, 1 = yes
Chronic diseases	0 = no, 1 = present at least one of eight chronic diseases (hypertension, diabetes, stroke, heart, dementia, osteoarthritis, paralysis, or hypercholesterol)
Disability	0 = no, 1 = present at least one of ten disabilities
Education	0 = any education, 1 = no education
Gender	0 = male, 1 = female
Living status	0 = living with other, 1 = living alone
Marital status	0 = married, 1 = single; single includes never married, divorced, widowed, and married but separated
Working status	0 = did not work, 1 = work

(x^2 = 142.50, $p < 0.001$), had OAA as the source of support (x^2 = 47.38, $p < 0.001$), had some type of disability (x^2 = 33.12, $p <$ 0.001), and had a chronic disease (x^2 = 4.07, p = 0.044) than those elderly in urban areas. ($\chi^2 = 47.38$, $p < 0.001$); they had some type of disability ($\chi^2 = 33.12$, $p < 0.001$), a chronic disease ($\chi^2 = 4.07$, p = 0.044), and were more likely to have caregivers ($\chi^2 = 142.50$, $p < 0.001$). Caregivers in the rural area were more likely to have primary education ($\chi^2 = 14.03$, p = 0.001), live with the elderly ($\chi^2 = 109.14$, $p < 0.001$), be workless ($\chi^2 = 12.54$, $p < 0.001$), and spend more time (13–24 hours) daily providing care ($\chi^2 = 35.57$, $p < 0.001$) (Tables 3 and 4).

3.2. Annual Cost and Use of Services. The annual cost and use of services are shown in Table 5. The total annual LTC spending was USD 7,285 for rural residents and USD 7,280.6 on average for urban residents.

For the rural area, the average spending on paid caregivers per year was USD 3,309.1 by men and USD 2,612.5 by women; these amounts were less than those for urban men (USD 4,005.8) and women (USD 3,134.9).

The informal care cost of rural residents was USD 2,065.2/year for men and USD 2,145.2/year for women; similarly, the informal care cost of urban residents was USD 2,192.3/year for men and USD 2,021.4/year for women. The cost of day/night care for rural residents was USD 2,717/year for men and USD 1,268.9/year for women.

The cost of daily supplies for rural men was USD 681.2/year and for rural women was USD 664/year. Similarly, the cost of daily supplies for urban men was USD 724.7/year and for urban women was USD 663.3/year.

The average spending on home renovation for the rural elderly was USD 42.7/year and that on medical devices for the rural elderly was USD 24.3/year. The average spending on home renovation for the urban elderly was USD 22.4/year and that on medical devices was USD 18.4/year.

3.3. Logistic Regression Analysis to Identify Factors That Influence LTC Utilization. The binary logistic regression analysis results are shown in Table 6. Age was positively associated with the cost of daily supplies (OR = 1.04, 95% CI: 1.01–1.06; p = 0.010) and that of medical devices (OR = 1.06, 95% CI: 1.03–1.09; $p < 0.001$). However, it was negatively associated with the institutional cost (OR = 0.92, 95% CI: 0.84–0.99; p = 0.033).

Living in an urban area was negatively associated with the cost of an institutional stay (OR = 0.09; 95% CI: 0.02–0.40; p = 0.002), the cost of home renovation (OR = 0.69; 95% CI: 0.49–0.94; p = 0.020), and the informal care cost (OR = 0.48; 95% CI: 0.30–0.77; p = 0.002).

Being female was negatively associated with the cost of formal care (OR = 0.12; 95% CI: 0.02–0.64; p = 0.013) and that of home renovation (OR = 1.56; 95% CI: 1.08–2.27; p = 0.019). Being single was negatively associated with the opportunity cost (OR = 0.59; 95% CI: 0.37–0.94; p = 0.026). Work was positively associated with the cost of daily supplies (OR = 1.48; 95% CI: 1.00–2.18; p = 0.048) but negatively associated with the opportunity cost (OR = 0.52; 95% CI: 0.32–0.86; p = 0.010).

An income of more than USD 4,354 per year was positively associated with the cost of medical devices (OR = 1.77; 95% CI: 1.15–2.73; p = 0.010) and the cost of home renovation for elderly (OR = 1.53; 95% CI: 1.04–2.26; p = 0.031).

The presence of at least one of eight chronic diseases was positively associated with the cost of daily supplies (OR = 3.98; 95% CI: 2.18–7.26; $p < 0.001$), the cost of medical devices (OR = 2.24; 95% CI: 1.33–3.80; p = 0.003), and the cost of home renovation (OR = 1.72; 95% CI: 1.13–2.63; p = 0.012). Some form of disability was positively associated with the cost of medical devices (OR = 3.44; 95% CI: 2.27–5.22; $p < 0.001$) but not significantly associated with the cost of daily supplies, the day/night care cost, the cost of formal care, the cost of home renovation for elderly, and informal cost.

4. Discussion

4.1. Annual LTC Costs per Person. This study focuses on the significance of social security and provision of care in costs for the elderly citizens living in the cities and villages of Thailand. Furthermore, this study seeks to explain some very critical determinants of care and its costs.

Noteworthy is the fact that the contribution of the rural areas on average yearly to the total amount of money estimated for this program was USD 7,285. A major share around USD 2,844.7 was distributed to formal care while

Table 3: Characteristics of elderly in study area ($N = 837$).

Care recipients	Rural, N (%)	Urban, N (%)	
N	437 (100)	400 (100)	
Mean age (SD)	71.44 ± 7.86	68.58 ± 5.71	
60–69	208 (47.6)	114 (59.3)	$\chi^2 = 50.32$, $p < 0.001$
70–79	156 (35.7)	154 (38.5)	
≥80	73 (16.7)	9 (2.3)	
Gender			$\chi^2 = 1.24$, $p = 0.266$
Female	302 (69.1)	262 (65.5)	
Marital status			$\chi^2 = 6.57$, $p = 0.037$
Never married	45 (10.3)	47 (11.8)	
Married living together	191 (43.7)	204 (51.0)	
Married not living together[a]	201 (46.0%)	149 (37.3)	
Education level			$\chi^2 = 44.93$, $p < 0.001$
Primary school and lower degree	365 (83.5)	253 (63.3)	
High school	44 (10.1)	82 (20.5)	
Diploma and higher degree	28 (6.4)	65 (16.3)	
Living arrangement			$\chi^2 = 0.11$, $p = 0.736$
Not alone	359 (82.2)	325 (81.3)	
Working status			$\chi^2 = 2.32$, $p = 0.128$
Did not work	294 (67.3)	249 (62.3)	
Annual income[b]			$\chi^2 = 50.79$, $p < 0.001$
No income	21 (5.3)	70 (18.7)	
<USD 4,354	311 (77.8)	208 (55.6)	
≥USD 4,354	68 (17.0)	96 (25.7)	
Source of support (not including work)[c]			
Old age allowance	388 (90.2)	284 (71.5)	$\chi^2 = 47.38$, $p < 0.001$
Children	154 (35.9)	120 (30.2)	$\chi^2 = 2.99$, $p = 0.084$
Pensions/lump sums	30 (7.0)	70 (17.6)	$\chi^2 = 22.05$, $p < 0.001$
Property income[d]	32 (7.4)	28 (7.1)	$\chi^2 = 0.05$, $p = 0.829$
Other	24 (5.6)	19 (4.8)	$\chi^2 = 0.27$, $p = 0.607$
Disability			$\chi^2 = 33.12$, $p < 0.001$
Any disabilities	109 (24.9)	39 (9.8)	
Chronic diseases[e]			$\chi^2 = 4.07$, $p = 0.044$
Any chronic disease	356 (81.5)	303 (75.8)	
Caregiver			$\chi^2 = 142.50$, $p < 0.001$
Have caregiver	327 (74.8)	135 (33.8)	

[a]Married not living together includes separated, widowed, and divorced. [b]Data were missing for some respondents for the yearly personal income (62). [c]One person may have more than one source of support. [d]Property income includes rental income, equity/fixed interest, and return from another investments. [e]Chronic diseases include hypertension, diabetes, stroke, heart problems, dementia, osteoarthritis, paralysis, and hypercholesterol.

USD 2,114 was allocated to informal care. The cities' LTC total yearly cost on average was USD 7,280.6. Additionally, the formal and informal sector's yearly economic value of USD 2,380.3 and USD 2,089, respectively, accounted for the bigger share of the total expenditure.

In this study, the hypothesis made is that the total expenditures of the rural elderly are higher than the urban elderly. However, this research does not completely reject the null hypothesis as the total average annual LTC expenditures for both rural and urban elderly are equivalent, according to this research.

This study arrives at a different finding than the several existing types of research, which hypothesized that the expenditure in urban areas is much higher than that of the rural [41, 42]. This observation can be ascribed to the fact that urban areas have better health care and medical facilities compared to the rural areas [14]. In addition, those living in urban areas, owing to their lifestyles, can afford better medical facilities and advanced treatments because they are economically endowed. The low-income people living in rural areas, however, might not be able to even afford low-cost health care [16, 18].

The 2014 Elderly Population survey evidenced 10 million elderly citizens in Thailand, of which 41% were urban residents [43]. In such a scenario, if every citizen were to access all kinds of care such as the ones included in this study, the

Table 4: Characteristics of caregivers ($N = 462$).

	Rural, N (%)	Urban, N (%)	
N	327 (100)	135 (100)	
Mean age (SD)	52.82 ± 15.11	52.50 ± 14.54	
<40	73 (22.3)	31 (23.0)	$\chi^2 = 0.78$, $p = 0.674$
40–59	146 (44.6)	65 (48.1)	
≥60	108 (33.0)	39 (28.9)	
Gender			$\chi^2 = 1.49$, $p = 0.222$
Female	232 (70.9)	88 (65.2)	
Marital status			$\chi^2 = 1.30$, $p = 0.523$
Never married	80 (24.5)	32 (23.7)	
Married living together	198 (24.2)	77 (57.0)	
Married not living together[a]	49 (15.0)	26 (19.3)	
Education level			$\chi^2 = 14.03$, $p = 0.001$
Primary school and lower degree	165 (50.5)	44 (32.6)	
High school	79 (24.2)	37 (27.4)	
Diploma and higher degree	83 (25.4)	54 (40.0)	
Relationship with care recipients			$\chi^2 = 3.86$, $p = 0.276$
Spouse	133 (40.7)	57 (42.2)	
Son/son-in-law	43 (13.1)	21 (15.6)	
Daughter/daughter-in-law	94 (28.7)	43 (31.9)	
Relatives	57 (17.4)	14 (10.4)	
Residence status			$\chi^2 = 109.14$, $p < 0.001$
Coresidence with elderly	280 (85.6)	112 (83)	
Working status			$\chi^2 = 12.54$, $p < 0.001$
Did not work	197 (60.2)	57 (42.2)	
Annual income			$\chi^2 = 77.21$, $p < 0.001$
No income	22 (7.3)	57 (42.2)	
<USD 4,354	190 (62.9)	50 (37.0)	
≥USD 4,354	90 (29.8)	28 (20.7)	
Reason for leaving a job[b]			$\chi^2 = 0.90$, $p = 0.636$
Care for an elderly	96 (55.8)	19 (47.5)	
Retirement	40 (23.3)	11 (27.5)	
Other	36 (20.9)	10 (25.0)	
Time spent in informal caregiving (hours/day)			$\chi^2 = 35.57$, $p < 0.001$
Less than 4	35 (11.5)	27 (20.8)	
5–8	134 (43.9)	78 (60.0)	
9–12	57 (18.7)	21 (15.6)	
13–24	79 (25.9)	4 (3.1)	

[a]Married not living together includes widowed and divorced. [b]Data were missing for some respondents for the reason for quitting their job (42).

total care expenditure's approximate value would be around USD 73 billion in average, per year, for the whole country.

The expenditures for both urban and rural contributors, in this study, were compared with six different types of LTC costs. The results showed that the expenditures, on average, on informal and formal care, health care devices, and home makers, were lower in urban areas in comparison to rural areas. However, the day and night care costs, as well as the costs of regular medical supplies in the cities, are higher than that of the rural areas. This could be largely attributed to the different settings in rural and urban areas [16].

When compared to women, the larger part of every category of the rural areas' expenditure is associated with men, save for the informal care. Whereas, in urban areas, men spend higher than women in a day or night care and informal care [21]. Also, according to sociology, this is attributed to a belief in conventional gender roles wherein every gender is culturally assigned roles, for instance, women being assigned families' caregiver roles [7].

Most senior citizens, despite having a choice of established LTC, prefer to remain at home and, thus, obtain support from the formal caregivers or informal programs

TABLE 5: Cost on services for rural and urban residents (person/year).

	Rural			Urban		
	Male	Female	Average	Male	Female	Average
Formal care (USD)	3,309.1	2,612.5	2,844.7	4,005.8	3,134.9	2,380.3
Service use (%)	37.4	38.7	39.1	42.7	41.2	32.7
Informal care (USD)	2,065.2	2,145.2	2,114	2,192.3	2,021.4	2,089
Service use (%)	23.4	31.7	29.0	23.3	26.6	28.7
Day/night care (USD)	2,717	1,268.9	1,590.7	2,438.3	1,741.6	2,090
Service use (%)	30.7	18.8	21.8	26.0	22.9	28.7
Daily supplies (USD)	681.2	664	668.7	724.7	663.3	680.6
Service use (%)	7.7	9.8	9.2	7.7	8.7	9.4
Home renovation (USD)	34.6	42.3	42.7	21.5	22.6	22.4
Service use (%)	0.5	0.6	0.6	0.2	0.3	0.3
Medical devices (USD)	25.0	23.8	24.3	10.5	20.7	18.4
Service use (%)	0.3	0.4	0.3	0.1	0.3	0.2
Total cost (USD)	8,841.2	6,756.6	7,285	5,387.4	7,604.7	7,280.6

The exchange rate of USD 1 = THB 34.45 (the exchange rate as of March 31, 2017).

[44, 45]. Noteworthy is the fact that in developed economies, there are well-sustained formal care expenditures for the senior citizens to access excellent medical and social services. Conversely, the dependent senior citizens of the low- and middle-income economies lack formal care assistance or social security and thereby are dependent on their families [7, 45, 46].

Owing to this situation, many policy initiatives suggest enhancement of abilities of families to provide health security and care to their elderly members. Yet, recent studies from low- and middle-income countries indicate that little attention has been accorded to dependent elderly citizens' informal caregivers as compared to certain informal care for certain diseases [47, 48].

This study concludes that around 70% of caregivers are females, which differed with other studies across Thailand that put it at 57–81% [49, 50]. These results further revealed that majority of the caregivers fall between the age group of 41 and 60 years. Of these statistics, the majority constitutes spouses accounting for 42.2% in urban areas and 40.7% in rural areas. In addition, daughters constitute 31.9% in urban areas and 28.7% in rural areas.

In consideration of sociodemographic variables, majority studies' variations regarding the informal caregivers are indicative of spouses and children to quit their careers towards taking care of the elderly [44, 48].

4.2. Factors Influencing LTC Utilization. The results of this study substantially linked the ages of the people to their expenditures on health care devices and regular supplies. The policy-makers' view point suggests that the process of aging could yield unwanted results like (i) higher consumption of health care, (ii) increased dependency, and (iii) higher expenditures on health care. The existing studies indicate that the medical services relating to LTC and acute care are costlier for seniors than it is for the young and the old [35, 51].

Also, an urban center dweller presented an inverse proportional to the use of informal health care, home renovation expenditures, and day and night care. This is evidenced by the fact that people from the rural areas use more of informal care than those from the urban. Additionally, the findings show that there are more home modifications in rural areas than there are in the urban areas. This scenario could be explained by the existence of higher rates of handicap zones (24.9%) in rural areas than in the urban (9.8%). In the past, being married or unmarried was inversely proportional to the use of informal care, which is one factor that affects the financial and mental well-being of people because it impacts on the provision of care and quality of the elderly life [37].

The potential risk of receiving informal care is considerably lower for the elderly who have jobs compared with those who are unemployed. This could be attributed to the fact that people facing health issues might have to quit their careers and need informal care. This means the elderly who are part of the workforce have better health than those who are not working [38].

On average, an elderly person who has an annual income exceeding USD 4,354 spends more on medical care and home renovation for elderly because they have an economical endowment to pay [52]. The study found that OAA assistance is a significant source of income for urban and rural elderly, offering USD 20–30 per month.

This study also found that living conditions and education have minimal effect on the use of health care services. The highly educated are assumed to be more aware of the chronic diseases than the uneducated [20, 40]. Moreover, some form of disability that some people have affects the use of medical devices. For instance, the elderly people having a functional disability often use acute care and formal LTC, leading to an increased health care costs [39, 53].

4.3. Strengths and Weaknesses. The major contribution of this study to the current knowledge lies in the provision of unique effects associated with the LTC in cities and villages. This study evaluates the expenditures related to factors which affect the

Table 6: Factors associated with LTC utilization from logistic regression analysis.

Independent variable	Formal care			Informal care		
	Coefficient	Odds ratio (95% CI)	p value	Coefficient	Odds ratio (95% CI)	p value
Age (years)	−0.01	0.99 (0.90–1.09)	0.869	0.03	1.03 (1.00–1.06)	0.078
Urban versus rural	−0.63	0.53 (0.12–2.44)	0.416	−0.74	0.48 (0.30–0.77)	0.002
Female versus male	−2.13	0.12 (0.02–0.64)	0.013	−0.17	0.84 (0.52–1.36)	0.479
Single[a] versus married living together	1.37	3.94 (0.78–19.99)	0.098	−0.53	0.59 (0.37–0.94)	0.026
No education versus any education	1.29	3.64 (0.31–42.78)	0.304	0.45	1.57 (0.67–3.65)	0.296
Living alone	0.21	1.24 (0.22–6.90)	0.809	0.04	1.04 (0.49–2.18)	0.923
Work versus not work	−1.41	0.25 (0.03–2.14)	0.203	−0.65	0.52 (0.32–0.86)	0.010
Annual income ≥ USD 4,354	0.99	2.69 (0.58–12.48)	0.208	0.20	1.22 (0.70–2.12)	0.479
Any chronic disease[b]	−0.72	0.49 (0.11–2.14)	0.342	−0.81	0.44 (0.25–0.80)	0.007
Any disability[c]	0.57	1.77 (0.38–8.38)	0.470	0.04	1.04 (0.62–1.74)	0.895
Constant	−3.20	0.04	0.375	−0.50	0.61	0.663
Independent variable	Day/night care			Daily supplies		
	Coefficient	Odds ratio (95% CI)	p value	Coefficient	Odds ratio (95% CI)	p value
Age (years)	−0.09	0.92 (0.84–0.99)	0.033	0.04	1.04 (1.01–1.06)	0.010
Urban versus rural	−2.41	0.09 (0.02–0.40)	0.002	0.05	1.05 (0.73–1.51)	0.787
Female versus male	0.09	1.09 (0.35–3.42)	0.884	0.09	1.09 (0.73–1.65)	0.668
Single[a] versus married living together	0.30	1.35 (0.47–3.85)	0.576	−0.01	0.99 (0.67–1.47)	0.960
No education versus any education	−0.56	0.57 (0.07–4.95)	0.597	−0.15	0.86 (0.42–1.76)	0.683
Living alone	−0.24	0.79 (0.24–2.61)	0.698	0.35	1.42 (0.90–2.24)	0.130
Work versus not work	−0.96	0.38 (0.13–1.15)	0.088	0.39	1.48 (1.00–2.18)	0.048
Annual income ≥ USD 4,354	−0.76	0.47 (0.10–2.15)	0.328	0.30	1.35 (0.87–2.09)	0.184
Any chronic disease[b]	0.89	2.42 (0.52–11.23)	0.258	1.38	3.98 (2.18–7.26)	<0.001
Any disability[c]	−1.84	0.16 (0.02–1.24)	0.080	0.39	1.48 (0.95–2.32)	0.086
Constant	2.71	15.03	0.356	−5.40	0.01	<0.001
Independent variable	Home renovation			Medical devices		
	Coefficient	Odds ratio (95% CI)	p value	Coefficient	Odds ratio (95% CI)	p value
Age (years)	−0.02	0.98 (0.96–1.00)	0.078	0.06	1.06 (1.03–1.09)	<0.001
Urban versus rural	−0.39	0.68 (0.49–0.94)	0.020	−0.11	0.90 (0.62–1.31)	0.577
Female versus male	0.45	1.56 (1.08–2.27)	0.019	−0.23	0.80 (0.53–1.20)	0.282
Single[a] versus married living together	−0.03	0.97 (0.68–1.37)	0.857	−0.11	0.90 (0.60–1.35)	0.612
No education versus any education	−0.72	0.49 (0.23–1.04)	0.062	0.09	1.10 (0.54–2.21)	0.797
Living alone	−0.26	0.77 (0.5–1.20)	0.245	−0.29	0.75 (0.44–1.27)	0.281
Work versus not work	0.01	1.01 (0.71–1.43)	0.960	−0.37	0.69 (0.45–1.05)	0.086
Annual income ≥ USD 4,354	0.43	1.53 (1.04–2.26)	0.031	0.57	1.77 (1.15–2.73)	0.010
Any chronic disease[b]	0.54	1.72 (1.13–2.63)	0.012	0.81	2.24 (1.33–3.80)	0.003
Any disability[c]	0.09	1.10 (0.72–1.68)	0.665	1.24	3.44 (2.27–5.22)	<0.001
Constant	−0.05	0.95	0.956	−5.86	0.00	<0.001

[a]Single includes never married, divorced, widowed, and married but not living together. [b]Any chronic disease includes hypertension, diabetes, stroke, heart problems, dementia, osteoarthritis, paralysis, and hypercholesterol. [c]Any disability includes personal hygiene, bathing, eating, toileting, upstairs 1-2 step, dressing, walking 200 meters, moving around the bed, urinary incontinence, and fecal incontinence.

prices of every care. The most desirable consequences of this research are those connected to social resources optimization such as promoting health care volunteer and measures to ensure institutionalization of the older people.

Though this study contributes significantly to the current knowledge in this field, it presents certain limitations. Firstly, this survey is rather cross-sectional and not longitudinal, which demands a cautious use of linkages. Secondly, this study has self-reported information and thereby is subject to bias. Thirdly, some of the important variables were neither optimally coded nor available. For instance, the lack of optimal coded levels of diseases and functional status, which may affect the perfection and thus the modification, may be imperfect. The regression process lacks consideration of the levels of disability. Lastly, the absence of the data on health care volunteer services and occupation details employed an average local formal care wage to derive the approximate value of the informal care. This was done as more than half of the caregivers were female, which might suggest an overestimation of this informal care expenditure.

Despite these limitations, this research will prove important to policy-makers and health workers in their quest to optimize social resources and determine ways of handling this situation and encouraging specific forms of home and community formal care. Moreover, from the social point of view, further studies on longitudinal approaches geared towards assessing the long-term economic effects must be conducted. In addition, further study of LTC policy under the National Health Security funding is desirable.

5. Conclusion

This study found the total average annual LTC expenditures between rural-urban residents to be similar. The rapid urban development in coastal areas drives Thailand's economic growth but threatens to leave the rural population behind. In contrast, rural areas surrounding the city are mainly concerned with agriculture that generates lower incomes and these populations are reported to have reduced access to LTC services. The superior ability to pay of urbanites enables them to access better quality health care services, whereas even small LTC expenditures can have a devastating impact on the household economy of rural residents. It is important that to reduce health inequality and to promote greater socioeconomic equality, Thailand must invest in health infrastructure in its rural regions. To meet the needs of increasing populations of disabled elderly people and rising expenditures, countries must restructure their delivery systems and find a balance between the costlier formal and cheaper informal care options.

Acknowledgments

The authors would like to express their sincere thanks to Dr. Robert S. Chapman, M.D., for his suggestions on the statistical analysis and gratefully acknowledge Dr. Suwit Wibulpolprasert, M.D., for his helpful advices. The authors also wish to express their appreciation to the staff in Muang and Bangmulnark subdistricts of Phichit Province for their assistance in data collection. This research has been supported by the National Research University Project, Office of Higher Education Commission (WCU-58-031-AS).

References

[1] S. Srithamrongsawat, K. Bundhamcharoen, S. Sasat, P. Odton, and S. Ratkjaroenkhajorn, *Projection of Demand and Expenditure for Institutional Long Term Care in Thailand*, Health Insurance System Research Office, Bangkok, Thailand, 2009.

[2] Y. Porapakkham, C. Rao, J. Pattaraarchachai et al., "Estimated causes of death in Thailand, 2005: implications for health policy," *Population Health Metrics*, vol. 8, no. 1, p. 14, 2010.

[3] A. Dans, N. Ng, C. Varghese, E. S. Tai, R. Firestone, and R. Bonita, "The rise of chronic non-communicable diseases in southeast Asia: time for action," *The Lancet*, vol. 377, no. 9766, pp. 680–689, 2011.

[4] WHO Study Group, *Home-Based Long-Term Care: Report of a WHO Study Group*, World Health Organization, Geneva, Switzerland, 2000.

[5] G. Damiani, V. Farelli, A. Anselmi et al., "Patterns of long term care in 29 European countries: evidence from an exploratory study," *BMC Health Services Research*, vol. 11, no. 1, p. 316, 2011.

[6] World Bank, "Long-term care in aging East Asia and Pacific," *Live Long and Prosper: Aging in East Asia and Pacific*, World Bank, Washington, DC, USA, 2016.

[7] N. Wongsawang, S. Lagampan, P. Lapvongwattana, and B. J. Bowers, "Family caregiving for dependent older adults in Thai families," *Journal of Nursing Scholarship*, vol. 45, no. 4, pp. 336–343, 2013.

[8] J. Knodel, J. Kespichayawattana, S. Wiwatwanich, and C. Saengtienchai, "The future of family support for Thai elderly: views of the populace," *Journal of Population and Social Studies*, vol. 21, no. 2, pp. 110–132, 2013.

[9] Hfocus, "Lamsonthi model: Family Care Team prototype," February 2017, https://www.hfocus.org/content/2016/04/12048.

[10] Isranew Agency, "NHSO set a budget 600 million baht for dependent elderly care for 1,000 subdistrict," February 2017, https://www.isranews.org/isranews/41355-nsho_41355.html.

[11] National Health Security Office, *Financial Management Framework for Severe Dependency Elderly Fiscal Year 2016*, National Health Security Office, Nonthaburi, Thailand, 2015.

[12] W. Suwanrada, S. Sasat, and S. Kumruangrit, *Financing Long Term Care Services for the Elderly in the Bangkok Metropolitan Administration*, Foundation of Thai Gerontology Research and Development Institute (TGRI) and Thai Health Promotion Foundation, Bangkok, Thailand, 2009.

[13] U. Wongsin, T. Sakunphanit, S. Labbenchakul, and D. Pongpattrachai, "Estimate unit cost per day of long term care for dependent elderly," *Journal of Health Systems Research*, vol. 8, no. 4, 2014.

[14] M. Liu, Q. Zhang, M. Lu, C. S. Kwon, and H. Quan, "Rural and urban disparity in health services utilization in China," *Medical Care*, vol. 45, no. 8, pp. 767–774, 2007.

[15] L. M. Goeres, A. Gille, J. P. Furuno et al., "Rural-urban differences in chronic disease and drug utilization in older oregonians," *Journal of Rural Health*, vol. 32, no. 3, pp. 269–279, 2016.

[16] T. Ikai, S. Yamtree, T. Takemoto et al., "Medical care ideals among urban and rural residents in Thailand: a qualitative study," *International Journal for Equity in Health*, vol. 15, no. 1, p. 2, 2016.

[17] H. Nishiura, S. Barua, S. Lawpoolsri et al., "Health inequalities in Thailand: geographic distribution of medical supplies in the provinces," *Southeast Asian Journal of Tropical Medicine and Public Health*, vol. 35, no. 3, pp. 735–740, 2004.

[18] S. Pannarunothai and A. Mills, "The poor pay more: health-related inequality in Thailand," *Social Science and Medicine*, vol. 44, no. 12, pp. 1781–1790, 1997.

[19] S. Kehusmaa, I. Autti-Ramo, H. Helenius, K. Hinkka, M. Valaste, and P. Rissanen, "Factors associated with the utilization and costs of health and social services in frail elderly patients," *BMC Health Services Research*, vol. 12, no. 1, 2012.

[20] C. Zyaambo, S. Siziya, and K. Fylkesnes, "Health status and socio-economic factors associated with health facility utilization in rural and urban areas in Zambia," *BMC Health Services Research*, vol. 12, no. 1, p. 389, 2012.

[21] N. Saikia, Moradhvaj, and J. K. Bora, "Gender difference in health-care expenditure: evidence from India Human Development Survey," *PLoS One*, vol. 11, no. 7, Article ID e0158332, 2016.

[22] K. Alam and A. Mahal, "Economic impacts of health shocks on households in low and middle income countries: a review of the literature," *Globalization and Health*, vol. 10, no. 1, p. 21, 2014.
[23] L. J. Ku, L. F. Liu, and M. J. Wen, "Trends and determinants of informal and formal caregiving in the community for disabled elderly people in Taiwan," *Archives of Gerontology and Geriatrics*, vol. 56, no. 2, pp. 370–376, 2013.
[24] J. Woo, S. C. Ho, J. Lau, and Y. K. Yuen, "Age and marital status are major factors associated with institutionalisation in elderly Hong Kong Chinese," *Journal of Epidemiology and Community Health*, vol. 48, no. 3, pp. 306–309, 1994.
[25] J. A. Oladipo, "Utilization of health care services in rural and urban areas: a determinant factor in planning and managing health care delivery systems," *African Health Sciences*, vol. 14, no. 2, pp. 322–333, 2014.
[26] W. Suwanrada, S. Sasat, N. Witvorapong, and S. Kumruangrit, "The cost of institutional Long Term Care for Older Persons: a case study of Thammapakorn Social Welfare Development Center for Older Persons, Chiang Mai Province," *Journal of Health Systems Research*, vol. 10, no. 2, 2016.
[27] National Health Security Office, *National Civil Registration System*, National Health Security Office, Nonthaburi, Thailand, 2015.
[28] T. Yamane, *Statistics, An Introductory Analysis*, Harper and Row Publishers, New York, NY, USA, 1973.
[29] K. Tisayaticom, W. Patcharanarumol, and V. Tangcharoensathien, *District Hospital Costing Manual (in Thai Language)*, International Health Policy Planning, Bangkok, Thailand, 2001.
[30] A. L. Creese and D. Parker, *Cost Analysis in Primary Health Care : A Training Manual for Programme Managers*, World Health Organization, Geneva, Switzerland, 1994.
[31] Bank of Thailand, *Foreign Exchange Rates*, Bank of Thailand, Bangkok, Thailand, March 2017, https://www.bot.or.th/English/Statistics/FinancialMarkets/ExchangeRate/_layouts/Application/ExchangeRate/ExchangeRate.aspx.
[32] P. Diehr, D. Yanez, A. Ash, M. Hornbrook, and D. Lin, "Methods for analyzing health care utilization and costs," *Annual Review of Public Health*, vol. 20, no. 1, pp. 125–144, 1999.
[33] T. P. Hofer, R. A. Wolfe, P. J. Tedeschi, L. F. McMahon, and J. R. Griffith, "Use of community versus individual socioeconomic data in predicting variation in hospital use," *Health Services Research*, vol. 33, no. 2, pp. 243–259, 1998.
[34] D. Gregori, M. Petrinco, S. Bo, A. Desideri, F. Merletti, and E. Pagano, "Regression models for analyzing costs and their determinants in health care: an introductory review," *International Journal for Quality in Health Care*, vol. 23, no. 3, pp. 331–341, 2011.
[35] J. X. Nie, L. Wang, C. S. Tracy, R. Moineddin, and R. E. Upshur, "Health care service utilization among the elderly: findings from the Study to Understand the Chronic Condition Experience of the Elderly and the Disabled (SUCCEED project)," *Journal of Evaluation in Clinical Practice*, vol. 14, no. 6, pp. 1044–1049, 2008.
[36] W. J. Baumol, "Health care, education and the cost of disease: a looming crisis for public choice," *Public Choice*, vol. 77, no. 1, pp. 17–28, 1993.
[37] K. Bolin, B. Lindgren, and P. Lundborg, "Informal and formal care among single-living elderly in Europe," *Health Economics*, vol. 17, no. 3, pp. 393–409, 2007.
[38] J. Lee and M. H. Kim, "The effect of employment transitions on physical health among the elderly in South Korea: a longitudinal analysis of the Korean Retirement and Income Study," *Social Science and Medicine*, vol. 181, pp. 122–130, 2017.
[39] T. R. Fried, E. H. Bradley, C. S. Williams, and M. E. Tinetti, "Functional disability and health care expenditures for older persons," *Archives of Internal Medicine*, vol. 161, no. 21, pp. 2602–2607, 2001.
[40] S. MacLeod, S. Musich, S. Gulyas et al., "The impact of inadequate health literacy on patient satisfaction, healthcare utilization, and expenditures among older adults," *Geriatric Nursing*, vol. 38, no. 4, pp. 334–341, 2017.
[41] M. Li, Y. Zhang, Z. Zhang, Y. Zhang, L. Zhou, and K. Chen, "Rural-urban differences in the long-term care of the disabled elderly in China," *PLoS One*, vol. 8, no. 11, Article ID e79955, 2013.
[42] C. E. McConnel and M. R. Zetzman, "Urban/rural differences in health service utilization by elderly persons in the United States," *Journal of Rural Health*, vol. 9, no. 4, pp. 270–280, 1993.
[43] National Statistical Office, *Survey of Elderly in Thailand 2014*, National Statistical Office (NSO), Thailand, 2014.
[44] C. Laubunjong, N. Phlainoi, S. Graisurapong, and W. Kongsuriyanavin, "The pattern of caregiving to the elderly by their families in rural communities of Suratthani Province," *ABAC Journal*, vol. 28, no. 2, pp. 64–74, 2008.
[45] S. Srithamrongsawat and K. Bundhamcharoen, *Synthesis of long-term care system for the elderly in Thailand*, Foundation of Thai Gerontology Research and the Development Institute, Bangkok, Thailand, 2010.
[46] U. Schneider, B. Trukeschitz, R. Muhlmann, and I. Ponocny, "Do I stay or do I go?"–job change and labor market exit intentions of employees providing informal care to older adults," *Health Economics*, vol. 22, no. 10, pp. 1230–1249, 2013.
[47] M. Zencir, N. Kuzu, N. G. Beser, A. Ergin, B. Catak, and T. Sahiner, "Cost of Alzheimer's disease in a developing country setting," *International Journal of Geriatric Psychiatry*, vol. 20, no. 7, pp. 616–622, 2005.
[48] A. Riewpaiboon, W. Riewpaiboon, K. Ponsoongnern, and B. Van den Berg, "Economic valuation of informal care in Asia: a case study of care for disabled stroke survivors in Thailand," *Social Science and Medicine*, vol. 69, no. 4, pp. 648–653, 2009.
[49] N. Sharma, S. Chakrabarti, and S. Grover, "Gender differences in caregiving among family-caregivers of people with mental illnesses," *World Journal of Psychiatry*, vol. 6, no. 1, pp. 7–17, 2016.
[50] R. del-Pino-Casado, A. Frias-Osuna, P. A. Palomino-Moral, and J. Ramon Martinez-Riera, "Gender differences regarding informal caregivers of older people," *Journal of Nursing Scholarship*, vol. 44, no. 4, pp. 349–357, 2012.
[51] C. de Meijer, M. Koopmanschap, T. B. d' Uva, and E. van Doorslaer, "Determinants of long-term care spending: age, time to death or disability?," *Journal of Health Economics*, vol. 30, no. 2, pp. 425–438, 2011.
[52] S. Limwattananon, V. Tangcharoensathien, K. Tisayaticom, T. Boonyapaisarncharoen, and P. Prakongsai, "Why has the Universal Coverage Scheme in Thailand achieved a pro-poor public subsidy for health care?," *BMC Public Health*, vol. 12, no. 1, p. S6, 2012.
[53] T. Lee, "The relationship between severity of physical impairment and costs of care in an elderly population," *Geriatric Nursing*, vol. 21, no. 2, pp. 102–106, 2000.

23

Knockout of Vasohibin-1 Gene in Mice Results in Healthy Longevity with Reduced Expression of Insulin Receptor, Insulin Receptor Substrate 1, and Insulin Receptor Substrate 2 in Their White Adipose Tissue

Eichi Takeda,[1] Yasuhiro Suzuki,[1] Tetsuya Yamada,[2] Hideki Katagiri,[2] and Yasufumi Sato[1]

[1]*Department of Vascular Biology, Institute of Development, Aging, and Cancer, Tohoku University, Sendai, Japan*
[2]*Department of Diabetes and Metabolism, Graduate School of Medicine, Tokyo University, Tokyo, Japan*

Correspondence should be addressed to Yasufumi Sato; yasufumi.sato.b3@tohoku.ac.jp

Academic Editor: Barbara Shukitt-Hale

Vasohibin-1 (Vashl), originally isolated as an endothelium-derived angiogenesis inhibitor, has a characteristic of promoting stress tolerance in endothelial cells (ECs). We therefore speculated that the lack of the *vashl* gene would result in a short lifespan. However, to our surprise, *vashl*$^{-/-}$ mice lived significantly longer with a milder senescence phenotype than wild-type (WT) mice. We sought the cause of this healthy longevity and found that *vashl*$^{-/-}$ mice exhibited mild insulin resistance along with reduced expression of the insulin receptor (insr), insulin receptor substrate 1 (irs-1), and insulin receptor substrate 2 (irs-2) in their white adipose tissue (WAT) but not in their liver or skeletal muscle. The expression of vashl dominated in the WAT among those 3 organs. Importantly, *vashl*$^{-/-}$ mice did not develop diabetes even when fed a high-fat diet. These results indicate that the expression of vashl was required for the normal insulin sensitivity of the WAT and that the target molecules for this activity were insr, irsl, and irs2. The lack of vashl caused mild insulin resistance without the outbreak of overt diabetes and might contribute to healthy longevity.

1. Introduction

The average human lifespan has been substantially elongated due to the improvement of public health and medical care in developed countries. Aging is associated with numerous changes to systemic physiology that affect physical function and performance. Moreover, aging is closely associated with various pathological conditions such as cancer and cardiovascular and neurodegenerative diseases. For this reason, aging has now become the greatest risk factor for disability and mortality, and healthy longevity has become one of the major objectives of medical research [1].

Numerous studies have being focused on the mechanism of aging [2], and so far they have revealed certain genes and signaling pathways that contribute to the regulation of the lifespan [3, 4]. Among them, insulin signaling plays a crucial and evolutionally conserved role in longevity [5, 6]. Decreased insulin signaling for longevity was first demonstrated in *C. elegance* [7] and next *Drosophila* [8] and further confirmed in mammals [9]. Indeed, the fat-tissue specific knockout of the *insulin receptor* gene in mice results in an extended lifespan [9]. However, as insulin signaling is essential for glucose homeostasis, this decreased insulin signaling should cause diabetes mellitus. Such a paradox has raised a challenging question as to how the preserved insulin signaling for glucose homeostasis and the reduced insulin signaling for longevity can be balanced [10].

The vascular system is one of the major target organs affected by aging [11, 12]. In order to maintain vascular integrity, vascular endothelial cells (ECs) should have self-defense systems. We previously reported that vasohibin-1 (Vashl) could be one of such systems [13]. Vashl was originally isolated as an angiogenesis inhibitor was preferentially expressed in ECs for negative-feedback regulation [14]. However, our subsequent analysis revealed that Vashl has an additional function that causes an upsurge in stress resistance of

ECs by increasing the expression of superoxide dismutase 2 (SOD2) and SIRT1 in ECs [15]. Along with this finding, we observed that the decreased expression of Vash1 promotes vascular diseases such as diabetic nephropathy and atherosclerosis [16, 17]. We then noticed that the expression of Vash1 in ECs is downregulated with aging due to an increase in the expression of a certain microRNA, namely, miR-22 [17]. This observation raised the question as to why nature would allow a decrease in the expression of such a valuable protein with aging.

Because of the protective role of Vash1 in the vasculature, in this present study we assumed that *vash1*$^{-/-}$ mice would have a short lifespan. However, to our surprise, *vash1*$^{-/-}$ mice lived significantly longer and looked healthier than wild-type (WT) mice. Therefore, we examined the reason for this unexpected healthy longevity in *vash1*$^{-/-}$ mice in relation to insulin signaling and further considered the meaning of this age-associated downregulation of vash1.

2. Materials and Methods

2.1. Quantitative Reverse Transcription Real-Time Polymerase Chain Reaction (qRT-PCR). Total RNA was prepared from mouse tissues by using ISOGEN II (Nippon Gene, Tokyo, Japan) according to the manufacturer's instructions. Single-stranded complementary DNA (cDNA) was synthesized by using ReverTra Ace (TOYOBO, Tokyo, Japan). PCR was performed with a thermal cycler system (CFX-96 Real-Time system, C1000 Thermal Cycler, Bio-Rad, Hercules, CA, USA) and SsoAdvanced Universal SYBR Green Supermix (BIO-Rad, Tokyo, Japan). β-actin was used as the reference gene. The primer pairs are shown in Table 2.

2.2. Animal Studies. All of the animal studies were approved by the Center for Laboratory Animal Research of Tohoku University. WT and *Vash1*$^{-/-}$ mice on a C57BL/6J background [18] were maintained under specific pathogen-free conditions with normal chow (CE-2; CLEA Japan Inc., Tokyo, Japan). WT and *Vash1*$^{-/-}$ mice were separately maintained for a certain period of time. To exclude the possible genetic events accumulated over time during separate inbreeding, we crossed *Vash1*$^{-/-}$ mice with WT mice, generated *Vash1*$^{+/-}$, *and then obtained Vash1*$^{-/-}$ again. We defined mice at the age of 8–10 weeks as young and those at 24–26 months as old.

2.2.1. Excision of Certain Mouse Tissues. Selected tissues such as white adipose tissue (epididymal fat pad), liver, and skeletal muscle were excised from the sacrificed mice, snap frozen, and stored at −80°C prior to examination.

2.2.2. High-Fat Diet (HFD) Feeding. Young WT and *Vash1*$^{-/-}$ mice were fed a HFD (D12079B, Research Diets, Inc., New Brunswick, NJ, USA) for 12 weeks. After the mice had been fasted for 10 hours (daytime), blood was collected via a tail vein every 2 weeks. Fasting blood glucose levels were measured by using a Glutest mint (Sanwa Kagaku Kenkyusho, Nagoya, Japan). Plasma insulin and leptin levels were measured with an Ultra-Sensitive Mouse Insulin ELISA Kit (Morinaga Institute of Biological Science, Yokohama, Japan). Plasma adiponectin levels were measured with Mouse/Rat Adiponectin ELISA Kit (Otsuka, Tokushima, Japan). The HOMA-IR index was calculated from the fasting insulin and glucose levels by using the following formula: 26 × fasting plasma insulin (μU/mL) × fasting blood glucose (mg/dL)/405.

2.2.3. Intraperitoneal Glucose Tolerance Test (IPGTT). IPGTT was performed for 10 hours (daytime) on fasted animals after 12 weeks of HFD feeding. The mice were injected with glucose (2 g/kg of body weight) intraperitoneally, after which blood glucose levels were measured at 0, 15, 30, 60, 90, and 120 min after injection.

2.2.4. Intraperitoneal Insulin Tolerance Test (IPITT). IPITT was performed on ad libitum-fed mice after 12 weeks of HFD feeding. The mice were injected with human regular insulin (0.5 or 0.75 U/kg body weight, Novolin R; Novo Nordisk, Bagsvaerd, Denmark) intraperitoneally, followed by measurement of blood glucose levels at 0, 10, 20, 40, 60, and 80 min after injection.

2.2.5. Biochemical Analysis of Serum Samples. Mice were sacrificed after a 16-hour fast; and blood samples were taken by cardiopuncture. The serum was prepared by centrifugation (2000g, 20 min, 4°C). For measuring certain parameters, samples were outsourced to ORIENTAL YEAST CO., LTD (Tokyo, Japan) for serum analysis.

2.2.6. Isolation of CD31-Positive ECs from the WAT. CD31-positive ECs were isolated from the WAT (epididymal fat pad) by the use of a Magnetic Cell Sorting System (MACS, Miltenyi Biotec, Auburn, CA). Tissues of WT or *Vash1*$^{-/-}$ mice were minced and digested with collagenase I and Dispase II (Wako). The cell suspensions were then filtered through a 70 μm cell strainer (BD) and treated with ACK Lysing Buffer (GIBCO) to remove erythrocytes. CD31-positive ECs were isolated by MACS with CD31 MicroBeads (Miltenyi Biotec) according to the manufacturer's instructions.

2.3. Quantification of vash1 Expression in Adipocytes. 3T3L1 preadipocytes were obtained from the Japanese Collection of Research Bioresources and cultured in Dulbecco's Modified Eagles Medium (DMEM)/low glucose media containing 10% fetal bovine serum (FBS; Sigma-Aldrich). Confluent 3T3L1 preadipocytes were cultured in differentiation medium consisting of DMEM, 10% FBS, 500 μM 3-isobutyl-1-methylxanthine (Wako), 10 μg/mL insulin (Wako), and 1 μM dexamethasone (Wako) for 3 days, after which the medium was aspirated and replaced with growth medium containing 10 μg/mL insulin. After 2 days, the medium was changed to growth medium for an additional 2 days to allow 3T3L1 cells to differentiate into mature adipocytes.

Total RNA was extracted from the cells by using an RNeasy plus mini-kit (QIAGEN). First-strand cDNA was synthesized from 1 μg of total RNA by use of ReverTra Ace (TOYOBO). QRT-PCR was carried out as described above. Reactions were carried out in triplicate and contained either

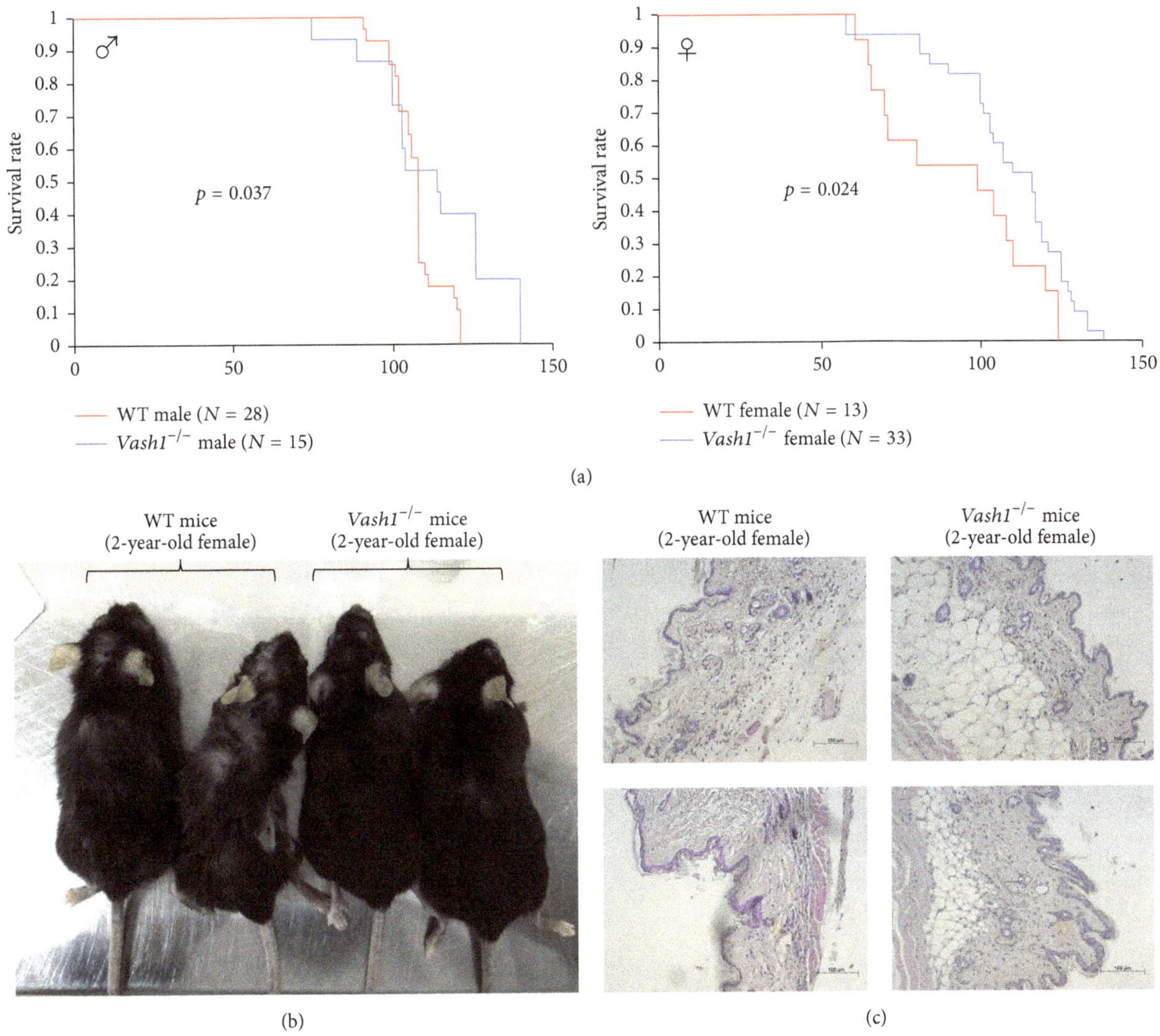

FIGURE 1: Healthy longevity of *vash1*$^{-/-}$ mice of both genders. (a) WT and *vash1*$^{-/-}$ mice of either gender were fed normal chow and compared for their survival rate. (b) Gross appearance of 2-year-old female WT and *vash1*$^{-/-}$ mice is shown. (c) Subcutaneous tissues from 2-year-old female WT and *vash1*$^{-/-}$ mice, stained with hematoxylin and eosin.

1 μL of the first-strand cDNA products or serially-diluted mouse *Vash1* cDNA standards (1 × 10 to 1 × 105 copies). PCR conditions consisted of an initial denaturation step at 95°C for 3 min, followed by 40 cycles of 10 sec at 95°C, 10 sec at 56°C, and 30 sec at 72°C. Quantification analysis was carried out with Bio-Rad CFX Manager software (Bio-Rad Laboratories).

2.4. Statistical Analysis. Data were expressed as the means ± SD. The statistical significance of differences between groups and p values were calculated by using unpaired Student's t-test or by one-way ANOVA followed by the Tukey post hoc test. A value of $p < 0.05$ was the criterion for significance. The significance of the difference between survival curves was analyzed by Kaplan-Meier survival analysis with log-rank testing. A value of $p < 0.05$ was the criterion for significance.

3. Results

3.1. Vash1$^{-/-}$ *Mice Live Longer with a Milder Senescence Phenotype.* We compared the lifespan of *vash1*$^{-/-}$ mice with that of wild-type (WT) mice. Mice were fed normal chow, and no growth retardation or abnormalities were observed in the *vash1*$^{-/-}$ mice. We initially speculated that the *vash1*$^{-/-}$ mice would have a short lifespan. However, to our surprise, *vash1*$^{-/-}$ mice lived significantly longer than the WT ones. This observation was made in both male and female knockout mice, but the difference appeared earlier in the female mice (Figure 1(a)). We also noticed obvious changes in their appearance. WT female mice at 2 years of age showed a senescence phenotype with missing hair, but such phenotype was scarcely observed in the *vash1*$^{-/-}$ female mice (Figure 1(b)).

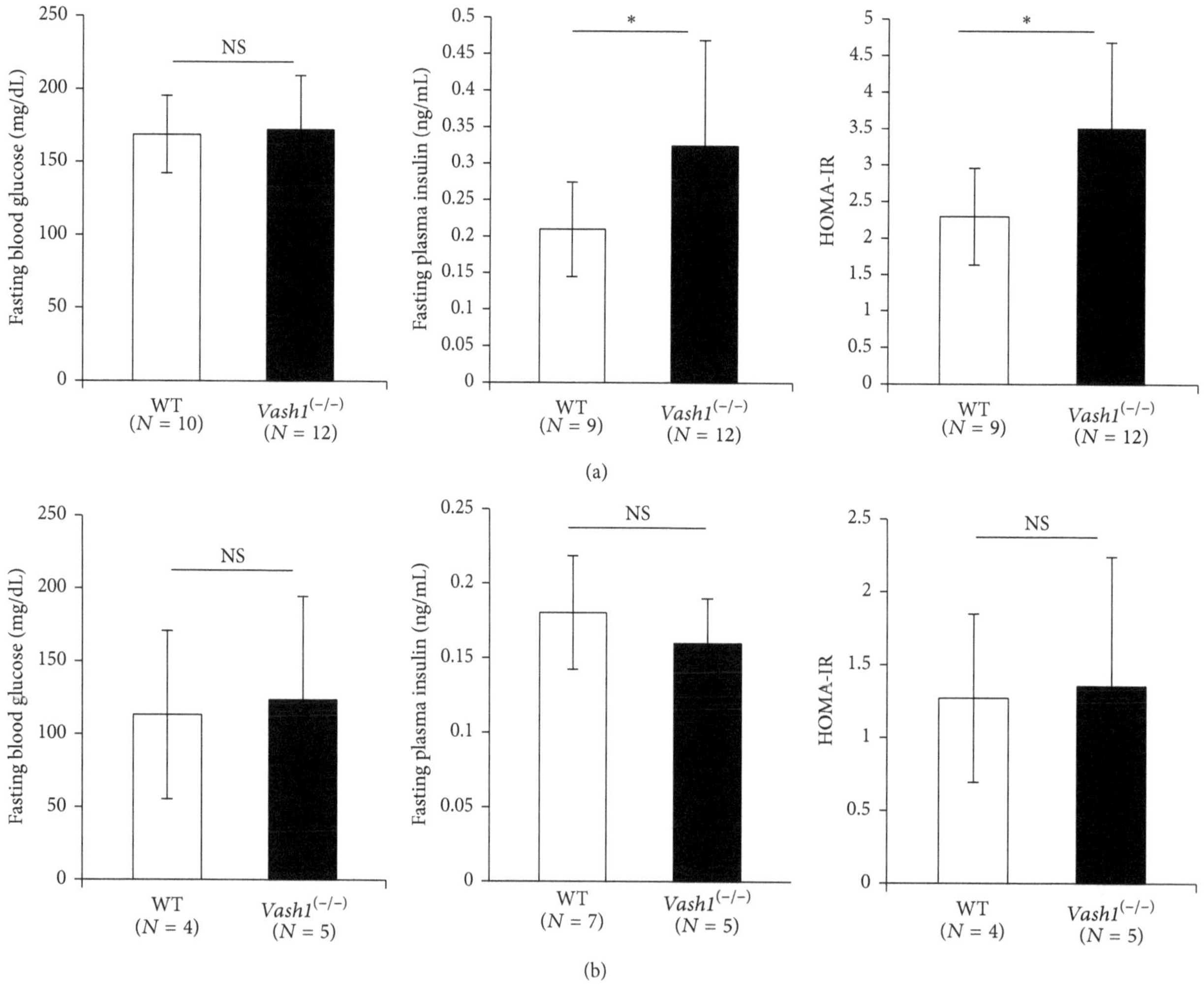

FIGURE 2: Insulin resistance in young *vashl*$^{-/-}$ mice. Fasting blood glucose, fasting plasma insulin, and HOMA-IR are compared between WT and *vashl*$^{-/-}$ of young (a) and old (b) male mice. Means ± SDs are shown. The statistical significance of differences was calculated by use of unpaired Student's t-test, and a value of $p < 0.05$ was the criterion for significance. $^*p < 0.05$.

Also, the subcutaneous fat tissue became thinner in the WT female mice, whereas it was preserved in the *vashl*$^{-/-}$ females (Figure 1(c)). Thus, *vashl*$^{-/-}$ mice exhibited healthy longevity.

3.2. Mild Insulin Resistance in vashl$^{-/-}$ *Mice in Their Early Life.* As insulin signaling is critically involved in the determination of lifespan; next we examined the metabolic status of the animals. *Vashl*$^{-/-}$ mice exhibited mild but apparent insulin resistance without elevation of their blood glucose in early life (Figure 2(a)), and such changes disappeared in late life (Figure 2(b)). Histological analysis revealed no obvious changes in pancreatic islet in their early life (see Supporting Figure 1 in Supplementary Material available online at https://doi.org/10.1155/2017/9851380). Serum biochemical analysis further revealed that there were no obvious abnormal findings in the *vashl*$^{-/-}$ mice, and besides, they had significantly lower levels of CRE, T-CHOL, F-CHOL, E-CHOL, PL, T-BIL, and D-BIL than the WT mice (Table 1).

3.3. Decreased Expression of insr, irs-1, and irs-2 in the WAT of vashl$^{-/-}$ *Mice.* Because of the presence of insulin resistance, we examined the major target organs of insulin and relevant genes that might cause insulin resistance. The expression of insulin receptor (insr), insulin receptor substrate 1 (irs-1), and insulin receptor substrate 2 (irs-2), but not that of Foxol, was significantly downregulated in the WAT of *vashl*$^{-/-}$ mice in their early life (Figure 3(a)). However, we could not find any significant differences in insr, irs-1, or irs-2 expression between the WT mice and *vashl*$^{-/-}$ mice in their skeletal muscle or liver (Figure 3(b)). In order to understand the cause of these differential changes in isnr, irs-1, and irs-2 expression between WT and *vashl*$^{-/-}$ mice among the 3 organs, we compared the level of vashl expression in them. As shown in Figure 3(c), the expression of vashl in the WT mice dominated in their WAT in early life. This expression pattern can be confirmed in human in the Genotype-Tissue Expression Portal (Supporting Figure 2). Thus, the distinctive expression

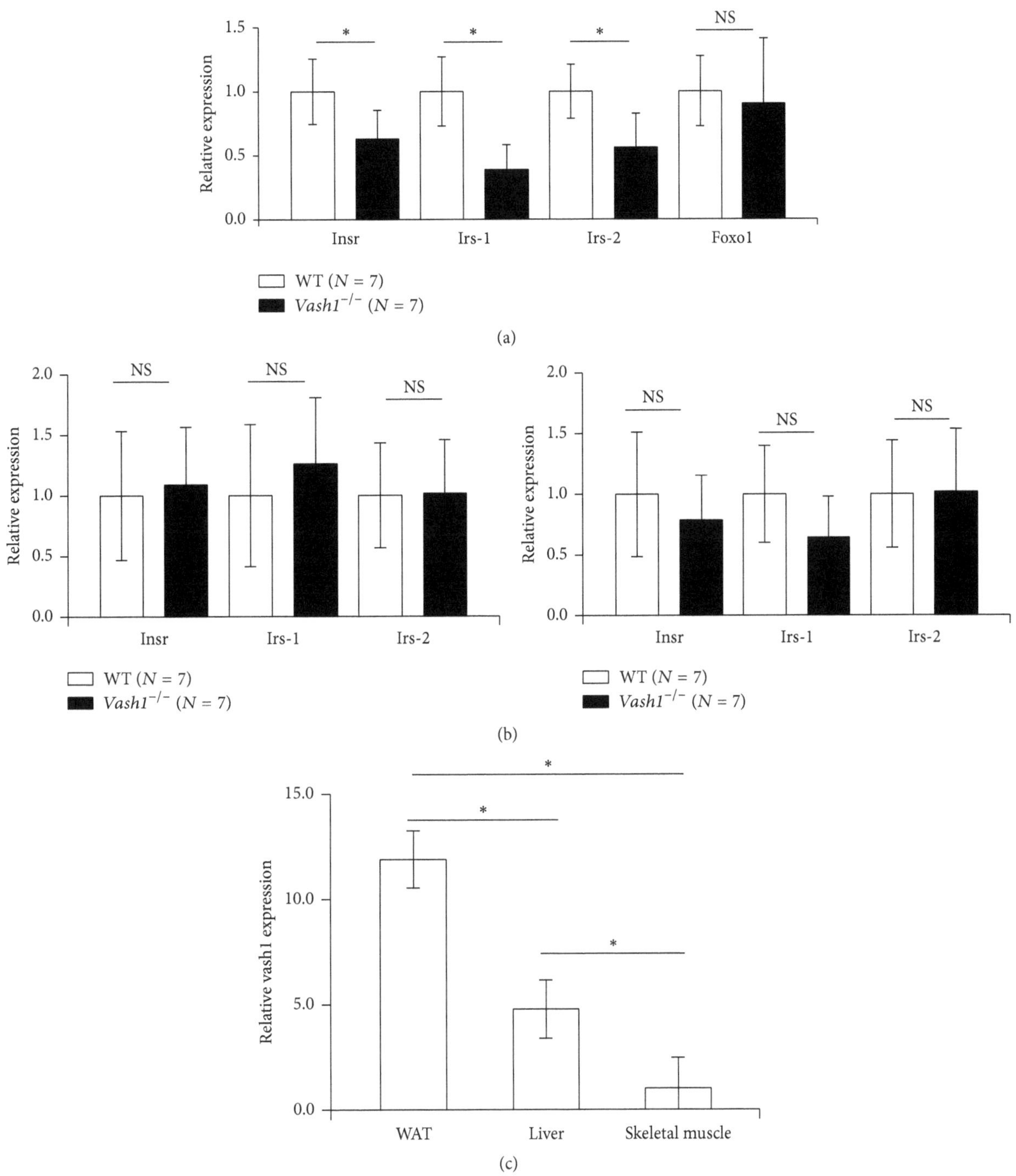

FIGURE 3: Downregulation of insr, irs-1, and irs-2 in WAT of young *vash1*$^{-/-}$ mice. (a) Total RNA was isolated from the WAT of WT and *vash1*$^{-/-}$ young male mice, and the expression of insr, irs-1, irs-2, and Foxo1 was compared between WT and *vash1*$^{-/-}$ mice. (b) Total RNA was isolated from skeletal muscle or liver of WT and *vash1*$^{-/-}$ young male mice; and the expression of insr, irs-1, and irs-2 was compared between WT and *vash1*$^{-/-}$ mouse tissues. (c) Total RNA was isolated from WAT, liver, and skeletal muscle of young WT male mice, and the expression of vash1 was compared. In (a)–(c), the means ± SDs are shown, the statistical significance of differences was calculated by use of the unpaired Student's t-test, and a value of $p < 0.05$ was the criterion for significance. $^*p < 0.05$.

pattern of vash1 among the 3 organs should explain such differential changes and further highlight the distinguishing role of vash1 in the WAT for the expression of insr, irs-1, and irs-2.

We further examined the expression of tnfα as an inflammatory cytokine responsible for insulin resistance, as well as sirt1 and sod2 as targets genes of Vash1 in ECs, but we could not find any differences in their expression levels between

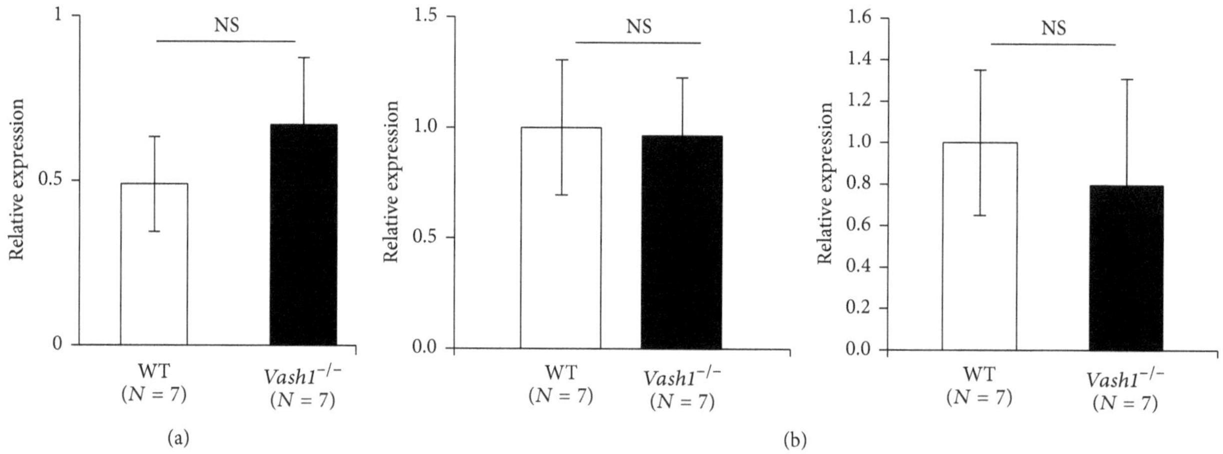

FIGURE 4: No alteration in the expression of tnfα, sod2, and sirtl in the WAT of young *vashl*$^{-/-}$ mice. (a) Total RNA was isolated from the WT and *vashl*$^{-/-}$ WAT of young male mice, and the expression of tnfα was compared between WT and *vashl*$^{-/-}$ mice. (b) Total RNA was isolated from WAT of WT and *vashl*$^{-/-}$ of young male mice, and the expression of sod2 and sirtl was compared between WT and *vashl*$^{-/-}$ mice. In (a) and (b), the means ± SDs are shown, the statistical significance of differences was calculated by use of the unpaired Student's t-test, and a value of $p < 0.05$ was taken as the criterion for significance.

WT mice and *vashl*$^{-/-}$ mice in their WAT (Figures 4(a) and 4(b)).

We reported previously that the expression of vashl is downregulated with aging [17]. We confirmed this age-associated downregulation of vashl in the WAT (Supporting Figure 3A). Therefore, the difference in vashl expression in WAT between WT mice and *vashl*$^{-/-}$ mice was large in their early life and minimized in their late life. Accordingly, the differences in the expression of insr, irs-1, and irs-2 in WAT disappeared in their late life (Supporting Figure 3B). We speculate this to be the reason why insulin resistance disappeared in their late life (Figure 2(b)).

Vashl is reported to be expressed preferentially in ECs ([14]; Shibuya et al., 2006). This was true in the WAT, as the expression of vashl was dominant in CD31-positive cells isolated from the WAT (Figure 5(a)). Moreover, the expression of vashl in in vitro differentiated adipocytes was comparable to the standard copy number of $1\text{–}10^2$ and was negligible (Figure 5(b)). These results highlight the particular role of endothelial vashl in the expression of insr, irs-1, and irs-2 in the WAT.

3.4. Lack of the vashl Gene Does Not Cause Diabetes Mellitus. Finally, we tested whether or not the lack of the vashl gene would be deleterious, causing diabetes. WT mice and *vashl*$^{-/-}$ mice were fed a high-fat diet (HFD) for 12 weeks, with various parameters being monitored. *Vashl*$^{-/-}$ mice were initially heavier than WT mice, but this difference disappeared later. Prior to HFD, we performed GTT and ITT and revealed the tendency of insulin resistance (Supporting Figure 4). We also could not find any differences in the fasting blood glucose level during the HFD feeding period (Figure 6(a)). Plasma adiponectin and leptin concentrations did not show any differences during the HFD feeding period (Supporting Figure 5). After a 12-week HFD feeding, we also performed GTT and ITT. Those examinations revealed that *vashl*$^{-/-}$ mice showed mild glucose intolerance and insulin resistance but never developed overt diabetes (Figures 6(b) and 6(c)).

4. Discussion

This is the first demonstration that conventional knockout of the *vashl* gene causes healthy longevity in mice. This finding was unexpected and surprising to us, because we regarded Vashl as an intrinsic factor that protects vascular ECs from cellular stresses. Indeed, when *vashl* knockout mice are exposed to various stresses, they develop vascular diseases such as diabetic nephropathy and atherosclerotic lesions [16, 17]. Moreover, extensive stresses induced by palaquat administration cause acute lung injury and kill more *vashl* knockout mice than WT mice [15]. Thus, the present unexpected findings forced us to evaluate how the lack of *vashl* gene caused this healthy longevity.

As described earlier, insulin signaling is essential for glucose homeostasis, but it is also involved in longevity. The principal target organs of insulin for glucose homeostasis are the skeletal muscle, the liver, and the adipose tissue. Insulin plays its role in an organ-specific manner: promotion of glucose and fatty acid uptake in the skeletal muscle, suppression of gluconeogenesis in the liver, and inhibition of lipolysis and stimulation of lipid biosynthesis in the adipose tissue [19]. Among these 3 organs, WAT-specific knockout of the *insr* gene results in longevity [9]. Here we revealed that the expression of vashl dominated in the WAT among these 3 organs and that gene knockout of *vashl* in mice caused significant downregulation of *insr, irs-1, and irs-2* genes in their WAT but not in their liver or skeletal muscle. Foxol, one of the most widely expressed members of the subfamilies of the family of winged helix forkhead transcription factors, is a downstream

TABLE 1: Biochemical analysis of sera from WT and *vash1*$^{-/-}$ mice.

	WT ($N = 8$)	*Vash1*$^{-/-}$ ($N = 6$)	p value
TP (g/dL)	4.838 ± 0.737	4.600 ± 1.197	0.6795
ALB (g/dL)	2.788 ± 0.557	2.783 ± 0.631	0.9900
BUN (mg/dL)	65.975 ± 47.696	57.850 ± 54.862	0.7779
CRE (mg/dL)	0.288 ± 0.162	0.108 ± 0.037	0.0164
Na (mEq/L)	153.75 ± 3.69	155.67 ± 4.13	0.3896
K (mEq/L)	6.250 ± 1.01	5.883 ± 2.054	0.6998
Cl (mEq/L)	107.63 ± 8.434	114.67 ± 7.005	0.1144
Ca (mg/dL)	9.913 ± 0.954	8.983 ± 0.708	0.0584
IP (mg/dL)	12.475 ± 0.774	11.833 ± 4.514	0.7440
Fe (mg/dL)	84.125 ± 26.712	116.00 ± 33.196	0.0842
AST (IU/L)	137.5 ± 37.4	171.5 ± 93.6	0.4317
ALT (IU/L)	22.875 ± 17.158	40.5 ± 31.15	0.2497
ALP (IU/L)	353.75 ± 86	357.83 ± 56.99	0.9168
LDH (IU/L)	518.5 ± 215.6	561.8 ± 503.4	0.8494
LAP (IU/L)	47.375 ± 7.963	41.333 ± 10.192	0.2590
AMY (IU/L)	3353.13 ± 584.42	4528.33 ± 4351.53	0.5394
CK (IU/L)	435.75 ± 326.84	491.67 ± 319.69	0.7544
ChE (IU/L)	37.625 ± 6.589	31.833 ± 10.722	0.2773
Lip (IU/L)	32.25 ± 27.92	17.33 ± 7.15	0.1844
T-CHOL (mg/dL)	113.875 ± 47.179	65.167 ± 30.656	0.0379
F-CHOL (mg/dL)	29.125 ± 13.840	16.167 ± 7.574	0.0464
E-CHOL (mg/dL)	84.75 ± 33.65	49.00 ± 23.45	0.0373
TG (mg/dL)	55.125 ± 26.867	29.667 ± 18.843	0.0594
PL (mg/dL)	218.25 ± 90.30	121.33 ± 59.51	0.0328
NEFA (mEq/L)	896.00 ± 409.70	937.00 ± 384.02	0.8519
LDL-C (mg/dL)	12.88 ± 7.41	7.00 ± 2.83	0.0689
HDL-C (mg/dL)	53.625 ± 22.507	32.833 ± 20.331	0.0968
T-BIL (mg/dL)	0.053 ± 0.021	0.105 ± 0.034	0.0114
D-BIL (mg/dL)	0.028 ± 0.013	0.057 ± 0.024	0.0311
I-BIL (mg/dL)	0.025 ± 0.020	0.048 ± 0.021	0.0631
TBA (mmol/L)	7.000 ± 7.010	12.667 ± 7.005	0.1626
TL (mg/dL)	325.50 ± 179.09	182.33 ± 89.35	0.2126
GLU (mg/dL)	101.625 ± 48.603	118.000 ± 68.667	0.6310
PA (mg/dL)	1.305 ± 0.351	1.515 ± 0.295	0.2482
LA (mg/dL)	52.063 ± 16.266	44.783 ± 15.497	0.4124
T-KB (mmol/L)	794.88 ± 504.14	937.83 ± 536.65	0.6232

Total protein (TP), albumin (ALB), blood urea nitrogen (BUN), creatinine (CRE), uric acid (UA), sodium (Na), potassium (K), chloride (Cl), calcium (Ca), inorganic phosphorous (IP), iron (Fe), aspartate aminotransferase (AST), alanine aminotransferase (ALT), alkaline phosphatase (ALP), lactate dehydrogenase (LDH), leucine aminopeptidase (LAP), amylase (AMY), creatine kinase (CK), choline esterase (ChE), lipase (Lip), total cholesterol (T-CHOL), free cholesterol (F-CHOL), esterified cholesterol (E-CHOL), triglyceride (TG), phospholipid (PL), nonesterified fatty acid (NEFA), low-density lipoprotein cholesterol (LDL-C), high-density lipoprotein cholesterol (HDL-C), total bilirubin (T-BIL), direct bilirubin (D-BIL), indirect bilirubin (I-BIL), total bile acid (TBA), total lipid (TL), blood glucose (GLU), pyruvic acid (PA), lactic acid (LA), and total ketone body (T-KB). Means ± SDs and p values are shown.

substrate of insulin signaling for the determination of lifespan [20], but its expression was not affected in the WAT of the *vash1*$^{-/-}$ mice. The expression of sirt1 and sod2, targets genes of Vash1 in ECs [15], was unchanged in the WAT, probably because their expressions were ubiquitous and not specific to ECs. Taking those findings into account, we propose that vash1 has a distinguishing role in the expression of insr, irs-1, and irs-2 in the WAT and that their expression may be at least one of the causes of longevity of *vash1*$^{-/-}$ mice.

Recent studies on insulin resistance emphasize the presence of inflammation and alteration of certain cytokines in the adipose tissue even when the focus is on the contribution of adipose ECs, and such insulin resistance rather results in a short life [21–25]. Our results on the expression of tnf*α* did not indicate the involvement of inflammation in the *vash1*$^{-/-}$ mice. Alternatively, because of the intimate anatomical arrangement between adipocytes and capillary networks, blood vessels may directly control the adipocyte

Table 2: Primer list.

Genes	Forward (5′ → 3′)	Reverse (5′ → 3′)
Vashl	GATTCCCATACCAAGTGTGCC	ATGTGGCGGAAGTAGTTCCC
Insr	ATGAGGCCAACCTTCCTGGAA	ACGGGACATTCTCCATGTCT
Irs-1	AGCCCAAAAGCCCAGGAGAATA	TTCCGAGCCAGTCTCTTCTCTA
Irs-2	AGTAAACGGAGGTGGCTACA	AAGCTGCTGAGAAGTCAGGT
Sod2	GGTCGCTTACAGATTGCT	CTCCCAGTTGATTACATTCC
Sirtl	AGTTCCAGCCGTCTCTGTGT	CTCCACGAACAGCTTCACAA
FoxOl	GCTGGGTGTCAGGCTAAGAG	TGGACTGCTCCTCAGTTCCT
Tnfα	GGGACAGTGACCTGGACTGT	AGGCTGTGCATTGCACCTCA
β-Actin	TCGTGCGTGACATCAAAGAG	TGGACAGTGAGGCCAGGATG

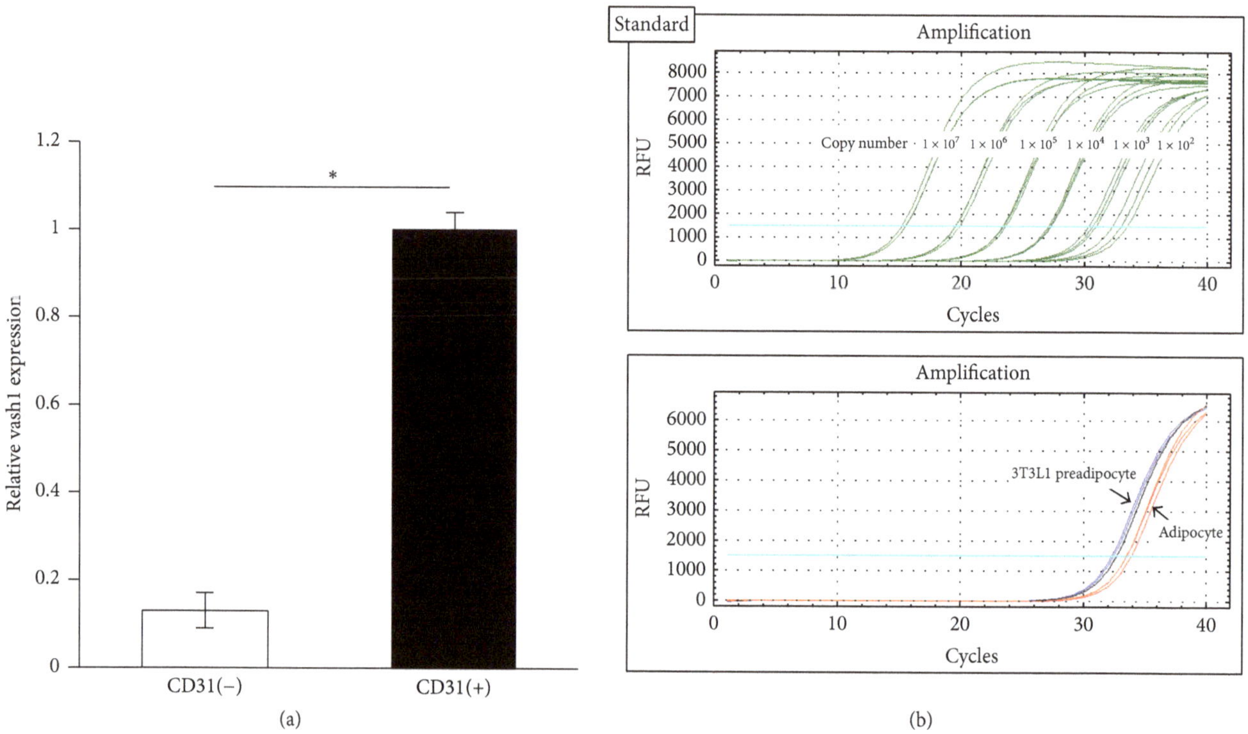

Figure 5: Vashl is expressed in ECs but not in adipocytes. (a) CD31-positive and -negative cells from the WAT of young WT male mice were separated as described in Materials and Methods, and the expression of vashl was compared. Means ± SDs are shown. The statistical significance of differences was calculated by use of the unpaired Student's t-test, and a value of $p < 0.05$ was the criterion for significance. (b) 3T3L1 preadipocytes were caused to differentiate into adipocyte in vitro, and the expression of vashl in those cells was quantified as described in Materials and Methods. $^*p < 0.05$.

function. Indeed, alterations in VEGF signaling modify vascular structure/function and change the insulin sensitivity of adipose tissue independent of inflammation [26–29]. But the lifespan and the status of insr, irs-1, and irs-2 expression were not characterized. The present study is the first to indicate the functional interaction between ECs and adipocytes, as vashl produced by adipose ECs influenced insulin sensitivity by modulating the expression of insr, irs-1, and irs-2 in the WAT. The molecular mechanism explaining how vashl regulates the expression of insr, irs-1, and irs-2 in the WAT is currently under investigation.

We previously reported that the expression of vashl decreases with aging [17]. Insulin resistance and the decreased expression of insr, irs-1, and irs-2 in the WAT of *vashl*$^{-/-}$ mice were evident in their early life but disappeared in their late life. These alterations could be explained by this age-associated downregulation of vashl in the WAT, as the difference in vashl expression between WT mice and *vashl*$^{-/-}$ mice was large in their early life but diminished in their late life. Then, the question is raised as to whether such changes in the early life of *vashl*$^{-/-}$ mice can influence longevity in their late life. An increasing amount of evidence indicates that nutritional events and/or hormonal alterations during development influence longevity in later life [30]. We therefore think it is possible that insulin resistance due to the decreased expression of insr, irs-1, and irs-2 in WAT in early life might influence the lifespan of *vashl*$^{-/-}$ mice.

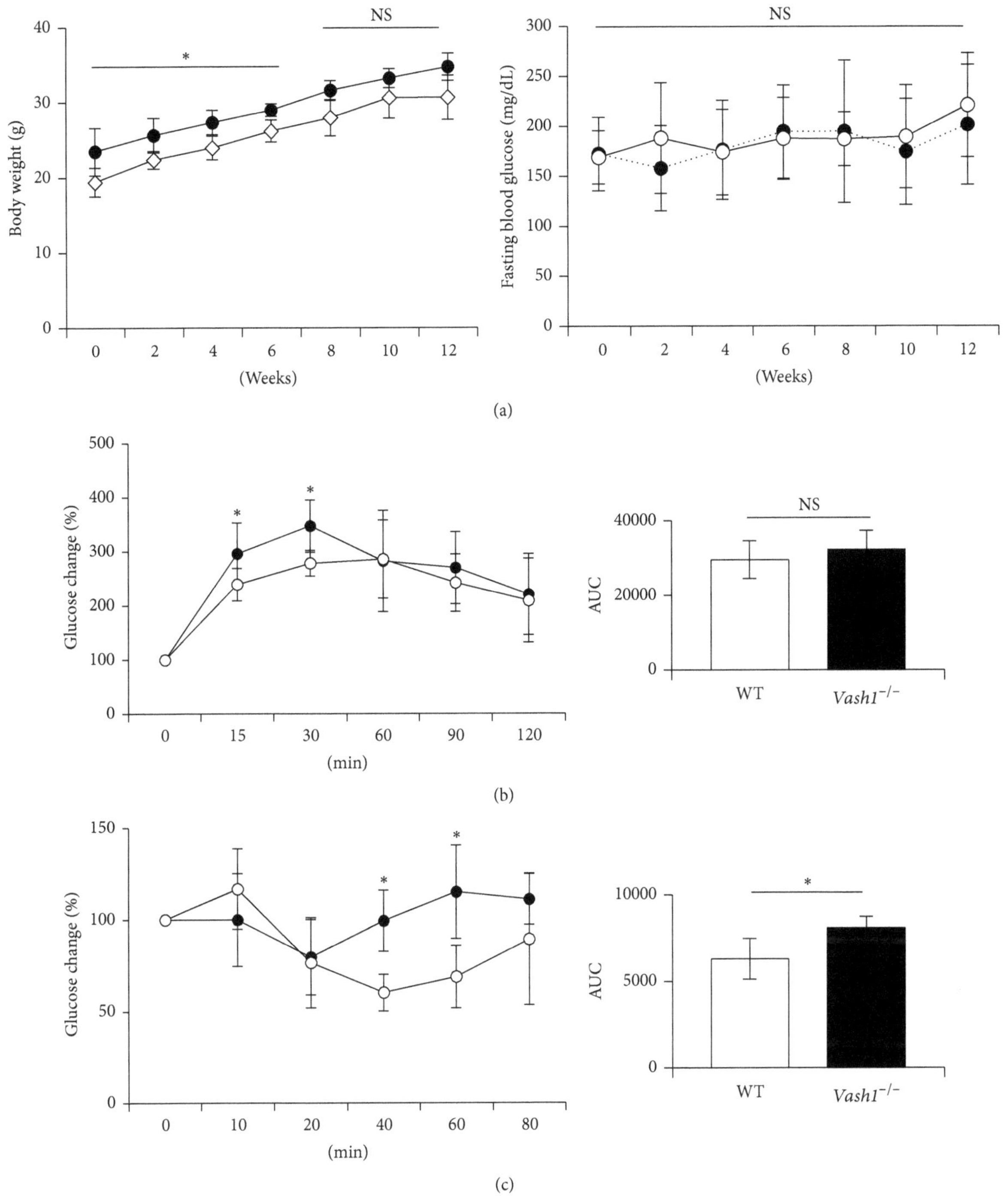

FIGURE 6: No outbreak of diabetes in *vash1*$^{-/-}$ mice. (a) WT and *vash1*$^{-/-}$ young male mice were fed a HFD, and body weight and fasting blood glucose were compared. Open circle, WT mice; closed circle, *vash1*$^{-/-}$ mice. Means ± SDs are shown ($N = 7$). The statistical significance of differences was calculated by use of the unpaired Student's t-test, and a value of $p < 0.05$ was the criterion for significance. (b) After a 12-week HFD feeding, the GTT was performed. Open circle, WT mice; closed circle, *vash1*$^{-/-}$ mice. Area under the curve (AUC) is shown on the right. Means ± SDs are given ($N = 7$). The statistical significance of differences was calculated by performing the unpaired Student's t-test, and a value of $p < 0.05$ was the criterion for significance. (c) After a 12-week HFD feeding, the ITT was performed. Open circle, WT mice; closed circle, *vash1*$^{-/-}$ mice. AUC is shown on the right. Means ± SDs are given ($N = 7$). The statistical significance of differences was calculated by use of the unpaired Student's t-test, and a value of $p < 0.05$ was taken as the criterion for significance. $^*p < 0.05$.

As a decrease in vash1 expression makes the vasculature vulnerable to cellular stresses, we were puzzled and wondered why nature would allow a decrease in the expression of such a valuable protein with aging [17]. There must be a reasonable explanation. In accordance with our present observations, we now speculate that vash1 influences not only tolerance toward vascular stresses but also insulin signaling, especially in the WAT, and that one purpose of age-associated downregulation of vash1 might be to afford healthy longevity.

Importantly, *vash1*$^{-/-}$ mice exhibited mild insulin resistance but never developed diabetes even when fed a HFD. This failure was probably because the downregulation of insr, irs-1, and irs-2 in the *vash1*$^{-/-}$ mice was limited to the WAT. As described earlier, there remains a challenging question as to how preserved insulin signaling for glucose homeostasis and reduced insulin signaling for longevity can be balanced in the body. We consider that the prominent function of vash1 in insulin signaling in WAT can be a promising answer to this question.

5. Conclusion

The expression of vash1 is involved in normal insulin sensitivity, and the targets of this effect are *insr, irs-1, and irs-2* genes in the WAT. The lack of the *vash1* gene causes mild insulin resistance and that might have contributed to healthy longevity without the development of overt diabetes. Our present findings should open a novel avenue for further research on healthy longevity.

Competing Interests

The authors declare no conflict of interests.

References

[1] M. Kaeberlein, P. S. Rabinovitch, and G. M. Martin, "Healthy aging: the ultimate preventative medicine," *Science*, vol. 350, no. 6265, pp. 1191–1193, 2015.

[2] C. López-Otín, M. A. Blasco, L. Partridge, M. Serrano, and G. Kroemer, "The hallmarks of aging," *Cell*, vol. 153, no. 6, pp. 1194–1217, 2013.

[3] S. J. Russell and C. R. Kahn, "Endocrine regulation of ageing," *Nature Reviews Molecular Cell Biology*, vol. 8, no. 9, pp. 681–691, 2007.

[4] C. J. Kenyon, "The genetics of ageing," *Nature*, vol. 464, no. 7288, pp. 504–512, 2010.

[5] M. Tatar, A. Bartke, and A. Antebi, "The endocrine regulation of aging by insulin-like signals," *Science*, vol. 299, no. 5611, pp. 1346–1351, 2003.

[6] C. E. Riera and A. Dillin, "Tipping the metabolic scales towards increased longevity in mammals," *Nature Cell Biology*, vol. 17, no. 3, pp. 196–203, 2015.

[7] C. Kenyon, J. Chang, E. Gensch, A. Rudner, and R. Tabtiang, "A C. elegans mutant that lives twice as long as wild type," *Nature*, vol. 366, no. 6454, pp. 461–464, 1993.

[8] M. Tatar, A. Kopelman, D. Epstein, M.-P. Tu, C.-M. Yin, and R. S. Garofalo, "A mutant *Drosophila* insulin receptor homolog that extends life-span and impairs neuroendocrine function," *Science*, vol. 292, no. 5514, pp. 107–110, 2001.

[9] M. Blüher, B. B. Kahn, and C. R. Kahn, "Extended longevity in mice lacking the insulin receptor in adipose tissue," *Science*, vol. 299, no. 5606, pp. 572–574, 2003.

[10] E. Cohen and A. Dillin, "The insulin paradox: aging, proteotoxicity and neurodegeneration," *Nature Reviews Neuroscience*, vol. 9, no. 10, pp. 759–767, 2008.

[11] J. C. Kovacic, P. Moreno, V. Hachinski, E. G. Nabel, and V. Fuster, "Cellular senescence, vascular disease, and aging: Part 1 of a 2-part review," *Circulation*, vol. 123, no. 15, pp. 1650–1660, 2011.

[12] J. C. Kovacic, P. Moreno, E. G. Nabel, V. Hachinski, and V. Fuster, "Cellular senescence, vascular disease, and aging: part 2 of a 2-part review: Clinical vascular disease in the elderly," *Circulation*, vol. 123, no. 17, pp. 1900–1910, 2011.

[13] Y. Sato, "Novel link between inhibition of angiogenesis and tolerance to vascular stress," *Journal of Atherosclerosis and Thrombosis*, vol. 22, no. 4, pp. 327–334, 2014.

[14] K. Watanabe, Y. Hasegawa, H. Yamashita et al., "Vasohibin as an endothelium-derived negative feedback regulator of angiogenesis," *Journal of Clinical Investigation*, vol. 114, no. 7, pp. 898–907, 2004.

[15] H. Miyashita, T. Watanabe, H. Hayashi et al., "Angiogenesis inhibitor vasohibin-1 enhances stress resistance of endothelial cells via induction of SOD2 and SIRT1," *PLoS ONE*, vol. 7, no. 10, Article ID e46459, 2012.

[16] N. Hinamoto, Y. Maeshima, H. Yamasaki et al., "Exacerbation of diabetic renal alterations in mice lacking vasohibin-1," *PLoS ONE*, vol. 9, no. 9, Article ID 0107934, 2014.

[17] E. Takeda, Y. Suzuki, and Y. Sato, "Age-associated downregulation of vasohibin-1 in vascular endothelial cells," *Aging Cell*, vol. 15, no. 5, pp. 885–892, 2016.

[18] H. Kimura, H. Miyashita, Y. Suzuki et al., "Distinctive localization and opposed roles of vasohibin-1 and vasohibin-2 in the regulation of angiogenesis," *Blood*, vol. 113, no. 19, pp. 4810–4818, 2009.

[19] J. Zhang and F. Liu, "Tissue-specific insulin signaling in the regulation of metabolism and aging," *IUBMB Life*, vol. 66, no. 7, pp. 485–495, 2014.

[20] R. Martins, G. J. Lithgow, and W. Link, "Long live FOXO: unraveling the role of FOXO proteins in aging and longevity," *Aging Cell*, vol. 15, no. 2, pp. 196–207, 2016.

[21] M. Tabata, T. Kadomatsu, S. Fukuhara et al., "Angiopoietin-like protein 2 promotes chronic adipose tissue inflammation and obesity-related systemic insulin resistance," *Cell Metabolism*, vol. 10, no. 3, pp. 178–188, 2009.

[22] A. Villaret, J. Galitzky, P. Decaunes et al., "Adipose tissue endothelial cells from obese human subjects: differences among depots in angiogenic, metabolic, and inflammatory gene expression and cellular senescence," *Diabetes*, vol. 59, no. 11, pp. 2755–2763, 2010.

[23] Y. Hasegawa, T. Saito, T. Ogihara et al., "Blockade of the nuclear factor-κB pathway in the endothelium prevents insulin resistance and prolongs life spans," *Circulation*, vol. 125, no. 9, pp. 1122–1133, 2012.

[24] N. J. Pillon, P. M. Azizi, Y. E. Li et al., "Palmitate-induced inflammatory pathways in human adipose microvascular endothelial cells promote monocyte adhesion and impair insulin transcytosis," *American Journal of Physiology—Endocrinology and Metabolism*, vol. 309, no. 1, pp. E35–E44, 2015.

[25] X. Sun, J. Lin, Y. Zhang et al., "MicroRNA-181b improves glucose homeostasis and insulin sensitivity by regulating endothelial function in white adipose tissue," *Circulation Research*, vol. 118, no. 5, pp. 810–821, 2016.

[26] I. Elias, S. Franckhauser, and F. Bosch, "New insights into adipose tissue VEGF-A actions in the control of obesity and insulin resistance," *Adipocyte*, vol. 2, no. 2, pp. 109–112, 2014.

[27] H.-K. Sung, K.-O. Doh, J. E. Son et al., "Adipose vascular endothelial growth factor regulates metabolic homeostasis through angiogenesis," *Cell Metabolism*, vol. 17, no. 1, pp. 61–72, 2013.

[28] J. Honek, T. Seki, H. Iwamoto et al., "Modulation of age-related insulin sensitivity by VEGF-dependent vascular plasticity in adipose tissues," *Proceedings of the National Academy of Sciences of the United States of America*, vol. 111, no. 41, pp. 14906–14911, 2014.

[29] M. R. Robciuc, R. Kivelä, I. M. Williams et al., "VEGFB/VEGFR1-induced expansion of adipose vasculature counteracts obesity and related metabolic complications," *Cell Metabolism*, vol. 23, no. 4, pp. 712–724, 2016.

[30] A. Bartke, "Early life events can shape aging and longevity," *Current Aging Science*, vol. 8, no. 1, pp. 11–13, 2015.

Permissions

All chapters in this book were first published in JAR, by Hindawi Publishing Corporation; hereby published with permission under the Creative Commons Attribution License or equivalent. Every chapter published in this book has been scrutinized by our experts. Their significance has been extensively debated. The topics covered herein carry significant findings which will fuel the growth of the discipline. They may even be implemented as practical applications or may be referred to as a beginning point for another development.

The contributors of this book come from diverse backgrounds, making this book a truly international effort. This book will bring forth new frontiers with its revolutionizing research information and detailed analysis of the nascent developments around the world.

We would like to thank all the contributing authors for lending their expertise to make the book truly unique. They have played a crucial role in the development of this book. Without their invaluable contributions this book wouldn't have been possible. They have made vital efforts to compile up to date information on the varied aspects of this subject to make this book a valuable addition to the collection of many professionals and students.

This book was conceptualized with the vision of imparting up-to-date information and advanced data in this field. To ensure the same, a matchless editorial board was set up. Every individual on the board went through rigorous rounds of assessment to prove their worth. After which they invested a large part of their time researching and compiling the most relevant data for our readers.

The editorial board has been involved in producing this book since its inception. They have spent rigorous hours researching and exploring the diverse topics which have resulted in the successful publishing of this book. They have passed on their knowledge of decades through this book. To expedite this challenging task, the publisher supported the team at every step. A small team of assistant editors was also appointed to further simplify the editing procedure and attain best results for the readers.

Apart from the editorial board, the designing team has also invested a significant amount of their time in understanding the subject and creating the most relevant covers. They scrutinized every image to scout for the most suitable representation of the subject and create an appropriate cover for the book.

The publishing team has been an ardent support to the editorial, designing and production team. Their endless efforts to recruit the best for this project, has resulted in the accomplishment of this book. They are a veteran in the field of academics and their pool of knowledge is as vast as their experience in printing. Their expertise and guidance has proved useful at every step. Their uncompromising quality standards have made this book an exceptional effort. Their encouragement from time to time has been an inspiration for everyone.

The publisher and the editorial board hope that this book will prove to be a valuable piece of knowledge for researchers, students, practitioners and scholars across the globe.

List of Contributors

Victoria F. Burns
Centre de Recherche et d'Expertise en Gérontologie Sociale (CREG´ES), C.S.S.S. Cavendish, 5800 Cavendish Boulevard, Montréal, QC, Canada H4W 2T5
School of Social Work, McGill University, Montréal, QC, Canada H3A 2A7

Jean-Pierre Lavoie
Centre de Recherche et d'Expertise en Gérontologie Sociale (CREGES), C.S.S.S. Cavendish, 5800 Cavendish Boulevard, Montréal, QC, Canada H4W 2T5
School of Social Work, McGill University, Montréal, QC, Canada H3A 2A7
Ecole de Travail social, Université du Québec Montréal, Montréal, QC, Canada H2L 4Y2

Damaris Rose
Centre Urbanisation Culture Société, Université INRS, 385 Rue Sherbrooke Est, Montréal, QC, Canada H2X 1E3

Kaycee M. Sink and Suzanne Craft
Department of Internal Medicine (Geriatrics), Wake Forest School of Medicine, Winston-Salem, NC 27157, USA

S. Carrie Smith, Donald W. Bowden and Jianzhao Xu
Department of Biochemistry, Wake Forest School of Medicine, Winston-Salem, NC 27157, USA

Joseph A. Maldjian
Department of Radiology, University of Texas Southwestern Medical Center, Dallas, TX 75390, USA

Barry I. Freedman
Department of Internal Medicine (Nephrology), Wake Forest School of Medicine, Winston-Salem, NC 27157, USA

Jasmin Divers
Department of Biostatistics, Wake Forest School of Medicine, Winston-Salem, NC 27157, USA

Adena M. Galinsky
Center on the Demography and Economics of Aging, NORC and the University of Chicago, 1155 E. 60th Street, Chicago, IL 60637, USA

Kathleen A. Cagney
Departments of Sociology and Health Studies, University of Chicago, 1155 E. 60th Street, Rm 238, Chicago, IL 60637, USA

Christopher R. Browning
Department of Sociology, Ohio State University, 214 Townshend Hall, 1885 Neil Avenue Mall, Columbus, OH 43210, USA

Göran Nilsson
Centre for Clinical Research, Västmanland County Hospital, Uppsala University, 721 89 Västerås, Sweden

Pär Hedberg
Department of Clinical Physiology, Västmanland County Hospital, 721 89 Västerås, Sweden

John Öhrvik
Department of Medicine, Karolinska Institutet, 171 76 Stockholm, Sweden

Geraldine Nosowska
Effective Practice Ltd., 8 Bridgetown, Totnes, Devon TQ95AB, UK

Kevin McKee
School of Education, Health and Social Studies, Dalarna University, 791 88 Falun, Sweden

Lena Dahlberg
School of Education, Health and Social Studies, Dalarna University, 791 88 Falun, Sweden
Aging Research Centre, Karolinska Institutet and Stockholm University, Gävlegatan 16, 113 30 Stockholm, Sweden

Charles A. Emlet
Social Work Program, University of Washington Tacoma, Tacoma, WA 98401, USA

Joane T. Moceri
Nursing Program, University of Washington Tacoma, Tacoma, WA 98401, USA

Kristina H. Lewis and Matthew W. Gillman
Obesity Prevention Program, Department of Population Medicine, Harvard Medical School, Harvard Pilgrim Health Care Institute, Boston, MA 02215, USA

Mary L. Greaney and Karen M. Emmons
Department of Medical Oncology / Population Sciences, Dana-Farber Cancer Institute, Boston, MA, USA

Elaine Puleo
Division of Biostatistics, Department of Public Health, University of Massachusetts, Amherst, MA 01003, USA

Gary G. Bennett
Department of Psychology and Neuroscience, Duke Global Health Institute, Duke University, Durham, NC 27708, USA

S. Morrison and K. M. Newell
School of Physical Therapy, Old Dominion University, Norfolk, VA 23529, USA
Department of Kinesiology, Pennsylvania State University, State College, PA 16801, USA

Myuri Ruthirakuhan, Angela C. Luedke, Angela Tam, Ankita Goel, Ayaz Kurji and Angeles Garcia
Department of Medicine (Geriatrics) and Centre for Neuroscience, Queen's University, Kingston, ON, Canada K7L 5A2

Ryuichi Hasegawa
Department of Occupational Therapy, College of Life and Health Sciences, Chubu University, 1200, Matsumoto, Kasugai, Aichi 487-8501, Japan

Mohammod Monirul Islam
Department of Rehabilitation, Yonaha General Hospital, 8-264-3 Izumi, Kuwana, Mie 511-0838, Japan

Ryuji Watanabe
Department of Rehabilitation, Tsushima City Hospital, 3-73 Tsubaki, Tsushima, Aichi 496-8537, Japan

Naoki Tomiyama
Division of Occupational Therapy, Faculty of Care and Rehabilitation, Seijoh University, 2-172 Fukinodai, Tokai, Aichi 476-8588, Japan

Dennis R. Taaffe
School of Environmental and Life Sciences, The University of Newcastle, 10 Chittaway Road, Ourimbah, NSW2258, Australia

Lídio Gonçalves Lima Neto, Aruanã Joaquim Matheus and Rodrigues Pinheiro
Laboratory of Immunology and Microbiology of Respiratory Infections, LAMIR, Universidade CEUMA, São Luis, MA, Brazil

Guilherme Borges Pereira
Undergraduate Program in Physical Education at the Catholic University of Brasilia, Brasília, Brazil

Richard Diego Leite
Department of Physical Education, Federal University of Espírito Santo (UFES), Vitória, ES, Brazil

Francisco Navarro, Janaina de Oliveira Brito Monzani and Cristiano Texeira Mostarda
Department of Physical Education, Federal University of Maranhão (UFMA), São Luis, MA, Brazil

Wandson Rodrigues Sousa
Postgraduate Program in Adult and Child Health, PPGSAC, UFMA, São Luis, MA, Brazil

Yoko Honda, Masashi Tanaka and Shuji Honda
Department of Genomics for Longevity and Health, Tokyo Metropolitan Institute of Gerontology, Sakaecho, Itabashiku, Tokyo 173-0015, Japan

Yoko Araki, Taketoshi Hata and Kenji Ichihara
Nagaragawa Research Center, Api Company Limited, Nagara, Gifu 502-0071, Japan

Masafumi Ito
Research Team for Mechanism of Aging, Tokyo Metropolitan Institute of Gerontology, Sakaecho, Itabashiku, Tokyo 173-0015, Japan

Kyle Y. Whitfield and Jason S. Daniels
Faculty of Extension, University of Alberta, Enterprise Square, Room 2-215, 10230 Jasper Avenue, Edmonton, Alberta, Canada T5J 4P6

Keri Flesaker
Department of Educational Psychology, University of Alberta, 6-102 Education North, Edmonton, Alberta, Canada T6G 2G5

Doneka Simmons
Senior Association of Greater Edmonton, 15 Sir Winston Churchill Square, Edmonton, Alberta, Canada T5J 2E5

Lindsay S. Nagamatsu and B. Peter Graf
Department of Psychology, University of British Columbia (UBC), 2136 West Mall, Vancouver, BC, Canada V6T 1Z4

Alison Chan, Jennifer C. Davis, Devika Sharma and Teresa Liu-Ambrose
Department of Physical Therapy, University of British Columbia (UBC), 212-2177 Wesbrook Mall, Vancouver, BC, Canada V6T 1Z3

Lynn Beattie
Alzheimer Clinic, G37 Purdy Pavilion, UBC Hospital, University of British Columbia (UBC), 2211 Wesbrook Mall, Vancouver, BC, Canada V6T 2B5
Brain Research Centre, University of British Columbia (UBC), 2211Wesbrook Mall, Vancouver, BC, Canada V6T 2B5

Michelle W. Voss
Department of Psychology, The University of Iowa, E11 Seashore Hall, Iowa City, IA 52242-1409, USA

Kelly A. Cotter
Department of Psychology, Sacramento State University, 6000 J Street, Sacramento, CA 95819, USA

Luis Miguel Rondón García
Faculty of Social Work, University of Granada, Granada, Spain

Jose Manuel Ramírez Navarrro
Faculty of Social Studies, University of Màlaga, Màlaga, Spain

Gianluigi Savarese
Department of Advanced Biomedical Science, University of Naples Federico II, 80131 Naples, Italy
Department of Clinical Medicine and Surgery, University of Naples Federico II, 80131 Naples, Italy

Vincenzo Mauriello
Arci Movie, 80147 Naples, Italy

Maria Quarto
Department of Physics, University of Naples Federico II, 80131 Naples, Italy

Annamaria Kisslinger
IEOS-CNR, Naples, Italy
Fondazione GENS Onlus, 80121 Naples, Italy

Donatella Tramontano
Fondazione GENS Onlus, 80121 Naples, Italy
Department of Molecular Medicine and Medical Biotechnology, University of Naples Federico II, 80131 Naples, Italy

Maddalena Illario
Department of Translational Medical Sciences, University of Naples Federico II, 80131 Naples, Italy
R&D Unit, Federico II University Hospital, 80131 Naples, Italy

Maulilio John Kipanyula and Wahabu Hamisi Kimaro
Department of Veterinary Anatomy, Faculty of Veterinary Medicine, Sokoine University of Agriculture, Chuo Kikuu, Morogoro, Tanzania

Paul F. Seke Etet
Department of Basic Health Sciences, Qassim University, Buraydah, Al-Qassim 51452, Saudi Arabia

Daniel Schniertshauer, Daniel Gebhard and Jörg Bergemann
Department of Life Sciences, Albstadt-Sigmaringen University of Applied Sciences, 72488 Sigmaringen, Germany

Sathirakorn Pongpanich
College of Public Health Sciences, Chulalongkorn University, Pathumwan, Bangkok 10330, ailand

Pattaraporn Khongboon
College of Public Health Sciences, Chulalongkorn University, Pathumwan, Bangkok 10330, ailand
Prince Mahidol Award Foundation under the Royal Patronage, Faculty of Medicine, Siriraj Hospital, Bangkoknoi, Bangkok 10700, ailand

Eichi Takeda, Yasuhiro Suzuki and Yasufumi Sato
Department of Vascular Biology, Institute of Development, Aging, and Cancer, Tohoku University, Sendai, Japan

Tetsuya Yamada and Hideki Katagiri,
Department of Diabetes and Metabolism, Graduate School of Medicine, Tokyo University, Tokyo, Japan

Index

CPSIA information can be obtained
at www.ICGtesting.com
Printed in the USA
LVHW062009100122
708212LV00002B/126

9 781639 270071